SPORTS & EXERCISE MASSAGE

Comprehensive Care in Athletics, Fitness, & Rehabilitation

SPORTS & EXERCISE MASSAGE

Comprehensive Care in Athletics, Fitness, & Rehabilitation

SANDY FRITZ, MS, NCTMB

Founder, Owner, Director, and Head Instructor
Health Enrichment Center
School of Therapeutic Massage and Bodywork
Lapeer, Michigan

With more than **700** illustrations

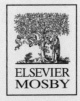

ELSEVIER
MOSBY

ELSEVIER
MOSBY

11830 Westline Industrial Drive
St. Louis, Missouri 63146

Notice

International Standard Book Number 0-323-02882-9

Publishing Director: Linda Duncan
Acquisitions Editor: Kellie Fitzpatrick
Developmental Editor: Jennifer Watrous
Publishing Services Manager: Melissa Lastarria
Project Manager: Rich Barber
Designer: Julia Dummitt
Editorial Assistant: Elizabeth Clark

Printed in Canada

Last digit is the print number: 9 8 7 6 5 4 3 2 1

This textbook is dedicated to all the athletes I have been privileged to work with, the Detroit Lions organization for their innovative approach to the care of their players, and to the future massage therapists—who will commit to dedicated and comprehensive study of therapeutic massage—and to those who will teach them.

In lieu of a formally written foreword, the following is a list of individuals for whom the author has provided therapeutic massage in support of their athletic endeavors or those who support her work. The following athletes, trainers, coaches, and support personnel have received massage from Sandy Fritz, have worked professionally with her, or both. They support the benefits of massage as described in this textbook. They sincerely hope this textbook will increase the competency of the massage therapists who serve this population and encourage beneficial and safe use of massage therapy in the sports and fitness community.

These individuals have provided permission to be included here:

National Football League (NFL)
Charlie Batch, Quarterback
Jerome Bettis, Running Back
Jeff Hartings, Center
Verron Haynes, Running Back
Chris Hope, Free Safety
Alonzo Jackson, Linebacker
Lee Mays, Wide Receiver
Brian Williams, Linebacker
Ray Brown, Offensive Tackle (19+ years)
Bill Schroeder, Wide Receiver
Michael Ricks, Tight End
Dewayne Washington, Cornerback
Eric Beverly, Guard/Center
Jason Gildon, Linebacker
Kevin Jones, Running Back
Charles Rogers, Wide Receiver
Olandis Gary, Running Back
Darrell Campbell, Defensive Tackle
Todd Fordham, Tackle
Wali Rainer, Linebacker
Scott Vines, Wide Receiver
Marcus Bell, Defensive Tackle
Scott Kowalkowski, Linebacker
Barrett Green, Linebacker
Ty Detmer, Quarterback
Larry Foster, Wide Receiver
Luther Elliss, Defensive End
John Jett, Punter

Jeff Backus, Tackle
Boss Bailey, Linebacker
Dre' Bly, Defensive Back
Jared DeVries, Defensive End
Eddie Drummond, Wide Receiver
Casey Fitzsimmons, Tight End
Andre' Goodman, Defensive Back
Az-Zahir Hakim, Wide Receiver
James Hall, Defensive End
Jason Hanson, Kicker
Matt Joyce, Offensive Line
David Kircus, Wide Receiver
David Loverne, Guard
Brock Marion, Free Safety
Nick Harris, Punter
Cory Redding, Defensive End
Shaun Rogers, Defensive Tackle
Cory Schlesinger, Running Back
Teddy Lehman, Linebacker
Tai Streets, Wide Receiver
Bracy Walker, Safety
Roy Williams, Wide Receiver
Damien Woody, Guard
Jody Littleton, Linebacker
Rick DeMulling, Tackle
Tyrone Hopson, Tackle
Paul Smith, Running Back
Robert Porcher, Defensive End

Major League Baseball (MLB)
Brian Tollberg, Pitcher
Lance Carter, Pitcher

National Basketball Association (NBA)
Antonio McDyess, Forward
Chauncey Billups, Point Guard

Professional Golfers Association (PGA)
Tom Gillis

Therapists, Trainers, and Others
David Hogarth, Physical Therapist
David Donatucci, Director of Performance
Craig Vandermause, NFL Football Administration
Kurt Schottenheimer, Coach, NFL
Charlie Sanders, Coach, NFL
Dan Henson, Coach, NFL
Malcolm Blacken, Strength Coach

Chris Curran, Assistant Athletic Trainer, NFL
Mark Glenn, Equipment Manager
Lee Levanduski, Physical Therapist
Andy Barnett, Strength Coach, NFL
Ken Crenshaw, Head Athletic Trainer, MLB
Joe Recknagel, Trainer, NFL
Al Bellamy, Athletic Trainer, NFL

This list of names has been compiled over the last several years. The positions listed next to the name reflect those that the individuals held at the time Sandy Fritz worked with them.

I am excited to present the first edition of this comprehensive textbook, which targets therapeutic massage for the sports and exercise community. As massage therapy evolves, there is a trend toward specialization based on career interests, specific populations, and massage modalities. The three main career tracks in massage are wellness/spa, medical/clinical, and sports and fitness. Specific populations include massage for prenatal care and the elderly, to name just a couple; modalities include methods such as lymphatic drain. Elsevier is providing comprehensive textbook and resource development in these areas. This sports and exercise text is a major development in advanced level training for massage therapists. The sports and fitness population is increasing its demand for highly trained massage therapists to address the specific needs of exercise and training protocols, including recovery and injury prevention. Massage is quickly becoming a supportive approach for addressing sports injuries. The information and skills involved in achieving these outcomes is over and above entry level training and conforms with the concept of a massage therapy specialty.

This textbook responds to the specific massage needs of professional, amateur, recreational, and rehabilitative sports and exercise participants. This is a broad scope of people with a variety of outcomes for massage, but they are all connected by their desire for efficient movement. Western society is currently overwhelmed with lifestyle-related health concerns such as weight management and cardiovascular disease. Exercise in not an option but a necessity in regaining and maintaining one's health. Physical exercise places demands on the body that, although beneficial, can result in discomfort. Delayed onset muscle soreness, which occurs when a new activity is undertaken or the intensity in the existing program is increased, is an example. As I write this preface in the spring of 2005, I am stiff and sore from raking the yard and getting the gardens ready. Massage can help with this aching and stiffness, making compliance with the exercise programs more likely. This is very important.

Providing massage, to the competing athlete–professional, amateur, or recreational–is an entirely different process than working with those striving to achieve fitness and to support healthy lifestyles. Athletes are all about performance, which places many more demands on the body than exercise for fitness. Recovery and injury prevention in this population is essential, as is knowing how to provide massage as part of injury treatment. With competitive athletes, it is not *if* they will get injured, but rather *when* and *how severely*.

Physical rehabilitation involves movement-related activity. General aerobic conditioning is necessary for cardiac rehabilitation. Rehabilitation is required for surgical procedures for joint injury or replacement. If surgery is involved, scar tissue management is important. Advancements in medical treatment are allowing athletes to compete longer at a higher level and letting the rest of us age while remaining active and productive without the pain and limitation of arthritic joints. If a person has experienced physical trauma, such as a car accident or playing football, the healing process in general, as well as the specifically targeted rehabilitation by the medical team, can be supported by the well-trained massage therapist.

That's what this book is about.

The textbook is divided into four units. Unit One is all about the world of the athlete and the background information needed to understand movement and fitness. Unit Two is a review of massage in relationship to this population, specific skills needed to address the conditions these people experience, and a comprehensive and detailed protocol as a foundation for working with this population. Unit Three is all about injury and treatment regimens, including specific massage protocols. The DVD that accompanies this text concentrates on demonstrating the skills presented in Units Two and Three. Unit Four is unique in that it provides detailed case studies for understanding how all information in the book fits together in a goal-oriented treatment process.

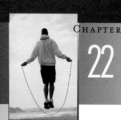

CHAPTER

22

CASE STUDIES

This unit is a unique perspective for a textbook. The unit is written more like a series of stories that chronicle the clinical practice of massage therapists specializing in sport and fitness massage. The content is technically correct and is presented in an interpersonal context of experienced massage therapists who are continually learning. The client profiles are often composite characters drawn from actual experience, designed to represent accurately the real-world application of information presented in this text. The goal is to involve the reader in a clinical reasoning outcome-based massage approach that is a realistic representation of the sport and rehabilitation environment and the persons involved. This is the best way for me, the author, to shift from teacher to mentor.

Each case in this unit is a composite of many different clients, but all the situations are ones with which I have been involved personally. As I reflect on all the sport stories I have read or watched, the underlying story is about the personal sacrifices and triumphs and the persons behind the scenes—the doctors, trainers, coaches, family, and massage therapist and others who contributed to the outcome, be it regaining fitness, ability to overcome injury, winning, and losing. Shakespeare coined the metaphor of the "play within the play," and these vignettes can be thought of as the play within the competition. I purposely have used a variety of formats for these case studies so that the reader can become familiar with different narrative and documentation style.

First, I will describe each of the clients, and then the text will follow a period of time using a charting format of the therapeutic massage session for

each client. Individual methods such as lymphatic drainage or joint play will not be described. Instead, the reader needs to refer to those areas in the text or other textbooks that are recommended to support this text. Because there is no way to develop precise protocols, a clinical reasoning model is used.

CASE ONE
MARGE—CARDIAC REHABILITATION

Marge is an 84-year-old woman with age-related cardiac insufficiency. The coronary arteries are somewhat blocked, but surgery is not the best option and the condition is being controlled with medication. Previously she underwent procedures to unblock arteries in her left leg and participated in a cardiac rehabilitation program.

Marge was a high school teacher for many years. She has been moderately active and basically healthy over her life span. She smoked for many years but quit in her 40s. When she was in her 60s, she fell and severely sprained her right wrist and left ankle and bruised her back. She did not receive rehabilitation after the fall and only had medical care for the acute phase of healing.

She cared for her husband during a long-term illness until he passed away. When Marge was in her mid-70s she found herself a widow, fatigued, and deconditioned. In addition, she had developed a kyphosis to which she is genetically predisposed and that had worsened during her years of caring for her husband. Being an intelligent and determined woman, she slowly began to reconstruct her

582

1 Explain the following statement and then justify why you agree or disagree with it. A star is born.

_____
_____
_____
_____
_____

2 Provide an example of the following movement strategies found in the activities of daily living.

Examples: Walking–going from one room to another; running–chasing a small child; hitting–knocking down cob webs; throwing–heaving trash into the trash can

A. Catching

B. Swinging

C. Kicking

D. Jumping

E. Turning

F. Cutting

3 Provide an example of an exercise or sport that involves each of the following movement strategies:

Examples: Walking–cardiovascular rehabilitation program; running–marathon racing

A. Hitting

B. Throwing

C. Catching

E. Swinging

E. Kicking

G. Jumping

H. Turning

I. Cutting

J. Pivoting

4 Pick an exercise activity or sport that you expect to have clients perform and identify the movement strategies involved.

Example: Basketball–running, throwing, catching, jumping, turning, cutting, pivoting.

_____
_____
_____
_____

5 For each of the following movement strategies, list the target areas for massage. (Hint: Do the movement and focus on which body area receives the most deceleration activity.)

Examples: Walking–calves; running–hips; hitting–shoulders and low back

A. Throwing

B. Catching

C. Swinging

D. Kicking

E. Jumping

F. Turning

G. Cutting

H. Pivoting

The workbook sections at the end of each chapter are not your typical fill-in-the-blank or labeling activities. The premise is that this is an advanced level study, and therefore the questions require the reader to manipulate the information from the chapter as well as integrate that information with the content of the entire book. It would be prudent to spend adequate time completing these workbook activities. They are not easy and that's appropriate for this level of study.

Real-life stories are included in section openers and are also spread throughout the text to maintain a focus on the people, and not just the sport they play or the condition they have. These stories help reinforce this broader base of understanding. I personally have lived these stories and have learned from every one of them. They are called *In My Experience* boxes.

A student DVD-ROM (that can be played on both set-top DVD players and personal computers) is included at the back of your textbook, as mentioned above. This supplement contains almost 2 hours of video demonstrating techniques presented in the book, as well as the general protocol. Whenever you see this DVD icon, there is a video clip demonstrating the technique being discussed.

IN MY EXPERIENCE...

Neutral Talk

Life is sometimes amusing, although I guess that depends on your perspective. Pets provide a never-ending source of amusement. There is Buttons the bull dog, Porkie the pig, Snoop and Nate, named after rappers, two little white fluffy dogs belonging to s big tough football player, and Killer the kitty. I recall a puffer fish with personality and a pet chicken named Kentucky Fried. There are more, but you get the idea. Pets, kids, and parents, are all part of the picture, especially if you see clients in their homes.

I especially enjoy the grandparents. They usually swing between being so proud of the athletic prowess of their grandchildren and treating them like little kids. I recall one athlete who was sound asleep while being massaged, when Grandma called. Still half-asleep, he jumped off the table, about lost the shorts he was wearing, ran up the stairs and answered her call with a "yes Ma'am."

Peoples' interests vary widely. Some people cook, others garden, and some watch movies. Pets, cooking, gardens, and movies make good neutral discussion topics as a segue into the massage, during that first 5 to10 minutes when settling down can be difficult.

Discussion about family is not so neutral. It is too easy to give advice. Because professional boundaries are a continuous concern, neutral discussion topics are important. The last thing an athlete wants to talk about is the "game" or competition. Usually the athlete don't want to talk at all, but the silence can be uncomfortable. If the TV is on, the program or movie being shown fills the gap. If the athlete is listening to music or talking on the phone, this also fills the space. I have watched a lot of TV that I might not have personally chosen and figured out how to time the massage so I am finished when the movie is finished. I always let the client choose the type music they want to hear. It is amazing how many different rhythms to which massage can be given.

If these void-filling activities aren't available or desired, I can always talk about my pets. I usually relate a funny story about how "Creature," my ferret, gets the best of my two dogs, or about events occurring in my little backyard garden habitat, such as the ongoing hummingbird fights and the summer-long saga of the poor male house wren who had a terrible time building a nest that suited a potential mate. When I was able to finally report success by the wren, my clients were thrilled and wanted a sequel.

I have shared a love of butterfly gardening with a professional wrestler who watched the life cycle of the Monarch butterfly with his young daughter, and of course I had to chuckle about the big tough football player with the two little white fluffy dogs.

Safe neutral talk, just for a few minutes, helps; then be quiet.

There is great additional support on the Evolve website that accompanies this book, such as news articles relating to hot topics in the sports industry and further resources to help in a sports massage practice or with clients. Throughout the text, if the Evolve icon pictured below appears, that content is enhanced by the Evolve website.

evolve The textbook, the DVD, the Evolve site, and the instructor support material (Instructor's Resource Manual and Test Bank) make this package the most comprehensive educational resource available for massage application targeting athletes and those in fitness and rehabilitation exercise programs.

The textbook is meant to be a teaching tool. In this advanced book, I took a little liberty in writing it in the style in which I teach my own students. This is also reflected on the accompanying DVD. It is possible to self-study the text and increase your skills and understanding of how massage supports the sports and fitness communities. The text is designed to be used in a formal classroom study with a skilled instructing staff. Chapter 1 talks about this in relationship to how such a course would be presented. Those that teach (like me) need to go the extra mile to understand the content and admit when they don't. It is impossible to know it all. It is true that some of the content in the text is based on my experience working with this population. I would expect that those teaching this material would respect that experience and then expand on the content of the textbook based on their own expertise with this population. The book does not have all the answers and requires the development of clinical reasoning skills. This means that the information can be challenged (make sure to justify the position taken) and even

more importantly, it can evolve into more effective massage application.

Finally, on a personal note, I love the massage profession. It has been my career path since the late 1970s. I have worked with thousands of clients (a lot of them athletes), taught massage since 1984, and raised three children with massage-related activity as my sole source of income. It has been a long, sometimes hard, but worthwhile journey. There are not many massage therapists around that have endured this long, and I intend to stick around for many more years and believe I owe it to the profession to give back a measure of what I have received. But I am over 50 years old and believe that it will take up to 10 years to prepare the next generation of massage therapists to take over. It just takes that much time to develop the necessary experience to be proficient in anything, including massage therapy. Massage in general, and this population specifically, has been a blessing for me. I did not seek out professional athletes as clients but ended up with a bunch of them. They are a demanding group, and I love it. I have been privileged to work with some of the greatest athletes of our time, and their support for massage will make an impact on future generations. It is important to return those blessings to those who will carry on—the future athletes, those striving to regain their physical fitness, and the massage therapists dedicated enough to take care of them. My contribution is this textbook, the students that I am able to personally teach, and the hope that there will be those who commit to excellence and evolve beyond me in skill, knowledge, and understanding.

Sandy Fritz
April 2005

ACKNOWLEDGMENTS

Writing a textbook is a team effort. Many thanks to my team:

My kids–Greg, Laura, and Luke

My staff at the Health Enrichment Center–Roxanne, Dianne, Dennis, their helpers, and all the instructors

My assistant–Amy Husted

My editors–Kellie Fitzpatrick, Jennifer Watrous, Elizabeth Clark, and Rich Barber

My designer–Julia Dummitt

My marketing representative–Julie Burchett and all the sales representatives

Many thanks to Stewart Halprin for producing the full-color photos in this book; Chris Roider for editing the video segments on the DVD; Chuck Le Roi, III for shooting the video segments; and Mike Silverman for writing and producing the music on the DVD.

The following individuals volunteered their time to participate in the photo and video shoots for this textbook. Their activities and sports of interest are also listed.

Kimberly Alvis
Personal fitness trainer
Aerobics instructor

Janet Blanner
Swimming
Running

Jay Criscione
Soccer
Volleyball
Snowboarding
Softball

J.R. Criscione
Walking (Treadmill)
Hiking

Sean Dorsey
Basketball

D.J. Frare
Gym owner
Personal trainer
Body building
Martial arts
Horseback riding

Teresa Frare
Pilates instructor
Personal fitness

Dottie Gray
Running

Sophia Gray
Running
Road biking

Deirdre Hughes
Soccer
Ballet
Tennis

Chris Jaeger
Volleyball
Triathlons
Hockey
Rock climbing

Karen McKie
Yoga
Pilates
Softball

Uan Nguyen
Martial arts
Biking

Jaleen Nowell
Running

Tom Pohlman
Bi-Athlete

Michael Townson
Basketball
Biking

CONTENTS

SPORTS & EXERCISE MASSAGE

Comprehensive Care in Athletics, Fitness, & Rehabilitation

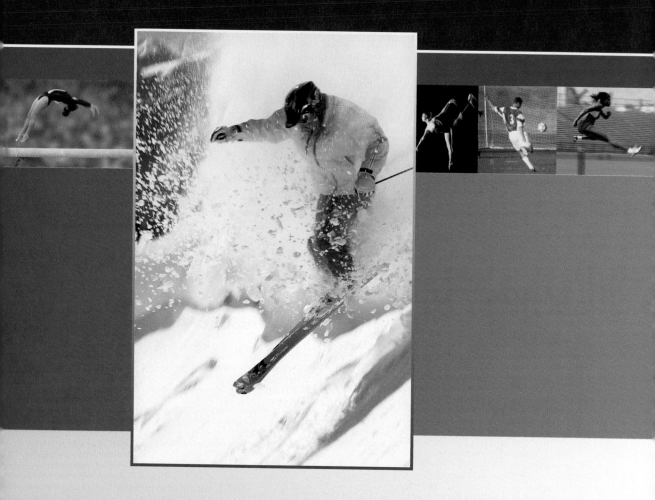

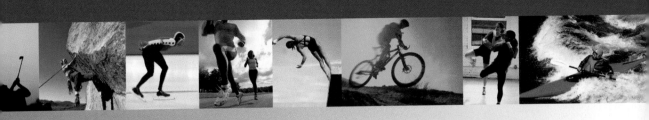

THEORY AND APPLICATION OF EXERCISE AND ATHLETIC PERFORMANCE

STORIES
from the field
JOSEPH
F. RECKNAGEL, ATC

All persons—athletes included—have a story. Each individual's story shapes his or her life. Because when working with so-called celebrities, one commonly focuses on what they do instead of who they are, I have included a few stories of individuals, who are also athletes, to put into perspective the importance of the professional relationship the massage therapist achieves and maintains with this type of client. We do not provide massage to a football player or basketball player or golfer. We support individuals in their own personal quest for achievement. The stories I have chosen to tell are about those with whom I have spent the most time and therefore know the best. The stories are from my point of view and with their permission.
—Sandy Fritz

I think one of my greatest teachers has been Joe. He has been part of the Detroit Lions organization for 25 years and an athletic trainer for 30 years.

Joe had a great teacher too. He had the opportunity to hone his professional skills from one of the most respected athletic trainers in professional sports—Kent Falb, ATC, PT, head athletic trainer for the Detroit Lions for 34 years.

Kent Falb also served as the president of the National Athletic Trainers Association (NATA). This is important in the ultimate influence Joe has had on me. The NATA, based in Dallas, provides the latest research and techniques to its 17,000-plus certified members, who are experts in providing quality health care for the physically active. The NATA is a not-for-profit organization with more than 23,000 members nationwide. The NATA is committed to advancing, encouraging, and improving the athletic training profession. Founded in 1950, the NATA has a membership of about 200 athletic trainers. Today, more than 92% of all certified athletic trainers in the nation are members of the NATA.

To become a certified athletic trainer, one must acquire a 4-year degree and pass a three-part exam administered by the NATA Board of Certification.

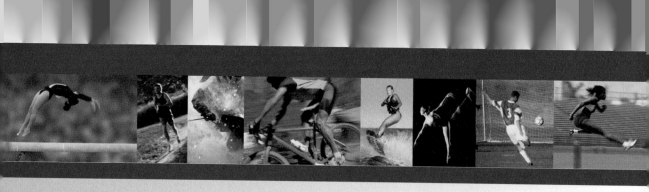

Nearly 100 colleges and universities offer an accredited athletic training curriculum.

In 1990 the American Medical Association (AMA) recognized athletic training as an allied health profession, and in 1998 the AMA recommended that certified athletic trainers be part of the health care unit at every high school.

I look at this small aspect of history and wonder about my own profession–therapeutic massage. For sure, Kent Falb lived professionalism and instilled it in Joe, and Joe expects this same level of professionalism from me and my students.

Joe's background in athletic training started in high school, and he has never looked back. After 4 years of undergraduate studies in athletic training and 1 year of graduate school, he spent a year as an assistant athletic trainer at the college level. Joe has been with the Detroit Lions ever since.

In the beginning of my relationship with the Detroit Lions, Kent was the head athletic trainer. Both he and Joe were supportive of massage but leery. They had had some bad experiences with massage practitioners (ethically and with players being hurt), and they held the massage program with tight constraints. I respected this and over time earned their respect.

Kent retired after the school's first year with the Lions, and before he left, he said, "Good job." These were the only words he ever said to me. This meant a lot. From the beginning Joe was the one put in charge of interfacing with the massage program and who did the talking such as, "be careful, don't stretch the area, leave it alone, make them feel better–don't hurt them."

Joe knows so much, and even though there was concern about massage being used effectively, once I proved myself (and this is key, I did have to prove myself), Joe became my main source of support

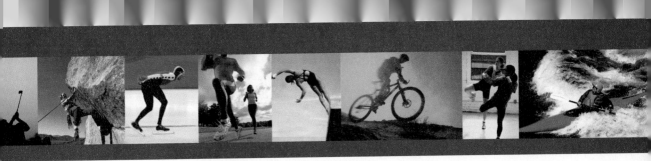

and information at the organization. He never made me feel stupid when I was asking stupid questions. He has seen many players come and go, has experienced many coaches and trends in football, and has seen and treated it all—from ingrown toenails (players have said he is the best!) to spinal cord injury—and literally has saved lives. I love it when he says that the most underrated treatment for athletes is rest, and I think he is correct.

I remember one time Joe came to me and said that it was really important for a particular young player who was injured to play—not just for the team, since he was likely to be let go at the end of the season—but for his career. If he had a good game, another team would pick him up. He asked me to work with him. He played—played well and thankfully did not get reinjured. He is still in the league. I am sure this young man never knew that Joe intervened and cared so much. This is just one example. I have seen this type of behavior from him many times.

Joe has talked to the massage students over the years and has shared the importance of professionalism and competency. I cannot overemphasize the importance of professionalism and respect for the trainers in these environments.

Often when Joe speaks publicly and privately, he mentions Kent Falb. You can hear the respect in his voice, and in his words, for his teacher and mentor. When I speak in the future about Joe, my mentor and teacher, you will hear the same things. ▪

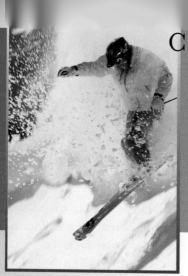

1

THE WORLD OF SPORTS AND EXERCISE MASSAGE

OBJECTIVES

Upon completion of this chapter, the reader will have the information necessary to:

1 Identify personal motivation for wanting to work with this population.

2 Explain realistic career expectations.

3 List the complexities of working with this population.

4 List the previous knowledge and experience needed to apply the information in the textbook.

5 Identify teachers, mentors, and resources for self-study in this career area.

6 Use this textbook for self- and classroom study.

7 Explain and list challenges and rewards for working with the population.

- What is it about working with sports and fitness issues that requires more learning and specific textbooks?
- What do I need to know to effectively work with athletes?
- Why do I want to work with athletes?
- Am I committed to putting as much time into my training and skills as athletes put into their training and skills?

These interesting questions are relevant for any massage therapist wishing to specialize and target his or her career toward a specific population. Substitute chronic illness, hospice, pre- and postnatal, elderly, infants, and so on, and the questions would be the same. It is important to identify the motivation for any course of study, especially at an advanced level.

This text targets the sports/fitness/physical rehabilitation client. These clients range from individuals involved in physical rehabilitation requiring exercise programs, including cardiovascular and cardiorespiratory rehabilitation, and physical therapy for orthopedic injury; persons incorporating exercise as part of a comprehensive fitness and wellness program, including weight management; and recreational and competitive athletes, both amateur and professional. Return to the questions above and really look at them. What is your motivation for wanting to learn how to use therapeutic massage to serve this population?

The sports, fitness, and rehabilitation community is using massage at an increased rate, which is admirable. However, there are many misconceptions, inaccurate information, and even dangerous methods being taught and practiced as sports massage. I have heard horror stories from athletes, trainers, doctors, and coaches and have told some myself. More commonly, I hear complaints from those who have received ineffective massage that was not worth the time and money. This is unacceptable. There is a professional responsibility to provide safe and effective massage care for all populations.

Please review the list in the foreword of this text of some of those with whom I have worked and who are involved in sports and fitness and support massage application as described in this book. These are the individuals who have been my information source for what athletes really expect from massage.

This text is written with many objectives. It should provide information to answer some of the questions listed at the beginning of this section, at least those about exercise, athletes, and what it takes to work with this group of clients. However, it cannot explain why you want to work in this realm. No textbook or teacher can answer that question for you. I am still figuring it out for myself. Many years of working with hundreds of athletes (for real), as well as with thousands of "ordinary" people, have blessed me with accumulated therapeutic massage experience, most of which has been learned independently of formal classroom training. One of the main purposes of this text is to consolidate this experience so that it won't take others over 20 years to become proficient at this type of massage application.

TEACHERS AND MENTORS

The textbook is designed to be a teacher, and I hope that it can be somewhat like a mentor. A **teacher** presents new information and skills and refines and targets previous learning. A **mentor** has professional experience, has achieved individual excellence, and wants to help others achieve their own success.

I have been fortunate in my career to have great teachers and mentors. One of these was Dr. David Gurevich–Russian physician, physical medicine specialist, soccer player, and tango dancer. It was an honor to learn from him for eight years. He taught me a practical and innovative application of massage, which he learned as a battlefield surgeon and long-time specialist in physical and rehabilitative medicine in Russia. Some of that knowledge was passed along to you through the textbooks *Mosby's Fundamentals of Therapeutic Massage* and *Mosby's Essential Sciences for Therapeutic Massage,* and even more is included in this text.

Dr. Leon Chaitow is also my teacher and mentor. His review and consolidation of research supporting soft tissue methods provide much of the foundation material for this book. All of his books should be read (in particular the texts I recommend in this book), to support the sports and exercise massage information in this book.

I admire the conceptual framework of Tom Myers, who integrates facial/muscular/structural function of the body. His textbook, *Anatomy Trains,* is recommended as a companion study with this text. The exacting, meticulous focus of Joe Muscolino's presentation of the musculoskeletal system in *The Muscular System Manual* is an ongoing study and reference. The serious massage therapist needs Donald Neuman's textbook–*Kinesiology of the Musculoskeletal System: Foundations for Physical Rehabilitation.* It beautifully describes human movement. I also respect Benny Vaughn, for his excellence in sports massage. His videotape series is a beneficial learning tool.

Since this text is not for the beginner, it is valuable to review and reflect on your therapeutic massage learning journey thus far, and take a realistic inventory of your skills, strengths, and weaknesses as you advance your educational experience. Who are your teachers and mentors? What authors, lecturers, and experts do you admire? What textbook and reference texts have been beneficial learning tools for you?

Athletes provide great learning experiences because, as a group, they present many different and complex problems that must be solved in order to help them reach and maintain their desired goals. Working with the sports population has challenged me to incorporate all my accumulated knowledge and experience, while maintaining my willingness to learn. My interface with other sports and exercise professionals has been immeasurably valuable. Each time I work alongside others I take in as much information as possible. Joe Recknagel and Tina Thompson are two athletic trainers who have taught me so much. Joe in particular has been in the trenches for years. I will never know as much as he knows, and I learn from him constantly.

Athletes themselves have been my best teachers. The world of athletics is culturally diverse and rich in cultural experience and has no room for prejudice. Other than the military, I don't think that multicultural interaction toward a common goal is displayed any better than in team sports. Most competing amateur and professional athletes are young, ranging from adolescence to 30 years old. As a 50-plus mom-type person, these interactions have kept me current and tolerant. When

working with cardiac rehabilitation, most of the clients are older than myself, giving me a picture of what my future may be. What clients teach you is impossible to learn in a classroom or a book. I think of the struggles I have had to find ways to help all the clients I have encountered over the years and how this motivation has challenged me to learn.

When I think of the athletes who have been my clients, and therefore my teachers, a few stand out. In particular I recall Charlie, the methods I improvised while working on his knees, and his persistence while working to reclaim his performance capacity in spite of challenges that would have overwhelmed others. Many persons have benefited from my experiences in helping Charlie.

There is Robert—a solid, 2-hour massage—week after week after week—it was a privilege watching him juggle the demands of professional sports and celebrity status while moving through his career as he changed from a kid to a man, maintaining his love for his family.

There is Barret's ability to only know how to go fast: he stops by running into something or someone. I never knew what I would find with him from day to day. I think also of Larry, Jimmy, and Chiti and the pain they endured, along with the tenacity of their determination. There is Scott, battling the problem in his neck plus everything else. The most important thing I learned from him,

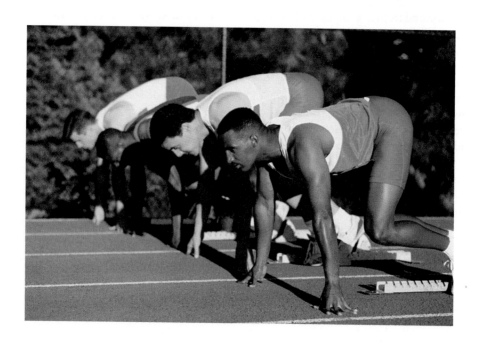

however, was the triumph of reclaiming one's self after the sports career is over.

There were lots of necks: Kyin's and Ron's ended their careers, and Korry's really big neck, to name a few. Lest I forget, there was James, who read the newspaper while getting a massage and who taught me to keep things in perspective. There was Jarrid's toe and John's psoas and willingness to be the demo.

There were also the backs. Steven's and Kurt's ended both careers. And there were dozens of coaches with the problematic back. It is common for coaches to have headaches (wonder why?).

I learned from Jason's routine and faith, Allen's pecs, Eddie's and Bryant's ankles, Michael's entire right side, Casey's concussion, Tony's shoulder (and just about everything else), Ray's fingers (but even more, his grace), Luther's elbow and compassion, Brock's and Drey's hamstrings, Zo's pain in the butt, and Eric's feet along with the laughs he provided, even when he was worried, sad, and scared. The list goes on and on. Those are just a few of my athlete teachers; there will be more. Every person you touch is your teacher—as a professional, you know this, right?

Of course each of my students has been my teacher as well. Those that commit to the time, intensity, and challenges of learning how to help athletes get my attention, be it patient and compassionate or brisk and to the point. There is not often time in some sports situations to be "nice." We all have to learn to toughen our hides, manage our emotions, and not take things personally. Of course, each student learns all the anatomy and physiology and massage methods—that's the easy part. The hard part is learning how to be a professional in the sports/fitness/rehabilitation environment. I will not tolerate groupies—no asking for autographs or any type of interaction with the athletes other than ultimate professionalism. **NO** makeup, fancy hairdos, long nails, jewelry, and especially NO ATTITUDE. I expect students to follow the rules, and of course I also have to comply with them. I learn from having to be the example. This is harder to teach and learn than one might expect.

Providing demo after demo, along with explaining my thought processes and skill applications during the demos, really integrates learning. I expect the athlete to learn while I'm explaining what is going on. After all, they will need to interview and screen qualified massage therapists as they move around the country. I expect my students to explain the massage application and outcome to each athlete with whom they work. Eventually (I hope), they will become their own self-teacher. In my mind, that is the mark of excellence: being able to teach yourself.

REALISTIC CAREER EXPECTATIONS

Working with athletes is hard, physical work. I remember teaching someone who weighed only 100 pounds how to provide enough pressure for a 350-pound lineman. She finally understood body mechanics. She did it, and others have benefited from her tenacity in spite of a few tears of frustration.

Helping students to learn to "let go" is important. The professional sports community is very mobile. You seldom work with this level of athlete for more than a season or two. Boundaries are a big deal. This population can be needy and demanding.

The reality check of building a professional practice with professional athletes is a wake-up call. The truth is that it does not happen very often and if it does, working with the professional athlete takes a lot of time, travel, and flexibility. There are not that many professional or Olympic athletes around. There are fewer than 400 NBA basketball players and less than 2500 NFL football players. The numbers for other team sports are somewhere in between. Individual professional athletes such as tennis players, golfers, and bowlers are also a small community.

Most massage therapists will serve the high school, collegiate, amateur, or semiprofessional athlete and also those in rehab or striving to achieve or maintain fitness. A common misconception is that professional athletes make millions and millions of dollars. Only a few are in that category. Most make far less, and amateurs generate no athletic income at all. Therefore, justifying the cost benefit of therapeutic massage is an ongoing issue, compared with its expense and regularity of use. Sports, fitness, and rehabilitation participation cost money, and often lots of it. If a person is going to use massage on a regular basis, the fees need to be manageable. How do I, as a mentor and teacher, instill the desire for excellence, awareness and acceptance of the time it takes, and the practice and persistence required to work with these types of issues and clients?

So, here is the reality: There is no such thing as "sports massage"—only appropriate massage application for each client. Whether your client is a runner, bowler, swimmer, surfer, or golfer; is a baseball, basketball, football, or soccer player; or has just completed a treadmill stress test–this is an important factor to consider as part of the treatment plan. This text also provides skill development for treating the general population: any client can sprain an ankle, develop post-exercise soreness, have a headache or backache. Do not limit the use of this text just to those considered athletes. We are all athletes in some form, anyway.

I believe that working with athletes is an advanced level career focus. It is expected that the readers of this text, whether as self-study or part of a formal course of study, are building upon the fundamentals of solid therapeutic massage practice, including anatomy, physiology, kinesiology, and pathology as presented in *Mosby's Fundamentals of Therapeutic Massage* and *Mosby's Essential Sciences for Therapeutic Massage*. These concepts will be reviewed in this text in the context of using therapeutic massage in the world of sports and exercise. You should already know about anatomy and physiology, sanitation, draping, massage manipulations, and techniques such as body mechanics, assessment, charting, and treatment plan development, as well as ethics and professionalism. These foundational skills and knowledge are even more important when specializing in a target population. The textbooks that I feel are necessary to really absorb the content of this text are listed in Box 1-1. It is from this base we will build to serve sports and exercise clients.

HOW THIS TEXTBOOK IS DESIGNED

This text is presented as an integrated **outcome-based** approach to massage. It is not based on specific modalities (Swedish massage, reflexology, shiatsu, deep tissue massage, and the seemingly never-ending list of others), because modalities do not support individual applications based on client goals. Instead, we will discuss the application of mechanical force to stimulate the neuro-endocrine/neuromuscular systems, to affect myofascial structure and function, to assist fluid movement, and to support homeostasis. The content should prepare the massage professional to interact effectively with various treatment, training, and rehabilitation protocols of the sports and fitness world. General lifestyle requirements such as sleep, nutrition, and stress management are an

Box 1-1   RECOMMENDED TEXTBOOKS

The following textbooks provide the foundation necessary to learn the material in this book.

Chaitow L, DeLany JW: *Clinical applications of neuromuscular techniques, vol 1, the upper body,* vol 1, Edinburgh, 2000, Churchill Livingstone.

Chaitow L, DeLany JW: *Clinical applications of neuromuscular techniques, vol 2, the lower body.* Edinburgh, 2002, Churchill Livingstone.

Fritz S: *Mosby's fundamentals of therapeutic massage,* ed 3. St. Louis, 2004, Mosby.

Fritz S: *Mosby's essential science for therapeutic massage: anatomy, physiology, biomechanics, and pathology,* ed 2. St. Louis, 2004, Mosby.

Ireland ML, Nattiv A: *The female athlete.* Philadelphia, 2002, Saunders.

Lowe W: *Orthopedic massage: theory and technique.* London, 2003, Mosby Ltd.

Muscolino JE: *The muscular system manual: the skeletal muscles of the human body,* ed 2. St. Louis, 2005, Elsevier.

Myers T: *Anatomy trains: myofascial meridians for manual and movement therapists.* Edinburgh, 2001, Churchill Livingstone.

Neumann D: *Kinesiology of the musculoskeletal system: foundations for physical rehabilitation.* St. Louis, 2002, Mosby.

important part of the athlete's world. These will be addressed as part of the knowledge foundation needed to be an effective massage practitioner with this type of client.

This text is surely not written from a conceptual framework. It is not only based on theory but is also more focused on practice. It is more about how than why. The practical application comes from years of working in the real world.

I have worked and continue to work with athletes: male, female, both human and animal, and young (7 years old) to mature (87 years young). There are few sports I have not worked with in the past 25 years. I teach advanced students and lead the massage program for a professional football team, the Detroit Lions (for more than 8 years), spanning four head coaches, three athletic trainers, and hundreds of football players, including rookies and 18-year veterans. I am also involved on an ongoing basis with both the International Management Group (IMG) and the International Performance Institute (IPI), with an advanced sports massage program serving elite athletes in football, golf, tennis, soccer, baseball, skating, and more. Years ago, I worked with professional wrestlers–that was fun! I have massaged golfers, dancers, acrobats, cheerleaders, rodeo riders, cyclists, bowlers, and musicians, as well as horses, dogs, and even performing parrots. I have worked with wheelchair athletes and those with various types of prostheses; with weekend warriors; and with amateur, Olympic, and professional athletes–individuals and collegiate, semi-pro and professional teams. I have worked in the areas of cardiovascular fitness; weight loss programs; pre- and post-pregnancy exercise; exercise protocols for depression, anxiety, and pain management; and physical rehabilitation. I have supported doctors, nurses, physical therapists, chiropractors, psychologists, athletic trainers, exercise physiologists, coaches, and parents of athlete kids.

It has been necessary to adapt and perform massage in the hospital; on the playing and practice field; in the locker room and training room; in game hotels; in the pool; on the floor; and with clients on their bed, on the couch, and just about everywhere else, including an actual massage room on rare occasions! I go to athlete's homes and have given massages in a furnace room (because it was warm, dark, and with no disturbances) complete with a water feature every time someone flushed the toilet; and in the garage (heated), family room, bedroom, and even the kitchen. I have worked in state-of-the-art training facilities as well as parking lots, offices, and airports; when working with a soccer team, we set up massage tables in the showers. One year the massage area for the Detroit Lions was the team racquet ball court–18 to 20 tables, 20 to 25 students, and that many football players. That was intense.

I have had experience with teams that win and teams that lose; individuals that win and individuals that lose; individuals that have potentials that they do not meet; and those that achieve far beyond what anyone expected. A few athletes have an attitude, but not very many. Almost all are great people, unlike what you hear and see in the media. I have worked with all colors, shapes, and sizes of athletes while they slept, watched practice tapes, received different treatment from the trainer, talked on the phone, watched TV, or fed their newborn baby. I have figured out how to give an entire full body massage while maintaining the athlete's view of the TV screen. Often, others were present, including athletes' kids on and under the massage table; their wives, husbands, mothers, fathers, grandparents, and friends on the table, mat or in a chair for a massage. Their dog has been under

the massage table and their cats on the table in my bag with all the linens.

I have seen professional athletes cry, complain, whine, and feel sorry for themselves. I have watched as they spent time with kids, the elderly, and others (mostly when the cameras weren't on), and when they were taking care of their family members. Athletes do laundry, take out the trash, and do the dishes just like everyone else. I know the tragedies of some of their lives and the determination it has taken to overcome the odds. They have asked me to massage them when they play while injured, lose their position or are cut from the team, and after their career is over, when they rebuild a life or when they don't and fall into destructive behavior. Many retired athletes suffer from the accumulated trauma, injury, and other residual effects following the end of their athletic careers.

I have seen athletes only once and then never again, or for a season, or, in the case of a few people, for their entire career and beyond. Athletes have sought my services on a weekly basis, daily basis, or 24 hours a day for weeks, to accelerate healing from surgery. Along the way, there have been a few very rich and many more not so rich athletes. I have laughed, cried, been ignored, angry, frustrated, tired, overwhelmed, and often clueless about what to do. I have also been proud, honored, and appreciated. I continue to laugh at the unexpected situations in which I find myself, in this crazy world of sports, fitness, and rehabilitation.

I have taught many students to work with various sport and fitness conditions. Over 50, fit but overweight, I look like a mom and am delighted to find that it works. I am very, very good at what I do and expect others to be so as well. The aim of this text is to share as much as I can about what works and what doesn't, why and how to fit into the various environments, and how to sustain this type of career. Sometimes I don't know how I do what I do. But usually it can be figured out and then taught to those willing to learn.

I will tell stories and give examples, all true–some with actual names, with permission and support, and others without, to protect confidentiality. Each story or example teaches a lesson–at least I learned one by living it. Out of necessity–the mother of invention–my students, fellow instructors, and I have figured out applications that you may not have considered but that work (usually). So, please keep an open mind and give these things a try before you judge. I share all this with you in this first chapter not to brag but to establish that I have been there, done that, made mistakes, and learned something from most of them and that I will not try to candy-coat this career track.

How did I end up with all these professional athletes as clients, especially since I am not athletically inclined? It just happened that way; it was not planned. Despite having a visual and balance problem that makes me clumsy, I still am effective with this population. You just never know where your career will lead you.

The immediacy and intensity of the athlete's world demand an integrated body/mind/spirit approach delivered by well-trained massage professionals. Exceptional demands are placed on professionals who work with athletes or those in physical rehabilitation because of the extraordinary circumstances of these individuals. The environment of competitive sports and physical rehabilitation makes for "bigger-than-life moments." There is the drama of win or lose, the trauma of injury, and the career-determining or even life-or-death situations of surgery and rehabilitation. Working in the world of sports and fitness can be like a roller coaster ride, but with a lot of monotony between the highs and lows. I have spent many hours waiting for athletes while they received treatment, slept, were interviewed, had meetings, or forgot appointments. Much of this text was written during this time. I wonder if research will ever be able to totally capture the multi-dimensional aspect of massage.

The massage therapist must not only be highly skilled in the massage application for the mode of sports or fitness activity but must also have motivation, maturity, reliability, compassion, tenacity, tolerance, stamina, flexibility, commitment, faith, hope, perseverance, humility, self-esteem, little need for personal glory, and the ability to work behind the scenes, to improvise, and above all else, to think and solve problems.

This book does not have all the answers or even all the information you will need to be a competent massage therapist. It is virtually impossible to describe in depth each and every sport in a single volume. However, this text does cover the general movement patterns used in sports and fitness: running, throwing, hitting, kicking, and so forth.

I recall working with students wanting to learn to work with surfers. I do not surf, so I had those students teach me how—not in the ocean, but on a table in the classroom. As I struggled to do the simple moves of sitting on the board, paddling, standing up, and maintaining my balance, I began to feel in my own body the areas of strain, repetitive movement, and physical skill required for this sport. With this information, I was able to target these areas in the surfer client. By teaching me about their particular sport, the students were able to better understand the soft tissue demands and target areas for massage application.

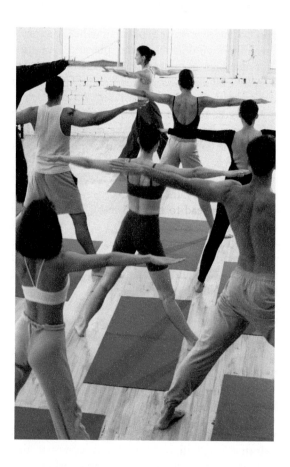

This is what I suggest for all of you. Each sport has an ideal performance form; superimposed on this is the form modified and adapted by the individual athlete. Now, I looked really silly on that table pretending to surf. I have also thrown a football, assumed the lineman's stance, tried to hit a baseball, served a volleyball, played golf, and attempted other related activities, although I was terrible at them. Looking silly doesn't matter if you can understand something better by experiencing it. There were rehab exercises and drills with various clients, when I rolled around in the wheel chair, examined the prosthesis, and put on the sports equipment and gear. By the way, pads and helmets are really heavy, and racing bike seats are not very comfortable!

The individual athlete is the best expert on his or her own situation. If you are going to be able to help individuals with massage, they need to be willing to teach you and you have to be willing to learn. You do not have to be proficient, just understand.

Primarily I am a teacher, so I wrote this text the same way that I teach a class. The approach that I use, and that seems to work best, is an integrated massage style based on valid scientific research coupled with the clinical success of some bodywork methods still awaiting validation. Research has identified massage benefits in relatively concrete terms based on physiologic mechanisms. Some sport-specific research will be presented later.

Basically, massage aims to produce three types of effect on the body systems: **structural, physiologic,** and **psychologic.** Although these effects are closely related, it is the initial mechanical effects brought about by the manual skills of a massage therapist that lead to the physiologic and psychologic effects. Hence, the stroking, squeezing, compression, rubbing, and so forth that are applied to the skin and underlying muscles not only produce physical benefits but also trigger physiologic and psychologic responses. To achieve the desired balance and results, it is vital to understand the principles behind the various massage techniques. The type and extent of effect on the body depend on the technique itself, the depth to which it is applied, and the area of the body being massaged.

Those involved in sports, fitness, and rehabilitation are often interested in adjunct therapies, including hydrotherapy, aromatherapy, Asian bodywork methods, magnets, and various forms of relaxation/meditation. Unit Two is devoted to this content. Understanding sports injuries and massage application requires a knowledge of tissue susceptibility to trauma and the mechanical forces involved. Unit Three is devoted to this content. The final unit of this text, Unit Four, combines all of the information in a series of case studies. By studying the various cases, the reader can integrate the textbook content into practical hands-on application.

This book is written as a textbook to support the classroom environment. It can also be used to self-teach. Once the information has been assimilated, then the text becomes a reference text because it is impossible to remember it all. The chapters are set up in typical textbook form with objectives and outlines. At the end of each chapter is a workbook section. Throughout the text are various commentaries by athletes and those involved in rehabilitation and associated professions, stories to illustrate a lesson or bring a concept alive, and helpful hints. It is logical to start at the beginning and work sequentially to the end of the text, since each chapter builds on the one before it. You can't just read this book. You need to do it, just as athletes do in training. They practice, over, and over, and over.

SUMMARY

It is unrealistic to think that the skills to professionally work both with the complexities of the athlete and those seeking fitness or function can be achieved overnight. It is realistic to expect that this is an advanced study requiring 500 hours or more of classroom study, and a minimum of 500 clinic hours. Whether you are in a formal course of study or self-teaching, expect to commit at least 12 to 24 months of concentrated study and practice with 500 to 1000 focused massage sessions to begin to achieve proficiency.

Your commitment to achieving this type of goal is a reflection of your desire for excellence. An athlete commits countless hours to practice and more hours of study to be excellent. A person in physical rehabilitation does the same. Why should they have any less of a commitment from the massage professional that they choose to work with them? Respect is earned, and this text provides part of the resources to achieve this respect. Some of the content in this text will be very technical because it needs to be. There is a lot to know, and this text has done some of the research for you, but it can't do it all—you must learn to do research, interpret data, and generate appropriate treatment plans yourself. Routines absolutely do not work in this arena. You must be able to think, have a purpose, be innovative, and continue to learn. Every client—not just an athlete—deserves this level of professionalism.

WORKBOOK

1 List common myths about athletes and then explain the more accurate view. Examples:

Myth–Most professional athletes are egocentric.
Accurate–Most athletes are polite and appreciative.
Myth–Sports massage is a specific modality.
Accurate–A person's physical activity needs to be considered as part of the treatment plan.

_____

_____

_____

_____

_____

2 List the necessary professional skills needed for working with this population. Example: stamina and patience.

_____

_____

_____

_____

_____

3 Using this textbook as a resource, develop a realistic list of knowledge and skills for massage application targeting this population. Example: sport injuries, body mechanics.

_____

_____

_____

_____

_____

_____

_____

4 Review the chapter objectives and then respond to each one. Repeat each objective.

_____

_____

_____

_____

_____

5 Respond to the following statement: If I were a competing athlete, I would expect my massage therapist to be able to

_____

_____

_____

_____

_____

6 Respond to the following statement: If I were beginning an exercise program, I would expect my massage therapist to be able to

_____

_____

_____

_____

_____

_____

_____

7 Respond to the following statement: If I were beginning a physical rehabilitation program, I would expect my massage therapist to be able to

_____

_____

_____

_____

_____

8 List at least three factors that make this population unique. Example: tendency to injury.

_____

_____

_____

_____

_____

9 List the professional skills you currently have that would support your proficiency in this area.

_____

_____

_____

_____

_____

10 List the professional skills you need to develop to competently serve this population.

_____

_____

_____

_____

_____

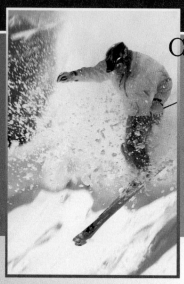

2

WHAT IS SPORTS MASSAGE?

OBJECTIVES

Upon completion of this chapter, the reader will have the information necessary to:

1 Define athletes and exercise.
2 Understand the cumulative effects of the strain of peak performance.
3 Identify the experts that work with athletes.
4 List the goals and outcomes common for this population.
5 Explain the categories of sports massage.

Who is an athlete? What is fitness? An **athlete** is a person who participates in sports as either an amateur or a professional. Athletes require precise use of their bodies. The athlete trains the nervous system and muscles to perform in a specific way. Often the activity involves repetitive use of one group of muscles more than others, which may result in hypertrophy, changes in strength, movement patterns, connective tissue formation, and compensation patterns in the rest of the body. These factors contribute to the soft tissue difficulties that often develop in athletes.

Fitness is a lifestyle. It is a body/mind/spirit endeavor. One who is fit typically lives a moderate life in a relatively simple way. Characteristics and behaviors enable a person to have the highest quality of life, an overall state of health, and the maximum degree of adaptive capacity to respond to the environment, as determined by genetic predisposition. Fitness and wellness are, relatively, the same realm. There is a continuum in the human experiences of energy expenditure and recovery, and the ease of this reflects one's fitness. Sports massage is targeted to support fitness, help reduce the demands the sport places on the body, increase the ability to perform the sport, and enhance and shorten recovery time.

Athlete
Athletic trainers
Exercise physiologists
Fitness
Intercompetition massage

Peak performance
Performance
Physical therapists
Promotional or event massage
Recovery/post-event/massage

Remedial/rehabilitation/orthopedic massage
Sports medicine physicians
Sports psychologists
Trauma
Traumatic injury

PERFORMANCE VS. FITNESS

Fitness is necessary for everyone's wellness, but the physical activity of an athlete goes beyond fitness; it is performance-based. **Performance** is the capacity to complete sport-specific activity with skill and competence. Because of the intense physical activity involved in sports, an athlete may be more prone to injury. Massage can be very beneficial for athletes if the professional performing the massage understands the biomechanics required by the sport. If the specific biomechanics are not understood, massage can impair optimal function in the athlete's performance.

When accumulated strain develops for any reason, the fitness/wellness balance is upset. Illness and/or injury can result. For competing athletes, a major strain is the demand of performance. Performance exceeds fitness, requiring increased energy expenditure, which in turn strains adaptive mechanisms and increases recovery time. Fitness must be achieved before performance, and fitness must be supported to endure the ongoing strain of **peak performance**, the highest level of skill execution.

Those who have become deconditioned and are unfit owing to a bad diet, lack of proper exercise, accelerated and multiple life stresses, as well as other lifestyle habits, will eventually also experience some sort of **illness** or injury. The injury/illness can be of a chronic nature, such as chronic fatigue. There seems to be a genetic tendency for a specific breakdown to occur; this can be considered a genetic weak link. It is likely that we all have these weak links, and that strain will affect this area first.

Traumatic injury is injury caused by an unexpected event. Accidents are a common cause of traumatic injury. Rehabilitation following this type of injury often requires physical training. A person may not consider himself or herself an athlete but may suffer the same results of stress common in athletes---post-activity soreness, fatigue, and joint pain, for example. The goal of rehabilitation is function. For peak performance, fitness is a prerequisite.

PEAK PERFORMANCE IS NOT PEAK FITNESS

Contrary to general beliefs, athletes, especially competing athletes, may not be fit or healthy. In fact, they may be quite fragile in their adaptive ability. This means that any demands to adapt, including massage, should be gauged by the athlete's adaptive capacity. A lack of understanding about the demands placed on athletes often leads to inappropriate massage care. The assumption is that these are strong, healthy, robust individuals, but this is not always true. They may be fatigued, injured, in pain, immunosuppressed, emotionally and physically stressed, and truly unable to adapt to one more stimulus in their life. Unless these stressors are recognized and principles of massage therapy are correctly applied, athletes may be subject to inappropriate massage that includes invasive methods that at the very least are fatiguing and, at worst, cause tissue damage.

Athletes experience body fatigue and brain fatigue. Massage can help restore balance if properly applied. If the body is tired, do not task it more; instead, help it rest. If the brain is tired, do not task it more; help it rest. Often the best massage approach is the general nonspecific massage that feels good, calms, and supports sleep. In physiologic terms, this produces parasympathetic dominance in the autonomic nervous system, which supports homeostasis, or self-healing.

The experts specializing in the care of athletes are **sports medicine physicians, physical thera-**

pists, athletic trainers, exercise physiologists, and sports psychologists (Box 2-1). It is especially important for athletes to work under the direction of these professionals to ensure proper sports form and training protocols. The professional athlete is more likely to have access to these professionals than recreational and amateur athletes, who may not have the financial resources to hire training personnel and can incur injury because of inappropriate training protocols.

Athletes depend on the effects of training and the resulting neurologic responses for precise functioning, such as the firing sequence of certain muscles. This is especially important prior to competition. Without the proper training and experience, it is easy for massage therapists to disorganize the neurologic responses if they do not understand the patterns required for efficient functioning in the sport. The effect is temporary, and unless the athlete is going to compete within 24 hours, it is usually not significant. However, if the massage is given just before competition, the results could be devastating. Any type of massage before a competition must be given carefully. If a massage professional plans to work with an athlete on a continuing basis, it is important that the practitioner really knows the athlete and becomes part of the entire training experience.

For the athlete, his or her psychologic state is crucial to performance; often the competition is won in the mind. Massage therapists are not sports psychologists. Remember that. However, athletes look to us for support, continuity, and feedback. Many athletes are very ritualistic about precompetition readiness. If massage has become part of that ritual and the massage professional is inconsistent in maintaining appointment schedules, an athlete's performance outcome can be adversely affected.

GOALS AND OUTCOMES FOR MASSAGE

Two of the most important goals of sports massage are to assist the athlete in achieving and maintaining peak performance and to support healing of injuries. Any massage professional should be able to recognize common sports injuries and should refer the athlete to the appropriate medical professional. Once a diagnosis has been made and a rehabilitation plan developed, the massage professional can support the athlete with general massage application and appropriate methods to enhance the healing process.

Many factors contribute to mechanical injuries and trauma in sports. **Trauma** is defined as a physical injury or wound sustained in sports that was produced by an external or internal force.

Healing mechanisms manifest as an inflammatory response and resolution of that response. Different tissues heal at different rates. For example, skin heals quickly, whereas ligaments heal slowly. Stress can influence healing by slowing the repair process. Sleep and proper nutrition are necessary for proper healing (Table 2-1).

Typically, post-trauma massage is focused on circulation enhancement as are other methods discussed. Contraindications may exist for deep transverse friction, specific myofascial release, and extensive trigger point work. Medication use, particularly analgesics and antiinflammatory drugs for pain is common, and their effects must be considered. (Refer to the *evolve* Evolve web site accompanying this book for a listing of common medications and their possible implications for massage.) Pain medication reduces pain perception so that the athlete can continue to perform before healing is complete. This interferes with successful healing. Antiinflammatory drugs may slow the healing process, particularly connective tissue healing.

TYPES OF SPORTS MASSAGE

In the past, massage for athletes has been categorized by when it is given and the reasons for the massage. Some of those categories are discussed

TABLE 2-1 STAGES OF TISSUE HEALING AND MASSAGE INTERVENTIONS		
STAGE 1: ACUTE INFLAMMATORY REACTION	**STAGE 2: SUBACUTE REPAIR AND HEALING**	**STAGE 3: CHRONIC AND MATURATION AND REMODELING**
Characteristics Vascular changes Inflammatory exudates Clot formation Phagocytosis, neutralization of irritants Early fibroblastic activity	Growth of capillary beds into area Collagen formation Granulation tissue; caution necessary Fragile, easily injured tissue	Maturation and remodeling of scar Contracture of scar tissue Alignment of collagen along lines of stress forces (tensegrity)
Clinical Signs Inflammation Pain prior to tissue resistance	Decreased inflammation Pain during tissue resistance	Absence of inflammation Pain after tissue resistance
Massage Intervention Protection Control and support of effects of inflammation (PRICE)* Passive movement mid-range General massage and lymphatic drainage with caution; support rest with full-body massage (3 to 7 days)	Controlled motion Promoting development of mobile scar Cautious and controlled soft tissue mobilization of scar tissue along fiber direction toward injury. Active and passive, open- and closed-chain range or motion, mid-range. Support healing with full-body massage (14 to 21 days)	Return to function Increase in strength and alignment of scar tissue Cross-fiber friction of scar tissue coupled with directional stroking along the lines of tension away from injury Progressive stretching and active and resisted range of motion; full-range. Support rehabilitation activities with full-body massage (3 to 12 months)

*Promoting healing and preventing compensation patterns.
From Fritz S: *Mosby's fundamentals of therapeutic massage,* ed. 3. St. Louis, 2004, Mosby.

here. However, if you are using outcome-based goals, then these categories become irrelevant. If massage is being used to assist pre-exercise warm-up, then it should be focused on those goals, but it is actually incorrect to call it pre-event massage. The same applies to massage focused to support the recovery process post competition. Does that really need to be called **post-event massage?** Currently some of the categories of sports massage are pre-event, intercompetition, remedial, medical or orthopedic, recovery, post-event, maintenance, and promotional or event massage.

PRE-EVENT MASSAGE

Pre-event massage is a stimulating, superficial, fast-paced, rhythmic massage that lasts for 10 to 15 minutes. The emphasis is on the muscles used in the sporting event, and the goal is for the athlete to feel that his or her body is "perfect" physically. Avoid uncomfortable techniques. This warm-up massage is given in addition to the physical warm-up; it is not a substitute. This style of massage can be used from 3 days before the event until imme-

diately preceding the event. Massage techniques that require extensive recovery time or are painful are strictly contraindicated. Focus on circulation enhancement and be very careful of overworking any area. Sports pre-event massage should be general, nonspecific, light, and warming. Avoid friction or deep, heavy strokes. Such a massage should be pain-free! It is suggested that only massage therapists who work on an ongoing basis with a particular athlete give the athlete a pre-event massage.

INTERCOMPETITION MASSAGE

Intercompetition massage, given during breaks in the event, concentrates on the muscles being used or those about to be used. The techniques are short, light, and focused. It is suggested that only massage therapists familiar with a particular athlete provide intercompetition massage.

POST-EVENT RECOVERY MASSAGE

Recovery massage focuses primarily on athletes who want to recover from a strenuous workout or competition when no injury is present. The method used to help an athlete recover from a workout or competition is similar to a generally focused, full-body massage, using any and all methods that support a return to homeostasis.

REMEDIAL/REHABILITATION/MEDICAL /ORTHOPEDIC MASSAGE

Remedial, rehabilitation, medical, and orthopedic massage are interrelated terms. **Remedial massage,** which is used for minor to moderate injuries, uses all methods presented in this text. In contrast, **rehabilitation massage** is used for more severe injury or as part of the postsurgical intervention plan. If the injury or surgery is related to the bones or joints, it can be considered **orthopedic massage.**

The methods of massage used in rehabilitation vary. Immediately after injury or surgery, relatively nonspecific, general stress reduction, and healing promotion massage techniques are implemented. Attention is given to the entire body while the area of injury or surgery heals. Any immobility, use of crutches, or changes in posture or gait during recovery will likely create compensation patterns. Massage can manage these compensation patterns while the physician, physical therapist, and trainer focus on the injured area. During active rehabilitation, massage can become part of the recovery process, supervised by an appropriately qualified professional, as part of a total treatment plan.

PROMOTIONAL OR EVENT MASSAGE

Promotional or event massage usually is given at events for amateur athletes and can be either the pre- or post-event massage style. These massages are offered as a public service to provide educational information. It is important to receive written documentation of informed consent from each person receiving a massage at these events (Figure 2-1). One way to do this is to include an informed consent statement with the sign-in sheet and have each participant read and sign it before receiving the massage. A short brochure or pamphlet explaining the benefits, contraindications, and cautions of sports massage is given to each participant. With permission from the organizer of the event, the brochure may include information allowing participating athletes to contact the massage professional at a later date.

The sports event massage lasts about 15 minutes and is quick-paced. This type of public, promotional environment is one area in which following

---

Sample Informed Consent Form for Use at Sporting Events

Name of massage practitioner or organization: _____

Sporting event: _____

Date: _____

I have received, read, and understand informational literature concerning the general benefits of massage and the contraindications for massage. I have disclosed to the massage practitioner any condition I have that would be contraindicated for massage. Other than to determine contraindications, I understand that no specific needs assessment will be performed. The qualifications of the massage practitioner and reporting measures for misconduct have been disclosed to me.

I understand that the massage given here is for the purpose of stress reduction. I understand that massage practitioners do not diagnose illness or disease, perform any spinal manipulations, or prescribe any medical treatments. I acknowledge that massage is not a substitute for medical examination or diagnosis, and it is recommended that I see a health care provider for those services.

I understand that an event sports massage is limited to providing a general, nonspecific massage approach using standard massage methods but does not include any methods to address specifically soft tissue structure or function.

Participant's Signature: _____   Date: _____

Participant's Signature: _____   Date: _____

Participant's Signature: _____   Date: _____

FIGURE 2-1 ■ An example of an informed consent form for use at sporting events. (From Fritz S: *Mosby's fundamentals of therapeutic massage,* ed 3. St. Louis, 2004, Mosby.)

a sports massage routine is especially important. The use of lubricants is optional; the massage practitioner may choose not to use them because of the risk of allergic reaction, staining of an athlete's uniform, or other unforeseen factors.

It is important to watch for any swelling that may indicate a sprain, strain, or stress fracture and refer the athlete to the medical tent for immediate evaluation. It also is important to watch for evidence of thermoregulatory disruption, such as hypothermia or hyperthermia, and refer the individual immediately to the medical tent if these are noted (being careful to avoid using any diagnostic terms or unduly alarming the individual).

If a massage professional is doing promotional work at sports massage events and is working with many unfamiliar athletes, it is best to perform post-event massage, because the effects of any neurologic disorganization caused by the post-event massage are not significant.

No connective tissue work, intense stretching, trigger point work, or other invasive work should be included in a massage of an athlete at a sporting event. The massage should be superficial, supportive, and focused mainly on circulation enhancement.

THE SPORTS MASSAGE TEAM

Often a group of massage professionals and supervised students work as a team at an event. A practitioner who is familiar with the sport usually is the team leader. All participating massage practitioners follow a similar routine. Remember, each member of a sports massage team represents the entire massage profession. Ethical, professional behavior is essential. This is why permission of the organizer is required if you plan to supply contact information in a brochure that you distribute at such an event.

ONGOING CARE OF THE ATHLETE

Regular massage allows the body to function with less restriction and accelerates recovery time. This is a major focus of this textbook. Most athletes require varying depths of pressure, from light to very deep; therefore, effective body mechanics by the massage practitioner is essential. Working with athletes can be very demanding. Their schedules may be erratic, and their bodies change almost daily in response to training, competition, or injury. Athletes can become dependent on massage; therefore, commitment by the massage professional is necessary.

SUMMARY

This chapter provides an overview and description of what sports massage entails. Also discussed are the various categories of sports massage. Currently the distinctions between the different categories are becoming blurred as the concept of outcome-based massage becomes more fully understood. For example, recovery massage is not presented here a method; rather, recovery is regarded as the goal of the client and the treatment objective of the therapist.

This chapter also compared performance and fitness and the relevance of differences between the two when developing the outcome for each massage session.

1 Compare and contrast an athlete's goal for peak performance with that of a person desiring fitness. Example: athletes target specific function; fitness is an overall state of health. Athletes strain their adaptive mechanism; fitness increases adaptive capacity.

_____

2 List contributing factors to adaptive strain. Example: deconditioning and injury.

_____

3 Give reasons why an athlete can be considered fragile. Example: peak performance predisposes to injury.

_____

4 Explain why athletes may receive inappropriate massage care. Example: athlete is physically tired and the massage is too aggressive.

_____

_____

_____

_____

_____

_____

_____

_____

_____

_____

_____

5 Reword the following categories of massage as outcome goals: pre-event, intercompetition, recovery, remedial, promotional. Example: pre-event: increase arterial flow to limbs.

_____

_____

_____

_____

_____

_____

_____

_____

_____

_____

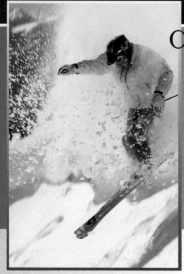

3

SCIENTIFIC VALIDATION OF SPORTS MASSAGE BENEFITS

OBJECTIVES

Upon completion of this chapter, the reader will have the information necessary to:

1 Identify commonly accepted outcomes for sports massage.

2 Apply research to develop outcome goals.

Validating the scientific basis of therapeutic massage is relatively easy. Research studies are beginning to consistently identify the underlying physiologic mechanisms of the body influenced by the application of mechanical stimuli and forces from massage. This is described in depth in Unit Two.

These benefits apply to everyone, and particularly to athletes, who may benefit even more owing to the stresses arising from training and competition. The specific research in sports and fitness massage is mixed in terms of benefits and underlying physiologic mechanisms.

Following is a brief review of some of the current sports massage research literature. All references for this book are listed at the end of each of the four parts and should be reviewed by the reader. It is difficult to identify the specific mechanisms that make massage application effective. Evidence-based research is scant, conflicting, and sometimes confusing. It is difficult to design studies of massage that meet the gold standard of being double-blind, and this affects acceptance by the traditional medical community. What once was thought to be true is being discounted, and we often do not know just why massage works. Time and more research may identify the mechanisms. Regardless, as professionals we are obligated to stay current with ongoing research results and be open to new ideas.

Analgesia
Breathing pattern disorders

Delayed onset muscle soreness
(DOMS)

Lymph flow

RESEARCH REVIEW

Research studies show that massage is being offered as part of medical and sports and fitness programs even though the knowledge of massage effectiveness is only partially corroborated by research. Many experts consider that the complex nature of the effects of massage make it difficult to define the exact mechanisms of these effects. It has become apparent that the desired effects of massage are dependent not on the modality—such as Swedish, deep tissue, or Asian—but rather on the type of mechanical forces used, and the intensity, tempo, and rhythm of the massage. For example, light, rapid massage will cause the athlete to be aroused and ready to compete. Slow, firm massage will instill a feeling of well-being and a state of relaxation. As stated in the majority of current literature, some of the common effects of massage include increased blood flow, increased lymphatic drainage, neural stimulation, encouragement of venous return, relief of pain, injury rehabilitation, and relaxation.

One topic subjected to multiple research studies is **delayed onset muscle soreness (DOMS).** The outcome of these studies varied, but a majority found that massage administered either immediately or 24 or 48 hours after exercise resulted in a reduction in DOMS. The best results were achieved when the massage was administered 2 hours post exercise, implying that timing is a factor. Although a scientific rationale has not been identified for these results, Russian sports therapists advocated that restorative massage be administered 1 to 3 hours after exercise.

Studies have shown that massage aimed at muscle relaxation can result in an increased range of motion in a joint. Muscles span joints, and if the individual muscles and/or groups of muscles are encouraged to relax, this has a direct effect in extending the limit to which the affected joint or joints can move. Kneading has been shown to decrease neuromuscular excitability, but only during the actual massage, and the effects are confined to the muscle(s) being massaged.

During warm-up protocols, stretching exercises produce the greatest flexibility in connective tissue around the joints, although massage has a significant beneficial effect as well. One study found that massage prior to activity could actually reduce the ability to generate force from muscle action. A different research study showed that maximal muscle power output during leg extension was significantly increased when athletes received massage beforehand. Such conflicting results make it difficult to arrive at absolute conclusions regarding the mechanisms and benefits of massage. Until the conflict is resolved, the determining factor should be the athlete's response. Performance experts strongly discourage athletes from receiving their first massage close to an important competition. When in doubt about the advisability of massage, wait until after the performance. It is also important that massage is carefully integrated into the athlete's entire training and competition programs. Random massage from multiple practitioners is less effective and could disrupt performance.

The effect of massage on **lymph flow** has been measured experimentally. There is a consensus within the literature demonstrating an increase in lymphatic flow. These data have implications for restorative massage outcomes and management of delayed onset muscle soreness. Lymph flow only increased with kneading and gliding massage and with active or passive exercise. Other studies, comparing massage to passive movement and electrical stimulation, again showed lymph flow to be greatest following massage.

Massage produces short-term **analgesia** by activating the gate-control mechanism through counterirritation and hyperstimulation analgesia. Cutaneous mechanoreceptors are stimulated by touch and rapidly transmit information within

23

large myelinated nerve fibers to the spinal cord. These impulses block the passage of painful stimuli entering the same spinal segment. Other physical therapies acting on this mechanism include thermal and electrical treatments and joint manipulation. Massage is a potent mechanical stimulus and a particularly effective trigger for the gate-control process.

Massage produces a warming effect on the tissue. There are many important therapeutic effects from heat. A mild degree of warming is effective in relieving pain. The proposed reason for this is the sedative effect on the sensory nerves. By virtue of relieving pain, associated muscle spasm and tension are also relieved. Heat also increases blood flow by dilating the capillaries and arterioles. Heating the tissues also causes an increase in muscle and ligament extensibility and ground substance pliability, enhancing stretching and facilitating muscle contractility.

Many researchers maintain that the recuperative benefits from massage may be more psychologic than physiologic. Massage promotes a feeling of well-being and even euphoria. The psychologic benefits of massage include controlled arousal before competition or training and positive mood states.

Physical relaxation can improve blood flow and reduce muscle tone and tension in connective tissue. Studies on fascia in humans using electron photomicroscopy found smooth muscle cells widely embedded within the collagen fibers and concluded that these intrafascial smooth muscle cells enable the autonomic nervous system to regulate a fascial pre-tension, independently of muscular tonus. The possible effects of active smooth muscle cell contractility may occur in the many fascial/connective tissue sites in which their presence has now been identified. Smooth muscle cells are found in ligaments, spinal discs, and the lumbodorsal fascia. They play a role in stability, impact on circulation to muscle and brain tissues by reducing blood vessel diameter, and therefore oxygenation. These responses are particularly relevant to the athlete. A further connective tissue consideration involves hypermobility, which has been shown to be a major risk factor in the evolution of low-back pain and joint injury. **Breathing pattern disorders** have been found to be much more common in hypermobile individuals in whom fascial stability is most needed and is often associated with chronic pain syndromes. Hypermobility, low-back pain, and breathing pattern disorders are common in the athletic population.

Cardiorespiratory adaptations to exercise are numerous. As a person exercises, the heart is effectively exercised. Changes in the intake, transport, and utilization of oxygen encompass adaptations in the heart, lungs, vascular tissue, and muscles. Massage targeted to normalizing and maintaining the breathing mechanism is beneficial in supporting cardiovascular adaptive functions and increases compliance in cardiorespiratory rehabilitation programs.

Massage is also used extensively in the area of injury rehabilitation. Inflammation is needed for tissue repair; however, too much is detrimental to the process. By the application of therapeutic modalities such as immobilization devices, exercises, and antiinflammatory medication, athletic trainers, physical therapists, and physicians attempt to control the inflammatory process. A knowledge of the inflammatory tissue repair process needs to be achieved in order to understand the rationale and principles behind massage. Fibroblasts are attracted to an injured site indirectly through chemotaxis by the presence of macrophages. Collagen is formed, making a seal over the injury site. Unfortunately the collagen fibers' organization is random and with little structure, causing the scar to be fragile. Stresses during the subacute phase, in the form of gentle movements of massage, may cause these fibers to rearrange themselves rapidly in a more orderly fashion, thus increasing their strength. The lack of movement during connective tissue repair can lead to exaggerated scar formation and increased pain when stretching the scar. Movement appears to inhibit scar formation by several means, including stimulating proteoglycan synthesis, which lubricates connective tissue and maintains distance between the fibers, orienting the laying down of new collagen fibers; and mechanical stress of fibers, which resist tensile forces, preventing intermolecular cross-linking from occurring. Not only does massage have a significant effect on collagen fibers; it also improves the extensibility of tissues. This information makes a strong case for the use of massage during injury rehabilitation.

It has been suggested that if an athlete has a massage at least once a week, the potential for injury is reduced and performance is enhanced. This is because the massage therapist performs a thorough examination of muscles and tissue and can identify and treat predisposing factors before injury occurs. This may be the most benefical aspect of massage.

Sports massage benefits people who exercise by assisting in the processes of compensation and adaptation. During and after exercise, the body's systems adapt to cope with the increased stresses placed on them by the activity. Regular exercise enables the body to cope with increased levels of stress, which allows the body to exercise at higher intensities or for longer durations. This is the body's reaction to conditioning and training activity. While the body is recovering from overload as a result of exercise, it overcompensates to increase its resistance to future stress. The manipulation of soft tissue prior to and after exercise promotes physiologic and psychologic changes that aid performance and recovery. (Refer to the Evolve site that accompanies this book for research articles showing the benefit of massage during and after exercise.)

SUMMARY

When comparing the various research studies of sports massage, one finds some areas of consensus along with opposing and contradictory opinions. Ongoing research will continue to clarify the physiologic mechanisms that underpin the various therapeutic effects of massage. The future of massage therapy depends on this research and its continued collaboration with medicine, physical therapy, and sports performance.

In the next chapter, we take a more in-depth look at the underlying anatomic structures and physiologic mechanisms identified in research studies and attempt to put into perspective the influence of massage application in relation to logical if not totally proven massage benefits.

1 List some research findings that support massage for relaxation. Example: Massage application is slow.

_____

_____

_____

_____

_____

_____

_____

_____

_____

2 List some current commonly accepted effects of massage. Example: neural stimulation.

_____

_____

_____

_____

_____

_____

_____

_____

_____

_____

3 Name specific conditions in which massage has been found beneficial. Example: delayed onset of muscle soreness.

_____

_____

_____

_____

_____

_____

_____

_____

_____

_____

_____

_____

4 Describe the interaction of relaxation, improved breathing, cardiorespiratory and vascular function, and changes in connective tissue pliability. Example: massage produces feelings of well-being that reduce physical awareness.

_____

_____

_____

_____

_____

_____

_____

_____

_____

_____

_____

_____

5 Explain how massage can prevent injury. Example: increases tissue pliability.

_____

_____

_____

_____

_____

_____

_____

_____

_____

_____

_____

_____

_____

_____

_____

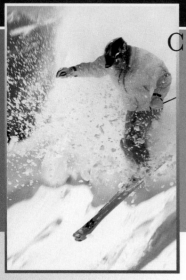

4

RELEVANT ANATOMY AND PHYSIOLOGY

OBJECTIVES

Upon completion of this chapter the reader will have the information necessary to:

1 Describe the fluid content of the body.

2 Create outcome goals for massage application that support beneficial fluid dynamics.

3 Describe neuroendocrine control of the body.

4 Create outcome goals for massage application that support effects of neuroendocrine function.

5 Describe the tensegretic and spiral design of the body as it is influenced by connective tissue.

6 Explain injury in relationship to tensegretic and spiral patterns of the body.

7 Describe joint function and its interrelationship with muscular balance.

8 Explain the relationship of muscle function to predictable patterns of dysfunction.

9 Explain how the kinetic chain relates to assessment and the development of treatment goals.

The effective and intelligent application of massage in sports and fitness and rehabilitation is dependent on comprehensive knowledge of anatomy, physiology, kinesiology, biomechanics, and relevant pathology. Sports and fitness massage produces a change in the structure and function of the client's body; therefore, assessment, treatment plan development, and massage implementation are made in relationship to this area of study.

Following is a review and discussion of relevant anatomy and physiology content as it relates to massage outcomes that commonly target this population group. It is expected that this section will be used in conjunction with the recommended reading listed in Box 1-1 in Chapter 1.

Acceleration
Anterior oblique subsystem
Bursa
Cartilage
Co-contraction
Concentric
Connective tissue
Core stabilization
Deceleration
Deep longitudinal subsystem
Dehydration
Eccentric
Edema
Electrolyte balance
Firing patterns
Force couples

Force stability
Form stability
Frontal plane movement
Global (outer unit) muscles
Hydrostatic force
Isometric
Joint mobilization
Joint stability
Kinetic chain
Lateral subsystem
Local (inner unit) muscles
Multiplanar movement
Muscle
Muscle length-tension relationship
Pain
Phasic/mover muscles

Posterior oblique subsystem
Pronation
Reflexive muscle action
Sagittal plane movement
Sensitization
Serial distortion pattern
Soft tissue
Spiral
Strength
Synergistic dominance
Tensegrity
Tonic/postural/stabilizing muscles
Transverse plane rotational movement
Upper crossed syndrome

The body structure we deal with consists of fluid and fibers. Their function is coordinated by chemicals and electrical signals. These chemicals and electrical signals control the body, and the fluid and fibers make up the soft tissue. **Soft tissue** includes the skin, fascia, muscles, tendons, and ligaments; cartilage, bursae, and joint capsules; nerves; vascular and lymphatic tubes; and various body fluids such as blood, lymph, and synovial fluid. Fibers (mostly connective tissue) provide structure for the body similar to the framework of a building. They provide the tension force to keep the body upright in gravity and transmit the forces from muscle cell contraction to create movement.

FLUID DYNAMICS

A major aspect of massage is support of the body's fluid dynamics.

The human body is approximately 70% water. This water, or fluid, is usually named for the tubes or compartments that contain it (e.g., lymph for lymph vessels). Fluids include the blood in the vessels and heart, lymph in the lymph vessels, synovial fluid in the joint capsules and bursa sacs, cerebrospinal fluid in the nervous system, and interstitial fluid that surrounds all soft tissue cells.

Water is found inside all cells (intracellular fluid). Water is bound with glycoproteins in connective tissue ground substance. The ratio of water in connective tissue helps to determine its consistency. Just as elsewhere, water in the body moves in waves by pumps, which include the heart, the respiratory diaphragm, the smooth muscle of the vascular and lymph system, and rhythmic movement of muscles and fascia. Water moves along paths of least resistance from high pressure to low pressure and flows downhill with gravity. Water moves at differing speeds according to other variables present, and its properties must be considered when applying massage methods.

Water is a constituent of all living things and often is referred to as the universal biologic solvent. It acts to minimize temperature changes throughout the body. Box 4-1 lists the many important functions of water in the body. The water content of body tissues varies. Adipose tissue (fat) has the lowest percentage of water; the skeleton has the second lowest water content. Skeletal muscle, skin, and blood have the highest content of water in the body (Table 4-1).

The total water content of the body decreases most dramatically during the first 10 years of life and continues to decline through old age, at which time water content may be only 45% of the total body weight. Men tend to have higher percentages

BOX 4-1   FUNCTIONS OF WATER IN HUMAN PHYSIOLOGY

- Provides medium for chemical reactions.
- Is crucial for regulating chemical and bioelectric distributions with cells.
- Transports substances such as hormones and nutrients.
- Aids oxygen transport from body cells to lungs.
- Aids carbon dioxide transport from body cells to lungs.
- Dilutes toxic substances and waste products and transports them to the kidneys and the liver.
- Distributes heat around the body.

TABLE 4-2   WHERE WATER IS LOST FROM THE BODY (HEALTHY ADULT)

ORGAN	MOOE OF LOSS	PERCENTAGE OF LOSS
Kidneys	Urine	62
Skin	Diffusion and sweat	19
Lungs	Water vapor	13
Gastrointestinal tract	Feces	6

From Fritz S: *Mosby's essential sciences for therapeutic massage: anatomy, physiology, biomechanics, and pathology*, ed 2. St. Louis, 2004, Mosby.

TABLE 4-1   PERCENTAGE OF WATER IN THE BODY TISSUES

TISSUE	PERCENTAGE OF WATER
Blood	83.0
Kidneys	82.7
Heart	79.2
Lungs	79.0
Spleen	75.8
Muscle	75.6
Brain	74.8
Intestine	74.5
Skin	72.0
Liver	68.3
Skeleton	22.0
Adipose tissue	10.0

From Fritz S: *Mosby's essential sciences for therapeutic massage: anatomy, physiology, biomechanics, and pathology*, ed 2. St. Louis, 2004, Mosby.

of water (about 65%) than women (about 55%), mainly because of their increased muscle mass and lower amount of subcutaneous fat.

Water is in a constant state of motion inside the body, shifting between the two major fluid compartments, the lymphatic and circulatory systems. Water is continuously lost from, and taken into, the body. In a normal healthy human, water input equals water output. Maintaining this equivalence is of prime importance in maintaining health. Approximately 90% of the water intake is via the gastrointestinal tract (food and liquids). The remaining 10% is called metabolic water and is produced as the result of various chemical reactions in the cells of the tissues.

Table 4-2 shows the routes by which the normal healthy adult loses water.

The amount of water lost via the kidneys is under hormonal control. The average amount of water lost and consumed per day is around 2.5 liters (approximately 4½ pints) in a healthy adult. Perspiration lost during exercise increases water loss and requires increased water consumption.

The walls of the blood vessels form a barrier to the free passage of fluid between interstitial areas and blood plasma. At the capillaries, these walls are only one cell thick. These capillary walls are generally permeable to water and small solutes but impermeable to large organic molecules such as proteins. Blood plasma tends to have a higher concentration of these molecules compared with the interstitial fluid. Much of the interstitial fluid is taken up by the lymphatic system and eventually finds its way back into the bloodstream. Increased interstitial fluid is a common form of edema found in athletes. Lymphatic drain massage methods support movement of interstitial fluid.

Water and small solutes such as sodium, potassium, and calcium can be exchanged freely between the blood plasma and the interstitial fluid. The action of the kidneys on the blood regulates these electrolytes. Electrolyte balance is essential for athletic performance. This exchange depends mainly on the hydrostatic and osmotic forces of these fluid compartments.

Force exerted by water is caused by the weight of water pushing against a surface, such as a dam in a river or the wall of a blood vessel. The pressure of blood in the capillaries serves as a major **hydrostatic force** (pressure caused by water) in the human body. Capillary hydrostatic pressure is a filtration force. This is because the pressure of the fluid is higher at the arterial end of the capillary than at the venous end. The pressure of the interstitial fluid is negative (−5 mm Hg) because the lymphatic system continuously takes up excess fluid forced out of the capillaries.

Osmotic pressure is the attraction of water to large molecules such as proteins. Proteins are more abundant in the blood vessels than outside them, so the concentration of proteins in the blood tends to attract water from the interstitial space.

Overall, near equilibrium exists between fluid forced out of the capillaries and the fluid reabsorbed, because the lymphatic system collects the excess fluid forced out at the artery end and eventually drains it back into the veins at the base of the neck.

A similar situation exists between the interstitial fluid and the intracellular fluid, although ion pumps and carriers complicate the process. Generally, water movement is substantial in both directions, but ion movement is restricted and depends on active transport via the pumps. Nutrients and oxygen, because they are dissolved in water, move passively into cells while waste products and carbon dioxide move out.

The mechanisms for regulating body fluids are centered in the hypothalamus. The hypothalamus also receives input from the digestive tract that helps to control thirst. Antidiuretic hormone (ADH) regulates body fluid volume and extracellular osmosis. ADH has many areas of influence in the body. One of the major functions of ADH is to increase the permeability of the collecting tubules in the kidneys, which allows more water to be reabsorbed in the kidneys. If the body is lacking fluid intake, such as during sleep or during heavy exercise, the result is a concentrated, darker-colored urine of reduced volume. Absence of ADH occurs when the individual is overhydrated. The urine is dilute, pale or colorless, and of high volume.

Primary factors involved in the triggering of ADH production are osmoreceptors and baroreceptors (pressure receptors). Secondary factors include, stress, pain, hypoxia, and severe exercise.

Dehydration is the result of water loss or lack of fluid intake. Relative dehydration occurs when the body loses no overall water content but rather gains sodium ions, which stimulate osmoreceptors.

The thirst response is connected to the osmoreceptors. How the response actually works is not yet completely understood. Moistening of the mucosal lining of the mouth and pharynx seems to initiate a neurologic response, which sends a message to the thirst center of the hypothalamus. Perhaps more important, stretch receptors in the gastrointestinal tract also appear to transmit nerve messages to the thirst center of the hypothalamus that inhibit the thirst response.

Changes in the circulating volume of body fluid also stimulate ADH secretion that results in an increase or decrease of internal pressure monitored by baroreceptors.

A reduction of 8% to 10% of the normal body volume of water because of hemorrhage or excess perspiration results in ADH secretion. Pressure receptors located in the atria of the heart and the pulmonary arteries and veins relay messages to the hypothalamus via the vagus nerve.

ELECTROLYTE BALANCE

An electrolyte is any chemical that dissociates into ions when dissolved in a solution. Ions can be positively charged (cations) or negatively charged (anions).

The major electrolytes and their charges found in the human body are:

Sodium (Na^+)
Potassium (K^+)
Calcium (Ca^{2+})
Magnesium (Mg^{2+})
Chloride (Cl^-)
Phosphate (HPO_4^{2-})
Sulfate (SO_4^-)
Bicarbonate (HCO_3^-)

Interstitial fluid and blood plasma are similar in their electrolyte makeup, sodium and chloride being the major electrolytes. In the intracellular fluid, potassium and phosphate are the major electrolytes.

Sodium Balance

Sodium balance plays an important role in the excitability of muscles and neurons and is also crucially important in regulating fluid balance in the body. The kidneys closely regulate sodium levels.

Potassium Balance

Potassium is the major electrolyte of intracellular fluid. Concentration within the cells is 28 times that of the extracellular fluids. As with sodium, potassium is important for the correct functioning of excitable cells such as muscles, neurons, and sensory receptors. Potassium also is involved in the regulation of fluid levels within the cell and in maintaining the correct pH balance within the body.

The pH balance of the body also affects potassium levels. In acidosis, potassium excretion decreases, whereas the opposite occurs in alkalosis.

Calcium and Phosphorus Balance

Calcium is found mainly in the extracellular fluids, whereas phosphorus is found mostly in the intracellular fluids. Both are important in the maintenance of healthy bones and teeth. Calcium is also important in the transmission of nerve impulses across synapses, the clotting of blood, and the contraction of muscles. If the levels of calcium fall below normal levels, muscles and nerves become more excitable. Phosphorus is required for the synthesis of nucleic acids and high-energy compounds such as adenosine triphosphate (ATP). Phosphorus is also important in the maintenance of pH balance.

Decreased levels of calcium in the body stimulate the parathyroid gland to secrete parathyroid hormone, causing an increase in calcium and phosphate levels of the interstitial fluids by releasing them from the reservoirs of these minerals lodged in the bones and the teeth. Parathyroid hormone also decreases calcium excretion by the kidneys. If the levels of calcium in the body become too high, the thyroid gland releases a hormone called calcitonin that inhibits the release of calcium and potassium from the bones. Calcitonin also inhibits the absorption of calcium from the gastrointestinal tract and increases calcium excretion by the kidneys.

Magnesium Balance

Most magnesium is found in intracellular fluid and in bone. Within cells, magnesium functions in the sodium-potassium pump and as an aid to enzyme action. Magnesium plays a role in muscle contraction, action potential conduction, and bone and teeth production. The hormone aldosterone controls magnesium concentration in extracellular fluid. Low magnesium levels result in an increased aldosterone secretion, and the aldosterone increases magnesium reabsorption by the kidneys.

Chloride Balance

Chloride is the most plentiful extracellular electrolyte, with an extracellular concentration 26 times that of its intracellular concentration. Chloride ions are able to diffuse easily across plasma membranes, and their transport is linked closely to sodium movement, which also explains the indirect role of aldosterone in chloride regulation. When sodium is reabsorbed, chloride follows passively. Chloride helps to regulate osmotic pressure differences between fluid compartments and is essential to pH balance. The chloride shift within the blood helps to move bicarbonate ions out of the red blood cells and into the plasma for transport. In the gastrointestinal system, chlorine and hydrogen combine to form hydrochloric acid.

pH Balance

pH is a measurement of the hydrogen concentration of a solution. Lower pH values indicate a higher hydrogen concentration, or higher acidity. Higher pH values indicate a lower hydrogen concentration, or higher alkalinity. Therefore hydrogen ion balance often is referred to as pH balance or acid-base balance. Hydrogen ion regulation in the fluid compartments of the body is critically important to health. Even a slight change in hydrogen ion concentration can result in a significant alteration in the rate of chemical reactions. Changes in hydrogen ion concentration also can affect the distribution of ions such as sodium, potassium, and calcium and the structure and function of proteins.

The normal pH of the arterial blood is 7.4; that of the venous blood is 7.35. The lower pH of the venous blood is caused by the higher concentration of carbon dioxide in the venous blood, which dissolves in water to make a weak acid called carbonic acid. When the pH changes in the arterial blood, two conditions may result: acidosis or alkalosis. Acidosis is a condition that occurs when the hydrogen ion concentration of the arterial blood increases and therefore the pH decreases. Alkalosis is the condition that occurs when the hydrogen ion concentration in the arterial blood decreases and the pH increases.

Sources of hydrogen ions in the body include carbonic acid (formed as previously mentioned), sulfuric acid (a by-product in the breakdown of proteins), phosphoric acid (a by-product of protein and phospholipid metabolism), ketone bodies (from fat metabolism), and lactic acid (formed in skeletal muscle during exercise).

About half of all the acid formed or introduced into the body is neutralized by the ingestion of alkaline foods. The remaining acid is neutralized by three mechanisms in the body: chemical buffers, the respiratory system, and the kidneys.

CLINICAL PROBLEMS WITH FLUID BALANCE

The fluid balance of the body can be upset in many ways, resulting in severe problems and even death. This problem is further described in Unit Three under thermoregulation and heat dysfunction.

DEHYDRATION

Dehydration obviously occurs in conditions in which water is unavailable (Figure 4-1). However, conditions such as diarrhea, severe vomiting, excessive sweating, bleeding, and surgical removal of body fluids also can result in dehydration. There are three types of dehydration:

1. Hypertonic dehydration occurs when fluid loss results in an increase in electrolyte levels, causing the blood pressure to fall and the blood

to become thicker, which can result in heart failure.

2. Isotonic dehydration results in no perceptible difference in the normal electrolyte balance, but it may lead to hypotonic dehydration, the third type.

3. Hypotonic dehydration occurs when fluid and electrolyte losses keep pace with each other and the intake of pure water alters the fluid electrolyte balance (too much water, not enough electrolytes). Thus in cases of severe diarrhea,

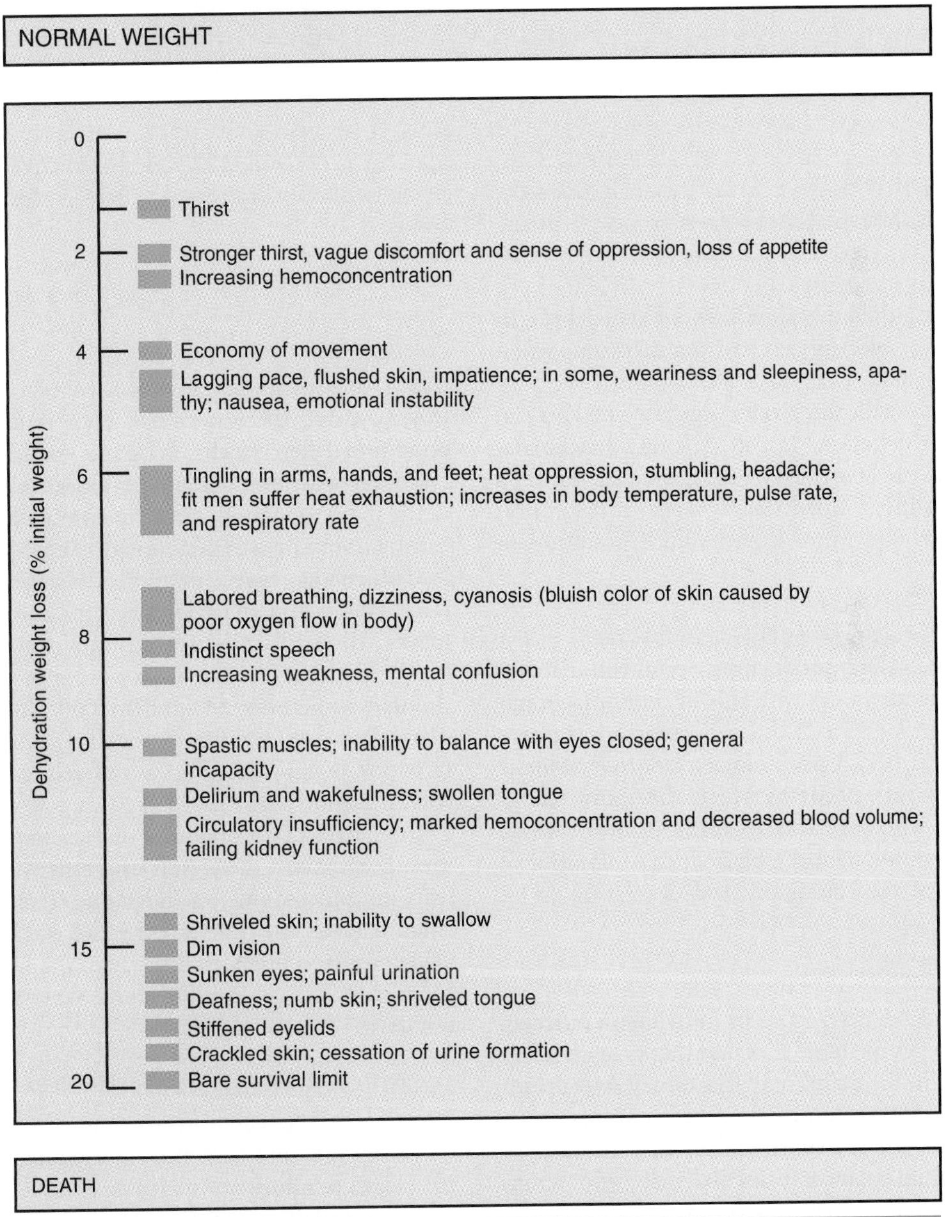

NORMAL WEIGHT

Dehydration weight loss (% initial weight)

- 0
- 1 Thirst
- 2 Stronger thirst, vague discomfort and sense of oppression, loss of appetite
  Increasing hemoconcentration
- 4 Economy of movement
  Lagging pace, flushed skin, impatience; in some, weariness and sleepiness, apathy; nausea, emotional instability
- 6 Tingling in arms, hands, and feet; heat oppression, stumbling, headache; fit men suffer heat exhaustion; increases in body temperature, pulse rate, and respiratory rate
- Labored breathing, dizziness, cyanosis (bluish color of skin caused by poor oxygen flow in body)
- 8 Indistinct speech
  Increasing weakness, mental confusion
- 10 Spastic muscles; inability to balance with eyes closed; general incapacity
  Delirium and wakefulness; swollen tongue
  Circulatory insufficiency; marked hemoconcentration and decreased blood volume; failing kidney function
- Shriveled skin; inability to swallow
- 15 Dim vision
  Sunken eyes; painful urination
  Deafness; numb skin; shriveled tongue
  Stiffened eyelids
  Crackled skin; cessation of urine formation
- 20 Bare survival limit

DEATH

FIGURE 4-1 ■ The effects of dehydration. (From Thibodeau GA, Patton KT: *Anatomy and physiology*, ed 5, St. Louis, 2003, Mosby.)

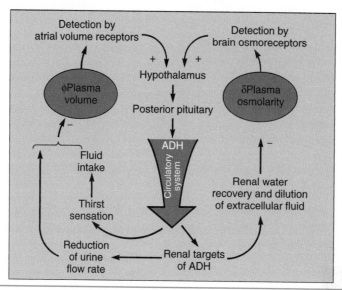

FIGURE 4-2 ■ Mechanisms of fluid and electrolyte regulation: the antidiuretic hormone system. (From Thibodeau GA, Patton KT: *Anatomy and physiology*, ed 5. St. Louis, 2003, Mosby.)

replacing the body fluid with a balanced preparation of electrolytes and water is important (Figure 4-2).

Problems with the production of urine also can lead to dehydration. Impaired ability to concentrate urine can be caused by damage to the medulla of the kidneys; inadequate water reabsorption occurs and the urine is too dilute, resulting in fluid loss.

Inadequate Antidiuretic Hormone Production

Inadequate ADH production occurs in diabetes insipidus. Individuals with this disorder may eliminate as much as 5 to 20 liters (8½ pints to 34 pints) of urine per day. A psychologic disorder known as polydipsia may occur in which the individual is obsessed with drinking (usually water), which results in dilution of the plasma, causing artificial lowering of the osmolarity and decreasing ADH secretion.

Solute Diuresis

Solute diuresis may occur in individuals suffering from diabetes mellitus. Elevated blood sugar levels can result in the inability of the kidney to reabsorb water, which then results in excess fluid loss.

The diabetic athlete should be monitored carefully for fluid balance. If fluid balance is not maintained, dehydration or even hypovolemic shock (because of insufficient volume of body fluid) may occur.

Edema

Edema is a condition in which an excess of fluid exists within the interstitial compartment. The condition often results in tissue swelling and is common whenever lymphatic blockage occurs or when the lymphatic system for some other reason cannot drain the area fast enough. Renal failure can lead to edema, especially the early stages of acute renal failure and the later stages of chronic renal failure. To test for edema, one applies steady pressure of the thumb onto the lower leg or other area thought to be affected for 10 to 20 seconds. If a depression remains after removal of pressure, fluid retention is indicated. This is referred to as pitting edema (Figure 4-3).

Edema may be a symptom of liver and heart failures. Liver failure can result in inefficient metabolism of aldosterone, a hormone that controls sodium levels. In heart failure, the production of aldosterone is enhanced because of the lowering of blood pressure. The result is the same as in liver failure.

Excessive Antidiuretic Hormone Secretion

Excessive ADH secretion is a rare condition that may occur because of tumors in the lung, brain, or pancreas, resulting in increased reabsorption of water. Local edema is part of the inflammatory response or can be a protective mechanism, especially in cases of joint dysfunction.

FIGURE 4-3

TESTING FOR EDEMA

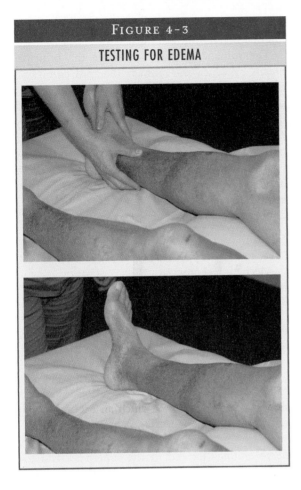

NEUROENDOCRINE CONTROL

The nervous system is anatomically and functionally connected throughout the entire body and may be structurally divided into the central nervous system (CNS) and the peripheral nervous system (PNS), which in turn is functionally divided into the somatic or motor nervous system and the autonomic nervous system. The endocrine hormone functions are interrelated as a mechanism of communication of homeostatic function. Massage affects every part of the nervous and endocrine systems. Sports massage targets all aspects of these functions. Proper function of the nervous and endocrine systems is especially important for athletes. Much of the training process for athletic performance is targeted to conditioning the nervous system reflexes. The endocrine system functions to sustain focus, endurance, and recovery.

CENTRAL NERVOUS SYSTEM

The CNS consists of the brain and spinal cord. The brain is divided into three sections: the cerebrum, brainstem, and cerebellum. The cerebrum is the largest portion of the brain and is generally responsible for higher mental functions and personality. The frontal-lobe area of the cerebrum also contains the motor cortex, which controls voluntary movements. Another area of the cerebrum is called the parietal lobe and contains the sensory cortex, which receives information about touch and proprioception. The brainstem is the center for the automatic control of respiration and heart rate. The cerebellum functions to control muscle coordination, the muscle's motor tone, and posture.

The limbic system and hypothalamus integrate emotional states, visceral responses, and the muscular system through endocrine and neurotransmitter chemicals. Emotions can alter muscular tone. States of anxiety create sustained increased tone, and depression creates loss of motor tone. It is well documented that the emotional state of the athlete influences performance. Athletes in rehabilitation programs often experience anxiety and depression.

The spinal cord is a continuation of the medulla portion of the brain and travels through the vertebral canal from the foramen magnum to the lumbar spine. The spinal cord becomes individual spinal nerves as they exit the vertebral column through openings between the sides of the vertebra called the intervertebral foramina. Anatomically, this is where the peripheral nervous system begins.

Information from all four classes of sensory receptors—mechanoreceptors, proprioceptors, chemoreceptors, and nociceptors—is sent to the spinal cord, which stimulates countless reflexive adjustments in the body.

PERIPHERAL NERVOUS SYSTEM

The PNS consists of 12 pairs of cranial nerves and 31 pairs of spinal nerves. The nerves are lubricated, and the fibers, fascicles, and gross nerves are designed to slide within the connective tissue spaces and grooves through which they run.

The peripheral nerves are vulnerable to compression and irritation at the nerve roots in the area of the intervertebral foramen and to entrapment, irritation, or compression in the extremities. They can become restricted or entrapped by adhesions in the connective tissue spaces or hypertonic muscles though which they travel. These restrictions prevent the normal gliding of the nerve. Nerves can become compressed in fibro-osseous tunnels such as the carpal tunnel. Nerves can become compressed, restricted, or irritated because of pressure from increased fluid or from inflammation caused by overuse or injury. Nerve pain tends to radiate and follow traceable pathways in the body.

SOMATIC NERVOUS SYSTEM

The somatic sensory nerves relay information from the skin to the CNS concerning pain, temperature, touch, and pressure. The sensory nervous system also conveys pain and proprioceptive information about position, as well as mechanoreceptor information about movement from the muscles, tendons, ligaments, joint capsules, and periosteum.

EPITHELIAL TISSUE

The epithelium and the nervous system are derived from the same embryologic tissue, the ectoderm. Therefore, the skin is an extension of the nervous system. The skin is the body's largest organ and contains blood vessels, glands, muscles, connective tissue, and nerve endings.

The skin contains four types of sensory nerve receptors called *mechanoreceptors*, which communicate with every other part of the body. Mechanoreceptors are sensitive to touch, pressure, movement, superficial proprioception, pain, and temperature. The skin provides sensation, information, and protection; assists with water balance; and regulates temperature.

Sensory information from the skin communicates to the spinal cord, where reflex connections are made to muscles, internal organs, and blood vessels. Skin pain can cause a contraction in the skeletal muscles or internal organs, and conversely, skeletal muscle and internal organs can refer pain to the skin.

Massage accesses the body through the skin and sends signals of pressure, movements, and stimulation for the body to process.

The somatic motor nerves relay information from the brain, through the spinal cord, and then to skeletal muscles. The visceral sensory nerves are part of the autonomic nervous system and send pain and pressure information from the internal organs to the CNS. The visceral motor nerves transmit impulses from the autonomic nervous system to the involuntary muscles, such as those found in internal organs and glandular tissue.

The somatic sensory nerves are the principal means by which the massage therapist communicates with the client. Each touch and movement sends a message to the CNS (spinal cord and brain), which, in turn, communicates with every other part of the body, including the centers of the person's emotions.

Soft tissue has four basic categories of sensory nerves. These receptors are stimulated by certain actions. Compression, irritation, or injury causes dysfunction of these sensory nerves. This is a common type of lingering sports injury.

The sensory receptors are:

Mechanoreceptors—touch, pressure, and movement.
Proprioceptors—changes in position and movement.
Chemoreceptors—sensitive to the acid/base balance, oxygen, and so forth
Nociceptors—irritation and pain.

Somatic sensory nerves are specialized receptors that relay information to the CNS about four types of information.

Touch and pressure originate from the sensory nerve endings located in the superficial and the deep layers of the skin, which communicate light touch, deep pressure, temperature, and pain. These nerve endings provide external information from the environment. Massage stimulation of the skin and superficial fascia is an effective communication with these sensors.

Proprioceptors and mechanoreceptors are located in muscles, tendons, and joints and communicate information about body position and movement. Massage interacts with these receptors through muscle energy methods, active and passive movements, and various mechanical forces of bend, shear, torsion, tension, and compression.

Chemoreceptors are stimulated when the body is inflamed and when a muscle is in a sustained contraction, decreasing the amount of oxygen in the tissue. These chemicals interact with fibroblasts, mast cells, and other cells to create a neurogenic inflammatory response called *neurogenic pain*. Massage may purposefully use controlled focused pain to release pain-inhibiting chemicals.

Pain is caused by the stimulation of nociceptors. These receptors are usually stimulated by chemicals such as substance P, bradykinin, and histamine, which excite the nerve endings. Pain is elicited by three different classes of stimuli: mechanical, chemical, and thermal. Soft tissue pain is caused by the chemicals released from an injury or from mechanical irritation caused by cumulative stress, microinflammation, or extreme hot or cold. Emotional or psychologic stress, called *autonomic disturbances*, can cause pain by causing hypertonic muscles and shifts in fluid flow affecting oxygen and nutrient delivery and waste removal.

Pain of somatic origin and from the viscera sends impulses to the limbic and hypothalamic areas of the brain and may be responsible for the reactions of anxiety, fear, anger, and depression. Also, the brain can inhibit or enhance a reaction to pain. This may explain how athletes in intense competition can ignore an injury and how fear and anxiety can exaggerate pain.

Touch, vibration, and joint and muscle movement stimulate mechanoreceptors, causing a decrease in the pain information received by the brain. Massage stimulates the entire region of the body being worked on, along with localized pain areas. A large number of mechanoreceptors are stimulated, dramatically reducing the discomfort of working deep into tissues. This is why full body massage is better for pain management than localized spot work.

Managing pain is discussed in detail in Unit Three.

Five types of sensory nerve receptors supply each muscle. These sensory nerves respond to pain, chemical stimuli, temperature, deep pressure, muscle length, the rate of muscle length changes, muscle tension, and the rate of change in tension.

Type 1a are primary muscle spindles.

Type 1b are Golgi tendon organs (GTOs).

Type 2 are secondary muscle spindles and include paciniform and pacinian corpuscles, which are sensitive to deep pressure.

Type 3 are free nerve endings, sensitive to pain, chemicals, and temperature.

Type 4 are nociceptors.

The two classes of sensory receptors that have a particular significance for the massage therapist are the muscle spindles and Golgi tendon organs. They detect the length and tension of the muscle and tendon, set the resting tone of the muscle, adjust the tension of a muscle for coordination and fine muscular control, and protect the muscles and joints through reflexes that contract or inhibit the muscle automatically. Muscle spindles are specialized muscle fibers called *intrafusal fibers*, located in a fluid-filled capsule embedded within each muscle. They respond to slow and rapid changes in muscle length; secondary endings respond to slow changes in muscle length and are sensitive to deep pressure. The spindles also play a role in joint position, muscle coordination and tone, and muscular control of movement.

Because muscle spindles detect changes in muscle length, stretching a muscle will increase their rate of signal discharge. The more refined the muscle's function, the greater the concentration of spindles. The greatest concentration of spindles is found in the lumbrical muscles of the hand, the suboccipital muscles, and the muscles that move the eyes.

States of anxiety or emotional or psychologic tension can cause an increase in the firing rate of the spindle cells. This increase causes the muscle tone to be "set" too high, creating hypertonicity and stiffness. If the motor tone is set too high, there are three ways to decrease the firing rate of a spindle cell and, therefore, cause the muscle to relax:

1. Decrease the muscle length by bringing the proximal and distal attachments toward each other.
2. Contract the muscle isometrically, as is done in contract and relax methods. This method causes the spindle activity to stop temporarily, allowing the muscle to be set to a new, more relaxed length.
3. Use inhibiting compression in the belly of the muscle to decrease firing.

Golgi tendon organs are sensory receptors in the form of slender capsules located along the muscle fiber at the musculotendinous junction. They sense changes in muscle tension and fire during minute changes in muscle tension. They have a protective function to prevent damage to a muscle being forcefully contracted. Discharge of the Golgi tendon organ stimulates nerves at the spinal cord, called *inhibitory interneurons*, causing the muscle to relax. Abnormal firing of the Golgi tendon organ can set the resting tone of the muscle too high, creating hypertonicity.

It is believed that all types of muscle energy methods can reset the muscle to its resting length and tone, but the exact mechanism is not fully understood. When a muscle voluntarily contracts isometrically, the Golgi tendon organs are stimulated to fire, which has an inhibiting effect on the muscle, causing it to relax. Inhibiting compression at the tendons can also decrease Golgi tendon organ activity.

AUTONOMIC NERVOUS SYSTEM

The autonomic nervous system is that part of the peripheral nervous system (PNS) that innervates the heart, blood vessels, diaphragm, internal organs, and the endocrine glands. It influences every other part of the body, including the muscular system. There are two main divisions, the sympathetic and the parasympathetic.

SYMPATHETIC NERVOUS SYSTEM

The sympathetic nervous system is responsible for the "fight or flight" response, excitement, anticipation, and performance, and is active when a person is under stress. It releases adrenaline into the blood, causes constriction of the peripheral blood vessels, increases the heart rate, and inhibits the normal movement of the intestines so that the blood is available to the skeletal muscles. When a person is under stress, as when competing in an athletic event, there is increased tension in the muscles because of the effects of the sympathetic nervous system, which uses energy. Stress from competition or trauma can lead to sympathetic dominance and a collection of problems including breathing disorders, slowed recovery and healing, emotional agitation, digestive upset, and more.

PARASYMPATHETIC NERVOUS SYSTEM

The parasympathetic nervous system is responsible for energy building, feeding, digestion, and assimilation. It functions to restore homeostasis and is active when the body is at rest and in recuperation. It causes a decrease in the heart rate, stimulates the normal peristaltic smooth muscle movement of the intestines, and promotes the secretion of all digestive juices and tropic hormones. A person can be in parasympathetic override (dominance), which contributes to lethargy and loss of normal motivation and depression.

Many athletes have an underactive parasympathetic nervous system and an overactive sympathetic nervous system. Because recovery is so important to the athlete, this is a major concern. One of the primary benefits of massage given in a relaxing manner is the stimulation of the parasympathetic nervous system. This induces a state of relaxation and promotes the healing and rejuvenating functions of the parasympathetic nervous system, which supports homeostasis.

SENSITIZATION OF NEUROENDOCRINE FUNCTION

The term **sensitization** is used to describe the phenomenon in the nervous system in which there is an exaggerated response to normal stimuli. There are two principal causes of sensitization.

The limbic areas of the brain can cause an emotional exaggeration of pain, which can trigger the CNS to cause the muscles to become either too tight or too loose. Concurrent stimulation of the hypothalamus in turn alters endocrine function. This emotional exaggeration is caused by many factors, including culture, family history, pain history, and individual psychology.

The second cause of sensitization occurs at the level of the spinal cord. The area in the spinal cord that receives information about pain is next to the receptive field for movement. Chronic inflammation can cause sensitization of mechanoreceptors, so that normal mechanical stimuli cause a mechanoreceptor to be a pain producer. Sensitization perpetuates pain patterns, such as chronic pain and lingering pain after injury. Massage applied over time may alter these pathways, decreasing chronic pain sensations.

EMOTIONAL STATES

The body tissues form a unified whole, and each tissue not only influences all other tissues, but also affects a person's emotions and psychology. Athletes must feel right to perform well. Performance is emotionally charged. Massage affects the autonomic nervous system, which regulates breathing, blood flow, heart rate, respiration, neurotransmitters, and endocrine functions, all of which are physiologic aspects of emotion.

The emotional roller coaster of performance—winning, losing—and the physical and emotional impact of trauma, repetitive injury, pain, and fatigue all have a psychologic impact that can manifest as part of traumatic stress syndrome and state-dependent memory.

The touch of the massage professional may trigger a memory pattern of an emotionally charged event. Each memory, including all the sensory information, nervous system functions, and endocrine functions in play at the time of the experience, is stored in a multidimensional way. When the body state changes, the memory becomes vague and less clear. Because massage produces changes in the nervous and endocrine systems and is a source of sensory stimulation, a state that holds a memory pattern for a client can be altered. This may help a person resolve and integrate a past experience, if appropriate professional support is available.

Often only pieces of a memory are retrieved. This is common with body memories. The massage may trigger a physiologic response, and yet no visual or sequential memory is retrievable. Compassion is required to support the client during these times. No verbal interaction is necessary. Referral to a psychologist may be necessary. Most professional sports organizations have access to sport psychologists, and rehabilitation programs are often multidisciplinary. The neurochemical aspect of the body/mind interaction is necessary for peak athletic performance, motivation for training and rehabilitation protocols, and physical and emotional healing.

SOFT TISSUE

THE BODY AS A TENSEGRITY STRUCTURE

Buckminster Fuller coined the word **tensegrity** to describe a structure that consists of tension parts like tent ropes and the tent canvas and compression units like tent poles. In the body, the myofascial unit is the tension part of the tensegretic form that transmits the force of muscle contraction to the connective tissue to move the body as well as to dynamically stabilize posture. The bones are the compression units and cannot keep the body upright without the muscle and connective tissue. It is the tension aspect of the structure, not the compression aspect, that holds the body upright. The human body depends on the soft tissues, including the tendons, ligaments, and joint capsules, for stability and movement.

The **spiral** is an essential pattern in the universe and is represented extensively in human form and function. The spiral form, coupled with concepts of tensegrity, conceptually unifies form and function of the body. This understanding is critical in athletic performance, because most athletic function is composed of twisting and untwisting of the body (Figure 4-4).

Muscles are composed of parallel fibers organized in spirals. Actin and myosin, the basic proteins that compose muscle fiber, form a double helix spiral. Microscopically, tendons, ligaments, joint

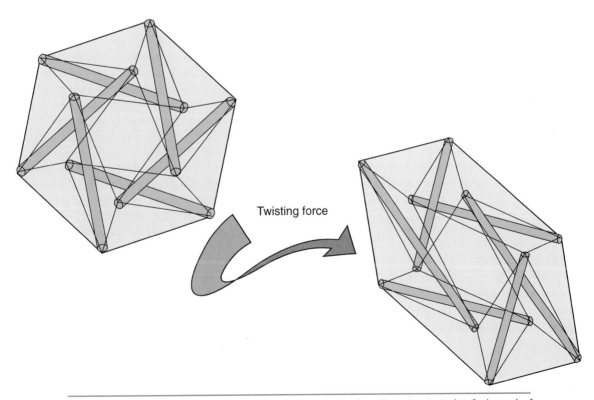

Twisting force

FIGURE 4-4 ■ Demonstration of the cell reacting to a twisting force. (From Fritz S: *Mosby's fundamentals of therapeutic massage*, ed 3. St. Louis, 2004, Mosby.)

capsules, and the fascia of muscles are composed of collagen molecules, which form a triple helix spiral. Soft tissue is organized around the joint in a spiral. Most famously, DNA, the code of instructions for cellular reproduction, is a double helix spiral. Soft tissue injury and dysfunction change the normal alignment of the soft tissue in multiple areas because of the tensegretic and spiral interconnective relationships of the body. These shifts influence function first and then form. Distortions in the tension units (soft tissues) create imbalances in the forces moving through the body, creating dysfunction. Muscles, tendons, and ligaments can misalign as the result of injury, repetitive use, and abnormal demands that often occur in athletic performance. If the soft tissue develops an abnormal position from dysfunction or injury, it introduces an abnormal torsion or twist into the tissue. This abnormal force decreases the water content of the tissue. If body fluids stagnate, mobility of the cells is decreased. The swelling following acute injury prevents normal fluid exchange.

Sustained muscle contraction and adhesions in chronic dysfunction and injury also create stagnation in the tissue. Stagnation reduces the tissue's ability to repair itself, owing to decreased cellular activity, decreased nutrition, and the accumulation of waste products. This tissue becomes fibrotic, nonpliable, and unelastic, so its ability to stretch and recoil is altered. Adhesions and abnormal function in the soft tissue and associated joint may develop as the result of decrease in water content. Layers of tissue begin to stick together, and function becomes strained and limited. A network of nerves is embedded within collagen. Adhesions, loss of the normal parallel alignment of the soft tissue fibers, abnormal position, torsion, and fluid stagnation all cause pain and create abnormal neurologic reflexes, which then affect function of somatic structures and internal organs.

During injury of soft tissue, the collagen fibers suffer both micro- and macroscopic tears. The fibers are repaired during the acute and subacute healing phase, with new collagen deposited in a random orientation. If there is no managed and appropriate remodeling of the fiber accumulation in the final stage of healing, the bundles of fibers or fascicles lose their ability to slide relative to each other and adhesions are formed. These adhesions prevent the normal broadening of the muscle fibers that occurs during muscle contraction.

Abnormal position and torsion of soft tissue contribute to abnormal forces moving through the joint, creating strain, compensation, and eventually degeneration. Joint dysfunction and degeneration cause irritation of the sensory nerve receptors in the soft tissue surrounding the joint. This irritation can create neurologic reflexes that inhibit or create hypertonicity in the surrounding muscles. For an athlete, this outcome compromises performance and contributes to continued injury and fatigue.

Soft tissues that can restrict joint motion are muscles, connective tissue, and skin. When stretching procedures are applied to these soft tissues, the velocity, intensity, and duration of the stretch force as well as the temperature of the soft tissues all affect the response of the different types of soft tissues. These elements are described as different qualities of touch applied during massage: depth of pressure, direction, duration, rhythm, speed, frequency, and drag.

Mechanical characteristics of contractile and noncontractile tissue as well as the neurophysiologic properties of contractile tissue all affect soft tissue lengthening.

When soft tissue is stretched, either elastic or plastic changes occur. *Elasticity* is the ability of soft tissue to return to its resting length after passive stretch. *Plasticity* is the tendency of soft tissue to assume a new and greater length after the stretch force has been removed. Both contractile and noncontractile tissues have elastic and plastic qualities. Muscle is primarily composed of contractile tissue but is attached to and interwoven with the noncontractile tissue of tendon and fascia. The connective tissue framework in muscle, not active contractile components, is the primary source of resistance to passive elongation of muscle. How massage and stretching increase tissue pliability is still not fully understood, but somehow the response of the tissue to impose mechanical force can result in injury as well as benefits.

Adhesions in the skin can develop following an impact injury, cut, or surgery. Because the superficial fascia in the dermis is connected to the underlying deep fascia coverings of the muscles, these adhesions decrease soft tissue mobility. Adhesions in the superficial fascia can also entrap the cutaneous nerves, leading to pain, numbing, and tingling. Protective uniforms and equipment for athletes attempt to shield the skin from injury, but skin injuries are common. Accumulative changes in skin pliability are problematic and can be managed with massage.

CONNECTIVE TISSUE

Connective tissue consists of hard and soft tissues. It forms the structure of the organs and blood vessels and bind joints together through ligaments and joint capsules. It transmits the pulls of the muscles through the connective tissue surrounding the muscles and the tendons. It forms tensegretic tension lines that transverse the body in many directions. Connective tissue is made up of ground substance and fibers. Strains and sprains of muscles, tendons, and ligaments are common in athletic activity and damage connective tissue.

Ground substance is a transparent, viscous fluid (like raw egg whites) that surrounds all the cells in the body. It is formed from glycosaminoglycans (GAGs) and water. GAGs act to draw water into the tissue and bind it. Water makes up approximately 70% of ground substance. Think of ground substance as "silly putty" or wallpaper paste or Jello. Ground substance is a source of nutrition and a carrier for waste products of cellular function. It is a lubricant and spacer between the collagen fibers, preventing the fibers from adhering to each other. Ground substance has a thixotropic quality. *Thixotropy* describes the property of a substance that becomes more fluid when agitated and more solid when still. Heat and agitation create a change in the ground substance from thick and stiff to a more fluid (pliable) state.

With disuse and immobilization, the tissues become cool and the ground substance becomes thicker and more gel-like. Stiffness and aching, decreased circulation and nutrition, and decreased lubrication result. Massage therapy can change the viscosity of ground substance from a gel to a more fluid state through the introduction of mechanical forces—that is, bend, shear, tension, compression, and torsion.

The active and passive tissue movement of massage stimulates the synthesis of ground substance and GAGs, promotes the circulation of blood and lymph, and supports ground substance pliability, creating greater lubrication to the tissue. Tissue movement also transports nutrients and promotes the exchange of waste products.

Chondrocytes, a type of cartilage cell, are found in the collagen matrix of cartilage. Chondrocytes synthesize new cartilage in the normal turnover of cells and in the repair of damaged cartilage. Joint injury and repair involve this cell type.

Osteocytes, or bone cells, transport materials to maintain the structure of the bones and are active in the repair of bone. Piezioelectric effects support bone repair and guide the tensegretic nature of bone formation.

Reticular fibers form a mesh network supporting organs and glands.

Elastin fibers are more elastic and are found in ligaments and the linings of arteries.

Collagen forms approximately 80% of tendons, ligaments, joint capsules, and a large percentage of cartilage and bone, giving shape to the soft tissue. It forms the structural support of the skin, muscles, blood vessels, and nerve fibers. Normal stresses, in the form of exercise and the activities of daily living, increase collagen synthesis and strengthen connective tissue. This is an important aspect of fitness, especially for the elderly.

Collagen stabilizes the joints through the ligaments, joint capsules, and periosteum by resisting the tension or pulling force transmitted through the joints by movement or gravity. Collagen transmits the pulling force of muscle contraction through the fascia within the muscle and the tendon attachment. The collagen fibers tend to orient to parallel and longitudinal alignment along the lines of mechanical stress imposed through loading of the tissue during activity. Normal gliding of collagen fibers is maintained by movement and lubrication from connective tissue ground substance.

Immobilization or lack of use decreases collagen production, leading to atrophy in the connective tissue and to osteoporosis in the bone. Without movement, collagen is laid down in a random orientation, packing the fibers close together and forming microadhesions. *Adhesions* are abnormal deposits of connective tissue between gliding surfaces. This atrophy and random orientation of fibers creates weakness in the tissue and instability of the associated joint. This condition is more common in those who are just beginning a fitness and performance regimen and increases injury potential. The aging process decreases the amount and quality of the collagen structure; therefore, exercise helps prevent age-related soft tissue dysfunction.

Excessive mechanical and repetitive stress results in excessive deposits of collagen, causing abnormal cross-fiber links and adhesions. The fibers pack closer together, lubrication is decreased, and the water content of ground substance is reduced. This in turn decreases the ability of the fibers and fascicles to slide relative to each other. This condition is often called *fibrosis*. Adhesions and fibrosis create a resistance to normal electrical flow. This decrease in electrical currents conducted in the connective tissues interferes with the normal repair and rejuvenation process.

Athletes are prone to excessive mechanical stress during practices and performance activity and to repetitive strain from the athlete's specific activities, such as throwing, hitting, jumping, and running. Massage mechanically deforms the collagen fibers by introducing bind, shear, torsion, compression, and tension forces. *Piezoelectricity* is the ability of a tissue to generate electrical potentials in response to pressure of mechanical deformation. It is a property of most, if not all, living tissues. Piezoelectric potentials direct collagen fiber formation. Also, the negative charge in the soft tissue is increased, which has a strong proliferative effect, stimulating the creation of new cells to repair an injured site.

Injury results in an acute inflammatory response. During the acute and subacute repair phase of the healing process, connective tissue fibers are laid down in a random orientation, instead of in normal lines of force. In essentially the same process of fibrotic change discussed above, the fibers pack closer together, forming abnormal cross-fiber links and adhesions. These adhesions can occur at every level of the soft tissue, including the ligament or tendon adhering to the bone, between the fascicles, the fibers themselves, or individual muscle layers. In athletes it is common to find first- and second-layer muscle adhesions, such as gastrocnemius/soleus and pectoralis major/pectoralis minor.

Because adhesions decrease tissue extensibility, the tissue becomes less elastic, thicker, and shorter. Clients will often feel stiff in the area of adhered and fibrotic tissue.

TENDONS

Tendons are a continuation of the connective tissue within the muscle. Tendons consist of long, spiraling bundles of parallel collagen fibers, oriented in a longitudinal pattern along the line of force stress, and are embedded in ground substance with a small number of fibroblasts. Tendons have a microscopic "crimp" or wavelike structure that acts like a spring, enabling them to withstand large internal forces. The junction where the muscle fibers end and the connective tissue that forms the tendon begins is called the *musculotendinous junction*. This area is vulnerable to injury.

Tendons may be cordlike, such as the Achilles tendon; a flattened band of tissue, such as the rotator cuff; or a broad sheet of tissue called an aponeurosis, such as the attachment of the latissimus dorsi. They are surrounded by a loose connective tissue sheath. In areas of high pressure or friction, such as where tendons rub over the bones of the wrist and ankle, the tendon sheath is lined with a synovial layer to facilitate gliding. Tendon attaches to bone by weaving into the connective tissue covering of the bone called the periosteum. Tendons attach muscle to bone and transmit the force of muscle contraction to the bone, thereby producing motion of the joint. They also help stabilize the joint and act as a sensory receptor through the Golgi tendon organs.

A strain is an injury to the tendon. It is a tearing of the collagen fibers at the musculotendinous junction, at the tenoperiosteal junction, or within the body of the tendon. Loss of normal motion in a tendon through injury or immobilization creates loss of collagen fibers and formation of adhesions between the tendon and the surrounding structures, including the tendon sheath.

LIGAMENTS

Ligaments attach bones at joints, help stabilize joints, help guide joint motion, prevent excessive motion, and act as sensory receptors. Ligaments are composed of dense, white, short bands of nearly parallel bundles of collagen fibers embedded in a matrix of ground substance and a small number of fibroblasts. They contain some elastic fibers and a "crimp" structure, giving them greater elasticity, and are pliable and flexible. All ligaments surrounding the joints contain proprioceptors, mechanoreceptors, and pain receptors that provide information about posture and movement, which plays an important role in joint function.

Under normal conditions, when the joint moves, the ligament is stretched and the crimp in the tissue straightens out. The ligament returns to its normal length when the joint returns to a neutral position.

If tension or force is slowly applied to a ligament consistently and sustained, the tissue will assume the new length because of its viscous nature. This condition can lead to overstretched, or lax, ligaments and compromises stability of the joint. Because ligaments stabilize joints and act as neurosensory structures, injuries to ligaments can create dysfunction of the joint and surrounding soft tissue. A reflex connection exists between the ligaments of a joint and the surrounding muscles that affects the motor tone of muscles. In the case of lax ligaments, tone in muscles reflexively increases to provide joint stability.

The joint capsule and ligaments typically respond to an injury by becoming stretched, with resulting joint instability. These structures can also shorten, creating loss of a joint's normal range of motion and joint stiffness. Immobilization causes ligaments to atrophy and weaken, changing the normal gliding motion of the joint. Ligaments can twist into abnormal positions. Irritation or injury of the ligaments usually causes a reflexive contraction or inhibition in the surrounding muscles. Muscle energy methods that address gait and firing pattern sequences can help restore normal function temporarily since the muscle is connected to the ligaments through a neurologic reflex. The condition will continue to occur because the instability of the joint is the underlying causal factor.

Injured ligaments can become thick and fibrous from increased collagen, abnormal cross-fiber links, and adhesions. This is especially common if inflammatory responses are slow to resolve or have remained chronic.

Massage applied to ligaments that have developed adhesions is performed across the direction of fibers to increase pliability and realign fiber structure. If ligaments are too lax, exercise rehabilitation can stimulate the production of new collagen and help restore normal integrity. Friction massage can be used to create small controlled inflammation in the ligament structure to stimulate collagen production as well.

PERIOSTEUM

Periosteum is a dense, fibrous connective tissue sheath covering the bones. The outer layer consists of collagen fibers parallel to the bone and contains arteries, veins, lymphatics, and sensory nerves. The inner layer contains osteoblasts (cells that generate new bone formation). Repetitive stress can stimu-late the inner layer of the periosteum to create bone outgrowths called spurs. This often occurs at the heel when the plantar fascia is short.

The periosteum weaves into ligaments and the joint capsule. Stretching of the periosteum provides mechanoreceptor information regarding joint function.

The periosteum also blends with the tendons, forming the tenoperiosteal junction where the muscle pulls on the bone during joint movement. The sensory nerves in periosteum are sensitive to tension forces.

A common site of soft tissue injury is the tenoperiosteal junction. An acute tear or cumulative microtearing of the periosteum can cause the orientation of the collagen in the area to become random, leading to the development of the abnormal cross-fiber links and adhesions. Massage can address this abnormal fibrotic developed at the tenoperiosteal junction. Friction is used to introduce small amounts of controlled inflammation. This results in an active acute healing process. When coupled with appropriate rehabilitation, a more functional healing is the outcome.

FASCIA

Fascia is a fibrous connective tissue arranged as sheets or tubes. Fascia can be thick and dense, or thin, filmy membranes. Fascia is connected throughout the body, creating a unified form. Think of fascia as duct tape or plastic wrap.

Superficial fascia lies under the dermis of the skin and is composed of loose, fatty connective tissue. Deep fascia is dense connective tissue that surrounds muscles and forms fascial compartments called septa, which contain muscles with similar functions. These compartments are well lubricated in the healthy state, allowing the muscles inside to move freely.

Fascia can tear, adhere, torque, shorten, or become lax, just as other connective tissue structures, and responds well to connective tissue massage methods described in Unit Two of this book.

Common sources of musculoskeletal pain are the deep somatic tissues, including the periosteum, joint capsule, ligaments, tendons, muscles, and fascia. The most pain-sensitive tissues are the periosteum and the joint capsule. Tendons and ligaments are moderately sensitive, and muscle is less sensitive. This is an important awareness for massage therapists, who are often overly focused on muscle function as opposed to the total soft tissue system.

In general, mechanical forces applied during massage create heat in the tissues. This heat stimulates cellular activity and improves the lubrication of the fibers by making the ground substance more fluid. Specific application of a massage approach to generate heat in the tissue can be used as a part of a warm-up activity.

Effectively focused massage can:

- Stimulate the fibroblasts to repair the injured collagen.
- Introduce mechanical forces to realign the collagen fibers to their normal parallel alignment.
- Lengthen shortened tissue and increase ground substance pliability.
- Stimulate fluid distribution and tissue layering to promote normal tissue gliding.
- Create controlled focused inflammation to increase collagen proliferation, especially in lax structures. Proper rehabilitation must be combined with this approach for a beneficial outcome. Otherwise the result can be increased adherence and scar tissue formation.

JOINT STRUCTURE AND FUNCTION

Joints are innervated by the articular nerves, which are branches of the PNS. Branches of these nerves also supply the muscles controlling the joints. This is important in understanding how muscles can cause joint dysfunction and how joint dysfunction can cause muscle problems.

Many sensory receptors surround the joint. There are four types of joint receptors, located in the joint capsule, ligaments, periosteum, and articular fat pads:

Type 1—located in the superficial layers of the superficial joint capsule. These mechanoreceptors provide information concerning the static and dynamic position of the joint.

Type 2—located in the deep layers of the fibrous joint capsule. These dynamic mechanoreceptors provide information about acceleration and deceleration movements.

Type 3—located in the intrinsic and extrinsic joint ligaments and articular fat pads. These dynamic mechanoreceptors monitor the

direction of movement and have a reflex effect on muscle tone to provide deceleration.

Type 4—located in joint capsules, ligaments, and periosteum. These pain receptors send information to the CNS about the functional status of the joint and its surrounding soft tissue.

The reflex control of the muscles surrounding the joint is called the *arthrokinematic reflex*. The CNS creates contraction or relaxation of the muscles to protect the joint. The arthrokinematic reflex coordinates agonists, antagonists, and synergists around the joint as well as other jointed areas for gross movements and fine muscular control. Proper function of these reflex mechanisms is extremely important in posture, coordination, and balance; direction and speed of movement; position of the joint and body; and pain in the joint.

Irritation of the pain receptors and mechanoreceptors typically causes the flexors of the joint to become facilitated and to become short, tight, and hypertonic, whereas the extensors of the joint become inhibited or weak and long.

Irritation of the joint receptors can lead to abnormalities in posture, muscle coordination, control of movement, balance, and awareness of body position. This is a major issue for athletes. Assessment and treatment of gait patterns and firing patterns, using massage, including muscle energy methods, can support normal reflex functions.

Joints are classified as:

- Fibrous joint—bones united by fibrous tissue that have little movement.
- Cartilaginous joint—bones united by fibrocartilage and the intervertebral discs of the spine and have slight movement.
- Synovial joint—bones are not united directly; instead, the joint has a cavity filled with synovial fluid. The two bones are surrounded by a joint capsule and move freely.

The joint capsule is composed of two layers, an outer layer composed of fibrous connective tissue, and an inner layer composed of synovial tissue.

The outer layer contains intrinsic ligaments that thicken within the body of the capsule and extrinsic ligaments that lie superficial to the capsule. Many of the tendinous insertions of muscles weave into the joint capsule. This layer helps to stabilize the joint, guide joint motion, and prevent excessive motion. The joint capsule is innervated with mechanoreceptors and pain fibers. The mechanoreceptors sense the rate and speed of motion and the joint position and have reflex connections to the muscles that affect the joint. Irritation or injury to the capsule can create muscle contractions designed to protect the joint. This is called *guarding*.

The inner layer of the joint capsule is a synovial membrane that secretes synovial fluid when it is stimulated by joint motion. Synovial fluid is thick, clear, and viscous and provides lubrication and nutrition for the joint.

Fibrosis or thickening of the outer layer of the joint capsule is caused by acute inflammation, irritation, inflammation caused by imbalanced stresses on the joint, and/or immobilization. A tight, fibrotic joint capsule results in compression of certain areas of the cartilage and degeneration of the joint surfaces. The capsule and supporting ligaments may also be stretched because of injury or excessive stretching during activity such as dancing and gymnastics. If there is a loss of adequate motion from immobilization, the fibrous layer of the joint capsule atrophies. and joint instability results.

The synovial membrane can become injured or dysfunctional because of acute trauma to the joint, cumulative stresses from chronic irritation caused by imbalanced forces on the joint, or immobilization. Joint swelling occurs during inflammation. The swelling typically causes abnormal muscle function controlling the joint. Immobilization, on the other hand, thickens the synovial fluid and causes an eventual decrease in the amount of synovial fluid. This leads to adhesions between the capsule and the articular cartilage, tendon sheaths, and bursae, contributing to stiffness and joint degeneration.

A fibrotic joint capsule is addressed by using massage to introduce mechanical forces into the tissue to increase pliability. The fibrotic capsule is treated with manual pressure on the capsule itself. The massage strokes are directed in all directions, addressing the irregular alignment of the collagen. Active and passive movement and stretching are used to reduce intraarticular adhesions.

A capsule that is too loose needs exercise rehabilitation to help lay down new collagen fibers and proprioception exercises to help restore neurologic function. Appropriate friction massage can stimulate an acute inflammatory response that stimulates collagen formation.

For an acute, swollen joint capsule, treat with gentle rhythmic compression and decompression of the joint and lymphatic drain to pump the excess fluid out of the capsule. Pain-free, passive range of motion is also used in the flexion/extension plane to act as a mechanical pump. If there is too little fluid in the joint, passive and active movement helps stimulate the synovial membrane, increasing synovial fluid and therefore lubrication and nutrition.

CARTILAGE

Cartilage is a dense, fibrous connective tissue composed of collagen, chondrocytes, or cartilage cells, and ground substance.

Hyaline or articular cartilage covers the ends of bones and provides a smooth gliding surface for opposing joint surfaces. Articular cartilage creates new cells with use and deteriorates with disuse. It has no nerve or blood supply and is composed mostly of water. It is elastic and porous and has the capacity to absorb and bind synovial fluid. Intermittent compression and decompression creates a pumping action, which causes the movement of synovial fluid in and out of the cartilage, which is self-lubricating as long as the joint moves. Normal joint movements open and close the joint surfaces, compress and decompress the cartilage, and tighten and loosen the and active forms of joint capsule and ligaments, all of which supports joint lubrication and nutrition.

Synovial joints generate compression and decompression through movement, intermittent contraction of the muscles, and twisting and untwisting of the joint capsule. Massage application that includes passive and active forms of joint movement introduces compression and decompression and supports joint health.

Athletes are particularly prone to cartilage damage. An arthritic joint is a joint with degeneration of the cartilage. Damage to articular cartilage may be caused by acute trauma or cumulative stresses. These stresses are often the result of imbalances in the muscles surrounding the joint, a tight joint capsule, or a loose joint capsule. A tight capsule creates a high-contact area in the cartilage and decreased lubrication. A loose capsule allows inappropriate joint laxity and rubbing. Imbalanced muscles that move the joint create excessive pressure on the cartilage. The cartilage degenerates, beginning with fracturing of the collagen fibers and depletion of the ground substance.

Recent studies show that cartilage cells can create new cartilage. The joint must be moved to stimulate the synthesis of chondrocytes and the secretion of synovial fluid. Compressing and decompressing the joint capsule pumps synovial fluid into and out of the cartilage, rehydrating the cartilage. In addition to appropriate exercise, massage including muscle energy methods supports joint health using the following methods: contract/relax, reciprocal inhibition, pulsed muscle, or a combination of these methods. Both active and passive movements of the joint, as well as compression and decompression (traction), promote fluid exchange.

Fibrocartilage consists of white fibrous connective tissue arranged in dense bundles or layered sheets. Fibrocartilage has great tensile strength combined with considerable elasticity. It functions to deepen a joint space, such as the labrum of the hip and shoulder, the menisci of the knee, and the intervertebral discs of the spine. It also lines bone grooves for tendons, such as in the bicipital groove for the long head of biceps brachii. Common sport injuries include various types of fibrocartilage damage.

BURSA

A **bursa** is a synovia-filled sac lined with a synovial membrane and is found in areas of increased friction. The function of bursae is to secrete synovial fluid, which decreases friction in the area.

Bursitis typically is caused by excessive friction of the muscles and connective tissue (tendons and fascia) that overlie the bursa. Massage can lengthen structures that are rubbing and drain excessive fluid from the area using lymphatic drain methods.

JOINT STABILITY

For a joint to perform a full and painless range of motion, it must be stable. A rule to follow is stability before mobility, mobility before agility. Otherwise, abnormal forces move through the joint, leading to excessive wear and tear on the articular surfaces. **Joint stability** is determined by:

- The shape of the bones that make up the joint. This is **form stability.**
- Passive stability provided by the ligaments and joint capsule. This is also form stability.
- Dynamic stability provided by the muscles to produce stability. This is **force stability.**

If instability in the joint is caused by the form (bones, ligaments) then soft tissue methods will only be palliative. However, if there is force instability in the joint as a result of muscle dysfunction, exercise and massage can be valuable.

It is important that the muscles that cross a joint are balanced with appropriate contraction ability; otherwise the forces on the joint will create uneven stresses, leading to dysfunction and eventual degeneration of the cartilage.

When a joint is in the close-packed position, the capsule and ligaments are tightest. In the least-packed position the joint is most open, and the capsule and ligaments are somewhat lax. Generally, extension closes and flexion opens the joint surfaces. Midrange of the joint is typically the least-packed position, and most vulnerable to joint injury (Tables 4-3 and 4-4).

John Mennell introduced the concept of "joint play," which describes movements in a joint that can be produced passively but not voluntarily. In most joint positions, a joint has some "play" in it that is essential for normal joint function. (See joint

TABLE 4-3	LEAST-PACKED POSITIONS OF JOINTS
JOINT(S)	**POSITION**
Spine	Midway between flexion and extension
Temporomandibular	Mouth slightly open
Glenohumeral	55° abduction, 30° horizontal adduction
Acromioclavicular	Arm resting by side in normal physiologic position
Sternoclavicular	Arm resting by side in normal physiologic position
Elbow	70° flexion, 10° supination
Radiohumeral	Full extension and full supination
Proximal radioulnar	70° flexion, 35° supination
Distal radioulnar	10° supination
Wrist	Neutral with slight ulnar deviation
Carpometacarpal	Midway between abduction/adduction and flexion/extension
Thumb	Slight flexion
Interphalangeal	Slight flexion
Hip	30° flexion, 30° abduction and slight lateral rotation
Knee	25° flexion
Ankle	10° plantar flexion, midway between maximum inversion and eversion
Subtalar	Midway between extremes of range of motion
Midtarsal	Midway between extremes of range of motion
Tarsometatarsal	Midway between extremes of range of motion
Metatarsophalangeal	Neutral
Interphalangeal	Slight flexion

From Magee DJ: *Orthopedic physical assessment*, ed 4. Philadelphia, 2002, Saunders.

TABLE 4-4	CLOSE-PACKED POSITIONS OF JOINTS

JOINT(S)	POSITION
Spine	Extension
Temporomandibular	Clenched teeth
Glenohumeral	Abduction and lateral rotation
Acromioclavicular	Arm abducted to 30°
Sternoclavicular	Maximum shoulder elevation
Elbow	Extension
Radiohumeral	Elbow flexed 90°, forearm supinated 5°
Proximal radioulnar	5° supination
Distal radioulnar	5° supination
Wrist	Extension with ulnar deviation
Carpometacarpal	Full flexion
Thumb	Full opposition
Interphalangeal	Full extension and medial rotation*
Hip	Full extension and lateral rotation of femur
Knee	Maximum extension
Ankle	10° plantar flexion, midway between maximum inversion and eversion
Subtalar	Supination
Midtarsal	Supination
Tarsometatarsal	Supination
Metatarsophalangeal	Full extension
Interphalangeal	Full extension

Some authors include abduction.
From Magee DJ: *Orthopedic physical assessment*, ed 4. Philadelphia, 2002, Saunders.

play methods for assessment and correction of joint play dysfunction in Unit Two.)

JOINT DEGENERATION

One common cause of joint degeneration is loss of normal function of the joint. This altered function can occur as a result of a prior trauma or cumulative stress on the joint and is common in athletic performance.

Most conditions called arthritis are in fact noninflammatory and should be referred to as *arthrosis*, meaning joint degeneration. The terms osteoarthritis and degenerative joint disease are typically used interchangeably to describe a chronic degeneration of a joint, although osteoarthritis may be used to describe an inflammatory condition. Many athletes will develop arthritis and arthrosis.

Appropriate massage addresses adhesions and tightening of the joint capsule or ligaments, sustained contraction of the muscle surrounding the joint, muscle imbalances across a joint, and irregular firing patterns of the muscles moving the joint.

Short and tight muscles must be lengthened and relaxed, and muscles that are weak and inhibited need to be reeducated and exercised to regain their normal strength. Muscle activation firing pattern sequences need to be normalized.

Joint mobilization is any active or passive attempt to increase movement at a joint. Joint mobilization within the normal range of motion is within the scope of practice for the massage therapist. The movement must not be forcefully abrupt or painful.

The goals of joint mobilization are:
- Restore the normal joint play
- Promote joint repair and regeneration
- Stimulate normal lubrication by stimulating synovial membranes to promote rehydration of articular cartilage
- Normalize neurologic function
- Decrease swelling
- Reduce pain

Joint manipulation can be valuable. The chiropractor, physical therapist, or other specialist can manipulate the joint structure.

MUSCLE

The structural unit of skeletal muscle is the muscle fiber. The fibers are arranged in parallel bundles called fascicles. Each fascicle is composed of many myofibrils. The myofibril is composed of thousands of strands of proteins, also arranged in parallel bundles called myofilaments, and these are further divided into actin and myosin, the basic proteins of contraction. Muscles contain satellite cells that can regenerate muscle fibers if injured. The muscle fibers are so interwoven with connective tissue that it is hard to separate the two. A more appropriate term might be myofascia.

The connective tissue of muscle transmits the pull of the contracting muscle cells to the bones and gives the muscle fibers organization and support. The collagen fibers (epimysium, perimysium, endomysium) and connective tissue converge to form the tendon. The tendon fibers weave into the connective tissue of the periosteum, joint capsule, and ligaments. All of these connective tissue layers are lubricated in the healthy state.

Muscles should slide over each other in relationship to each other; when this does not happen, function is altered. This commonly occurs in athletes and as part of the aging process.

Muscles are dynamic stabilizers of the joints because they actively hold the joints in a stable position for posture and movement. Muscles sense joint movement and body position.

Muscles are connected to the nerves in the skin and to the nerves in the neighboring joint's capsule and ligaments through neurologic reflexes. If the skin or joint is irritated or injured, the muscle may go into a reflexive spasm or into inhibition. Muscles have pain receptors that fire with chemical or mechanical irritation.

Muscles act as a musculovenous pump because the contracting skeletal muscle compresses the veins and moves blood toward the heart. A similar process assists lymphatic movement.

MUSCLE FUNCTION TYPES

Muscles exert a pull when the actin/myosin is stimulated to contract. There are three types of muscle functions, all involving contraction:

1. Isometric—In an **isometric** contraction, the muscle contracts, but its constant length is maintained. The main outcome is stabilization.
2. Concentric—**Concentric** contraction is the shortening of muscle fibers while it contracts. The main outcome is movement/acceleration.
3. Eccentric—**Eccentric** function is the moving apart of the proximal and distal attachments while muscle fibers contract. The main outcome is control of movement and deceleration.

Muscles that contract concentrically to perform a certain movement are called agonists. This action is called **acceleration**, and the muscle is called the prime mover. For example, the biceps muscle is an agonist for elbow flexion. All movements in the body are accomplished by more than one muscle. The muscles that perform the opposite movements of the agonists are called the antagonists, and they provide control through deceleration during eccentric function. The triceps is the antagonist for the biceps, because the triceps extends the elbow. The muscle that works with another muscle to accomplish a particular motion is called a synergist. The term *synergist* includes stabilizers and neutralizers.

Typically, when the agonist is working concentrically, the antagonist is functioning eccentrically.

Sherrington's law of reciprocal inhibition states that there is a neurologic inhibition of the antagonist when the agonist is working. When we contract the biceps to flex the elbow, the triceps is being neurologically inhibited, which allows it to lengthen during elbow flexion. Co-contraction is an exception to this rule. **Co-contraction** occurs when the agonist and antagonist are working together. For example, when you make a fist, the flexors and extensors of the wrist are co-contracting to keep the wrist in a position that ensures the greatest strength of the fingers.

Human movement seldom involves pure forms of isolated concentric, eccentric, or isometric actions. This is because the body segments are periodically subjected to impact forces, as in running or jumping, or because some external force such as gravity causes the muscle to lengthen. In many situations, the muscles first act eccentrically, with a concentric action following immediately, mixed in with isometric stability function.

Two types of motor nerves supply each muscle: Alpha nerves fire during voluntary contraction of a muscle. Gamma nerves have voluntary and involuntary functions and unconsciously help to set the motor tone of the muscle, its resting length, and its function during voluntary activities for fine muscular control.

As previously discussed, five types of sensory nerve receptors supply each muscle. The sensory nerves are sensitive to pain, chemical stimuli, temperature, deep pressure, and mechanoreceptor stimuli. Two specialized receptors, the muscle spindle and the Golgi tendon organ, detect muscle length and changes in length and muscle tension. Muscle spindles detect length, and Golgi tendon organs detect tension in the muscle.

Muscle Length-Tension Relationship

A muscle develops its maximum strength or tension at its resting length or just short of its resting length because the actin and myosin filaments have the maximum ability to slide. When a muscle is excessively shortened or lengthened it loses its ability to perform a strong contraction. This is called the length-tension relationship (Figure 4-5). A muscle can develop only moderate tension in the lengthened position and minimum tension in the shortened position. Often athletes overtrain, thinking it will make them stronger, but what really happens is that the length-tension relationship is disturbed and strength is decreased. Massage can effectively normalize this situation.

Length-tension relationship

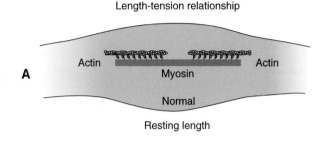

A

Actin   Actin

Myosin

Normal

Resting length

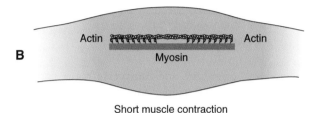

B

Actin   Actin

Myosin

Short muscle contraction

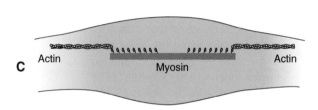

C

Actin   Actin

Myosin

Long muscle contraction

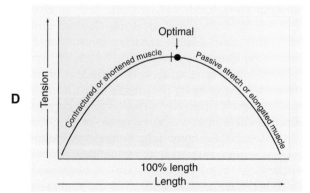

D

FIGURE 4-5 ■ Length-tension relationship. **A,** Normal resting length. When the muscle is stimulated to contract actin in an appropriate position to attach to myosin cause maximal contraction. **B,** Short muscle. Contraction ability is limited because actin has no space to "crawl" and cause contraction. **C,** Long muscle. Contraction ability is limited because actin is too far away to attach to myosin to begin contraction. **D,** Optimal length-tension relationship.

REFLEXIVE MUSCLE ACTION

Protective coordinated **reflexive muscle action** is an important consideration when providin massage, which is influenced by the following reflexive actions:

- Withdrawal reflexes, such as pulling away from a hot stove, involve instantaneous muscle contraction.
- Righting reflexes, such as tonic neck reflex and oculopelvic reflexes from the eyes, ears, ligaments, and joint capsules, communicate with the muscle and stimulate instantaneous contraction for protection of the joint and associated soft tissue, as well as support upright posture.
- Arthrokinematic reflexes are unconscious muscle contractions of muscles surrounding a joint that are caused by irritation in the joint.
- Splinting, guarding, and involuntary muscle contraction can be caused by a muscle injury.
- Emotional or psychologic stress creates excessive and sustained muscle tension.
- Viscerosomatic reflexes occur when an irritation or inflammation in a visceral organ causes a muscle spasm.

KINETIC CHAIN

Muscles do not function independently; instead, a body-wide interactive network is involved. This network is called the **kinetic chain** (Figure 4-6). The kinetic chain influences training, conditioning, rehabilitation, and massage application. It consists of the muscular/fascia system (functional anatomy), the articular joint system (functional biomechanics), and the neural/chemical system (motor behavior).

Each of these systems works interdependently to allow structural and functional efficiency. If any of the systems do not work efficiently, compensations and adaptation occur in the other systems. These compensations and adaptation lead to tissue overload, decreased performance, and predictable patterns of injury.

Normal or maximally efficient function is an effectively integrated, **multiplanar** (frontal, sagittal, transverse) **movement** process that involves acceleration, deceleration, and stabilization of muscle and fascial tissue and joint structures. Many strength and conditioning programs involve only uniplanar force movement. Very little time is spent on core stabilization, neuromuscular stabilization, and eccentric training in all three planes of motion (sagittal, frontal, and transverse). This situation predisposes an athlete for neuromuscular dysfunc-

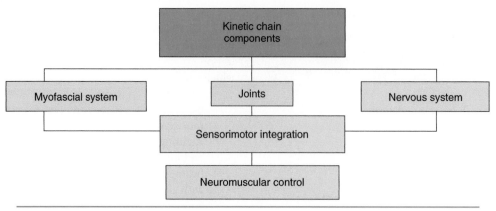

FIGURE 4-6 ■ Kinetic chain components. (Modified from Fritz S: *Mosby's essential sciences for therapeutic massage: anatomy, physiology, biomechanics, and pathology*, ed 2. St. Louis, 2004, Mosby.)

tion. The massage professional can manage or assist in reversal of the dysfunctional patterns that occur from these types of exercise and training regimens.

Conditioning programs and fitness protocols need to follow a sequence. Stability must develop before effective mobility. The core is considered the lumbar-pelvic-hip complex, thoracic spine, and cervical spine. The core operates as an integrated functional unit to dynamically stabilize the body during functional movements. The stabilization system has to function optimally to effectively utilize the strength and power in the prime movers. Many low back pain and hamstring problems are directly related to problems with core stability.

There are many types of strength including maximal strength, absolute strength, relative strength, strength endurance (stamina), speed strength, stabilization strength, and functional strength.

During movement, muscles must eccentrically function to decelerate gravity, ground reaction forces, and momentum, before concentric contraction causes acceleration to produce movement. Stabilization strength, core strength, and neuromuscular efficiency control the time between the eccentric function and the preceding concentric contraction. Therefore, eccentric neuromuscular control and stabilization strength exercises should begin to make up a larger portion of any fitness program. Since eccentric movement has a greater potential to result in delayed-onset muscle soreness, the massage application needs to effectively manage this response to exercise and training and ensure that compliance and performance are sustained. Functional movement patterns involve acceleration, stabilization, and deceleration, which occur at every joint.

Frontal plane movement includes adduction and abduction. **Sagittal plane movement** includes

flexion and extension, and **transverse plane rotational movement** includes internal and external rotation (Figures 4-7 and 4-8).

Muscles must adjust to gravity, momentum, ground reaction forces, and forces created by other functioning muscles. During functional movement, the transversus abdominis, internal oblique, multifidus, and deep erector spinae muscles stabilize the lumbar-pelvic-hip complex, whereas the prime movers perform the actual functional activities.

Muscles function synergistically in groups called force couples to produce force, reduce force, and dynamically stabilize the kinetic chain. **Force couples** are integrated muscle groups that provide neuromuscular control during functional movements.

When viewing the movement of the body as an integrated functional system, muscles can be classified as either local or global. Muscles that cross one joint are considered **local muscles** and form the inner unit. **Global muscles** cross multiple joints and form the outer unit.

The local musculature and connective tissue (inner unit) structurally consist of soft tissue that is predominately involved in joint support or stabilization. The joint support system of the core (lumbar-pelvic-hip complex) are muscles that either originate from or insert into the lumbar spine and include the transversus abdominis, lumbar multifidus, and internal oblique muscles, the diaphragm, and the muscles of the pelvic floor.

Local musculature also forms peripheral joint support systems of the shoulder, pelvic girdles, and limbs that consists of muscles that are not movement-specific but provide stability to allow movement of a joint. They also have attachments to the joint's passive elements, such as ligaments and capsules, that make them ideal for increasing joint stability. A common example of a

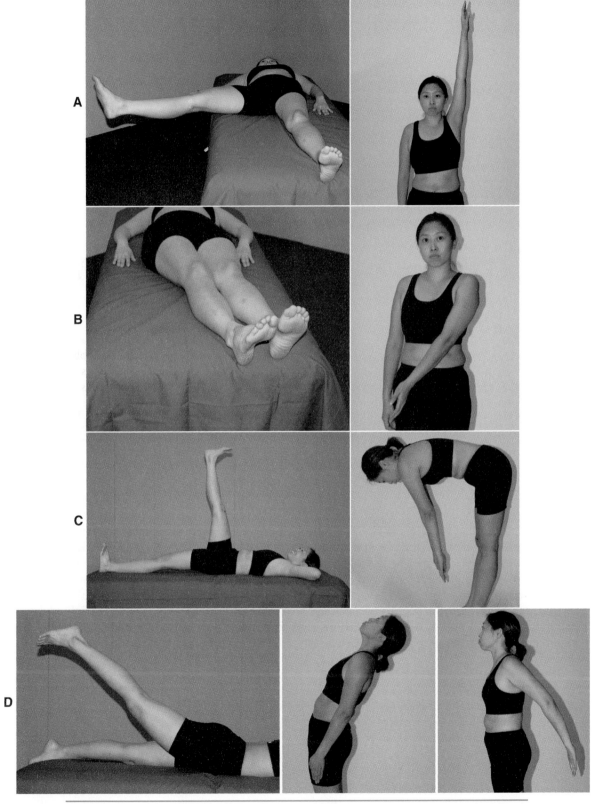

FIGURE 4-7 ■ Examples of range of motion. **A,** Frontal plane—abduction. **B,** Frontal plane—adduction. **C,** Sagittal plane—flexion. **D,** Sagittal plane—extension.

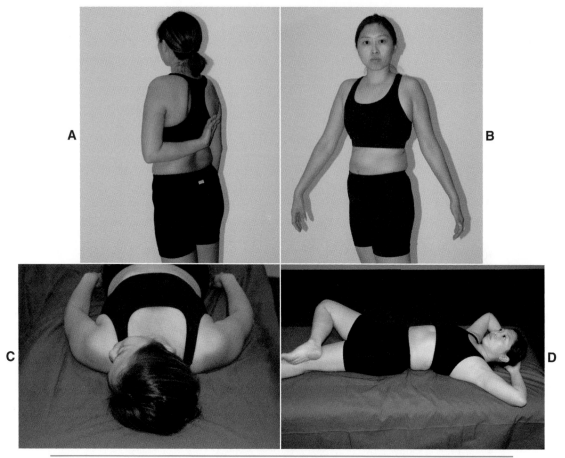

FIGURE 4-8 ■ Examples of transverse movement. **A,** Internal rotation. **B,** Trunk rotation. **C,** Transverse plane rotation (cervical). **D,** External rotation.

peripheral joint support system (local muscles/ inner unit) is the rotator cuff of the glenohumeral joint that provides dynamic stabilization for the humeral head in relation to the glenoid fossa during movement. Other joint support systems include the posterior fibers of the gluteus medius and the external rotators of the hip that perform pelvic-femoral stabilization, and the vastus medialis oblique muscles that provide patellar stabilization at the knee.

The global muscles (outer unit) cross multiple joints and are predominately responsible for movement. This group consists of more superficial muscles. The outer unit muscles are predominantly larger and associated with movement of the trunk and limbs and equalize external loads placed upon the body. The major ones include the rectus abdominis, external oblique, erector spinae, gluteus maximus, latissimus dorsi, adductors, hamstrings, quadriceps, and biceps and triceps brachii. They also are important because they work together in complementary patterns to transfer and absorb forces from the upper and lower extremities to the pelvis.

evolve Log on to the Evolve website that accompanies this book to see illustrations depicting these concepts.

The outer unit musculature has been broken down and described as force couples working in four subsystems. As described by Mike Clark, these subsystems include the deep longitudinal, posterior oblique, anterior oblique, and lateral. Tom Myers describes similar patterns as myofascial unit meridians.* Regardless, these muscle/fascial groups operate as an integrated functional unit because the central nervous system processes patterns of movement, not isolated muscles, and massage needs to address the system, not individual muscles.

---

*See Myers T: *Anatomy trains: myofascial meridians for manual and movement therapists.* Edinburgh, 2001, Churchill Livingstone.

DEEP LONGITUDINAL SUBSYSTEM

The major soft tissue components of the **deep longitudinal subsystem** are the erector spinae and biceps femoris muscles, thoracolumbar fascia, and sacrotuberous ligament. The long head of the biceps femoris attaches to the sacrotuberous ligament at the ischium. The sacrotuberous ligament in turn attaches from the ischium to the sacrum. The erector spinae attaches from the sacrum and ilium up to the ribs and cervical spine. Activation of the biceps femoris increases tension in the sacrotuberous ligament, which transmits force across the sacrum, stabilizing the sacroiliac joint, and allows force transference up through the erector spinae to the upper body. The functional interaction provides one pathway of force transmission longitudinally from the trunk to the ground. This muscle and fascia system functions mostly in the sagittal plane.

This transfer of force is necessary for normal gait. Prior to heel strike, the biceps femoris activates to eccentrically decelerate hip flexion and knee extension. Just after heel strike, the biceps femoris is further loaded through the lower leg via inferior movement of the fibula. This tension from the lower leg, up through the biceps femoris, into the sacrotuberous ligament and up the erector spinae creates a force that assists in stabilizing the **evolve** sacroiliac joint.

Another group of muscles acting as a force couple consists of the superficial erector spinae, psoas, transversus abdominis, lumbar, multifidus, and internal obliques and the muscles of the diaphragm and pelvic floor. Dysfunction of any structure can lead to sacroiliac joint instability and low-back pain. The weakening of the gluteus maximus (often inhibited by the psoas and other related muscles) and structures of the deep longitudinal subsystem and/or latissimus dorsi may also lead to increased tension in the hamstring and therefore cause recurring hamstring strains.

Dysfunction in any of these structures can lead to sacroiliac joint instability and low back pain. These areas need to be addressed as one functional unit, not individual muscles.

POSTERIOR OBLIQUE SUBSYSTEM

The muscles and fascia of the **posterior oblique subsystem** function in the transverse plane. The major muscles are the latissimus dorsi and the gluteus maximus. When the contralateral gluteus maximus and latissimus dorsi muscles contract, this creates a stabilizing force for the sacroiliac joint.

Just prior to heel strike, the latissimus dorsi and the contralateral gluteus maximus are eccentrically loaded. At heel strike, each muscle accelerates its respective limb and creates tension in the thoracolumbar fascia. This tension creates a force couple that assists in the stability of the sacroiliac joint. **evolve** .

The posterior oblique subsystem is important for other rotation activities such as swinging a golf club or a baseball bat and throwing a ball.

ANTERIOR OBLIQUE SUBSYSTEM

The **anterior oblique subsystem** functions in a transverse plane orientation very similarly to the posterior oblique subsystem but on the front of the body. The functional muscles include the internal and external oblique muscles, adductor complex muscle, and hip external rotators. These muscles function as an aid in the stability and rotation of the pelvis, as well as contributing to leg swing. The pelvis must rotate in the transverse plane in order to create a swinging motion for the legs. This rotation comes in part from the posterior muscle and anterior muscle groups. The fiber arrangements of the muscles involved—latissimus dorsi, gluteus maximus, internal and external obliques, adductors, and hip rotators—indicate this type of function. The obliques and adductors complex produce rotational and flexion movements and stabilize the **evolve** lumbar-pelvic-hip complex.

LATERAL SUBSYSTEM

The **lateral subsystem,** which is composed of the gluteus medius, tensor fasciae latae, adductor complex, and quadratus lumborum muscles, creates frontal plane stability. This system is responsible for pelvic femoral stability, such as during single leg functional movements when walking or climbing stairs. The ipsilateral gluteus medius, tensor fasciae latae, and adductors combine with the contralateral quadratus lumborum to control the pelvis and femur in the frontal plane. **evolve** .

Dysfunction in the lateral subsystem increases pronation (flexion, internal rotation, and adduction) of the knee, hip, and/or feet during walking, squats, lunges, or when climbing stairs.

When in a closed kinetic chain, full body *pronation* is multiplanar (frontal, sagittal, and transverse) synchronized joint motion that occurs with eccentric muscle function. *Supination* is multiplanar (frontal, sagittal, and transverse) synchronized joint motion that occurs with concentric muscle function (Box 4-2). This means that for one joint pattern to move effectively, all the involved joints have to move. Movement can be initiated at any joint in the pattern, and restriction of any joint in the pattern will restrict motion or increase motion in interconnected joints.

To briefly describe functional biomechanics, the gait cycle is reviewed here. During walking or other locomotor activities such as running, motion at the subtalar joint is linked to the transverse plane rotations of the bone segments of the entire lower extremity. During the initial contact phase of the gait cycle, the subtalar joint pronates, which creates internal rotation of the tibia, femur, and pelvis. At mid-stance, the subtalar joint supinates, which creates external rotation of the tibia, femur, and pelvis. Poor control of pronation decreases the ability to eccentrically decelerate multisegmental motion and can lead to muscle imbalances, joint dysfunction, and injury. Poor production of supination decreases the ability of the kinetic chain

to concentrically produce the appropriate force during functional activities and can lead to synergistic dominance. During functional movement patterns, almost every muscle has the same synergistic function: to eccentrically decelerate pronation or to concentrically accelerate supination. The CNS recruits the appropriate muscles in an optimal muscle activator firing pattern sequence during specific movement patterns.

Joint arthokinematics refers to roll, slide, glide, and translation movements that occur between two articular partners. *Joint play* is defined as the involuntary movement that occurs between articular surfaces that are separate from the range of motion of a joint produced by muscles. It is an essential component of joint motion and must occur for normal functioning of the joint. Predictable patterns of joint arthrokinematics occur during normal movement patterns. Optimum length-tension and force couple relationships ensure maintenance of normal joint kinematics.

Optimal posture enables the development of high levels of functional strength and neuromuscular efficiency. Functional strength is the ability of the neuromuscular system to perform dynamic eccentric, isometric, and concentric actions efficiently in a multiplanar environment. This process allows the appropriate motor program (muscle activator sequence) to be chosen to perform an activity, thus ensuring that the right muscle contracts at the right joint, with the right amount of force, and at the right time. If any component of the kinetic chain is dysfunctional (such as short muscle, weak muscle, joint dysfunction), then neuromuscular control is altered. This decreases force production, force reduction, and stabilization.

If the kinetic chain is out of alignment, the individual will have decreased structural efficiency, functional efficiency, and performance. For example, if one muscle is tight (altered length-tension relationships), the force couples around that particular joint are altered. If the force couples are altered, the normal arthrokinematics is altered.

Arthrokinematic inhibition is the neuromuscular phenomenon that occurs when a joint dysfunction inhibits the muscles that surround the joint. For example, a sacroiliac joint dysfunction causes arthrokinematic inhibition of the deep stabilization mechanism of the lumbo-pelvic-hip complex (transversus abdominis, internal oblique, multifidus, and lumbar transversospinalis). All of these neuromuscular phenomena occur secondary to postural dysfunctions.

Box 4-2 JOINT MOVEMENT INVOLVED WITH PRONATION AND SUPINATION

Pronation	Supination
Foot	*Foot*
1. Dorsiflexion	1. Plantar flexion
2. Eversion	2. Inversion
3. Abduction	3. Adduction
Ankle	*Ankle*
1. Dorsiflexion	1. Plantar flexion
2. Eversion	2. Inversion
3. Abduction	3. Adduction
Knee	*Knee*
1. Flexion	1. Extension
2. Adduction	2. Abduction
3. Internal rotation	3. External rotation
Hip	*Hip*
1. Flexion	1. Extension
2. Adduction	2. Abduction
3. Internal rotation	3. External rotation

DEVELOPMENT OF MUSCLE IMBALANCES

Muscle imbalances are caused by postural stress, pattern overload, repetitive movement, lack of core stability, and lack of neuromuscular efficiency.

SERIAL DISTORTION PATTERNS

Kinetic chain dysfunction typically results in predictable patterns. Although each individual will display the pattern somewhat differently, the following information provides a conceptual way of understanding integrated function and dysfunction. Vladimir Janda discovered that muscles react to pain or excessive stress in predictable patterns. He found that certain muscles tend to become overactive, short, and tight, and describes these muscles as having a postural or stabilizing function. He found that other muscles tend to become inhibited and weak, and noticed that most of these muscles were concerned with movement rather than stability. Many terms are used to describe these muscle functions. Two more accurate terms that have been suggested for these groups are tightness-prone stabilizer (postural) and inhibition-prone mover (phasic). The muscles of the body can be classified on the basis of which muscles have primarily a stabilizing role, and which muscles have primarily movement roles. These categorizations are controversial, because most muscles can function in both roles (Box 4-3). **Tonic/postural/stabilizing muscles** play a primary role in maintenance of posture and joint stability. The primary role of the phasic/mover muscles is quick movement. Tonic/postural/stabilizing muscles react to stress by becoming short and tight, and phasic/mover muscles react to stress by becoming inhibited and weak.

The phasic/mover group is characterized as being prone to developing tightness, readily activated during most functional movements, and overactive in fatigue situations or during new movement patterns. The stabilization group is prone to weakness and inhibition, is less activated in most functional movement patterns, and fatigues easily during dynamic activities. If the phasic/mover group is prone to tightness and overuse, this can cause reciprocal inhibition of its functional antagonists. This inhibition leads to poor neuromuscular efficiency and further postural dysfunction. Furthermore, if the stabilization group is prone to weakness, then synergistic dominance (discussed later) can result.

Box 4-3 MOVERS AND STABILIZERS IN MUSCLES OF THE HUMAN BODY

Movement Group	Stabilization Group
Gastrocnemius/soleus	Peroneals
Adductors	Anterior tibialis
Hamstrings	Posterior tibialis
Psoas	Vastus medialis oblique
Tensor fasciae latae	Gluteus maximus/medius
Rectus femoris	Transversus abdominis
Piriformis	Internal oblique
Erector spinae	Multifidus
Pectoralis minor/major	Deep erector spinae
Latissimus dorsi	Transversospinalis
Teres major	Serratus anterior
Upper trapezius	Middle/lower trapezius
Levator scapulae	Rhomboids
Sternocleidomastoid	Teres minor
Scalenes	Infraspinatus
Teres major	Posterior deltoid
	Longus colli/capitis
	Deep cervical stabilizers

An important difference between the two muscle groups is that a small reduction in strength of an inhibition-prone muscle initiates a disproportionately larger contraction of the antagonist tightness-prone muscle. Because work and recreational activities favor tightness-prone muscles getting stronger, tighter, and shorter as the inhibition-prone muscles become weaker and more inhibited, unless fitness programs are balanced, dysfunctional patterns are exacerbated, and the length-tension relationship becomes important. Some muscles, such as the quadratus lumborum and scalenes, can react with either tightness or weakness.

In addition to the causes of muscle dysfunction listed previously, muscle injury, training protocols, reduced recovery time, chronic pain, and inflammation create disturbances in normal muscle function and may stimulate a neurologic-based tightness or weakness in a muscle. In a force couple relationship, muscles work together to produce movement or dynamic force joint stability. Serial distortion patterns in the kinetic chain disrupt force couple relationships.

A **serial distortion pattern** is the state in which the functional and structural integrity of the kinetic chain is altered and in which compensations and adaptations occur (Figure 4-9). These distortion patterns can be described as:

- Upper crossed syndrome (Figure 4-10)
- Lower crossed syndrome (Figure 4-11)
- Pronation distortion syndrome (Figure 4-12)

A short, tight muscle is held in a sustained contraction. The muscle is constantly working and consumes more oxygen and energy, and generates more waste products than a muscle at rest. Circulation is decreased because the muscle is not performing its normal function as a pump, which can lead to ischemia and cause the pain receptors to fire. The sustained tension in the muscle pulls on its attachments to the periosteum, joint capsule, and ligaments, creating increased pressure, uneven forces, and excessive wear in the joint. Short, tight muscles often compress nerves between muscles or through a muscle, a form of impingement syndrome.

Long weak muscles are unable to support joint stability and contribute to poor posture, excessive tension and compression, and abnormal joint movements. Muscle activator firing pattern sequences and gait reflexes are disturbed.

Inhibited muscles interfere with vascular and lymphatic movement.

Massage application as described in this book is particularly effective in dealing with these conditions and supports other professional treatments. Massage lengthens short tight muscles, normalizes firing patterns, and increases tissue pliability. These benefits support therapeutic exercise to treat the long weak and inhibited muscles. In other words, treatment involves massage and stretching of short tight muscles, and exercise for long weak muscles.

Reciprocal inhibition is the process whereby a tight muscle, the psoas for example, causes decreased neural stimulus in its functional

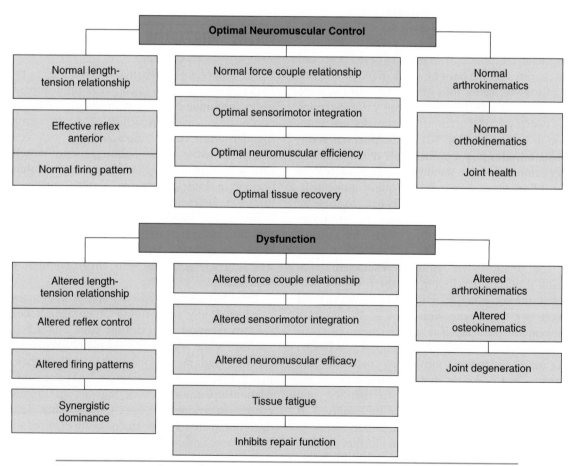

FIGURE 4-9 ■ Overview of neuromuscular control. (Data from Chaitow L, DeLany JW: *Clinical applications of neuromuscular techniques, vol 1, the upper body.* Edinburgh, 2001, Churchill Livingstone.)

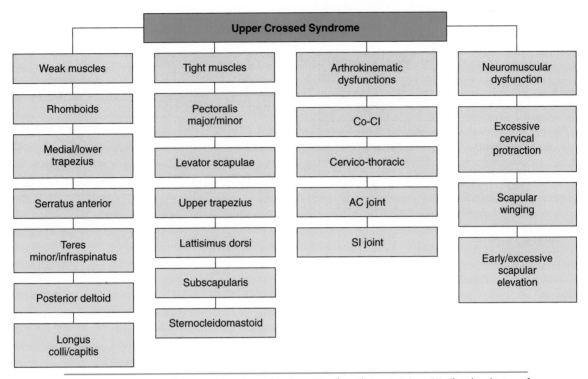

FIGURE 4-10 ■ Upper crossed syndrome flow chart. (Data from Chaitow L, DeLany JW: *Clinical applications of neuromuscular techniques, vol 1, the upper body*. Edinburgh, 2001, Churchill Livingstone.)

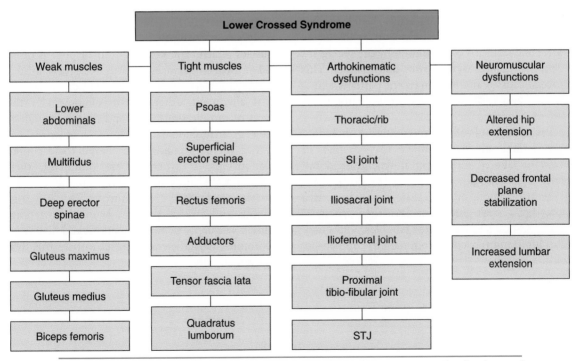

FIGURE 4-11 ■ Lower crossed syndrome flow chart. (Data from Chaitow L, DeLany JW: *Clinical applications of neuromuscular techniques, vol 1, the upper body*. Edinburgh, 2001, Churchill Livingstone.)

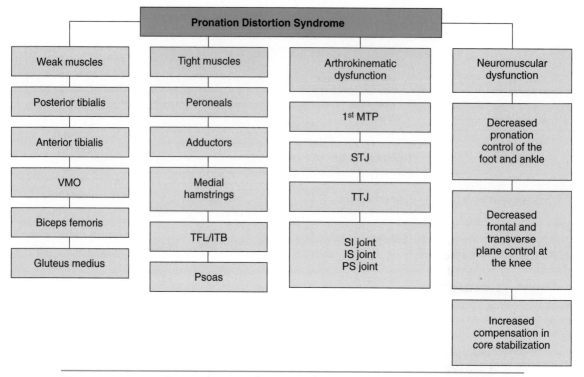

FIGURE 4-12 ■ Pronation distortion syndrome. (From Chaitow L, DeLany JW: *Clinical applications of neuromuscular techniques, vol 1, the upper body.* Edinburgh, 2001, Churchill Livingstone.)

antagonist the gluteus maximus. This process results in decreased force production by the prime mover and leads to compensation by the synergists, a process called **synergistic dominance.** This process leads to altered movement patterns and is assessed and treated with muscle activator firing pattern sequences. Synergistic dominance often occurs as the result of improper training, including overtraining, and fatigue. Athletes may complain of heavy or labored movement if synergistic dominance is occurring.

As an example of synergistic dominance, if a client has a weak gluteus medius, then synergists (tensor fasciae latae, adductor complex, and quadratus lumborum) become dominant to compensate for the weakness. This alters normal joint alignment, which further alters the normal length-tension relationships around the joint where the muscles attach. The combination of poor posture and muscle imbalances causing reciprocal inhibition and synergistic dominance leads to altered joint alignment. Altered joint alignment is the result of muscle shortening and muscle weakness. Altered arthrokinematics (joint movement) is further altered secondary to altered force couple relationships. If synergists are dominant, then normal joint movements are altered because muscles are firing out of sequence. This is a continuous and cyclical process. Muscle shortening, muscle weakness, joint dysfunction, and decreased neuromuscular efficiency can all initiate this dysfunctional pattern.

IN MY EXPERIENCE...

Consider the knee as one of the most used and abused joints in athletic activity. An injury to the knee typically causes the joint to be held in a sustained flexion during the acute phase. This position is the least-packed joint position, can accommodate increased fluid, and is the most comfortable. This position pulls the soft tissue on the medial and lateral aspects of the knee into an abnormal posterior alignment, with the posterior short and anterior long. This misalignment creates abnormal torsion in the skin, muscles, tendons, and ligaments of the medial and lateral aspects of the knee, shortening of structure at the back of the knee, and weakening of the medial quadriceps, particularly the vastus medialis oblique. The increased torsion causes a decreased flow of fluids in the area, leading to a decreased ability for repair and the tendency for tissue layers to stick together and form adhesions. The sustained position eventually becomes fibrotic, and the knee ends up stuck in flexion and unable to fully extend. At the very least, performance is diminished. Compromised patterns body-wide will begin to occur and reinjury is likely. Also, compensation patterns in other parts of the body become prone to injury, including a tendency for tissue layers to stick together and for adhesions to develop. So what is the next step? There is no defined recipe; clinical reasoning is essential and revolves around the following concepts:

Apply therapeutic massage with an intelligent focus.

Normalize soft tissue structures by reintroducing the normal spiral orientation to the soft tissue and increase pliability and separation of the tissue layers.

Massage can:

Create a mechanical force—tension, bind, shear or torsion —on the fibers to encourage relaxation.

Reintroduce controlled acute inflammation to signal regeneration of connective tissue structures.

Create a piezoelectric effect, (mechanical energy is transformed into electrical energy). The piezoelectric effect increases cellular activity, tissue repair, and alignment.

Normalize fluid movement, rhythmic cycles of joint compression and decompression (traction), rocking, and specific methods such as lymphatic drain to restore the natural rhythmic movement of the body's fluids.

Normalize autonomic nervous system, neurotransmitter, and the endocrine function. Deliberate use of stimulation or inhibition and pressure levels encourage appropriate neurochemical function.

SUMMARY

Massage targets both the connective tissue and neuromuscular aspect of muscle tissue function because tension in a muscle and its fascia is created by both active and passive elements. Passive elements include collagen fibers and ground substance, which are influenced by massage introduction of various mechanical forces. Because muscle contains ground substance, it demonstrates viscous behavior. It becomes thicker and stiff when it is stretched quickly, is cold, or is immobilized. It becomes more fluid-like when it is stretched slowly or when it is heated. Active components include the contractile proteins actin and myosin and the nerves' massage interactions with the neurochemical stimulus.

The most important signs of impaired muscle function are:

- Increased muscle motor tone–This occurs when muscles are held in a sustained contraction.
- Muscle inhibition–A muscle may be functionally weak, which creates joint instability and causes others to become hypertonic in compensation.
- Muscle imbalance–This change in function in the muscles crossing a joint occurs when certain muscles react to stress by getting shorter and tight and others become longer and weak. This is an important factor in chronic pain syndromes because this imbalance alters the movement pattern of the joint.
- Joint dysfunction–Muscle dysfunction creates uneven distribution of forces on the weight-bearing surfaces of the joint.
- Abnormal muscle firing pattern sequences–Muscle dysfunction is often expressed by improper contraction sequences.

The reader is strongly encouraged to maintain active study of anatomy and physiology. Unit Two discusses this information in relation to massage benefits, assessment, and treatment plan development. Unit Three explores the related issues of sport pathology and uses this base to build treatment plans.

1 Locate and summarize the various contents in this book that relate to fluid dynamics. Include concepts of assessment, treatment, outcomes, contraindications, and benefits (list page numbers).

_____

_____

_____

_____

_____

_____

2 Locate and summarize the various contents in this book related to neuroendocrine control of the body. Include concepts of assessment, treatment outcomes, contraindications, and benefits (list page numbers).

_____

_____

_____

_____

_____

_____

_____

_____

3 Locate and summarize the various contents in this book related to connective tissue and function. Include concepts of assessment, treatment outcomes, contraindications, and benefits (list page numbers).

_____

_____

_____

_____

_____

_____

_____

_____

_____

_____

4 Locate and summarize the various content in this book related to joint function. Include concepts of assessment, treatment outcomes, contraindications, and benefits (list page numbers).

_____

_____

_____

_____

_____

_____

_____

_____

5 Locate and summarize the various content in this book related to muscular function. Include concepts of assessment, treatment outcomes, contraindications, and benefits (list page numbers).

_____

_____

_____

_____

_____

_____

_____

_____

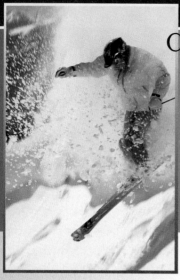

CHAPTER

5

FITNESS FIRST

OBJECTIVES

Upon completion of this chapter the reader will have the information necessary to:

1 List the benefits of exercise.

2 Describe how exercise is part of a fitness program.

3 Explain the importance of proper breathing to fitness.

4 List and explain the components of a fitness program.

5 Explain intensity, duration, and frequency as these terms relate to a conditioning program.

6 Define force, work, power, and torque.

7 Explain why it is important to include endurance, aerobic exercise, adaptation, and training stimulus threshold in a therapeutic exercise program.

8 List the major energy-producing systems in the body and their implications for fitness programs.

9 Identify the physiologic changes that occur with exercise.

10 Explain the importance of core strength as it relates to fitness.

11 List and describe the three main components of an exercise program that targets fitness.

12 Describe how flexibility supports an exercise program.

13 Develop massage outcomes to support a fitness program.

Fitness is essential. Regular physical activity helps keep us healthy, mobile, strong, and flexible. The outcome of appropriate exercise, proper nutrition, and emotional and spiritual balance is the foundation for fitness.

Benefits from physical activity include:

• Decreased risk of death from coronary heart disease and of developing hypertension, colon cancer, and diabetes

Adaptation
Aerobic exercise
Aerobic exercise training
Aerobic (oxygen) system
Anaerobic glycolytic system
Breathing dysfunction
Circuit-interval training
Circuit training
Conditioning
Continuous training
Cool-down

Core strength
Core training
Deconditioning
Duration
Endurance
Energy
Energy systems
Exercise
Exercise intensity
Flexibility training
Force

Frequency
Interval training
Overload principle
Phosphagen system
Physical fitness program
Specificity principle
Strength training
Stretching
Therapeutic exercise
Torque
Warm-up

- Improved muscle strength and stamina
- Improved mood and increased general feeling of well-being
- Decreased symptoms of anxiety and depression
- Increased control of pain and joint swelling associated with arthritis/arthrosis

Exercise is essential in maintaining the body's overall well-being. Even modest amounts of exercise can substantially diminish the chances of dying from heart problems, cancer, or other diseases.

Deconditioning occurs with prolonged inactivity. Its effects are frequently seen in someone who has had an extended illness. These effects are also seen, although possibly to a lesser degree, in the individual who is sedentary because of lifestyle or increasing age. Decrease in maximal oxygen consumption, cardiac output, and muscular strength occurs very rapidly. There needs to be a balance between training and recovery to prevent both overtraining and deconditioning. People with disabilities require regular physical activity just as much as others without disabilities.

There are additional benefits that are especially important for people with disabilities, because regular physical activity can lessen the probability of developing other physical or mental conditions associated with the disability. These secondary conditions include obesity, pressure sores, infections, fatigue, depression, and osteoporosis. Such conditions can lead to further disability and possible loss of physical independence.

Many people with disabilities are more prone than the general population to underuse, overuse, or misuse of various muscle groups. For instance, a person who uses a wheelchair may have very well-developed anterior muscles from pushing the chair but may need to develop the upper back muscles. Structured exercise and massage can help to balance out these differences. Because of the adaptation of the body to compensate for a disability, other body areas are overused. If the lower extremities are affected, fluid movement (circulation and lymphatic) is compromised. Massage can target both these areas and support the fitness program.

Developing the physical capacity and strength to move around and perform daily life activities can assist those with disabilities to accomplish or sustain their independence. Physical fitness programs can also help lessen or even reverse some of the physiologic changes that are associated with aging, including loss of:

- Lean muscle tissue and strength
- Aerobic capacity
- Flexibility
- Balance
- Bone density
- Cognitive functions, especially the speed of memory

Staying active also often helps if activity is limited because of medical conditions, such as arthritis/arthrosis or osteoporosis, that may impair the ability to perform important daily activities such as driving, walking up stairs, and lifting groceries more comfortably.

Regular physical activity can prevent and in some cases reverse some of these changes. It can also help to prevent many conditions associated with aging, such as coronary artery disease, high blood pressure, stroke, diabetes, depression, and some cancers.

What used to be considered diseases of middle age are now showing up in adolescents. This is a major concern. These problems usually occur in conjunction with childhood and adolescent obesity.

Certain well-known risk factors lead to heart disease, including obesity, high blood pressure, high cholesterol, low levels of "good" (high-density-lipoprotein [HDL]) and high levels of "bad" (low-density-lipoprotein [LDL]), cholesterol, diabetes, cigarette smoking, and family history of heart disease. Exercise has a dramatic effect on almost all of these risk factors by:

- Promoting weight loss as a result of increasing calories burned.
- Controlling blood pressure through exercise and diet.
- Improving cholesterol levels. In particular, aerobic exercise raises blood levels of HDL cholesterol. HDL cholesterol carries LDL cholesterol to the liver, preventing it from clogging arteries.
- Reducing the tendency for smoking and other detrimental behaviors, because exercise calms nervous tension.

Any muscle, including the heart, is strengthened by exercise. A well-conditioned heart has a low resting heart rate. The fewer times it has to beat each minute, the longer it rests between beats and the less strain is put on it.

Conditioning the heart involves identifying a safe and normal heart rate and determining an appropriate training range. The predicted maximum heart rate is the highest number of beats per minute that is safe during the exercise session. There are two ways to determine this rate. An exercise stress test can determine the heart rate by calculating it with a simple formula: 220 minus the person's age. For example, a person 30 years old would have a predicted maximum heart rate of 190 beats per minute.

During exercise, the heart rate must be brought into the training range, which is 70% to 85% of the maximum rate. This is the heart rate that best conditions the heart. The 30-year-old individual, with a predicted maximum heart rate of 190, would have a training range of 125 to 160 beats per minute.

Heart rate monitors are available, or you can take the pulse manually. The easiest place to take the pulse rate during exercise is at the side of the throat on the carotid artery. Place the index and middle fingers at the base of the neck on either side

of the windpipe and count the heartbeats for 15 seconds. Multiply this number by 4. This yields the number of heartbeats per minute.

The type of aerobic activity makes no difference as long as a training range is reached. Ideally, the heart rate is maintained in the training range for at least 20 minutes three times a week. However, research shows that even less exercise—12 minutes three times a week—can produce health benefits. A little exercise is better than none at all.

BREATHING

Proper breathing at all times is important. If breathing is not effective, the ability to exercise is compromised. Breathing patterns, both functional and dysfunctional, are a direct link to altering autonomic nervous system patterns, which in turn affect endocrine function and mood, feelings, and behavior. Especially when working with athletes, the breathing function may be a causal factor in many soft tissue symptoms.

The shoulders should not move during normal relaxed breathing. The accessory muscles of respiration located in the neck area should be active only when increased oxygen is required during physical activity. These muscles (scalenes, sternocleidomastoid, serratus posterior superior, levator scapulae, rhomboids, abdominals, and quadratus lumborum) may be constantly activated for breathing when forced inhalation and expiration are not needed. This will result in dysfunctional muscle patterns and therefore dysfunctional breathing. This is the pattern for *sympathetic dominance* breathing.

If the athlete does not balance the oxygen/carbon dioxide levels through increased activity levels, overbreathing in excess of physical demand can occur. Patterns of **breathing dysfunction** (overbreathing) are quite common in the athletic population. This can occur for a variety of reasons, including inability to achieve *parasympathetic dominance* (relaxation) after training or competition; dysfunction of respiratory muscles (Box 5-1); or restricted structure, particularly the ribs and thoracic vertebrae.

Appropriate massage is effective in treating soft tissue dysfunction, whereas joint manipulation of some type (e.g., chiropractic) may be necessary for treating facet and costal rib restrictions.

Overbreathing affects performance and decision making. Chronic breathing dysfunction patterns interfere with training by causing fatigue and inter-

Box 5-1 BREATHING PATTERN DISORDER

Breathing pattern disorder is a complex set of behaviors that leads to overbreathing despite the absence of a pathologic condition. It is considered a functional syndrome because all the parts are working effectively, and therefore a specific pathologic condition does not exist. Instead, the breathing pattern is inappropriate for the situation, resulting in confused signals to the CNS, which sets up a whole chain of events.

Increased ventilation is a common component of fight-or-flight responses. However, when our breathing rate increases but our actions and movements are restricted or do not increase accordingly, we are breathing in excess of our metabolic needs. Blood levels of carbon dioxide (CO_2) fall, and symptoms may occur. Because we exhale too much CO_2 too quickly, our blood becomes more acidotic. These biochemical changes can cause many of the following signs and symptoms:

Cardiovascular: Palpitations, missed beats, tachycardia, sharp or dull atypical chest pain, "angina," vasomotor instability, cold extremities, Raynaud's phenomenon, blotchy flushing or blush area, capillary vasoconstriction (face, arms, hands)

Neurologic: Dizziness; unsteadiness or instability; sensation of faintness or giddiness (rarely actual fainting); visual disturbances (blurred or tunnel vision); headache (often migraine); paresthesia (numbness, uselessness, heaviness, pins and needles, burning, limbs feeling out of proportion or as if they "don't belong"), commonly of hands, feet, or face but sometimes of scalp or whole body; intolerance to light or noise; enlarged pupils (wearing dark glasses on a dull day)

Respiratory: Shortness of breath, typically after exertion; irritable cough; tightness or oppression of chest; difficulty breathing, "asthma"; air hunger; inability to take a satisfying breath; excessive sighing, yawning, and sniffing

Gastrointestinal: Difficulty swallowing, dry mouth and throat, acid regurgitation, heartburn; hiatal hernia; nausea, flatulence, belching, air swallowing, abdominal discomfort, bloating

Muscular: Cramps, muscle pain (particularly occipital, neck, shoulders, and between scapulae; less commonly the lower back and limbs), tremors, twitching, weakness, stiffness, tetany (seizing up)

Psychologic: Tension, anxiety, "unreal" feelings, depersonalization, feeling "out of body," hallucinations, fear of insanity, panic, phobias, agoraphobia

General: Feelings of weakness, exhaustion; impaired concentration, memory, and performance; disturbed sleep, including nightmares; emotional sweating (axillae, palms, and sometimes whole body); woolly or thick head

Cerebral vascular constriction, a primary response to breathing pattern disorder, can reduce the oxygen available to the brain by about one half. Among the resulting symptoms are dizziness, blurring of consciousness, and possibly because of a decrease in cortical inhibition, tearfulness and emotional instability.

Other effects of breathing pattern disorder that therapists should watch for are generalized body tension and chronic inability to relax. In addition, individuals with breathing pattern disorder are particularly prone to spasm (tetany) in muscles involved in "attack posture"; they hunch their shoulders, thrust the head and neck forward, scowl, and clench their teeth.

(From Fritz S: *Mosby's fundamentals of therapeutic massage*, ed 3. St. Louis, 2004, Mosby.)

fering with sleep and recovery. Because overbreathing perpetuates the fight-or-flight response (sympathetic dominance), any performance or cognitive process requiring controlled and calculated movement and decision making is compromised. Athletes in general may have difficulty managing aggressive behavior. Sympathetic dominance may result in behavior such as a golfer hitting a putt too hard, a football player jumping offside because his timing is off, a quarterback overthrowing to receivers, and a receiver being a little ahead of the football. Baseball pitchers, fielders, and batters are affected when visual perceptions are altered. Basketball players are especially vulnerable, and shooting accuracy is affected by sympathetic dominance and overbreathing.

Assessment for functional breathing problems is very important. If breathing issues are apparent, the athlete should be referred to his or her physician for evaluation to rule out a serious pathology such as asthma, chronic bronchitis, and cardiac and endocrine disorders. Those with cardiac and/or respiratory conditions are prone to breathing dysfunction. In order to recognize and then develop an appropriate treatment plan, a brief overview of breathing functions is presented here, and an assessment and treatment plan is suggested with a basic protocol in Unit Two. It is strongly suggested that the text *Multidisciplinary Approaches to Breathing Pattern Disorders** be obtained and studied thoroughly.

---

*Chaitow L, Bradley D, Gilbert C: *Multidisciplinary approaches to breathing pattern disorders*, Edinburgh, 2002, Churchill Livingstone.

OVERVIEW OF BREATHING FUNCTION

PHASES OF BREATHING

Breathing includes three categories of the phase of inspiration (bringing air into the body) and two categories of the phase of expiration (moving air out of the body).

Quiet inspiration takes place when an individual is resting or sitting quietly. The diaphragm and external intercostals are the prime movers. When *deep inspiration* occurs, the actions of quiet inspiration are intensified. When people need more oxygen, they breathe harder. Any muscles that can pull the ribs up are called into action. *Forced inspiration* occurs when an individual is working very hard and needs a great deal of oxygen, such as during aerobic exercise. Not only are the muscles of quiet and deep inspiration working, but also the muscles that stabilize and/or elevate the shoulder girdle to lift the ribs directly or indirectly.

The expiration phase is divided into two categories—quiet expiration and forced expiration. *Quiet expiration* is mostly passive. It occurs through relaxation of the external intercostals and the elastic recoil of the thoracic wall and tissues of the lungs and bronchi, with gravity pulling the rib cage down from its elevated position. Essentially no muscle action is occurring. *Forced expiration* uses muscles that can pull down the ribs and muscles that can compress the abdomen, forcing the diaphragm upward.

Normal breathing consists of a shorter inhale in relation to a longer exhale. The ratio of inhale to exhale is 1 count inhale and 4 counts exhale. The ideal pattern ranges between 2 to 4 counts for the inhale and 8 to 16 counts for the exhale. Reversal of this pattern, in which the exhale is shorter and the inhale longer, is the basis of breathing pattern dysfunction. Massage methods, along with retraining breathing, can help restore normal function.

Observation indicates whether the client is using accessory muscles to breathe; in this case, the chest movement is concentrated in the upper chest instead of the lower ribs and abdomen. The shoulders should not move up and down during relaxed breathing. The accessory breathing muscles will show increased tension and a tendency toward the development of trigger points if the breathing pattern is dysfunctional. These situations can be identified by palpation. Connective tissue changes are common because breathing dysfunction is often chronic.

Therapeutic massage can normalize many of these conditions and support more effective breathing. It is difficult to breathe well if the mechanical mechanisms are not working efficiently. Many who have attempted breathing retraining have become frustrated by their inability to accomplish the exercises. They may have more success after the soft tissue and mechanisms of breathing are more normal. Specific protocols to assess and address breathing dysfunction are discussed in Unit Three.

THE PHYSICAL FITNESS PROGRAM

Exercise and stretching programs are important parts of any comprehensive fitness program because they provide the activity the body was designed to perform. Exercise has become an essential purpose unto itself. A physical fitness program needs to be appropriate; it is important to modify exercise systems and stretching programs to fit individual needs. Age, maturation, body composition, muscular strength, cardiovascular endurance, state of heat acclimation, nutritional status, and psychological and emotional condition should all be considered when designing programs for different populations.

A physical examination should be conducted before starting an exercise program. The increase in energy requirements during exercise requires circulatory and respiratory adjustments to meet the increased need for oxygen and nutrients; to remove the end products of metabolism, such as carbon dioxide and lactic acid; and to dissipate excess heat. The shift in body metabolism occurs through a coordinated activity of all the systems of the body—neuromuscular, respiratory, cardiovascular, metabolic, and hormonal.

Age is not as much a risk as is straining an unconditioned heart. If a sedentary person's heart is only borderline healthy, a conditioning program could put him or her at risk for a heart attack. Appropriate exercise prescriptions should be developed and monitored by those with specialized training such as exercise physiologists and athletic trainers. The massage therapist does not develop exercise protocols but does need to understand the aspects of an exercise program and to support the process with appropriate massage application.

Often people will overtrain, or attempt to proceed too fast. If this happens, there is an increase risk for fatigue, muscle injury, and stress. It is common for the person to seek massage for these symptoms. However, the problem is more than the massage therapist can handle without additional professional support.

When beginning an exercise program, the client should start slowly and gradually increase the duration of exercise up to 20 minutes or more during each session. The exercise should not be a long, strenuous workout on the very first day. However, many overtrain and find instead of benefits that they are sore and become discouraged.

Overtraining may decrease immune function, which increases susceptibility to colds and infections. Several studies have shown that intense daily training reduces resistance to infectious diseases such as colds and the flu. The massage therapist should be aware that infection is a symptom of overtraining.

Long training sessions can decrease exercise effectiveness. Although exercise is a great way to reduce stress and anxiety and to lift mood, high-intensity training may counteract the pleasurable and mood-normalizing effects. Research has shown that an increased training intensity can create feeling of tenseness, depression, and anger.

Peak athletic performance is achieved from a base of physical fitness. Those who are deconditioned; are rehabilitating from an injury, cardiac event, or stroke; or who have experienced prolonged inactivity have to regain fitness. Whether a person is a competing athlete or is exercising as part of weight reduction program, massage can assist in achieving and maintaining fitness.

All sports differ in the relative importance of the agility, speed, aerobic endurance, anaerobic power and capacity, strength, flexibility, balance, and coordination required to excel. These factors must be taken into account when designing successful strength and conditioning programs for individual athletes. A strength and conditioning program should prioritize the importance of each of these athletic demands.

Training for a particular sport or event is dependent on the **specificity principle.** That is, the individual improves in the exercise task used for training and may not improve in other tasks. For example, swimming may enhance one's performance in swimming events but may not improve one's performance in treadmill running. The athlete should train as if competing in the targeted sport. It is probably detrimental to performance for sprinters and interior linemen to train by running distance miles and lifting light weights for 50 repetitions. Conversely, endurance athletes such as

marathon runners, need to train for sustained activity. Therapeutic massage should address the appropriate recovery period required for each sport.

It is important to consider the body parts of the athlete that are most prone to injury in a particular sport. These body parts need to be strengthened, not only to improve the performance of the muscles used in the sport but also to minimize the risk of injury to these muscles and joints. This is sometimes called *prehabilitation training* and is supported by appropriate sports massage application to prevent injury. The large muscle groups of the back, abdomen, shoulders, and hips, commonly called the *core*, should be included as part of strength-training sessions.

Mature and more experienced athletes can tolerate more intensive strength and conditioning programs. Programs for young and/or inexperienced athletes need to be carefully designed and implemented.

Factors considered in conditioning programs are:

- Strength and endurance required for the particular sport
- Movements required to perform the activity
- The athlete's strength-to-body-weight ratio
- Positional/sport needs
- Training history
- Body composition
- Aerobic and anaerobic fitness
- Injury-prone or previously injured sites that require special attention

If the massage professional is going to effectively support strength and conditioning programs and the performance demands of the athlete, he or she must understand these issues and the roles of the athlete, and the therapeutic exercise that the professional uses.

CONDITIONING

Effective endurance training must produce a conditioning, or cardiovascular, response. **Conditioning** is dependent on three critical elements of exercise: intensity, duration, and frequency.

Exercise is any and all activity involving force generation by activated skeletal muscles. Exercise consists of physical concepts of force, work, power, torque, and energy.

Force changes or tends to change the state of rest or motion in matter or it changes or tends to change the velocity of an object. In sport, the object may be an opposing player or a ball. In rehabilitation programs, the object may be a weight machine. Force may increase or decrease velocity in a moving object, initiate movement in a stationary object, or decrease an object's velocity to zero.

Torque is a force to produce rotation of an object about an axis. Torque is an important concept in understanding all of the body movements because each joint serves as an axis of rotation. (Recall the spiral formation of the body discussion in Chapter 2.) The principal purpose of a muscle is to produce torque about the joint(s) over which it functions. This concept is rather simple when applied to the knee and elbow joints, which perform in similar fashion to a door hinge. Assessment becomes more complicated when analyzing a joint such as the shoulder, which is capable of a variety of movements, or the vertebral column, in which many muscles and numerous adjacent joints are involved.

Energy is needed to produce work or heat. During exercise, all the energy released in the muscle that does not produce work results in heat. The energy of physical exercise can be considered in terms of the potential energy of the biochemical substances utilized for muscular actions (adenosine triphosphate [ATP], carbohydrate, and fat. The actual release of this energy occurs as muscle cells develop force; heat is generated, and the kinetic energy works on the human body or objects used in an exercise routine or in a competitive sport.

THERAPEUTIC EXERCISE

Performing physical work requires cardiorespiratory functioning, muscular strength and endurance, and musculoskeletal flexibility. To become physically fit, individuals must participate regularly in **therapeutic exercise**—that is, some form of physical activity that challenges all large muscle groups and the cardiorespiratory system, and promotes postural balance.

Any exercise and stretching program must begin slowly. Activity levels can be increased gradually each week. It takes about 8 weeks for those who are new to a program to reach a level of comfort. Additional activities may be added gradually once the body adapts.

ENDURANCE

Endurance is the ability to work for prolonged periods of time and to resist fatigue. Stamina is another term used to describe endurance. It includes muscular endurance and cardiovascular endurance. Muscular endurance refers to the ability of an iso-

lated muscle group to perform repeated contractions over a period of time, whereas cardiovascular endurance refers to the ability to perform large-muscle dynamic exercise, such as walking, running, swimming, and biking, for long periods of time.

AEROBIC EXERCISE TRAINING

Aerobic exercise training is an exercise program focused on increasing cardiorespiratory fitness and endurance. Training is dependent on exercise of sufficient intensity, duration, and frequency to produce cardiovascular and muscular adaptation in an individual's endurance. This is different from training for a particular sport or event in which an individual improves in the exercise task used and may not improve in other tasks or whole-body conditioning.

ADAPTATION

Adaptation results in increased efficiency of body function and represents a variety of neurologic, physical, and biochemical changes within the cardiovascular, neuromuscular, and myofascial systems. Athletic performance will increase as a result of these changes and these systems will adapt to the training stimulus over time. Significant changes in fitness can be measured in 10 to 12 weeks.

Adaptation is dependent on:
- The ability of the organism to change
- The training stimulus threshold (the stimulus that elicits a training response)

The person with a low level of fitness will have more potential to improve than the one who has a high level of fitness. However, the adaptive capacity of the former may be strained, so change usually needs to occur gradually.

The higher the initial level of fitness, the greater the intensity of exercise needed to elicit a significant change. Here again, the person with a low level of fitness will have more potential to improve than the one who has high levels of fitness. For example, a person who has not engaged in regular exercise and now is exercising to manage blood pressure will adapt more readily than an active tennis player getting ready for competition.

Regardless, fitness must be achieved before performance. In some instances, an athlete may be overtraining and undermining fitness. An athletic trainer, exercise physiologist, or physical therapist is best qualified to assess what is the appropriate training stimulating threshold. These specialists can also monitor progression in achieving fitness and then indicate when the athlete is ready for performance-based training.

ENERGY USE AND RECOVERY

Individuals engaging in physical activity expend energy. Activities can be categorized as light or heavy by determining the energy cost. Most daily activities are light and are aerobic (oxygen-based) because they require little power but occur over prolonged periods. Heavy work usually requires energy supplied by both the aerobic and anaerobic systems (non–oxygen-based).

Energy systems are metabolic systems involving a series of biochemical reactions resulting in the formation of ATP, carbon dioxide, and water. The cell uses the energy produced from the conversion of ATP to adenosine diphosphate (ADP) and phosphate to perform metabolic activities. Muscle cells use this energy for actin-myosin cross-bridge formation when contracting.

During fitness and performance training, three major energy systems are activated. These are the phosphagen system, the aerobic (oxygen) system, and the "in-between" system (anaerobic glycolytic system). The intensity and duration of activity determine when and to what extent each metabolic system contributes.

The body functions somewhat like an internal combustion engine. It burns fuel (nutrients) and oxygen for energy just as a car engine burns gasoline mixed with oxygen and gives off heat as it burns energy. Temperature rises during exercise and waste products are produced as the body uses energy.

The body utilizes carbohydrates in the diet as its energy source. It converts complex carbohydrates and sugars in the diet to a fuel substance called glycogen. Glycogen is found in large amounts in the liver as well as in muscle cells. The glycogen in muscles combines with oxygen, brought in by the circulating blood from the lungs, and releases energy; this is known as the *aerobic energy cycle*. The waste products are carbon dioxide and water.

Once the muscle glycogen is exhausted from prolonged exercise, reserve glycogen is released from the liver and carried to muscle cells so that they can continue working. This glycogen release continues until the body's supply of glycogen is totally depleted. At this point, if demand continues, the body changes fuels and begins to burn fat instead of glycogen. This is a whole new energy cycle, called the *anaerobic energy cycle*. The waste product produced is lactic acid.

The body can easily rid itself of carbon dioxide and water, but it has difficulty getting rid of lactic acid. As exercise continues, lactic acid begins to build up in the muscles, causing fatigue. This buildup of lactic acid is what causes the burning pain in exhausted muscles. When exercise ends, the lactic acid is dissipated.

THE PHOSPHAGEN SYSTEM

The **phosphagen system** supplies energy for brief, high-power events such as the sprints, jumps, vaults, and throws in track and field; batting, base-running, and fielding in baseball; power lifting and Olympic weight lifting; and much of the blocking and tackling done by linemen in football. Each of these activities lasts only a few seconds, and the energy is provided mostly by the breakdown of phosphocreatine stored in the muscles. Oxygen is not required during the exertion, so the energy is supplied anaerobically.

If the athlete is using mostly the phosphagen system, the focus of strength and conditioning is brief, near-maximal exertion. Massage targets breathing and fluid movement and parasympathetic dominance to support recovery.

THE AEROBIC (OXYGEN) SYSTEM

The **aerobic (oxygen) system** provides most of the energy for activities that last longer than a couple of minutes and for recovery between repeats of brief, high-intensity activities. Daily life activities are aerobic. Other than sprints at the beginning and end of the race, distance runners and swimmers and road cyclists rely almost entirely on aerobic metabolism.

The aerobic system has the following characteristics:

- Glycogen, fats, and proteins are fuel sources.
- Oxygen is required.
- ATP is resynthesized in the mitochondria of the muscle cell. The ability to metabolize oxygen and other substrates is related to the number and concentration of the mitochondria and cells.
- The system predominates over the other energy systems after the second minute of exercise.

Aerobic activity focuses on the cardiovascular system and the aerobic capacity of the muscles to perform longer-duration activities that require less than maximal intensities of exertion. In the weight room, focus should be on lifting relatively light weights and more repetitions. This is the type of fitness program used for cardiorespiratory rehabilitation and weight management. Again, massage should support recovery. The focus of massage would include parasympathetic dominance and arterial circulation.

ANAEROBIC GLYCOGEN BREAKDOWN: THE "IN-BETWEEN" SYSTEM

For activities that last longer than about 10 seconds but less than 2 minutes, the majority of the energy is supplied by the anaerobic breakdown of glycogen (a carbohydrate) stored in the muscles. This is sometimes called the "lactic acid" system or the **anaerobic glycolytic system.** Events such as a 400-meter run in track, a 50-meter swim, a series of fast breaks in basketball, or a series of sprints down the soccer or football field would require energy from this system. Strength and conditioning activities would be intermediate between those recommended for the phosphagen system and those for the aerobic system.

The anaerobic glycolytic system has the following characteristics:

- Glycogen (glucose) is the fuel source.
- No oxygen is required.
- ATP is resynthesized in the muscle cell.
- Lactic acid is produced.
- The systems provide energy for activity of moderate intensity and short duration.
- It is the major source of energy from the 30th to 90th second of exercise.

In sports such as soccer, basketball, wrestling, lacrosse, rugby, tennis, ice hockey, field hockey, and rollerblading, and during daily life activities, people use both anaerobic and aerobic metabolism to produce energy. This means that the optimal training for fitness should include a combination of brief, high-intensity activities along with more prolonged, lesser-intensity exertion.

To improve fitness, it is important to increase the supply of oxygen to the muscles and prevent the exhaustion of glycogen reserves.

Recruitment of muscle motor units is dependent on the rate of work. Fibers are recruited selectively during exercise. Slow-twitch fibers (type I) are characterized by a slow contractile response, are rich in myoglobin and mitochondria, have a high oxidative capacity and a low anaerobic capacity, and are recruited for activities demanding endurance. These fibers are supplied by small neurons with a low threshold of activation and are used preferentially in low-intensity exercise.

Fast-twitch fibers (type IIb) are characterized by a fast contractile response, have a low myoglobin content and few mitochondria, have a high glocolytic capacity, and are recruited for activities requiring power.

Fast-twitch fibers (type IIa) have characteristics of both type I and type IIb fibers and are recruited for both anaerobic and aerobic activities.

FUNCTIONAL IMPLICATIONS

Bursts of intense activity lasting up to 50 seconds develop muscle strength and stronger tendons and ligaments. ATP is supplied by the phosphagen system.

Intense activity for 1 to 2 minutes, repeated after 4 minutes of rest or mild exercise, provides anaerobic power. ATP is supplied by the phosphagen and anaerobic glycolytic system.

Activity using the large muscles at less than maximal intensity for 3 to 5 minutes, repeated after rest or mild exercise of similar duration, may develop aerobic power and endurance capabilities. ATP is supplied by the phosphagen, anaerobic glycolytic, and aerobic systems.

Activity of submaximal intensity, lasting 30 minutes or more, taxes a high percentage of the aerobic system and develops endurance.

An understanding of the metabolic demands imposed by the sport and the biomechanics of every task executed by the athlete is necessary. A particular sport does not usually fall cleanly into one energy-system category or another but rather involves all three (phosphagen system, glycolytic system, oxidative system) to a greater or lesser extent. In soccer, for example, all three energy systems are used. Soccer players must explode to the ball or to mark an opposing player or go up high for a header, but they also must cover a total distance of approximately six miles by the end of the game, with rest periods of about 3 seconds every 2 minutes of play.

The energy system that is primarily used will determine the optimal types of conditioning and strength training for the sport. For example, jumpers and vaulters don't need to spend a lot of time running distances of over 400 meters or doing multiple sets in the weight room of 12 and 15 repetitions. The combinations of sets and repetitions used in strength training should be consistent with the energy requirements and movement patterns of the sport or desired activity, dictating that a strength and conditioning program for an offensive tackle in football, a shortstop in baseball, and an elderly woman struggling with daily care activities are very different. For the offensive tackle, conditioning should develop strength, muscle mass, power, quickness, three-step speed, and anaerobic conditioning capacity. For the baseball shortstop, strength and muscle mass are not so critical. His or her training should improve speed, explosive power and quickness, and the ability to change movement direction instantly. The elderly woman needs balance and leg strength to prevent falling.

The physical therapist or strength and conditioning and positional coaches make the decisions regarding the appropriate type of training and implement these programs. The athlete's training history is crucial. An individual who has never followed any kind of strength and conditioning program must be brought along much more slowly and carefully than an athlete with advanced training experience. Each athlete is unique; therefore, performance segments need to be individually developed. Massage can support the athlete by managing any discomfort that accompanies an exercise training program.

PHYSIOLOGIC CHANGES THAT OCCUR WITH EXERCISE

The cardiovascular system and the muscles used will adapt to the training stimulus over time. Significant changes can be measured in a minimum of 10 to 12 weeks. Adaptation results in increased efficiency of the cardiovascular system and the active muscles. Adaptation represents a variety of neurologic, physical, and biochemical changes within the cardiovascular and muscular systems. Performance increases as a result of these changes.

Changes in the cardiovascular and respiratory systems as well as changes in muscle metabolism occur with exercise. These changes happen at rest and during exercise. It is important to note that all of the following training effects cannot result from one training program. A regular ongoing process of exercise with a variety of activities is necessary to achieve and maintain fitness.

CARDIOVASCULAR RESPONSE TO EXERCISE

Stimulation of small myelinated and unmyelinated fibers in skeletal muscle involves a sympathetic nervous system response. The sympathetic nervous system response includes generalized peripheral vasoconstriction and increased myocardial con-

tractility, increased heart rate, and hypertension. This results in a marked increase and redistribution of cardiac output.

Frequency of sinoatrial node depolarization increases and heart rate increases; there is a decrease in vagal stimuli as well as an increase in sympathetic stimulation. Generalized vasoconstriction occurs that allows blood to be shunted from the nonworking muscles, kidneys, liver, and spleen to the working muscles. The veins of the working as well as the nonworking muscles remain constricted.

Cardiac output increases because of the increase in myocardial contractility, heart rate, and blood flow through the working muscle.

A change at rest involves a reduction in the resting pulse rate with a decrease in sympathetic dominance and lower levels of norepinephrine and epinephrine. There is an increase in parasympathetic restoration mechanisms. A decrease in blood pressure can occur. There is often an increase in blood volume and hemoglobin, which facilitates the oxygen delivery capacity of the system.

During exercise there is a reduction in the pulse rate and decrease of norepinephrine and epinephrine. There is an increase in cardiac function and an increased extraction of oxygen by the working muscle.

RESPIRATORY RESPONSE TO EXERCISE

Respiratory changes occur rapidly, with an increase in gas exchange by the first or second breath, an increase in body temperature, increased epinephrine levels, and increased stimulation of receptors of the joints and muscles. Baroreceptor reflexes, protective reflexes, pain, emotion, and voluntary control of respiration may also contribute to the increase in respiration.

Alveolar ventilation, occurring with the diffusion of gases across the capillary alveolar membrane, increases 10-fold to 20-fold in heavy exercise to supply the additional oxygen needed and excrete the excess carbon dioxide produced.

The increased blood flow to the working muscle previously discussed provides additional oxygen. There is also extraction of more oxygen from each liter of blood.

Changes that happen at rest include larger lung volumes because of improved pulmonary function. Changes with exercise occur because of a larger diffusion capacity in the lungs because of the larger lung volumes and greater alveolar-capillary surface area. Breathing is deeper and more efficient.

METABOLIC CHANGES

Muscle hypertrophy and increased capillary density are observed at rest and with exercise following endurance training. There is a noticeable increase in the number and size of mitochondria, which increases the capacity to generate ATP aerobically.

There is a decreased rate of depletion of muscle glycogen and lower blood lactate levels at submaximal work levels as the result of an increased capacity to mobilize and oxidize.

OTHER SYSTEM CHANGES

Changes in other systems that occur with exercise training include:

- A decrease in body fat, blood cholesterol, and triglyceride levels and an increase in heat acclimatization
- An increase in breaking strength of bones, ligaments, and tendons

CORE STRENGTH

All people need **core strength,** or core stabilization training to achieve physical fitness. The athlete's success is related to how strong and flexible his or her muscles are in the midsection. Core strengthening should be an essential part of all fitness programs. The trunk is the platform around which all multijoint and multiplanar motions occur. Exercising with a weak or dynamically unstable core is like running on a surface covered with marbles. Being out of control or off balance in the trunk increases the need for compensatory strained motions in adjacent joints. Recent evidence suggests that female athletes with a weak core are more likely to sustain tears of the anterior cruciate ligaments. Lack of core strength is a cause of falls leading to injury in the elderly.

A strength-training program cannot be effective without training core muscles in the body. The body is an integrated system, not just an accumulation of parts and pieces that can be individually sport-trained.

CORE TRAINING

Core training is essential for fitness and performance. **Core training** is an attempt to centralize the strength, flexibility, coordination, and power of the body into the most powerful region of the body, the hips and torso. The intent is to strengthen the muscle groups that stabilize the skeletal structure. These are primarily the muscles in the thoracic area that determine posture and link the upper and lower body. The muscle groups that are strengthened with core training generally do not have the range of motion needed for movement, but they are the stable "platform" from which the arms and legs work.

When the abdominal muscles work in isolation, they bend the spine forward and flex it or twist it to one side, but when they work in conjunction with the powerful hips and extensor muscles of the back, they create spine stability. When the muscles of the hips and trunk work together, they form a functionally stabilizing unit.

Core training is not about strength. Rather, it is about stability, stamina, and coordination. Strength is the ability to produce force, whereas stability is the act of controlling force. This is an extremely important distinction. The word *core* represents the central part of the body, the torso and hips. The core is the powerhouse of the body. Even though the abdominal muscles are an important part of the core, core training is not about abdominal conditioning. The abdominals should never be totally isolated in training because they are never totally isolated in movement. Abdominal muscles work in coordination with the adductor and hip muscles during activity.

The center of mass is the midsection and is the point of stability. When the midsection is off balance, the body is off balance. If this area is strong and stable, the body has a platform from which to generate coordinated activity.

If mobility and stability are inadequate, then the core will compensate in some way. The core functions through reflex reactions based on movement, balance, and task. These reflexes cannot function normally if the core must compensate for hip tightness, poor abdominal strength, poor balance when standing on one foot, or tightness with torso rotation.

Examples of core training are basic yoga and the mat work developed by Joseph Pilates. These are basic, no-nonsense approaches that demand more strength from the core than from the extremities if done correctly. Many athletes are able to move large amounts of weight in relationship to their body weight but have a very hard time getting through some of the basic core movements of yoga or Pilates. It may appear that this happens because of a lack of flexibility, but actually core stability is the determining factor. These people are not weak, and they have been successful in the weight room, but they are unsuccessful in balancing the body by developing the core. The strength of the extremities is not supposed to exceed the strength of the core. The core is the foundation of power and strength.

Almost every movement in sports requires a transfer of energy—from arm to arm, from arm to leg, from leg to arm, or from leg to leg—and the core is the common denominator. Core training should lay the foundation for strength, power, speed, and agility training. The core balances the network of forces acting on the body and redistributes those forces appropriately. The core attempts to compensate for differences between right and left shoulder flexibility, right and left hip flexibility, and poor flexibility in the spine. Without proper flexibility, the core ends up absorbing some of those forces. This can cause injury and loss of power. Serious athletes cannot afford either.

The definition of stability is the ability to control movement and force, not the production of movement or the generation of force. Therefore the best core training programs require the spine to be held in a natural or neutral position while breathing and while moving the arms and legs in motions that mimic the functional ways in which the core will be a stressed in a given sport or activity.

Core training targets individual muscles and small groups of muscles. This awareness of specific muscles or muscle groups is the first step in improving various posture and form issues. Massage supports core training by reducing tension in muscles that may be sending reciprocal inhibition signals to the core muscles. Massage that lengthens the short muscles reduces inhibition signals, allowing exercise to be effective.

Core training focuses on muscular areas of the abdominals including obliques and transverse abdominals, upper and lower back muscles, hips (gluteals, hip flexors, psoas), outer and inner thighs (abductors and adductors), hamstrings, and even pectoralis and triceps.

The athlete is actually only as strong as the weakest muscular link. For example, the quads of a bodybuilder must have strength in the upper body to control the force the quads can develop.

When a person is riding a bike, gravity dictates that all downward force generated at maximum output is limited to the person's body weight and the opposing force of pulling up by the opposite crank arm. An additional downward force can be created by pulling up on the handlebars, thus opposing the tendency for the body to rise as the legs push down on the pedals with the quads. Because the legs are attached at the hips, and not at the arms, the stable platform the arms create must be extended to the hips and legs through a stable torso.

Similar dynamic examples apply to running and swimming. Having a strong torso helps hold the form together in the latter stages of an endurance effort when fatigue occurs.

One misconception about core stability concerns the activity of the rectus abdominis. Because it is not a major core muscle, if it is or was dominant it can inhibit the obliques and transversus abdominis, setting up a chain of events as follows:

Rectus abdominis is dominant, which results in inhibition of abdominal obliques and transversus abdominis;
Psoas shortens and inhibits gluteus maximus;
Hamstring and lumbar muscles must dominate in hip extension—hamstrings shorten and become injury prone;
Calf muscles, particularly gastrocnemius, shorten;
Tension increases in Achilles tendon and plantar fascia.

This is a fairly consistent pattern. The massage professional can support core training effectiveness by using massage to inhibit inappropriate muscle dominance patterns and by assessing and treating muscle activation firing pattern sequences.

A short sequence of core movements is shown in Figure 5–1. These can all be done without any special equipment; only a floor with a little padding is needed. The ball is a beneficial additional to core training.

Also recommended is the draw-in maneuver in which the abdomen is "hollowed" by drawing the obliques toward the lumbar area.

EXERCISE INTENSITY

Exercise intensity is based on the **overload principle,** which is stress on an organism that is greater than that regularly encountered during everyday life. To improve cardiovascular and muscular endurance, an overload must be applied to these systems. For adaptation to occur, the exercise intensity load must be just above the training stimulus threshold. Once adaptation to a given load has

FIGURE 5-1

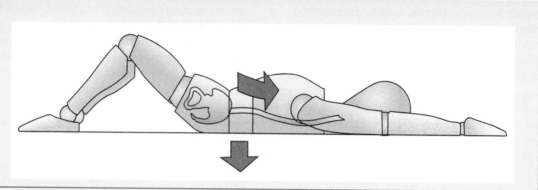

A Draw-in maneuver.

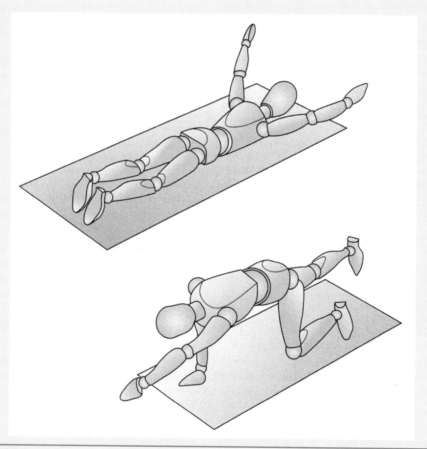

B Prone core exercises.

FIGURE 5-1, CONT'D

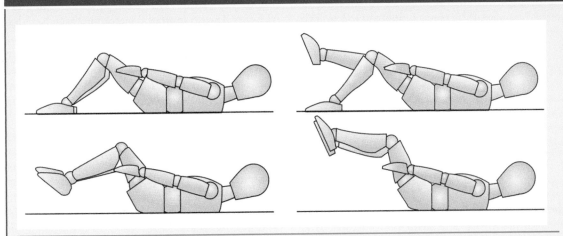

C Supine core exercises.

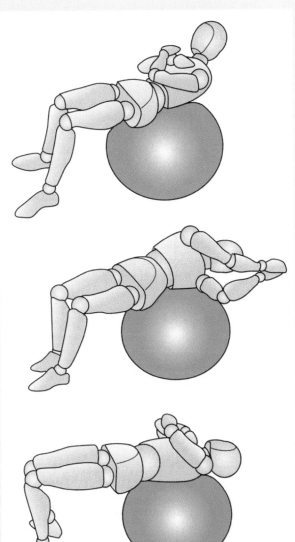

D Ball curl exercises. (From Fritz S: *Mosby's fundamentals of therapeutic massage,* ed. 3. St. Louis, 2004, Mosby.)

taken place, for the individual to achieve further improvement the training intensity (exercise load) must be increased. Increasing intensity too quickly can result in injury. Training stimulus thresholds are variable, depending on the individual's level of health, level of activity, age, and gender.

Appropriate intensity during exercise does result in conditions that may be uncomfortable for the average person. Delayed onset muscle soreness, general stiffness, and mild fatigue are common and expected. Massage can be used to minimize the discomfort and therefore supports training.

DURATION

The optimal **duration** of exercise for cardiovascular conditioning is dependent on the total work done, exercise intensity and frequency, and fitness level. Generally speaking, the greater the intensity of the exercise, the shorter the duration needed for adaptation; the lower the intensity of exercise, the longer the duration needed. A 20- to 30-minute session is generally optimal at 70% of maximum heart rate. When the intensity is below the heart rate threshold, a 45-minute continuous exercise period may provide the appropriate overload. With high-intensity exercise, 10- to 15-minute exercise periods are adequate. Three 5-minute daily periods may be effective in someone who is deconditioned. Exercise for periods longer than 45 minutes increases the risk of musculoskeletal injury and soreness. If the duration must exceed 45 minutes, massage can minimize the discomfort at least temporarily through symptom management of pain, aching, and stiffness.

FREQUENCY

Optimal **frequency** of fitness training is generally three to four times a week. Frequency varies, dependent on the health and age of the person. If training is at a low intensity, greater frequency may be beneficial. A frequency of two times a week does not generally evoke cardiovascular changes, although individuals who are deconditioned may initially benefit from a program of that frequency. For those who are in good general health, exercising 30 to 45 minutes at least three times a week appears to protect against coronary heart disease. As frequency increases beyond the optimal range, the risk of musculoskeletal injury and soreness increases. This may occur during initial stages of rehabilitation protocols. The competing athlete will often exercise and train every day, which actually works contrary to achieving fitness and increases injury potential.

Many types of activities provide the stimulus for improving cardiovascular and cardiorespiratory fitness. The important factor is exercise that involves large muscle groups that are activated in a rhythmic, aerobic way. For specific aerobic activities such as cycling and running, the overload must use the muscles required by the activity as well as stress the cardiorespiratory system (specificity principle). If endurance of the upper extremities is needed to perform activities, then the upper extremity muscles must be targeted in the exercise program. The muscles trained develop a greater oxidative capacity, with an increase in blood flow to the area. The increase in blood flow is due to increased microcirculation and more effective distribution of the cardiac output. Training benefits are optimized when programs are planned to meet the individual needs and capacities of the participants. The skill of the individual, variations among individuals in competitiveness and aggressiveness, and variation in environmental conditions all must be considered.

MAINTAINING FITNESS

The frequency or duration of physical activity required to maintain a certain level of aerobic fitness is less than that required to improve it. The beneficial effects of exercise training are reversible. The process of deconditioning occurs rapidly when a person stops exercising. After only 2 weeks of reduced activity, significant reductions in work capacity can be measured, and improvements can be lost within several months. A progressive reconditioning program is required. This is the task of the strength and conditioning coach.

THE EXERCISE PROGRAM

There are three components of the exercise program: (1) warm-up, (2) aerobic exercise, and (3) cool-down. Performance training for athletes can occur as part of the aerobic portion of the program or directly following it.

WARM-UP

The purpose of the **warm-up** period is to enhance the numerous physiologic adjustments that must take place before physical activity. Physiologically, a time lag exists between the onset of activity and the need for bodily adjustments to meet the physical requirements of the body.

Warm-up results in an increase in muscle temperature. The higher temperature increases the efficiency of muscular contraction by reducing connective tissue viscosity and increasing the rate of nerve conduction.

Warm-up literally means warming up muscle fibers by increasing the body temperature. When breaking into a sweat, body temperature elevates by about 2°F, which is appropriate for warming. This leads to a wide variety of beneficial physiologic changes:

- The warmer muscle fibers get, the softer and more fluid they become. They are then able to stretch more easily and to contract more rapidly. The faster a muscle contracts, the stronger it is.
- The higher the temperature of muscle cells, the faster they are able to metabolize the oxygen and fuel they need.
- As muscles warm, the response to nerve impulses quickens, causing faster contraction and, therefore, a quicker response.
- Warming joints lubricates them, allowing them to move more freely with less energy expended. This protects the joints from excessive wear.
- Warm-up gradually increases the heart rate and prevents abnormal heart rhythms. Sudden strenuous exercise can cause the heart to demand more oxygen than the circulatory system can provide, resulting in a strain on the heart. Studies show that warming up may help prevent the heart attacks that result from abnormal heart rhythms.
- Oxygen extraction from hemoglobin is greater at higher muscle temperatures, supporting the aerobic process. Dilation of constricted capillaries, which increases the circulation, increases oxygen delivery to the active muscles and minimizes oxygen deficit and formation of lactic acid. An increase in venous return occurs. Adaptation in sensitivity of the neural respiratory center increases respiratory rate.

Warm-up activities include rhythmic movement of the large muscles of the body and should be related to the sport performance requirements. Regardless of whether a person is engaging in fitness or wishes to increase or maintain athletic performance, the warm-up period is critical for preventing injury and supporting training per performance during competition.

Massage as Part of Warm-Up

Massage before a workout can make athletes feel weak and unmotivated. They may not even want to do their workout after the session, so be cautious. Work to increase flexibility and range of motion. Shaking, rolling tissue gently, and muscle energy techniques can be appropriate. Duration time is short, about 15 to 20 minutes.

AEROBIC EXERCISE

The **aerobic exercise** period is the conditioning part of the exercise program. Attention to the intensity, frequency, and duration will have an impact on the program's effectiveness. The main considerations when choosing a specific method of training is that the method:

- Stimulates increased cardiac output.
- Enhances local circulation.
- Increases aerobic metabolism within the appropriate muscle groups.
- Does not cause injury.
- Is weight-bearing, to support bone health.
- Is above the threshold level for adaptation to occur.
- Is below the level of exercise that evokes fatigue symptoms.

In aerobic exercise, submaximal, rhythmic, repetitive, dynamic exercise of large muscle groups is emphasized. There are four methods of training that will condition the aerobic system: continuous, interval, circuit, and circuit-interval.

CONTINUOUS TRAINING

Continuous training involves a submaximal energy requirement sustained throughout the exercise period. Once the steady state is achieved, the muscle obtains energy by means of aerobic metabolism. Stress is placed primarily on the slow-twitch muscle fibers. The activity can be prolonged for 20 to 60 minutes without exhausting the oxygen transport system. Work rate is increased progressively as training improvements are achieved. Overload can be accomplished by increasing the exercise duration. In the healthy individual, continuous training is the most effective way to improve endurance. Brisk walking is an excellent example of continuous training.

INTERVAL TRAINING

In this type of exercise program, the exercise period is interspersed with a relief interval. **Interval training** is generally less demanding than continuous training. In the healthy individual, interval training tends to improve strength and power more than endurance. The relief interval is either a rest relief (passive recovery) or a work relief (active recovery), and its duration ranges from a few seconds to several minutes. Work recovery involves continuing the exercise, but at a reduced level from that of the work period. During the relief period, a portion of the muscular stores of ATP and the oxygen associated with myoglobin that were depleted during the work period are replenished by the aerobic system.

The longer and more intense the work interval, the more the aerobic system is stressed. With a short work interval, the duration of the rest interval is critical if the aerobic system is to be stressed. A rest interval equal to one and a half times the work interval allows the succeeding exercise interval to begin before recovery is complete and stresses the aerobic system.

A significant amount of high-intensity exercise can be achieved with interval or intermittent work if there is appropriate spacing of the work-relief intervals. Examples are lap swimming with rest periods and race walking or sprinting short distances with periods of slower walking interspersed.

CIRCUIT TRAINING

Circuit training employs a series of exercise activities. At the end of the last activity, the individual starts again from the beginning and moves through the circuit. The series of activities is repeated several times. Several exercise modes can be used involving large and small muscle groups and a mix of static or dynamic effort.

Use of circuit training can improve strength and endurance by stressing both the aerobic and anaerobic systems. Often a combination of aerobic activities and weight training is included in the exercise program. Core training that strengthens the postural muscles of the torso can be included in circuit training. Activities using various sizes of exercise balls promote postural balance and core strength.

CIRCUIT-INTERVAL TRAINING

Circuit-interval training, in which the two types are combined, is effective because of the interaction of aerobic and anaerobic production of ATP. In addition to the aerobic and anaerobic systems being stressed by the various activities, with the relief interval there is a delay in the need for anaerobic processes and the production of lactic acid, because the rest period allows blood oxygen levels to be replenished.

Head Massage as Part of Aerobic Training

Massage may be used during aerobic training in targeted areas that interfere with the ability to exercise. Examples are localized muscle cramp and isolated muscle tension.

COOL-DOWN

A **cool-down** period is necessary following the aerobic exercise and performance-training period. The cool-down period prevents pooling of blood in the extremities by continuing to use the muscles to maintain venous return. It enhances the recovery period with the oxidation of metabolic waste and replacement of energy stores and prevents myocardial ischemia, arrhythmias, and other cardiovascular conditions.

Characteristics of the cool-down period are similar to those of the warm-up period. A total-body exercise such as calisthenics or brisk walking that decreases in intensity is appropriate. The cool-down period should last for 5 to 10 minutes. Flexibility programs are used after the cool-down period. Cool-down massage is used after the cool-down and can be part of a flexibility program if stretching is included in the massage.

STRENGTH TRAINING

Strength training involves muscle contraction against resistance. There are many forms of strength training: weight machines, free weights, and resistance bands. To prevent injury, it is important to be properly trained in whatever strength program is used.

Most sports require overall strength training, but exercise programs should be adjusted to meet the specific requirements of a given sport. In football, linebackers and defensive backs make most of the tackles and need to improve upper-body as well as lower-body strength. Running backs and wide receivers should concentrate on lower-body strength training to develop their legs.

Similarly, runners, dancers, and soccer players need lower-body strength; baseball players, golfers, swimmers, and gymnasts need to work more on upper-body strength; and basketball players and wrestlers need both upper- and lower-body strength.

Tennis players require lower-body strength to develop their legs but also need to pay particular attention to upper-body strength. Strengthening the shoulder helps prevent rotator cuff injuries. If tennis players would strengthen their forearm and wrist muscles, they wouldn't be as prone to tennis elbow.

Typically, strength training programs target different muscles on different days, and intersperse light and heavy repetitions. For example, follow a light "Day 1" program on Monday and a light "Day 2" program on Tuesday; rest on Wednesday; on Thursday and Friday, alternate heavy programs.

STRENGTH TRAINING INFLUENCES ON CHILDREN

Traditionally, sports experts thought that strength training by children didn't accomplish anything. Both boys and girls supposedly lacked the boost of testosterone in their blood needed to add muscle bulk. It was believed that until a child had gone through puberty and developed secondary sexual characteristics, there was no point in strength training. Strength training was also thought to put undue stress on the growth plate in a young child's bones and stunt the child's growth. By speeding up maturation, strength training theoretically would prevent the bones from growing to their full, natural length.

It is now known that preteens, even though they lack the testosterone necessary to increase muscle bulk, can increase their strength without injuring themselves. A major study by the Sports Medicine section of the American Academy of Orthopedic Surgeons proved that strength training does not injure the growth plate or stunt a child's growth. The American Academy of Pediatrics now agrees that children as young as 11 years of age can begin a well-supervised weight-training program.

Unfortunately, all too frequently 6- and 7-year-olds are being pushed into weight training by their overeager parents. Young children typically lack sufficient concentration and regimentation for weight training to be beneficial. They often do themselves harm because they don't have the coordination to handle weights and are not mature enough to understand what they are doing or why. Any child interested in strength training needs to be closely supervised.

Starting around age 12, a child can begin lifting light weights with many repetitions in order to learn the proper techniques. More weight can be added as the child gets stronger and grows. With an adequately supervised program, there is room for great improvement in a child's strength without the threat of injury.

STRENGTH TRAINING FOR WOMEN

Strength training is essential for women. The big difference between a man's and a woman's strength is in the upper body. In fact, a woman's lower-body strength is pound-for-pound about the same as a man's. Women runners know that the longer the distance to be covered, the more closely they can compete with men because they don't have to propel as much weight.

MASSAGE AS PART OF STRENGTH TRAINING

Strength training involves both concentric and eccentric movement, increasing the potential for delayed onset muscle soreness. Lymph drain-type massage is helpful. Do not use deep compression after strength training. The tissues are taut from increased blood and lymph in the areas. This is a fluid issue, not a tensor issue. Deep compression can damage fluid-filled tissue.

FLEXIBILITY TRAINING

Flexibility is the ability to move a single joint or a series of joints through a normal, unrestricted, pain-free range of motion. It is dependent upon the extensibility of muscle, which allows muscles that cross a joint to relax, lengthen, and yield to a stretch force. The arthrokinematics of the moving joint as well as the ability of connective tissues associated with the joint to deform also affect joint range of motion (ROM), and an individual's overall flexibility.

Dynamic flexibility refers to the active ROM of a joint. This aspect of flexibility is dependent on the degree to which a joint can be moved by a muscle contraction and the amount of tissue resistance met during the active movement. *Passive flexibility* is the degree to which a joint can be passively moved through the available ROM and is dependent upon the extensibility of muscles and connective tissues that cross and surround a joint. Passive flexibility is a prerequisite for, but does not ensure, dynamic flexibility.

Muscle tissue and fascial shortening causes a change in the length-tension relationship of the muscle. As the muscle shortens, it is no longer able to produce peak tension. The result is a muscle that is weak but short and tight. Loss of flexibility, for whatever reason, can cause pain arising from muscle, connective tissue, or the periosteum. This in turn decreases muscle strength.

Flexibility is the ability to elongate a muscle, as when the hamstrings are stretched during a forward bend; however, mobility is a broader concept. Mobility involves the muscle and joint freedom of movement. A good example of mobility is the ability to keep the heels flat while squatting past the point where the thighs are parallel to the floor. Note that a squat involves multiple joints and muscles. Strength can be defined as the ability to produce force or movement; stability is the ability to control force or movement. In most cases, stability is a precursor to strength. When stability and strength are functioning, then mobility is possible.

STRETCHING

Stretching is a general term that describes any therapeutic modality designed to lengthen (elongate) pathologically shortened soft tissue, particularly connective tissue structures, to increase range of motion. The end result is increased flexibility.

The main components of a flexibility program include a controlled sustained load on the muscles and connective tissue components without straining the joint structure. Many types of flexibility programs exist. Yoga is an excellent example of a flexibility program.

When a muscle is passively stretched, initial lengthening occurs in the neuromuscular component and tension in the muscle rises sharply. After a point, there is a mechanical disruption of the cross-bridges of actin and myosin as the filaments slide apart, and an abrupt lengthening of the sarcomeres occurs (called sarcomere give). Various applications of muscle energy methods support this process. When the stretch force is released, the individual sacromeres return to their resting length instead of the shortened position. The tendency of muscle to return to its resting length after short-term stretch is called *elasticity*.

Stretching specifically targets the connective tissue structures. The increase in connective tissue's pliability and length is called *plasticity*.

To get the most from stretching, a customized routine to fit the needs of the individual is most effective. For example, in one routine, you stretch until feeling a slight pull without pain. As the stretch is held, the muscle will relax. As less tension is felt, increase the stretch again until the same slight pull is felt. This position should be held until no further increase is felt. If range of motion is not gained using this technique, consider holding the stretch longer (up to 60 seconds).

Bouncing while stretching, or ballistic stretching, can do more damage than no stretching at all. With each bounce, muscle fibers fire and shorten the muscle—the opposite of what the activity is trying to accomplish. Bouncing actually reduces flexibility. A static stretch—holding the muscle still for 10 to 20 seconds—is much better. The muscle responds by lengthening slowly. Each stretch should be gradual and gentle.

Stretching is enhanced by incorporating various muscle energy methods and increasing the muscle's tolerance to stretching.

Studies indicate that continuous stretching without rest may be better than cyclic stretching (applying a stretch, relaxing, and reapplying the stretch); however some research shows no difference. Massage is effective in normalizing muscle tone and motion. It is also effective in assisting the athlete to achieve and maintain flexibility.

In addition to improving range of motion, stretching is extremely relaxing, and most athletes use stretching exercises to maintain a balance in body mechanics. One of the biggest benefits of stretching may be something that research cannot quantify: it just feels good. Whether the massage therapist stretches the client or the trainer or physical therapist does, the focus of stretching depends on the individual's athletic activities to lengthen shortened tissues. Massage is an excellent way to support flexibility programs especially if the methods used address both the elasticity and plasticity of the soft tissue.

SUMMARY

This chapter presents information about physical fitness and conditioning programs. Therapeutic exercise provides benefit. The exercise program needs to be individually designed for each client. Depending on the client's physical condition, variables that are considered for each fitness program include intensity, duration, frequency, and type of activity. These variables target both anaerobic and aerobic energy systems.

The three main parts of a therapeutic exercise program are warm-up, aerobic activity, and cooldown. Strength training, especially core strength training, is important. Flexibility rounds out the fitness program. Massage support is appropriate during all aspects of a fitness program.

1 Design an exercise program for the following people:

A. A 19-year-old male in a weight management program.

_____

_____

_____

_____

_____

B. A 28-year-old female training for a marathon.

_____

_____

_____

_____

C. A 49-year-old female wishing to increase fitness and management of age-related changes.

_____

_____

_____

_____

D. A 71-year-old male for cardiovascular fitness.

_____

_____

_____

_____

E. Yourself.

_____

_____

_____

_____

_____

2 Describe massage support for each one of the exercise programs developed above.

A.

_____

_____

_____

B.

_____

_____

_____

C.

_____

_____

_____

D.

_____

_____

_____

E.

_____

_____

_____

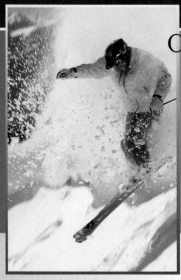

6

SPORT-SPECIFIC MOVEMENT

OBJECTIVES

Upon completion of this chapter the reader will have the information necessary to:

1 Identify elements that influence performance skill.
2 Describe the importance of coordinated movement strategies.
3 Describe the movement strategies of:

catching	running
cutting	swinging
hitting	throwing
jumping	turning
kicking	walking
pivoting	

4 Compare and contrast acceleration and deceleration.
5 Explain why massage application is movement-generated rather than sport-generated.

Each sports activity consists of a combination of functional movements. Because therapeutic massage is targeted to support effective functional movement, in general it is more important for the massage therapist to understand the movements required to accomplish a task, as opposed to the movements required for proficiency in a specific sport. Assessment can then be focused on the combination of movements that constitutes a sport-specific or activity-specific pattern. It is the role of the performance coach to develop sport-specific skills in the athlete or performer and of the physical therapist or similar professional to target skill achievement in those in rehabilitation. It is the responsibility of the massage therapist to identify the demands of the client's activities and the sequence of the movements required for performance, and then to

Catching
Cutting
Functional movement development
Gait cycle
Hitting
Jumping

Kicking
Movement strategies
Pivoting
Reaction time
Rotation
Running

Swinging
Throwing
Turning
Walking

apply appropriate massage treatment both to support performance and to correct dysfunction.

As discussed in the previous chapter, mobility and stability must coexist to create efficient movement in the human body. If a movement problem exists because of reduced mobility (soft tissue shortening or joint stiffness) or reduced ability (poor strength, coordination, control, or deconditioning), then the movement pattern is altered to compensate.

Mobility and stability are the functional building blocks of strength, endurance, speed, power, and agility. When these building blocks are not in place, the athlete compensates, developing bad biomechanical habits that allow him or her to continue performing a skill, but in a nonoptimal way. Compensations increase the chances of poor performance as well as injury.

Physical performance is about **functional movement development,** which is not the same as fitness or muscular strength development. It involves integration of all aspects of training working together without conscious effort. In the field of education, this unconscious effort is referred to as *automaticity.* Automaticity is an important factor in the performance of athletes; for the brain and muscles to habitually perform a movement, the brain and muscles must be consistently trained in the way in which they will be used in a specific sport or activity.

Sport skills are learned. Talent is a combination of physical ability, perception, and dedication to repetitive training. People can be born with a tendency toward a particular set of skill development. There is a genetic predisposition to muscle mass, muscle fiber type, neuromuscular sensitivity, height, cognitive processing, and so forth. Genetic predisposition can be enhanced or deterred by

lifestyle (diet, substance use, activity), environment (air quality, sanitation, water quality, training facility, economic opportunity, social support), and motivation (drive, determination, and training commitment).

BASIC FUNCTIONAL MOVEMENTS AND MOVEMENT STRATEGIES

Certain combinations of basic functional movements equal sport-specific skills. These basic movements include walking/running, jumping, kicking, and throwing. These can be further categorized as rotation, swinging, catching, hitting, cutting, pivoting, and turning. Therapeutic massage targets the physical capacity to execute these movements.

These combined movements begin in the core and progress through the limbs to the distal joints. These patterns are called **movement strategies.**

Factors important for optimal movement include the following: stable head position with eyes oriented to the horizon, body oriented to a vertical upright position with center of gravity over a base of support, core stability, limb position, velocity, and coordination. These factors are monitored by reflex patterns in the eye, ear, head, neck, vestibular network, and foot-ankle complex.

The speed of **reaction time** determines the speed of movement. Visual stimuli trigger the oculomotor response, which translates to visual and auditory strategies for movement. These reflex responses decrease with fatigue, pain, illness, injury, stress, and age. The skilled athlete is able to scan the environment by looking and listening and responds with appropriate movement faster than nonathletes, indicating both genetic tendency as well as learned ability support performance.

The body can move in many different ways. Some are efficient and some are not. Sometimes what feels natural is incorrect and what feels extremely awkward is correct. Bad performance habits increase potential for injury.

Muscles do not get short or weak for just any reason. If muscles are short it is because the individual has used them in a shortened range, and the activities performed do not lengthen them. As a result, over time the athlete adapts and uses movement patterns that rely on short muscles. Because these patterns are habitual, if a muscle is stretched one day it will likely return to the length that it is most familiar with (the short position) and that is are used most often. Weak muscles, particularly muscles that are used infrequently or that may at one time have been injured, respond similarly. Following an injury, movement patterns are altered to avoid using the injured area. By the time healing occurs, a habitual movement pattern has developed that is familiar and difficult to change.

Often fatigue, weakness, and tightness will challenge or affect postural and core stability. Optimal functional movement is impossible with faulty posture and an unstable core. Remember—stability first, then mobility, agility, and finally sport-specific skill.

GAIT CYCLE (WALKING AND RUNNING)

Aspects that influence gait are the number of steps per minute, called the step rate; and the time it takes to complete the full **gait cycle,** called the stride time (Figures 6-1 and 6-2). Walking speed is increased by increasing either step rate or stride length (Figure 6-3).

As gait speed increases, the time of double limb support decreases. During running, the periods of double limb support disappear and are replaced by periods of both feet being off the ground.

Usually the transition from walking to running occurs when the speed is greater than 4 miles per hour. During running, the arms also do more than counterbalance rotation during walking. The shoulder/arm movement becomes part of the propulsion process as well.

The arms automatically counterbalance the legs. The swing of one arm creates a counter-rotation between the hip and shoulders that complements the work of the core stabilizers. Swinging the arms faster and farther produces greater stability

throughout the core, which typically results in greater mobility of the hips, improving stride, cadence, symmetry, and rhythm.

ROTATION, THROWING, AND SWINGING

Hitting a ball and swinging a racket or club are examples of swinging movements that involve rotation (Figure 6-4). **Rotation** and **swinging** movements occur in many sports, including those that require throwing, such as baseball, and tennis.

Throwing, striking, and swinging in most cases are the result of two types of force: linear and rotational. The athlete shifts weight away from and then toward the target with the lower body. He can remain still, step, or stride. A coiling spiral movement is followed by an uncoiling movement that starts at the hips and then moves to the shoulders and arms. The weight shift is the source of power. The goal is not to generate rotational power but rather to transform linear or weight-shifting power into rotational power.

Simple rotation and swinging involve both arms working together; throwing and striking focus all energy into the movement of one arm. Weight shifting, balance, and coordination are all important in what appears to be a simple upper-body movement. To propel the arm for throwing, striking, and swinging, an athlete needs to have a coordinated action of the lower body and trunk. It is more common to have a dynamic lower body by taking a step in a throw or a strike than remain still. A weight shift from one foot to the other provides the linear component of power, which is transformed into rotational power if there is no step involved, like in golf. Processing of visual and auditory stimuli provides accuracy during throwing.

Another important element to consider in rotation or swinging is symmetry. Whether the movements of the sport are asymmetric (one-sided), (golfers, baseball players, and rowers use swing or rotation of the body in one direction of movement), or symmetric (two-sided) (lacrosse, tennis, and racquetball players and kayakers use swing in rotation from both sides of the body), it is important to maintain symmetry while also supporting dominant performance–based movement.

CATCHING AND HITTING

Catching and **hitting** require visual and auditory tracking of a moving object and precise movement for contact with the object (Figure 6-5). Catching

Heel strike = Initial contact

Hip	25° Flexion	Hip extensors eccentric
Knee	0°	Quadriceps concentric
Ankle	0°	Tibials concentric

A

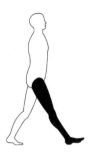

Foot Flat = Loading Response

Hip	26° Flexion	Hip extensors eccentric and hip abductors isometric
Knee	15° Flexion	Quadriceps eccentric
Ankle	10° Plantar flexion	Pretibials eccentric

Midstance = Midstance

• The body (center of gravity) reaches its highest point in the gait cycle

Hip	0°	Hip abductors isometric
Knee	0°	Quadriceps concentric initially, then no muscle activity
Ankle	0°	Plantar flexors (calf) eccentric

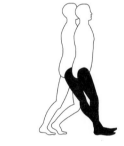

B

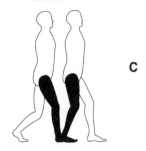

C

Heel-Off = Terminal Stance

Hip	20° Hip hyperextension	No muscle activity
Knee	0°	No muscle activity
Ankle	10° Dorsiflexion	Plantar flexors (calf) eccentric

Toe-Off = Preswing

Hip	0°	Adductor longus
Knee	40° Knee flexion	No muscle activity
Ankle	20° Plantar flexion	Plantar flexors concentric initially, then no muscle activity

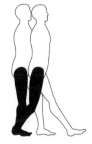

D

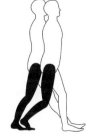

E

FIGURE 6-1 ■ **A** to **E,** Components of the stance phase. (Modified from *Fritz S: Mosby's essential sciences for therapeutic massage,* ed 2. St. Louis, 2004, Mosby.)

Acceleration = Initial swing

Hip	15° Hip flexion	Hip flexors concentric
Knee	60° Knee flexion	Knee flexors concentric
Ankle	10° Plantar flexion	Tibials concentric

A

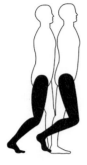

Midswing = Midswing

Hip	25° Hip flexion	Hip flexors concentric initially, then hamstrings eccentric
Knee	25° Knee flexion	Knee extension is created by momentum and gravity and short head of biceps femoris control rate of knee extension through eccentric control
Ankle	0°	Tibials concentric

B

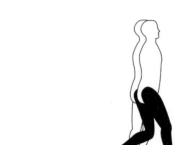

Deceleration = Terminal swing

Hip	25° Flexion	Hamstrings eccentric
Knee	0°	Quadriceps concentric to insure knee extension and hamstrings are active eccentrically to decelerate the leg
Ankle	0°	Tibials concentric

C

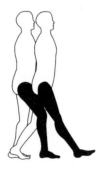

Arm swing

- The upper extremities serve an important role in counterbalancing the shifts of the center of gravity.

- A reciprocal arm swing is seen in a mature gait (e.g., the left arm swings forward as the right leg swings forward and vice versa).

- As the shoulder girdle advances, the pelvis and limb trail behind. With each step, this is reversed.

D

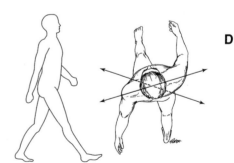

FIGURE 6-2 ■ **A** to **F,** Components of the swing phase. (Modified from Fritz S: *Mosby's essential sciences for therapeutic massage,* ed. 2 St. Louis, 2004, Mosby.)

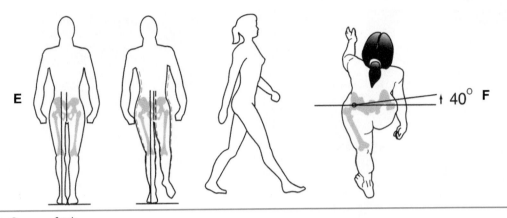

FIGURE 6-2 ■ CONT'D

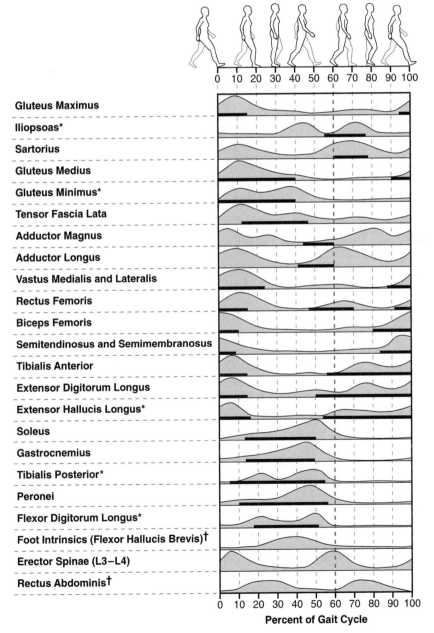

FIGURE 6-3 ■ Timing-intensity activator sequence and amount of time used during gait cycle for individual muscles. (From Neumann DA: *Kinesiology of the musculoskeletal system: foundations for physical rehabilitation.* St. Louis, 2002, Mosby. Muscle timing data from Knutson, Soderberg, 1995; Relative intensity of muscle activation data from Winter, 1991. *Bechtol, 1975; †Carlsoo, 1972.)

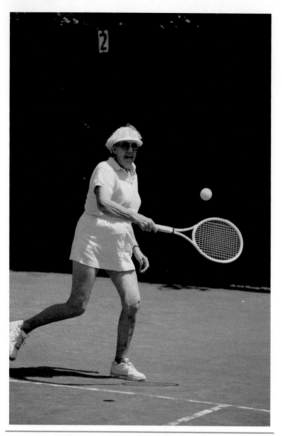

FIGURE 6-4 ■ Example of rotation and swinging.

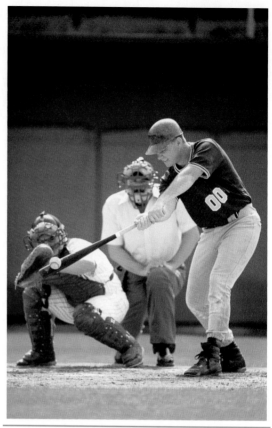

FIGURE 6-5 ■ Example of catching and hitting.

and hitting are typically the end result of rotational and swing movement strategies. It is the added component of visual and auditory tracking of the object that provides accuracy to actually hit or catch the ball or other object as it comes toward the individual.

If part of the sport requires grab and then push or pull movements, the athlete needs grip, torso, core, and arm strength.

KICKING AND JUMPING

When propelling the leg through the air in a kick or the body through the air with a jump, unrestricted and free movement is necessary (Figure 6-6). Mobility, stability, and power create balance in performance. If strength and power are not balanced by flexibility, power will be wasted on overcoming tightness.

Jumping consists of taking off and landing. Jumping does not usually require equal effort by both legs, with both legs performing the same movement. A vertical leap, such as that used for assessment, is an example of a perfect double leg

jumping situation; however, this movement rarely occurs in sports.

In **kicking,** all movements rely on stability, strength, balance, and coordination while standing on one leg to provide a foundation of power. Most jumping movements also require the movement to occur predominately off one leg. During kicking movements, one leg usually remains on the ground to generate the power for the kick.

Jumping is an effort of both legs moving in different directions. The propulsion leg, typically the last one to leave the ground, generates the push in a jump. A skilled jumper also creates pull with the other leg by accelerating one leg up when flexing the hip and knee. The weight and momentum of this leg pulls the body up as the strength and power of the other leg pushes the body up. Both legs work together in opposite directions.

An athlete may prefer to jump off one leg and kick with another, or a particular sport may dictate the movement, as with the specialty position of kicking in football. An athlete such as a martial artist, soccer player, or dancer may need to be able to

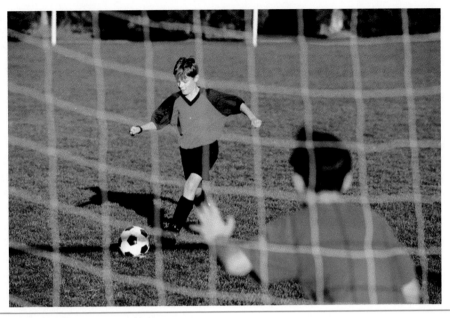

FIGURE 6-6 ■ Example of kicking.

perform a wide array of kicks. Even if the athlete never plans to kick with the nondominant leg, it is important to have balance between the left and right sides.

The length-tension relationship and muscle firing activator sequence and gait patterns become critical during performance of jumping or kicking, and this is an area that the massage therapist can directly influence.

Every kicker has a favorite style. Performance demand will create some asymmetry of function, but this should not compromise general function. The hip range of motion should be similar on the left and right. The ability to stand, balance, and demonstrate control on one leg should be similar as well.

CUTTING AND TURNING/PIVOTING

Changing direction—**cutting** and **turning/pivoting**—requires the ability to lower the center of gravity, decelerate, and accelerate in a controlled function (Figure 6-7). Quickness is often thought of as the ability to start a movement in a short amount of time. Actually, true quickness involves the ability to stop a movement in a short amount of time. Quickness improves as deceleration develops, because when an athlete is able to stop more efficiently and with better control, there is more time to set up, change direction, and accelerate in a new direction.

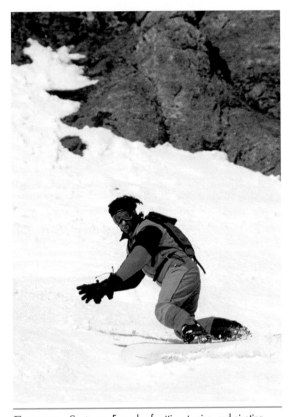

FIGURE 6-7 ■ Example of cutting, turning, and pivoting.

A low center of gravity is safe and productive in situations in which control is not possible. However, control is needed even in situations in which a low center of gravity cannot be achieved. The athlete needs to be able to lunge and squat to lower the center of gravity. The illusion of quickness is a demonstration of both of these factors. Quickness on the field or court also looks like above-average acceleration, but most of the time acceleration is not the issue. Deceleration is the key, because it sets up the rest of the movement. When one athlete is able to break away from another, it often is done with a cutting or turning movement. This movement is the result of deceleration with direction change, followed by acceleration. It is important for athletes to train for deceleration using eccentric muscle functions.

Acceleration is created by concentric muscle function and deceleration by eccentric muscle function. There is more potential for post-exercise soreness, disrupted muscle firing activation sequences, and an altered length-tension relationship with eccentric movement. Unit Two discusses this in-depth and how massage can be beneficial.

Deceleration places much greater stress on the joints and muscles than when they are accelerated. When an athlete tries to change direction without properly decelerating, the joints and muscles are off-balance, which slows down the athlete and increases the potential for injury. Deceleration training ultimately will reduce the risk of injury from deceleration-type movements such as landing, stopping, or changing direction.

SUMMARY

This chapter develops the understanding necessary to separate sport-specific movements into fundamental movement strategies. With this knowledge, all movement and sport activities can be understood. Assessment and treatment plans are based on movement efficiency or inefficiency. By comparing the optimal movement processes with those the client displays during assessment, the areas best addressed by massage are identified.

It is unrealistic to expect any text to thoroughly cover specifics of each and every sport or fitness and rehabilitation movement. However, massage practitioners work with a variety of clients participating in many different recreational, professional, fitness areas, as well as in activities of daily living, all of which are movement-dependent. The strategies described in this chapter are the ABCs of movement; by understanding these movement patterns, massage can be outcome-targeted and therefore sport-specific or activity-specific.

1 Explain the following statement and then justify why you agree or disagree with it. A star is born.

_____

_____

_____

_____

_____

_____ .

2 Provide an example of the following movement strategies found in the activities of daily living.

Examples: Walking–going from one room to another; running–chasing a small child; hitting–knocking down cob webs; throwing–heaving trash into the trash can

A. Catching

_____

B. Swinging

_____

C. Kicking

_____

D. Jumping

_____

E. Turning

_____

F. Cutting

_____

3 Provide an example of an exercise or sport that involves each of the following movement strategies:

Examples: Walking–cardiovascular rehabilitation program; running–marathon racing

A. Hitting

_____

B. Throwing

_____

C. Catching

_____

E. Swinging

_____

F. Kicking

_____

G. Jumping

_____

H. Turning

_____

I. Cutting

_____

J. Pivoting

_____

4 Pick an exercise activity or sport and identify the movement strategies involved.

Example: Basketball–running, throwing, catching, jumping, turning, cutting, pivoting.

_____

_____

_____

5 For each of the following movement strategies, list the target areas for massage. (Hint: Do the movement and focus on which body area receives the most deceleration activity.)

Examples: Walking–calves; running–hips; hitting–shoulders and low back

A. Throwing

_____

B. Catching

_____

C. Swinging

_____

D. Kicking

_____

E. Jumping

_____

F. Turning

_____

G. Cutting

_____

H. Pivoting

_____

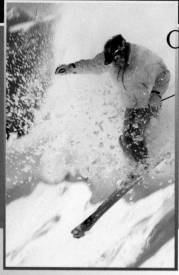

CHAPTER

7

NUTRITIONAL SUPPORT AND BANNED SUBSTANCES

OUTLINE

OBJECTIVES

Upon completion of this chapter the reader will have the information necessary to:

1 Explain general dieting recommendations.
2 Describe an antiinflammatory diet.
3 Describe the sport performance–related diet.
4 Explain why fluid intake is important.
5 List the components necessary for weight management.
6 Describe nutritional supplements.
7 List the risks and benefits of using nutritional supplements by athletes.
8 List banned substances.
9 Explain the relationship between eating disorders and exercise or sport performance.
10 Define the three major eating disorders of athletes.
11 List the symptoms of eating disorders.
12 Report life-threatening substance abuse behavior and eating disorders to the appropriate professional.

The massage therapist needs to understand the nutritional needs of the athletic client. Nutrients and/or the use of nutritional supplements and banned substances can influence massage outcomes and present contraindications. Proper nutrition is necessary for recovery, healing, and performance. Appropriate use of various nutritional supplements can support, but not replace, a nutritious diet.

Unfortunately, much dietary advice in the sport and fitness world is exaggerated, inaccurate, and can be downright harmful. Certain substances are illegal and their use can jeopardize an athlete's career.

Nutrition is not an exact science. The massage therapist is not usually a nutritional expert. Therefore, it is important for the athlete to consult a reputable person, such as a registered dietitian,

Alcohol
Anabolic steroids
Anorexia athletica
Anorexia nervosa
Banned substances
Beta blockers
Bulimia nervosa
Caffeine
Cannabinoids
Creatine

Disordered eating
Diuretics
Eating disorders
Ephedrine
Fluid intake
Glucocorticosteroids
Glucosamine
Healthy diet
Hormones
International Olympic Committee

Local anesthetics
Narcotics
Nutritional antioxidants
Nutritional supplements
Protein
Ribose
Sport performance—related diet
Stimulants
United States Anti-Doping Agency
Weight control

preferably one who specializes in sports and cardio-vascular nutrition. For a reliable reference, contact the American Dietetic Association, which lists more than 3000 specialized dietitians across the country.

GENERAL DIETARY RECOMMENDATIONS

A **healthy diet** consists of appropriate portions of healthy fats such as olive, grapeseed, and flaxseed oils and healthy carbohydrates (whole-grain foods) such as whole wheat bread, oatmeal, and brown rice. Vegetables and fruits should be eaten in abundance. A balanced diet includes moderate amounts of healthy sources of protein such as nuts, legumes, fish, poultry, lean meat, eggs, and dairy products.

A healthy diet minimizes the consumption of fatty red meat, refined grains including white bread, white rice and pasta made with white flour, and sugar. It eliminates food containing trans fat, which includes many fast foods and prepared food. A high-quality multiple vitamin that breaks down quickly in the digestive system is suggested for most people.

evolve Visit the Evolve website that accompanies this book for more information on dietary recommendations.

Fruits and vegetables reduce the risk of cardio-vascular disease. Folic acid and potassium appear to contribute to this effect, which has been confirmed in several epidemiologic studies. Inadequate consumption of folic acid is responsible for higher risks of serious birth defects, and low intake of lutein, a pigment in leafy green vegetables, is associated with increased risk for cataracts and degeneration of the retina. Fruits and vegetables are also the primary source of many vitamins needed for good health.

High consumption of red meat has been associated with an increased risk of coronary heart disease (probably because of red meat's high saturated fat content) and of type 2 diabetes and colon cancer. It may aggravate the inflammatory response and may increase pain sensitivity. The elevated risk of colon cancer may be related in part to the carcinogens produced during cooking and to the chemicals found in processed meats such as salami and bologna.

Poultry and fish, in contrast, contain less saturated fat and more unsaturated fat than red meat does. Fish is a rich source of the essential omega-3 fatty acids as well. Eggs do not appear to have adverse effects on heart disease risk, probably because the effects of a slightly higher cholesterol level are counterbalanced by nutritional benefits. This is especially true of eggs from chickens fed special vegetarian diets to increase nutritional value. Many people avoid nuts because of their high fat content, but the fat in nuts, including peanuts, is mainly unsaturated, and walnuts in particular are a good source of omega-3 fatty acids. Also, people who eat nuts are actually less likely to be obese. Nuts are more satisfying to the appetite, and eating them seems to have the effect of significantly reducing the intake of other foods.

People need to eat clean and fresh food as much as possible. Organic foods and free-range/hormone-free meat, poultry, and fish are becoming easier to obtain. Even though the cost is higher, the value is usually worth the investment.

An important aspect of caring for the athlete and for those in various rehabilitation programs is management of inflammation. Therefore eating a diet targeted to reducing inflammation is prudent. An antiinflammatory diet follows the recommendations given in this section. In addition, foods especially high in antioxidants are valuable.

SPORT PERFORMANCE–RELATED DIET

Various opinions exist about the components of a diet needed to support athletic performance and recovery. The amount of carbohydrates included in a **sport performance–related diet** is one area of discussion. In one research study, volunteers were placed on a normal diet composed of 50% carbohydrates, 34% fats, and 16% proteins. The maximum amount of time their muscles could work continuously was 114 minutes. On a noncarbohydrate diet composed of 46% fats and 54% proteins, the maximum was 57 minutes. However, on a high-carbohydrate diet of 82% carbohydrates and 18% proteins, the maximum was 167 minutes, nearly three times as long as for the noncarbohydrate diet.

Endurance athletes know that a high-carbohydrate diet helps performance by storing more fuel (glycogen) in the muscle, but a high-carbohydrate diet seems to be relevant to all sports. People in stop-and-start sports, such as tennis, after consecutive days of hard training also deplete their muscle glycogen stores. After each day's workout, a diet that contains sufficient carbohydrates is necessary to replace the glycogen used during activity.

A diet high in complex carbohydrates, moderate in proteins, and adequate in good fats can also help keep the energy level up during a weight loss program. Complex carbohydrates also have a fair amount of fiber, so the calories are more filling with fewer calories consumed. Many foods high in carbohydrates have small amounts of protein and a large number of vitamins and minerals. Sources of complex carbohydrates include whole-grain breads, cereals, and grains; legumes such as beans, peas, and lentils; fruits; and vegetables.

Children need a relatively high level of protein in their diets because they are still growing, whereas adults need only enough protein to maintain tissue repair. Although protein cannot be metabolized for energy, it contains amino acids, the building blocks

for body tissue. During exercise, there is a breakdown of body tissue, especially during contact sports such as football, but this also occurs during general exercise such as jogging. Continued use of muscle fibers breaks them down, and the body needs protein to repair them.

Eating foods high in fats and proteins slows down the stomach-emptying process. Therefore, it makes sense to eliminate high-fat, high-protein foods from pre-event meals. Instead, an athlete may benefit from eating high complex-carbohydrate, low-fat foods, such as whole-grain breads and pasta, at least 2 hours before a workout or competition so that the stomach empties before exercising. The athlete should allow 3 to 4½ hours between eating and an upcoming competition, because competition anticipation slows down digestion and an upset stomach may occur.

If a person has not eaten for 6 to 8 hours, his or her blood sugar level will be low. Symptoms of low blood sugar include dizziness, inability to think clearly, shakiness or weakness, and difficulty concentrating. Eating carbohydrates can restore and maintain blood sugar levels during exercise and prevent hunger and exhaustion after a workout. All people should avoid eating foods with high sugar content such as candy because they cause a sharp increase in blood sugar levels. The body responds to this increase by releasing insulin, which burns up blood sugar reserves and depletes overall energy rather than providing an extra boost.

High-potassium foods such as leafy dark green vegetables, citrus fruits, bananas, and melons are good for athletes because they are great sources of carbohydrates and proteins, contain no fat, and provide lots of vitamins and minerals.

Fluid intake is important because people can suffer heat problems from inadequate fluid replacement. Heat exhaustion or heat stroke can be life-threatening for both professional and amateur athletes. To prevent dehydration, 16 ounces of water should be consumed 15 minutes prior to a workout. Replenish fluids with water, electrolyte drinks, and diluted 50/50 fruit juices after exercise, and eat salty and high-potassium foods such as pickles. Thirst is not a good guide for fluid replacement.

During the 2 hours before exercise, it is best to drink only plain, noncarbonated water. The bubbles in carbonated water make a person feel full, so plain water is better. During warm-up, cold water is always appropriate. Cold water empties from the stomach faster than warm water. If an

Box 7-1	DIETARY SOURCES OF ANTIOXIDANT VITAMINS
Antioxidant Vitamin	**Dietary Sources**
Vitamin E	Plant oils (e.g., corn, soybean), grains, nuts, asparagus, eggs
Vitamin C	Citrus fruits, tomatoes, potatoes, green vegetables
Carotenoids (Provitamin A)	Carrots, broccoli, spinach, sweet potatoes, peaches

athlete has stomach cramps, it's probably from taking too much water at once. If an athlete experiences muscle cramps, an electrolyte sport drink diluted (50/50) with warm water may help.

The athlete should drink 4 to 8 ounces of water every 15 minutes during demanding performance, especially if he or she is sweating.

After a workout, cold water or a watered-down electrolyte drink is advisable. Within 2 hours after exercise, and preferably within 15 minutes, a high-carbohydrate snack is appropriate. Ingesting carbohydrates within that time frame seems to accelerate the replacement of muscle glycogen reserves.

Because high-carbohydrate drinks slow fluid replacement, it is best to get some fluid replacement underway first. A good rule of thumb is to take:

1. Water
2. An electrolyte replacement drink
3. A high-carbohydrate sport drink within 2 hours, and as close to 15 minutes as possible, after exercise

Limit caffeinated drinks such as coffee, cola, and iced tea. Although caffeine produces a feeling of increased energy, too much caffeine is a diuretic, and fluids are lost because of excessive urination. The same goes for alcohol. Athletes should limit intake of caffeine or alcohol to two drinks or less daily because both promote water loss.

WEIGHT CONTROL

Weight control includes weight gain, weight loss, and weight maintenance. Body weight and body composition should be evaluated as part of a weight control program. With a diet or exercise program, the scale is not what determines the progress made. Muscle weighs more than fat, and as muscle mass is increased with exercise, body weight may increase, even though total body fat is decreasing.

An athlete's weight may stay the same during off-season training, but during training 10 pounds of muscle may be added and 10 pounds of fat may be lost. The athlete will not see a change on the scale but will see a dramatic change in body composition.

The gold standard for determining body fat is hydrostatic weighing. This is a rather complicated procedure that involves full-body immersion in water. A simple yet reliable method is to have a trained professional measure skin thickness in several areas of the body using calipers. This provides a reading of body fat percentage within a narrow range under controlled conditions.

Many people who exercise are overweight but not overfat. Being overweight alone is not a health risk, but being overfat is. A "thin" person may have lower than normal weight for his or her age and sex owing to one or more of the following factors: shorter height (shorter bones), a smaller frame (smaller, lighter bones), less muscle, and less body fat. A "heavy" person's weight could be the result of one or more of these same factors if he or she is heavier than normal. Once the current body weight versus body fat is calculated, an ideal body weight goal can be established.

The more muscle and less fat, the faster and quicker an athlete. A higher tolerance for exercising in the heat should also be true. The heart and muscles will not have to work as hard, and a thin individual will be less prone to injury because he or she carries less dead weight on the lower back, hip, knee, and ankle joints.

Athletes who are trying to lower body fat levels must maintain a certain level for general health. The essential body fat level for men is at least 3%, with 6% body fat being optimal because of possible hydration problems. For women the optimal body fat level is between 9% and 12% for elite athletes and about 15% for amateur athletes. Some women athletes, particularly runners and gymnasts, try to get their body fat levels as low as a man's. This can be dangerous. A woman needs a higher level of body fat to maintain normal menstrual function and reproductive capabilities.

Optimal body fat levels differ depending on the activity and the goal (fitness or performance). Activities that require more speed and quickness and less body contact require lower levels of body fat. In some sports, athletes need body fat for protection. For example, hockey and football players need body fat to be protected from the pounding they take during contact. Football receivers and defensive backs do not need a lot of excess body fat because it will slow them down, but defensive linemen need the extra bulk provided by more body fat.

If a person is 20% over the ideal body weight, doctors would consider him or her obese. Obesity can lead to heart disease, high cholesterol levels, diabetes, and cancer of the breast, prostate, and colon. Overweight and obesity have become an epidemic in the general population. Weight control in this population can be accomplished by exercising daily and avoiding an excessive total intake of calories. Cardiovascular rehabilitation management in persons with diabetes or arthritis/arthrosis and those with many other health concerns also involves weight loss.

Because exercise is a required component of a weight management program, sport and fitness massage becomes an important component as well. The massage therapist can support the weight loss program by supporting the necessary exercise program and providing pleasure sensations to replace those provided by food.

There is no magic formula for weight loss. The best way to lose body fat is to decrease the intake of food and increase aerobic exercise. This dynamic duo is not only the best program for training, performance, and weight control, but for overall fitness as well.

NUTRITIONAL SUPPLEMENTS

A nutritional, or dietary, supplement, by definition, is a substance added to the diet to make up for a nutritional deficiency. It is not intended as a substitute for eating well. Nutritional supplements include the following:

- Vitamins
- Amino acids
- Minerals
- Herbs
- Other botanicals

Anything classified as a dietary supplement is not required to meet FDA or other standards. There are no regulations that guarantee the safety or purity of something sold as a supplement. With so much contradictory information regarding health and performance benefits of the many supplements available, it is difficult to make an informed decision about what actually works and what could be harmful. Products that have a USP (United States

Pharmacopeia) stamp on the label and that are eligible for the Consumer Lab seal of approval are the most reliable.

Because supplements are substances added to the diet to make up for a nutritional deficiency, an athlete would be wise to have a nutritional specialist evaluate his or her diet before developing a supplement program. Ideally, everything an athlete requires for energy and high performance can be obtained through a well-balanced diet, a high-quality multivitamin and mineral supplement, additional antioxidants, and glucosamine.

ANTIOXIDANTS

It is now clear that **nutritional antioxidants** work as a team to protect cells from free radical–mediated damage. It is possible that supplementation with nutritional antioxidants provides protection for the heart (cardioprotection). Cardiovascular disease is a major cause of death throughout the world. Therefore, finding ways to reduce the risk of developing cardiovascular disease and protecting the heart in the event of a heart attack is important. Regular exercise and dietary intake of adequate nutritional antioxidants are two lifestyle factors within our control that have been shown to provide cardioprotection.

Numerous antioxidants have been studied, and three naturally occurring antioxidants have been linked individually or in combination to protection against cardiac injury. These same antioxidants function as anti-inflammatory agents.

Vitamin E. Vitamin E is the most widely distributed antioxidant found in nature. Vitamin E, a generic term, refers to eight different structural variants of tocopherols or tocotrienols. They are lipid-soluble antioxidants that protect against free radical–mediated damage to cell membranes.

Vitamin C. Vitamin C is another naturally occurring antioxidant. It is water-soluble and has a twofold role as an antioxidant: it recycles vitamin E, and it directly scavenges free radicals.

Alpha Lipoic Acid. Alpha lipoic acid is a naturally occurring, water-soluble antioxidant that can recycle vitamin C. It is also capable of directly scavenging radicals within the cell.

Given that some antioxidants can be toxic when consumed in very large doses, the decision to use dietary antioxidant supplements should be approached with caution and made only on the advice of a well-trained nutritionist. See Box 7-1 for dietary sources of antioxidant vitamins.

A general rule is that most vitamin and mineral dietary requirements are best met by eating foods containing them rather than by ingesting a supplement, and this rule should be followed for antioxidants as well. A prudent dietary goal is to obtain most antioxidant vitamins (e.g., vitamins A, E, and C) and minerals (e.g., zinc, copper, magnesium, and selenium) through a varied diet. A diet rich in fruits and vegetables is a sound approach toward obtaining the maximum health benefits from antioxidants.

SUPPLEMENTS OFTEN USED BY ATHLETES

Creatine

To meet the demands of high-intensity exercise, such as sprinting or power sports, muscles generate energy from chemical reactions involving adenosine triphosphate (ATP), phosphocreatine (PCr), adenosine diphosphate (ADP), and creatine. Stored PCr can fuel the first 4 to 5 seconds of a high-intensity effort, but after that, another source of energy is needed. Creatine supplements seem to work by increasing the storage of PCr, thus making more ATP available to fuel the working muscles and enable them to work harder before becoming fatigued.

Creatine has been used by athletes for over 10 years; yet there is very little research regarding safety or long-term effects. Increasingly, research is looking at possible benefits of this supplement. What little research there is suggests that creatine works to build muscle in those who, through illness or disease, have a compromised muscle mass and strength. Athletes with high creatine stores don't appear to benefit from supplementation, whereas individuals with the lowest levels, such as vegetarians, have the most pronounced results following supplementation. Creatine might enable a healthy athlete to maintain a higher training load.

Claims for creatine:
- Improves high-power performance of short duration.
- Increases muscle mass.
- Delays fatigue.
- Increases creatine and creatine phosphate levels in muscles.

Valid research indicates that creatine can improve high-power performance during a series of repetitive high-power output exercise sessions. It may augment gains in muscle hypertrophy during resistance training, especially in those with compromised

skeletal muscle mass due to injury or disease. It does not increase endurance or anabolic effect.

Cautions for creatine use:
- Causes muscle cramping, strains, and pulls.
- Causes renal stress/damage.
- Increases risk of heat illness (athletes should increase fluid intake when taking creatine).

Caffeine

Caffeine has been used by endurance athletes for years as a way to stay alert and improve endurance. It is one of the best-researched nutritional supplements, and the overwhelming scientific evidence suggests that, in moderation, it has no adverse health effects. Caffeine use is fairly common among athletes at all levels of competition. However, keep in mind that caffeine is on the International Olympic Committee (IOC) banned substance list.

Claims for caffeine:
- Improves athletic performance.
- Increases energy.
- Delays fatigue.
- Improves fat burning.
- Spares muscle glycogen.
- Promotes body fat loss.

Valid research indicates that caffeine can act as a central nervous system (CNS) stimulant, raise epinephrine levels, increase alertness, delay fatigue, and may slightly spare muscle glycogen. It does not promote body fat loss.

Cautions for caffeine use:
- Causes side effects such as nausea, muscle tremor, palpitations, and headache, including withdrawal headache.
- Potentiates ephedrine side effects (should not be taken together).
- Acts as a diuretic, so adequate fluid intake is crucial.

Protein

High-protein/low-carbohydrate diets are popular, promising quick and easy weight loss. Power athletes have argued for years that high-protein diets lead to increased muscle mass and strength gains. Research on both athletes and sedentary individuals has failed to support these claims.

Claims for high-protein diet:
- Protein supports muscle growth.
- Protein increases muscle strength and mass.
- Weight training increases protein requirements dramatically.
- Protein improves recovery.

Valid research indicates that **protein** intake of greater than 2 grams/kg of body weight per day does nothing to increase muscle growth and does not enhance recovery.

Cautions for high-protein diet:

- Increases risk of certain cancers.
- Increases calcium excretion and increase risk of osteoporosis.
- Leads to reduced intake of vitamins, minerals, fiber, and phytochemicals

Glucosamine

In the laboratory, **glucosamine** stimulates cartilage cells to synthesize glycosaminoglycans and proteoglycans. In animal models, oral glucosamine sulfate has a beneficial effect on inflammation. Used as a supplement, glucosamine appears safe; however, more long-term research is needed to determine its effectiveness.

Claims for glucosamine:

- Protects cartilage from damage during weight-bearing exercise.
- Slows cartilage breakdown.
- Stimulates growth of cartilage.
- Reverses clinical course of arthritis.

Valid research indicates that glucosamine does play a role in maintenance and repair of cartilage and stimulates cartilage cells to synthesize cartilage building blocks. It also may have an antiinflammatory action by interfering with cartilage breakdown.

Glucosamine is most effective for early arthritis when cartilage is still present; it is less effective for severe arthritis. Supplements appear to be safe. Glucosamine is recommended if physical activity stresses the joints.

Cautions for glucosamine are minimal if dosage recommendations are followed.

Ribose

Ribose has many important roles in physiology. For example, ribose is a necessary substrate for synthesis of nucleotides, and it is part of the building blocks that form DNA and RNA molecules.

There is still a great deal of research to be done before any claims of athletic performance benefits can be made for ribose.

Claims for ribose:

- Increases synthesis and reformation of ATP.
- Improves high-power performance.
- Improves recovery and muscle growth.
- Increased cardiac muscle tolerance to ischemia.

Valid research indicates that ribose does improve the heart's tolerance to ischemia, but no research published in peer-reviewed journals shows benefits in athletic performance. The only research that supports ribose supplementation shows benefits in patients with heart conditions who lack the ability to synthesize ribose.

Ephedrine

Ephedrine, now banned by most sport organizations, is a drug derived from the plant *Ephedra equisetina*. It has been used for hundreds of years as a CNS stimulant and decongestant. A synthetic form of the drug, pseudoephedrine, is a common ingredient in over-the-counter and prescription cold and allergy products. Structurally similar to amphetamines, it increases blood pressure and heart rate. The mechanisms behind ephedrine's effect on weight loss appear to be those of increasing energy expenditure through increased lipolysis; increasing basal metabolic rate through thyroxine; and decreasing food intake by suppressing appetite.

Ma huang is an herbal form of ephedrine called ephedra that is contained in many herbal products available in health food stores (often along with chromium). Ma huang has been blamed for the deaths of several high school students who used it as a stimulant or aphrodisiac; the deaths presumably resulted from CNS dysregulation or cardiac arrhythmia. Sports-related deaths associated with ephedra use have been reported.

Claims for ephedrine:

- Increases body fat loss.
- Improves athletic performance.
- Improves concentration.

Valid research indicates that ephedrine has no effect on strength, endurance, reaction time, anaerobic capacity, or recovery time after prolonged exercise.

Caffeine increases the effect of ephedrine, and the combination can be dangerous.

Cautions for ephedrine are extensive. It is strongly suggested that it not be used. Ephedrine is banned by the National Collegiate Athletic Association (NCAA) and the IOC. The FDA has documented 40 deaths and more than 800 side effects linked with ephedrine use.

Side effects vary and do not correlate with the amount consumed. They include:

- Irregular heart rate
- Elevated blood pressure
- Dizziness
- Headache

- Heart attack
- Stroke
- Seizure
- Psychosis
- Death

BANNED SUBSTANCES, INCLUDING DRUGS

Athletes become vulnerable to using banned substances when they reach a plateau at some point in their training and the substances help them move beyond it. Some athletes may become curious and take banned substances just to see what will happen or may give in to peer pressure to try them. The psychological effects of some banned substances, such as greater aggression and feelings of invincibility and euphoria may be pleasurable enough that an athlete doesn't want to stop taking a banned drug. Athletes know that banned drugs enhance performance and that some of their competitors and fellow athletes take them.

The massage therapist may recognize the signs of banned substance use. Knowing what to do with this knowledge can be a very difficult ethical dilemma. Massage therapists must not recommend or provide supplements or other substances to athletes.

The terms **banned drug** and **banned substance** refer to compounds that are prohibited for use during athletic training and competition. The body naturally produces some of these compounds, such as testosterone and growth hormone, in small amounts. Other compounds, including some anabolic steroids, are created only in the laboratory. **evolve** (Visit the Evolve website that accompanies this book for more information on banned substances.) To make things more complicated, different sport organizations ban different substances—if they ban anything at all. Athletes who compete in Olympic sports must avoid taking compounds listed on the IOC list of banned substances. If they test positive for any such drugs, they may not compete for a short time (e.g., a few months) or for as long as the rest of their lives.

At the time that this book was being written, Major League Baseball finally banned performance-enhancing drugs such as androstenedione and steroids. The IOC, National Football League (NFL), National Basketball Association (NBA), and NCAA all prohibit the use of androstenedione. The NFL, NBA, and IOC prohibit steroids and test for them.

Even if a substance is not classified as a drug, it can still be banned. Some substances that are banned by the IOC are sold in the United States as nutritional supplements rather than as drugs. They can be bought at some health food stores and pharmacies. This category includes dehydroepiandrosterone (DHEA), androstenedione, and creatine.

Various vitamins and herbal mixtures sold through catalogs and advertised in muscle magazines purportedly improve strength. There is absolutely no evidence that any of them work. An illegal drug called gamma hydroxybutyrate is being sold in body-building and athletic clubs and in some health food stores. The FDA has issued a public health warning stating that this potent drug has serious side effects, including coma, seizures, and severe breathing problems.

The IOC also bans certain practices that achieve the same results as banned drugs. Blood doping is one such practice. This involves removing and storing a small quantity of blood, and then administering it immediately before a competition. The additional red blood cells increase the amount of oxygen that the blood carries to the muscles, and thereby increase the amount of work the athlete can do before performance starts to wane.

The list of substances banned by the International Olympic Committee is the most comprehensive used by an agency governing sports. The types of drugs and substances included have many common medical uses, so it is important for athletes to check the list before entering a sanctioned competition.

Anabolic Steroids

Anabolic steroids are probably the best known of the IOC's banned substances. Anabolic steroids have several medical uses. They improve the symptoms of arthritis, and they may help people infected with the human immunodeficiency virus (HIV) gain and maintain muscle mass and reduce the wasting that occurs with acquired immunodeficiency syndrome (AIDS).

This group of drugs includes synthetic derivatives of testosterone, a male sex hormone. Men who are testosterone-deficient due to endocrine disease may take steroids to supply the missing testosterone. Some of the most common steroids include dehydrochlormethyl testosterone (Turnibol), metandienone (Dianabol), methyltestosterone (Android), nandrolone phenpropionate (Durabolin), oxandrolone (Oxandrin), oxymetholone (Anadrol), and stanozolol (Winstrol).

Some athletes take anabolic steroids to increase their muscle mass and strength. The drugs may help athletes recover from a hard workout more quickly by reducing the amount of muscle damage that occurs during the session. Some like the aggressive feelings that occur when the drugs are taken over several weeks or months. Athletes usually take anabolic steroids at doses that are much higher than those prescribed for either AIDS wasting or testosterone replacement therapy. The effects of taking steroids at very high doses have not been well studied.

Steroid use has potentially life-threatening side effects. Men may develop prominent breasts and shrunken testicles. Women may develop a deeper voice and enlargement of the clitoris. Severe acne, liver abnormalities and tumors, increased low-density lipoprotein (LDL) and lower high-density lipoprotein (HDL) cholesterol levels, psychiatric disorders, and dependence may occur in both sexes. If an injected form is used, there is a higher risk of infections and diseases that are transmitted in blood, including HIV and hepatitis. Use of steroids by adolescents can halt their normal pattern of growth and development and put them at risk for future health problems.

Steroid users may develop a severe form of acne over the upper torso and become prematurely bald. They also are more susceptible to injuries of the bones and tendons because these support structures aren't strong enough to anchor overdeveloped muscles.

A relatively new group of steroid users are female body builders. More muscular female body builders tend to win more competitions. Women can strengthen their upper bodies with weight training, but the only way to bulk up these muscles is by taking male hormones.

Female body builders not only suffer the same side effects as men, but they also lose breast tissue, develop deeper voices, undergo changes in the structure of their reproductive organs, and grow increased facial and body hair. None of these changes is reversible. Women on steroids also stop menstruating, which is reversible when the steroids are discontinued.

Beta-2 Agonists

Drugs in another class, the **beta-2 agonists**, also are considered anabolic agents. This group includes drugs such as salmeterol (Serevent) and metaproterenol (Alupent). Beta-2 agonists may be prescribed for athletes if they have asthma and administer them with an inhaler.

Stimulants

Stimulants may reduce fatigue, suppress appetite, and increase alertness and aggressiveness. They stimulate the CNS, increasing heart rate, blood pressure, body temperature, and metabolism.

The most common stimulants include caffeine and amphetamines such as Dexedrine and Benzedrine. Cold remedies often contain the stimulants ephedrine, pseudoephedrine hydrochloride (Sudafed), and phenylpropanolamine (Acutrim). Illegal drugs such as cocaine and methamphetamine also belong to this group.

Although stimulants can boost physical performance and promote aggressiveness on the field, they have side effects that can impair athletic performance. Athletes may become psychologically addicted or develop tolerance and need greater amounts to achieve the desired effects. Nervousness and irritability make it hard to concentrate. Insomnia prevents an athlete from getting needed rest. Heart palpitations, weight loss, hypertension, hallucinations, convulsions, brain hemorrhage, heart attack and other circulatory problems may result.

Narcotics

Narcotics are synthetic compounds and drugs derived from the poppy, such as morphine, codeine, and heroin. In conventional medicine they're used to ease pain, and injured athletes may use them for that purpose. Narcotics act as a sedative and decrease bowel activity. Some people experience elation or euphoria when taking narcotics. Adverse effects include nausea and vomiting, mental clouding, dizziness, delirium, constipation, respiratory depression, muscle rigidity, and low blood pressure. Dependence and addiction are common among those who abuse narcotics.

Diuretics

Diuretics change the body's natural balance of fluids and salts (electrolytes) and can lead to dehydration. This loss of water may allow an athlete to compete in a lighter weight class, which many athletes prefer. Diuretics also help athletes pass banned substance drug testing by diluting their urine.

Diuretics are commonly used to treat high blood pressure and conditions that cause fluid retention (edema), such as congestive heart failure. When taken in small amounts, they have relatively few side effects, although electrolyte disturbances can occur.

When taken at the higher doses preferred by some athletes, however, the adverse effects may be significant. Using diuretics to achieve weight loss may cause muscle cramps, exhaustion, decreased ability to regulate body temperature, potassium deficiency, and heart arrhythmias.

Some of the most common diuretics are acetazolamide (Diamox, Storzolamide), benzthiazide (Marazide, Aquastat), spironolactone (Aldactone), dichlorfenamide (Daranide), chlorothiazide (Diuril), and furosemide (Lasix, Fumide).

Hormones, Mimetics, and Analogues

This class of drugs includes several **hormones** naturally produced by the body that can enhance performance. The IOC banned substance list includes:

Human chorionic gonadotropin (HCG). A hormone of early pregnancy that stimulates secretion of testosterone by the fetus (prohibited only in men).

Luteinizing hormone (LH). A hormone that stimulates the secretion of sex hormones by the ovaries and testes (prohibited only in men).

Adrenocorticotropic hormone (ACTH). A hormone that stimulates secretion of other hormones by the adrenal cortex.

Tetracosactide (corticotropin). A hormone that stimulates growth of the adrenal cortex or secretion of its hormones.

Human growth hormone (HGH). A hormone that indirectly stimulates the transport of amino acids (protein) into cells, thereby increasing body size.

Insulin-like growth factor (IGF-1). A peptide that mimics many of the functions of insulin on tissues, such as stimulation of amino acid uptake, and all the substances associated with it.

Erythropoietin (EPO). A hormone that stimulates the formation of red blood cells.

Insulin. A hormone that stimulates the absorption of sugars, fats, and proteins into cells (permitted in athletes with documented type 1 diabetes—formerly called juvenile or insulin-dependent diabetes).

Many sports authorities believe that HGH and EPO are the most commonly abused compounds in this category.

SUBSTANCES BANNED BY OTHER AGENCIES

The IOC permits individual sport-governing agencies to ban some classes of drugs. These classes include alcohol, cannabinoids, local anesthetics, glucocorticosteroids, and beta blockers.

Alcohol

Alcohol may impair judgment and cause a loss of coordination.

Cannabinoids

Cannabinoids, the active compounds in plants such as marijuana, may decrease awareness of the athlete's surroundings, impair judgment, and reduce reaction time.

Local Anesthetics

The regular use of local anesthetics is prohibited because they may mask the pain of injury and permit an athlete to injure himself or herself more seriously or put others at risk. They may be used when medically necessary, such as when treating an injury.

Glucocorticosteroids

Systemic use of **glucocorticosteroids** is prohibited because they alter metabolism, circulation, muscle tone, arterial blood pressure, and other body functions. They may be used when medically necessary, such as after an injury.

Beta Blockers

Beta blockers slow the heart rate and are used to treat high blood pressure and some heart disease. In sports that require precision rather than speed, strength, or endurance, a lower heart rate can be an advantage. Shooters, biathletes, and modern pentathletes may take these drugs so that they can shoot between heartbeats to improve accuracy. Beta blockers also help steady the hands of shooters and archers. Some of the more common banned beta blockers include acebutolol (Sectral), atenolol (Tenormin), metoprolol tartrate (Lopressor), and propranolol (Inderal).

IDENTIFICATION OF BANNED SUBSTANCE USERS

Determining which athletes use banned substances is not easy. There are no accurate tests for some banned drugs, such as human growth hormone. Many athletes have learned how to avoid testing positive for drugs.

The **United States Anti-Doping Agency** (USADA) is responsible for coordinating drug testing of U.S. athletes. (See Box 7-2 for information about Olympic drug testing.)

A urine test for EPO and a test for HGH are in development. Because of the serious consequences of using banned substances, the massage therapist must never recommend the use of any such product.

EATING DISORDERS

Eating disorders have been associated with athletic participation in various sports. Prolonged nutrient inadequacies and impaired psychological functioning that are associated with eating disorders can affect physical performance and, if uncorrected, can be life-threatening. Massage therapists should be aware of the signs and symptoms that accompany disordered eating patterns and should know how to respond when they suspect that they are dealing with an eating-disordered athlete.

Eating disorders manifest as a refusal to maintain a minimal healthy body weight (i.e., 85% of expected body weight), dramatic weight loss, fear of gaining weight even when underweight, abnormal preoccupation with food, abnormal food-

consumption patterns, and binge eating associated with loss of control and feelings of guilt.

Eating disorders common in the athlete are anorexia athletica, anorexia nervosa, and bulimia nervosa.

Anorexia athletica has been proposed as a classification of athletes who show significant symptoms of eating disorders but who do not meet the diagnostic criteria for anorexia nervosa or bulimia nervosa.

Anorexia nervosa is characterized by a refusal to maintain weight at or above a minimal normal level for height and age; an intense fear of gaining weight or becoming fat; a disturbance in the way in which one's body weight, size, or shape is perceived by the individual; and, in females, absence of at least three menstrual cycles when otherwise expected to occur.

Bulimia nervosa is characterized by recurrent episodes of binge eating, a feeling of lack of control over eating behavior, regularly engaging in self-induced vomiting, strict fasting, use of laxatives, excessive vigorous exercise, and a minimum average of two binge eating episodes per week for at least 3 months.

There is a spectrum of abnormal eating patterns, varying from mild to severe. There are nonclinically defined disorders such as the relentless effort to eliminate all fat from the diet, an unnecessary and unhealthful practice that can certainly have a negative impact on physical performance, among other things. "**Disordered eating**" is differentiated from an "eating disorder" by the degree and frequency of the aberrant eating behaviors.

There are few controlled studies on the prevalence of eating disorders among athletes. However, several smaller studies suggest that the prevalence of "disordered eating" among female athletes may be as high as 62% in sports such as gymnastics, and as high as 31% in men who participate in sports requiring a specified weight in order to compete, such as wrestling and rowing. It is important to emphasize that athletes in all sports can develop disordered eating behaviors, but sports associated with higher rates of disordered eating problems can be classified into three distinct groups: "appearance sports" such as gymnastics, body building, figure skating, and ballet; sports in which low body weight is considered advantageous, such as distance running and horse racing; and "weight category" sports such as wrestling and boxing.

Studies have provided numbers that suggest a higher incidence of eating disorders among athletes in sports or performers in which the strength: weight ratio is a premium and body fat is expected to be low (gymnastics, ballet, long-distance running).

Females tend to have a smaller percentage of lean body mass than males and therefore have a reduced calorie need. To be thinner, females generally have to eat considerably less than males. In female athletes, this reduced food intake may not be sufficient to satisfy hunger and, when combined with the desire to lose weight, may result in disordered eating patterns. Many reports on the female triad—eating disorders, amenorrhea, and osteoporosis—have been published that provide a hint of the health-related consequences of inadequate consumption of food.

Muscle power and endurance will be affected, and the athlete with a disordered eating pattern is likely to become ill more frequently. Severe and prolonged disordered eating can negatively affect every organ system in the body.

Endocrine abnormalities are common in persons with anorexia nervosa, and more subtle endocrine abnormalities have been described in those with bulimia nervosa as well. Furthermore, eating disorders can lead to gastrointestinal complications such as esophagitis, esophageal tears, and pancreatitis.

Fluid and electrolyte disturbances can increase the risk of cardiac arrhythmias, renal damage, impaired temperature regulation, and loss of endurance and coordination.

Swelling of the parotid glands as a result of frequent stimulation of the salivary glands caused by repeated vomiting can produce a "chipmunk-like" appearance in individuals with bulimia. Although this condition is painless and of no significant medical consequence, it does distort facial features. This may have no direct effect on athletic performance, but it is disfiguring and it can be emotionally upsetting to the individual searching for the unrealistic "ideal body."

The massage professional will often identify eating problems before anyone else. Concerns should be expressed to a coach or athletic trainer if necessary. Eating disorders lead to life-threatening conditions that should not be overlooked. Dieting, weight loss, and pre-event diet rituals do not mean that an athlete has an eating disorder. However, if any of the following signs or behaviors are recognized, they should not be ignored:

- Repeated comments about being or feeling fat
- Weight loss below ideal competitive weight that continues during the off-season
- Secretive eating or disappearing immediately after meals
- Excessive exercise that is not part of the team training regimen
- Weakness, headaches, and dizziness with no apparent medical cause

In anorectics, the most obvious physical symptom is an emaciated appearance. The anorectic's shoulder blades, backbone, and hip bones protrude, and muscle groups are clearly visible. However, keep in mind that the athlete with anorexia may not be as thin or light as the non-athletic anorectic because physical training will generally increase muscle mass to a certain extent. Anorectics may also suffer from cold intolerance, dress in layers or baggy clothes, and have persistent rashes, thin hair and nails, and gum disease.

It is important for the massage therapist to remain supportive of an individual that is suspected of suffering from an eating disorder, but the behavior should not be condoned. Be aware of mood swings and do not attempt to challenge the athlete about the logic or significance of the abnormal behavior. Eating disorders are often rooted in psychological disturbances, cultural myths, and body image distortion. They are serious conditions that require referral for professional intervention.

During treatment for an eating disorder, the athlete should have access to a physician, mental health worker, and nutrition therapist (generally a registered dietitian) who have been trained to work with eating-disordered patients. Massage has been shown to be beneficial in the treatment of eating disorders (Tiffany Fields).

SUMMARY

The massage therapist can support recommended dietary plans but should never recommend or provide supplements to clients. The massage therapist may be the first to notice dietary problems, eating disorders, or the use of banned substances. These behaviors have serious consequences and can be life threatening. They require referral and reporting to the supervising medical professional. Because this population is vulnerable to various internal and external pressures, the massage therapist should remain vigilant for the development of potentially destructive behavior.

1 Analyze your own diet in relationship to general dietary recommendations.

_____

_____

_____

_____

_____

_____

_____

_____

_____

_____

_____

_____

_____

_____

_____

3 Develop a recommended fluid intake protocol.

2 List the differences between the general dietary recommendations and the sport performance diet.

_____

_____

_____

_____

_____

_____

_____

_____

_____

_____

_____

_____

4 List the claims of supplements that are invalid.

_____
_____
_____
_____
_____
_____
_____
_____
_____

5 Develop a reporting plan for banned substance use and eating disorders.

_____
_____
_____
_____
_____
_____
_____
_____
_____
_____
_____

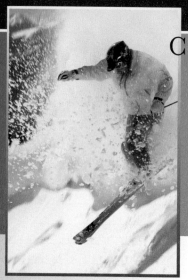

INFLUENCES OF THE MIND AND BODY

OBJECTIVES

Upon completion of this chapter the reader will have the information necessary to:

1 Define sport psychology.

2 Identify qualifed sport psychologists.

3 Explain how massage supports the sport psychologist.

4 List ways in which massage supports the zone experiences—mental toughness, ideal performance state, and peak performance.

5 Explain the importance of sport psychology during injury rehabilitation.

6 Identify the signs of mental and emotional strain requiring referral to the medical team or sport psychologist.

7 List the five stages of the response to injury.

8 Describe the role of the massage therapist during emotional and mental strain.

9 List factors that interfere with restorative sleep.

10 List behaviors that support restorative sleep.

S port psychology is the study of the psychological and mental factors that influence, and are influenced by, participation and performance in sport, exercise, and physical activity, and the application of the knowledge gained through this study to everyday settings.

Sport psychology professionals are interested in how participation in sport, exercise, and physical activity may enhance personal development and well-being throughout the life span.

Sport psychology involves several different components: mental training, performance enhancement, social interactions, learning, motivation, leadership, anxiety and stress management, cognitive rehearsal techniques (including hypnosis), intentional control training, injury treatment, cognitive intervention strategies, aggression management, and cohesion/congruency.

Acute stress

Coping skills

Chronic stress

Insomnia

Mental toughness

Peak performance

Restorative sleep

Secondary gain

Sport psychologist

The zone

Sport psychology professionals may be trained primarily in the sport sciences, with additional training in counseling or clinical psychology, or they may be trained primarily in psychology, with supplemental training in the sport sciences.

The activities of a particular sport psychology professional will vary based on the practitioner's specific interests and training. Some may primarily conduct research and educate others about sport psychology. These individuals teach at colleges and universities and, in some cases, also work with athletes, coaches, or athletic administrators. They provide education as well as develop and implement programs designed to maximize the overall well-being of sport, exercise, and physical activity participants.

Other professionals may focus primarily on applying sport psychology knowledge. These individuals are more interested in the enhancement of sport, exercise, and physical activity performance or enjoyment. They may consult with a broader range of clients and may serve in an educational or counseling role.

Only those individuals with specialized training and, with certain limited exceptions, only those with appropriate certification and/or licensure may call themselves a *sport psychologist.* A sport psychologist should be a member of a professional organization such as the Association for the Advancement of Applied Sport Psychology (AAASP) and/or the American Psychological Association (APA). A growing number of sport psychology professionals are certified by the AAASP. These professionals–who earn the designation Certified Consultant, AAASP (or CC, AAASP)–have met a minimum standard of education and training in the sport sciences and in psychology. They have also undergone an extensive review process. The AAASP certification process encourages sport psychology professionals who complete it to maintain high standards of professional conduct.

Some sport psychology professionals may be listed on the U.S. Olympic Committee (USOC) Sport Psychology Registry, meaning that they are approved to work with Olympic athletes and national teams. To be on the Registry, a professional must be a CC, AAASP and a member of the APA.

WHY SPORT PSYCHOLOGY?

During the last two decades sport psychology has received significant and increasing attention from athletes, coaches, parents, and the media. A growing number of elite, amateur, and professional athletes acknowledge working with sport psychology professionals.

Exercise specialists, athletic trainers, youth sport directors, corporations, and psychologists are using knowledge and techniques developed by sport psychology professionals to assist with improving exercise compliance, rehabilitation programs, educating coaches, building self-esteem, teaching group dynamics, and increasing performance effectiveness.

Almost all sports are based on competition. Striving to reach peak performance is appropriate until athletes push themselves beyond their capacity. Exercise is very helpful in alleviating stress, releasing tensions, and producing a relaxing kind of fatigue. However, some people go far beyond this normal response and become overly dependent on daily exercise.

One of the by-products of exercise is the production of naturally occurring brain chemicals that influence mood. Endorphins are morphine-like substances that produce a sense of well-being and relaxation and are responsible for the "runner's high." Some people become addicted to daily exercise because of the production of these chemicals. If they don't exercise, they become depressed and irritable, and they may actually have withdrawal symptoms. If they become injured, they will make life miserable for everyone around them until they can get back to exercising daily. Many athletes refuse to take time off because of their drive to keep pushing themselves. It can be difficult to get the message across that an injury, like a hamstring pull, may take three or more months to heal. This mental outlook often interferes with even the best treatment because the athlete will try to play before he or she is ready.

Muscles may be held in sustained tension due to overuse, poor posture, and/or psychological or emotional stress. States of anxiety and anger, for example, can create sustained muscular hypertonicity. Emotional stress, such as depression, can also create a decrease in muscular tone and a loss of sensory motor communication.

Appropriate massage can support the work of the sport psychologist by calming anxiety, reducing increased motor tone of muscles, and to a lesser extent, addressing mild depression. Massage affects the same mood-altering neurochemicals as exercise.

WHAT IS THE ZONE?

Studies of athletes, artists, and others have shown that being "in **the zone**" generally means a state in which the mind and body are working in harmony. When in the zone, an individual is calm yet energized, challenged yet confident, focused yet instinctive. Different parts of the brain are working together smoothly to automate the movement or skill. This is comparable to the massage practitioner's being "centered."

Training the mind is an important step toward getting in the zone. Aspects of mental training for some sports and positions include increasing concentration and focus, controlling emotions, feeling relaxed but energized, being calm and positive, and aiming to feel challenged and confident. A person who is in the zone is free of worries and is confident and relaxed so that the best performance just occurs automatically.

Getting in the zone combines physical and mental training. When the body is conditioned, skills are well practiced, or habituated, and mental conditioning is congruent; a zone experience is then possible.

The implications for massage supporting "zone" functions are vast. Physical sensations of relaxation can help relieve anxiety and tension and improve concentration and focus. Various progressive relaxation methods that involve contracting and releasing the tension in large muscles are used. Massage can induce deep relaxation and support zone functions.

Guided imagery can help reduce anxiety, increase concentration and confidence, and serve as mental practice or rehearsal. Imagery techniques work well in conjunction with relaxation techniques such as massage because the relaxation can help the client better imagine performing the skill required. During massage or other induced relaxation states, the athlete can picture mentally himself or herself performing a specific sport or activity. He or she can visualize being dressed, getting ready to perform, hearing the sounds and smells—feeling the muscles and emotions and envisioning doing the activity, practicing skills, running the race—whatever it might be.

Negative thoughts can get in the way of concentration and confidence. The massage therapist must not be negative during the massage and must support positive and productive thought processes.

Although training the mind and body can lead to more skillful and enjoyable play, it is important to understand that the athlete might not get in the zone all the time. The zone experience does not happen nearly as often as people like to think it does. Do not overfocus on the zone experience during the massage.

There are several names for states of being similar to the zone. Each is slightly different, but the basic concepts are the same.

Mental toughness is the ability to perform near the athlete's best no matter what the competitive circumstance—to maintain a calmness of thought, thinking positively, being realistic, and remaining focused.

Ideal performance state is the level of physical and mental excitement ideal for performing at the top. Key elements include being confident, relaxed yet energized, positive, challenged, focused, and automatic.

Peak performance describes one's very best performance, although a person need not necessarily be in the zone while achieving it. Key elements include being focused, relaxed, confident, and energized.

INJURY AND SPORT PSYCHOLOGY

Whether the athlete is a competitive or a recreational exerciser, recovering from an injury can present a challenge. How the athlete understands and responds to pain and limitation is a very individual experience based on many factors. There are, however, certain responses and psychological skills that can help most people take an active role in their own recovery.

People often initially feel overwhelmed by an injury. The ability to cope will greatly improve if the athlete works closely with the doctor and other health care providers to develop a clear plan for recovery.

Successful rehabilitation begins with becoming informed about the injury. It's important to know the extent of the injury, anticipated recovery time, and understand the rehabilitation plan required to recover safely and effectively.

It is important that the injured person considers himself or herself as an active participant in rehabilitation planning and treatment. An individual may not understand the scientific aspects of recovery, but he or she is the expert on his or her own experience—a reality that may either help or hinder rehabilitation.

How the athlete responds to the injury is also very important. Although certain sports or activities have greater risk for injury than others, an injury is usually not expected or planned for. Athletes are rarely prepared for the emotional response to an injury.

Injuries have very different meaning for different people. For some, an injury might be life-threatening or career-ending. For others, an injury might take them away from a team or social structure that gives them a sense of identity and community. An injury can also interfere with a job or responsibilities at home. It's important, therefore, that the athlete acquire **coping skills** required to help through the loss—with professional help if necessary.

Athletes should try to maintain a sense of identity and importance through activities that help them feel good. They should express their needs and concerns to the health care team. It is helpful to identify any negative mental responses to injury, then reframe them to promote a positive approach to healing: being aware of the current level of function and of what function is lost, and then moving beyond those limitations to envision the future level of function.

The athlete needs to ask for and receive help and to be surrounded by emotionally and physically supportive people. Interaction with those who hinder the healing process should be eliminated or minimized.

Athletes in today's society have many things to deal with, including multiple personal and professional demands, increased stress, and injury. Some athletes know how to successfully deal with injury and others have a hard time coping with it. The athlete may need professional help getting through the injury healing process, and the massage therapist needs to be supportive.

Injury can negatively impact the mind, emotions, and body. Rehabilitation is often a time of emotional distress.

Signs that an athlete is having some problems include:
- Depression
- Feeling of being helpless
- Mood swings
- Dwelling on minor complaints
- Denial

Injury rehabilitation impacts a person in many ways, including:
- Change in status relative to peers
- Dealing with pain
- The need for discipline and compliance with rehabilitation programs
- Decreased independence and control
- Resultant worries about finances
- Changes in self-esteem or self-image

When these issues are recognized by the massage therapist, a referral is necessary. Avoid the tendency to try to fix them. Ultimately, therapeutic massage is secondary to, although supportive of, the medical team, including the sport psychologist. Respect for professional boundaries and honoring scope of practice are essential. However, because of the time massage therapists spend with athletes and the compassionate quality of the professional interaction, we may be the first to notice difficulties. Athletes may also share information with massage professionals that was not provided to others working with them.

As massage professionals interested in the sports massage career specialty, understanding and helping an athlete through an injury are very important. We need to understand the demands placed on the whole person as well as addressing the injury.

Sport psychology interventions can minimize negative experiences and maximize recovery from injury. Mental training enhances performance in rehabilitation and sport, improving the ability to return to play. The outcome of an injury, degree of pain, and expected performance are important factors in determining how fast rehabilitation occurs.

When coaches or trainers adopt an attitude that injured athletes are worthless, they create an environment in which athletes will continue to participate while hiding their injuries, increasing the likelihood of further injury. Similarly, coaches who emphasize a strong will to compete and win, no matter what the athlete's physical status, promote the idea of sacrificing one's body for the team, which can cause players to take unhealthy risks and become injured.

All athletes should understand that the nature of participation in sports dictates that at some time, pain and injury are very likely to occur. However, instead of stressing the inherent risks associated with sport, the focus should be on doing those things that can minimize the chances of injury, such as making certain that the athlete is fit, is practicing safe sport techniques, and is learning to recognize when his or her body is saying that something is wrong. If athletes develop the confidence that they have done as much as they can to reduce the likelihood of injury, perhaps their risk of injury will indeed be minimized. Teaching athletes how to distinguish between the "normal" pain and discomfort associated with training and "injury" pain is of vital importance. Athletes who do not learn to make this distinction often become seriously injured because they do not recognize the onset of minor injuries and do not modify their training regimens accordingly.

The individual's current medical status must also be addressed. Conditions such as diabetes, asthma, and high blood pressure, as well as orthopedic concerns, must also be factored into the exercise prescription for rehabilitation or fitness-based programs for performance.

Learning stress management skills is important for athletes—both for enhancing performance and for reducing injury risk. Psychological stress has been shown to predict increases in injury. Stress is thought to increase the risk of injury because of the unwanted disruption in concentration or attention and increased muscle tension associated with heightened stress. Athletes especially prone to injury seem to be those who experience considerable life stress. They have little social support from others, possess few psychological coping skills and are apprehensive, detached, and overly sensitive.

Sport massage therapists should learn to treat the whole athlete, not just the injury. They must communicate effectively and factually without instilling fear or unrealistic expectations and with concern for the athlete's feelings.

No one can work closely with human beings without becoming involved with their emotions and, at times, their personal problems. The sport massage therapist is placed in numerous daily situations in which close interpersonal relationships are important. Understanding an athlete's fears, frustrations, and daily crises is essential, along with knowing when to refer individuals with emotional problems to the proper professionals. Injury prevention includes dealing with both psychological and physiologic attributes of the athlete. The athlete who competes while angry, frustrated, or discouraged or while suffering from some other emotional disturbance is more prone to injury than one who is better adjusted emotionally. Because of the emotional intensity surrounding competing athletes, the massage therapist working with this population needs to attend to his or her own mental health.

IN MY EXPERIENCE...

I remember working with a rookie football player who was extremely homesick. He came from a large family and was the "baby." It was unclear if he really wanted to play football at a professional level. The transition from the college game to the demands of "going to work" seemed to overwhelm him.

He had a turf toe injury that just would not heal to his satisfaction. The pain and functional limitations exceeded the typical time usually indicated for being excused from practice. The coach became impatient with him and the athletic trainer was unable to provide further treatment.

I was working with the young man for the turf toe injury and for general massage. He became attached to me and began saying things like "you remind me of my mom." Eventually I talked with the trainer about this, who then talked with the coach.

Intervention was provided. Voluntarily, the young man's mom began to schedule more frequent visits, and the situation improved. He did play professional football and was moderately successful, lasting for about 5 years in the league. When the constant moving around and separation from his family became too difficult, he left the league. He is currently teaching and coaching football at a high school near his family and is married and has a family of his own.

MASSAGE APPLICATION

Generally speaking, injured athletes can experience feelings of vulnerability, isolation, and low self-worth. Denial of the reality of the injury also comes into play. All of these feelings can adversely affect the athlete and his rehabilitation. The injured athlete may experience a number of personal reactions besides a sense of loss. These may include physical, emotional, and social reactions. A fairly predictable response to injury often occurs in five sequential stages: (1) denial, (2) anger, (3) grief, (4) depression, and (5) reintegration. Athletes who fail to move through these five stages may suffer adverse psychological effects related to the injury. Such adverse effects are more likely to occur if the injury is season-ending or career-ending.

Some degree of psychological distress and discomfort accompanies most major athletic injuries. However, more serious problems of poor psychological adjustment to injury are often preceded by the following warning signs:

- Feelings of anger and confusion
- An obsession with the question of returning to play
- Denial of the injury
- Exaggerated bragging about accomplishments
- Guilt about letting one's team down
- Withdrawal from significant others
- Rapid mood swings
- Pessimistic attitude about the prognosis for recovery

When these warning signs are detected, the athlete should be referred to a sport psychologist or other mental health professional.

Certain factors are commonly seen among athletes going through adjustment to injury and rehabilitation. Severity of injury usually determines length of rehabilitation. Regardless of length of rehabilitation, the injured athlete has to deal with three reactive phases of the injury and rehabilitation process:

- Reaction to injury
- Reaction to rehabilitation
- Reaction to return to competition or career termination

Other factors that influence reactions to injury and rehabilitation are the athlete's coping skills, past history of injury, social support, and personality traits. All athletes do not necessarily have all of these reactions nor do all reactions fall into the suggested sequence.

Athletes who deal with their feelings and focus on the future rather than the past have a tendency to advance through rehabilitation at an accelerated rate. Those who have a high degree of hardiness, well-developed self-concept, good coping strategies, and mental skills are more likely to recover rapidly and fully from injury than athletes who lack these qualities.

Athletes who lack motivation and are depressed or in denial have difficulty with the rehabilitation process

Following injury, particularly one that requires long-term rehabilitation, the athlete may have problems adjusting socially and may feel alienated from the rest of the team. The athlete may believe that there has been little support from coaches and teammates. The athletic trainer is responsible for rehabilitation and becomes the primary source of social support. The massage therapist can play an important part of this support process only if the professionals work together. Conflict among professionals can adversely affect this process.

One of the outcomes of an injury may be **secondary gain.** This can be a beneficial "time-out" (time to rest and refocus) and a decrease in pressures and expectations. Secondary gain can both support and interfere with the healing process.

Psychological strategies and communicative skills used by the sport psychologist help the athlete move successfully through a rehabilitation process. Care needs to be taken to maintain appropriate boundaries during this vulnerable time for the athlete.

The following strategies are used by the massage therapist to support the medical staff:

Coping skills. The massage professional has a limited role in this area. Teaching self-help is appropriate as long as it does not conflict with other treatment being provided.

Education about the injury. Make sure the information is correct and not in conflict with other professionals before sharing it.

Coping with non-participant status and other changes. These changes include separation from family, friends, and teammates. The massage therapist is supportive but defers to the medical and coaching staff.

Managing emotional reactions to injury and regaining sense of control. The massage therapist can target the massage to address the physical effects of emotional turmoil and refers to the sport psychologist for additional mental support.

Pain management. The massage therapist can play an active role in helping the athlete to cope with pain related to injury, surgery, and rehabilitation after returning to play.

During injury rehabilitation, management of the emotional demands of treatment and rehabilitation includes:

- Adhering to physical therapy
- Maintaining motivation for rehabilitation
- Tolerating pain
- Goal-setting and achievement
- Consultation with medical and rehabilitation staff as needed
- Coping with chronic pain
- Coping with issues associated with returning to sport activity such as fear of reinjury, intrusive or disruptive thinking regarding the injury, and loss of confidence

The massage therapist plays an important supportive role during this phase of rehabilitation and reinforces the awareness of physical healing to support rehabilitation.

STRESS

Stress is often associated with situations or events that are difficult to handle. How a person views things also affects the level of stress. Unrealistic or high expectations increase the stress response.

Stress may be linked to external factors, such as:

- Community
- Unpredictable events
- Environment
- Work
- Family

Stress can also come from internal factors, such as:

- Irresponsible behavior
- Poor health habits
- Negative attitudes and feelings
- Unrealistic expectations

It is one thing to be aware of stress in daily life, but it is another to know how to change it. Stress is not just in the mind. It is a physical response to an undesirable situation, and it has the potential to control one's life. Stress has many sources. Mild stress can result from being caught in a traffic jam,

standing in line at a store, or getting a parking ticket. Stress also can be severe and cause major health problems. Divorce, family problems, and the death of a loved one can be devastating.

Stress can be short-term (acute) or long-term (chronic). **Acute stress** is a reaction to an immediate or perceived threat. Everyday life sometimes poses situations that aren't short-lived, such as relationship problems, loneliness, and financial or health worries. The pressures may seem unrelenting and can cause chronic stress.

When a person's coping behavior is ineffective, a physical stress response occurs to meet the energy demands of the situation. First the stress hormone adrenaline is released. Then the heart beats faster, breathing quickens, and blood pressure rises. The liver increases its output of blood sugar, and blood flow is diverted to the brain and large muscles. The massage therapist should recognize signs and symptoms of nonproductive sympathetic dominance.

After the threat or anger passes, the body relaxes again. One may be able to handle an occasional stressful event, but when it happens repeatedly, such as with chronic stress, the effects multiply and are compounded over time.

For example, a football player endures week after week of hits in a season, or a source of pain, and may reach a point of not being able to handle it anymore.

It is evident that there is too much stress for a person to cope with when the following telltale signs appear:

- Irritability
- Sleep problems (sleeps all the time or can't sleep at all)
- Lack of joy
- Loss of appetite or can't stop eating
- Trouble with relationships (e.g., no longer gets along with friends and family members)
- Illness, infertility, or fatigue

Signs of **chronic stress,** which can damage overall health, include:

- Uneasiness and vigilance
- Anxiety and panic attacks
- Sadness or a heightened sense of energy
- Depression or melancholia
- Loss of appetite
- Anorexia or overeating
- Alertness
- Irritability
- Suppression of the immune system
- Lowered resistance to infections

- Increased metabolism
- Diabetes or hypertension
- Infertility
- Fatigue
- Absence of menstruation (amenorrhea), loss of sex drive, or performance ability

COPING WITH STRESS

The following measures can help in coping with stress.

Sleep well. Sleep is very important and can provide the athlete with the energy needed to face each day. Going to sleep and awakening at a consistent time also may help the person sleep more soundly. Restorative sleep should be a major goal for massage.

Eat a balanced diet that includes a variety of foods and provides the right mix of nutrients to keep the body systems working well. When healthy, the athlete will be better able to control stress and pain

Change the pace of your daily routine.

Be positive. It helps to spend time with people who have a positive outlook and a sense of humor. Laughter actually helps ease pain because it releases the chemicals in the brain that give a sense of well-being.

Physical relaxation helps manage stress by:

- Reducing anxiety and conserving energy
- Increasing self-control when dealing with stress
- Helping to recognize the difference between tense muscles and relaxed ones
- Helping to remain alert, energetic, and productive

Massage is a major relaxation modality. It supports techniques such as deep breathing, progressive muscle relaxation, word repetition, and guided imagery.

Progressive Muscle Relaxation

This technique involves relaxing a series of muscles, one at a time. First, raise the tension level in a group of muscles, such as in a leg or an arm, by tightening the muscles and then relaxing them. Concentrate on letting the tension go out of each muscle. Then move on to the next muscle group. Do not tense muscles near the pain sites. Massage supports the practice of progressive muscle relaxation.

Word Repetition

Choose a word or phrase that is a cue for relaxing, and then repeat it. While repeating the word or

Box 8-1	LIFESTYLE ADJUSTMENTS TO STRESS

- Simplify life.
- View negative situations as positive and a chance to improve life.
- Use humor to reduce or relieve tension.
- Exercise.
- Get more sleep.
- Eat a good breakfast and lunch.
- Reduce or eliminate caffeine consumption. Caffeine is a stimulant.
- Get a regular massage.
- Don't take work problems home or home problems to work.
- Call a friend and strengthen or establish a support network.
- Hug your family and friends.
- Do volunteer work or start a hobby.
- Pray or meditate.
- Practice relaxation techniques, such as deep breathing and self-hypnosis.
- Take a vacation.

phrase, breathe deeply and slowly and think of something that gives pleasant sensations of warmth and heaviness.

Guided Imagery

Also known as visualization, this technique involves lying quietly and picturing yourself in a pleasant and peaceful setting. Try to experience the setting with all of the senses, as if you are actually there. For instance, imagine lying on the beach. Picture the beautiful blue sky, smell the salt water, hear the waves, and feel the warm breeze on your skin. The messages your brain receives as you experience these sensations help you to relax (Box 8-1).

RESTORATIVE SLEEP

Restorative sleep is extremely important for anyone who is an athlete or in rehabilitation. Almost everyone has occasional sleepless nights, perhaps due to stress, heartburn, or drinking too much caffeine or alcohol. How much sleep is enough varies for different individuals. Although $7\frac{1}{2}$ hours of sleep is about average, some people do fine on only 5 or 6 hours of sleep, while others need 9 or 10 hours a night.

IN MY EXPERIENCE...

Neutral Talk

Life is sometimes amusing, although I guess that depends on your perspective. Athletes' pets provide a never-ending source of amusement. There is Butkus the bull dog, Porkie the pig, Snoop and Nate, named after rappers, (two little white fluffy dogs belonging to a big tough football player), and Killer the kitty. I recall a puffer fish with personality and a pet chicken named Kentucky Fried. There are more, but you get the idea. Pets, kids, and parents are all part of the picture, especially if you see clients in their homes.

I especially enjoy the grandparents. They usually swing between being so proud of the athletic prowess of their grandchildren and treating them like little kids. I recall one athlete who was sound asleep while being massaged, when Grandma called. Still half-asleep, he jumped off the table, about lost the shorts he was wearing, ran up the stairs, and answered her call with a "yes Ma'am."

Peoples' interests vary widely. Some people cook, others garden, and some watch movies. Pets, cooking, gardens, and movies make good neutral discussion topics during that first 5 to 10 minutes of the massage when settling down can be difficult.

Discussion about family is not so neutral. It is too easy to give advice. Because professional boundaries are a continuous concern, neutral discussion topics are important. The last thing an athlete wants to talk about is the "game" or competition. Usually the athlete doesn't want to talk at all, but the silence gap can be uncomfortable. If the TV is on, the program or movie being shown fills the gap. If the athlete is listening to music or talking on the phone, this also fills the space. I have watched a lot of TV that I might not have personally chosen and figured out how to time the massage so I am finished when the movie is finished. I always let the client choose the type of music they want to hear. It is amazing how many different rhythms to which massage can be given.

If these void-filling activities aren't available or desired, I can always talk about my pets. I usually relate a funny story about how "Creature," my ferret, gets the best of my two dogs, or about events occurring in my little backyard garden habitat, such as the ongoing hummingbird fights and the summer-long saga of the poor male house wren who had a terrible time building a nest that suited a potential mate. When I was able to finally report success by the wren, my clients were thrilled and wanted a sequel.

I have shared a love of butterfly gardening with a professional wrestler who watched the life cycle of the Monarch butterfly with his young daughter, and of course I had to chuckle about the big tough football player with the two little white fluffy dogs.
Safe neutral talk, just for a few minutes, helps; then be quiet.

Lack of restorative sleep can affect energy levels, and restorative sleep helps bolster the immune system, fighting off viruses and bacteria.

Insomnia is the most common of all sleep disorders. Insomnia includes difficulty going to sleep, staying asleep, or going back to sleep when awakened early. It may be temporary or chronic. About one out of three people have insomnia at some point in their lives. Simple changes in one's daily routine, lifestyle, and habits may result in better sleep (Box 8-2).

Insomnia becomes more prevalent with age. As a person gets older, the following changes often occur that may affect sleep.

Between the ages of 50 and 70, more time is spent in stages 1 and 2 of non–rapid eye movement (NREM) sleep and less time in stages 3 and 4. Stage 1 is *transitional sleep*, stage 2 is *light sleep*, and stages 3 and 4 are *deep (delta) sleep*, the most restful kind. Because one is sleeping lighter in stages 1 and 2, one is more likely to wake up. With age, the internal clock often speeds up and a person may get tired earlier in the evening and consequently wake up earlier in the morning.

A change in daily activity can disrupt sleep patterns regardless of whether the client is less or more physically or socially active. Consistent activity as part of daily activities helps promote a good night's sleep. The retired client may also have more free time and, because of that, drink more caffeine or alcohol or take a daily nap. These things can also interfere with sleep at night.

A change in health can affect sleep patterns. The chronic pain in conditions such as arthritis and back problems as well as depression, anxiety, and stress can interfere with sleep. Older men often develop noncancerous enlargement of the prostate gland (benign prostatic hyperplasia), which can cause the need to urinate frequently, interrupting sleep. In women, hot flashes and urinary urgency that accompany menopause can be equally disruptive. Other sleep-related disorders, such as sleep apnea and restless legs syndrome, also become more common with age. Sleep apnea causes one to stop breathing periodically throughout the night and awaken. Restless legs syndrome causes an unpleasant sensation in the legs and an uncontrollable desire to move them, which may awaken one or prevent one from falling asleep. Nutritional depletions may be the reason for the restless legs syndrome, and therefore nutritional supplements may help. A nutritionist or physician can help make recommendations.

Box 8-2   COMMON CAUSES OF INSOMNIA

Stress. Realistic and unrealistic concerns about work, school, health, or family keep the mind too active and unable to relax for sleep. The busy brain and excessive boredom can create stress and interfere with sleep.

Anxiety. Everyday anxieties as well as severe anxiety disorders may keep the mind too alert to fall asleep at the beginning or in the middle of the night.

Depression. People either sleep too much or have trouble sleeping if depressed. This may be due to chemical imbalances in the brain or because worries that accompany depression may keep them from relaxing enough to fall asleep when needed.

Stimulants. Prescription drugs, including some antidepressant, high blood pressure, and steroid medications, can interfere with sleep. Many over-the-counter medications, including some brands of aspirin, decongestants, and weight-loss products, contain caffeine and other stimulants. Antihistamines may initially make one groggy, and they can worsen urinary problems, making it necessary to get up more during the night.

Changes in the environment or work schedule. Travel or working a late or early shift can disrupt the body's circadian rhythms, making it difficult to get to sleep. Circadian rhythms act as internal clocks, guiding the wake-sleep cycle, body metabolism, and body temperature.

Long-term use of sleep medications. Doctors generally recommend using sleeping pills only for up to 4 weeks until the person notices benefits from self-help measures. If someone needs sleep medications longer, they should be used no more than 2 to 4 times a week so that they don't become habit-forming. Sleeping pills often become less effective over time.

Medical conditions that cause pain. These include arthritis, fibromyalgia, and neuropathies that result in nerve pain. Many people with fibromyalgia experience higher-frequency brain waves than normally expected when they sleep. The higher-frequency brain waves may interfere with the restfulness of sleep.

Behavioral insomnia. This may occur when people worry excessively about not being able to sleep and try too hard to fall asleep. Most people with this condition sleep better when they're away from their usual sleep environment or when they don't try to sleep, such as when they're watching TV.

Eating too much too late in the evening. Having a light snack before bedtime is OK, but eating too much may cause the person to feel physically uncomfortable when lying down, making it difficult to get to sleep. Many people also experience heartburn, or reflux, which is a back flow of food from the stomach to the esophagus after eating. This uncomfortable feeling may keep a person awake.

The following strategies promote restorative sleep:

- Stick to a schedule. Keep bedtime and wake time routines on as constant a schedule as possible.
- Limit time in bed. Too much time in bed can promote shallow, unrestful sleep. Try to get up at the same time each morning, regardless of when going to bed.
- Avoid "trying" to sleep. The harder a person tries, the more awake the person becomes. Reading or listening to music until drowsy helps one to fall asleep naturally.
- Avoid or limit caffeine, alcohol, and nicotine. Caffeine and nicotine can keep a person from falling asleep. Alcohol can cause unrestful sleep and frequent awakenings.
- Reset the body's clock. If falling asleep too early, use light to push back the internal clock. In the evenings, if it still light, go outside in the sun or sit near a bright light.
- Check medications. If medications are taken regularly, check with the doctor to see if the medications may be contributing to sleep disturbances. Also check the labels of over-the-counter products to see if they contain caffeine or other stimulants such as pseudoephedrine.
- Don't put up with pain. Make sure that any pain reliever being taken is effective enough to control pain while sleeping.
- Find ways to relax. A warm bath or light snack before bedtime may help prepare for sleep. Massage also may help promote relaxation.
- Limit naps. Naps can make it harder to fall asleep at night.
- Minimize sleep interruptions. Close the bedroom door or create a subtle background noise, such as running a fan, to help drown out other noises. Sleep in a different room if the bed partner snores.
- Adjust bedroom temperatures. The room should be comfortably cool.
- Limit nighttime use of the bathroom by drinking less toward the evening.

The training and competing athlete needs an appropriate amount of restorative sleep. This is typically 8 to 9 hours at night and a 1-hour nap. Playing schedules and travel to different time zones disrupt an athlete's sleep patterns. Sleeping in a different bed when traveling can also be a problem.

SUMMARY

This chapter briefly describes the mental and emotional world of the athlete. The role of the sport psychologist is becoming increasingly important. More people are seeking professional assistance for coping and performance, especially in managing stress. Stress is both mental and physical. It is in this area that massage is most beneficial.

The massage therapist must not take on the role of psychologist. Instead, the massage professional provides a skilled and compassionate touch, a nonjudgmental and no-advice giving presence, and a supportive and quiet experience.

1 Write a case study (fictional or real) about the circumstances that would indicate that a client needs a referral to help with mental and emotional coping.

Example: A 29 year old golfer has played in eight tournaments and he hasn't made the cut (got into the final money-making rounds). He is not sleeping and has been experiencing headaches and an "upset stomach."

_____

_____

_____

_____

_____

_____

2 Using the case study you wrote about in Question 1 and the approach used by sport psychologists, identify at least three methods that would be appropriate to help the client.

Example: visualization, hypnosis, progressive relaxation.

_____

_____

_____

_____

_____

_____

_____

_____

_____

3 Again, using the case study from Question 1, develop a massage treatment plan that would complement the treatment of a sport psychologist.

Example: parasympathetic dominance, deep pressure, nonspecific massage with attention to breathing function.

_____

_____

_____

_____

_____

_____

_____

_____

_____

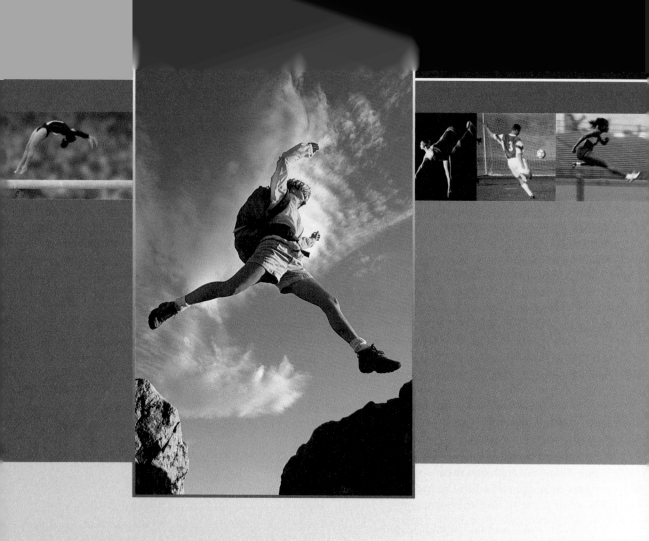

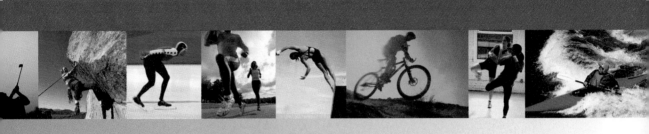

UNIT TWO

SPORTS MASSAGE: THEORY AND APPLICATION

STORIES
from the field
ROBERT PORCHER

All persons—athletes included—have a story. Each individual's story shapes his or her life. Because when working with so-called celebrities, one commonly focuses on what they do instead of who they are, I have included a few stories of individuals, who are also athletes, to put into perspective the importance of the professional relationship the massage therapist achieves and maintains with this type of client. We do not provide massage to a football player or basketball player or golfer. We support individuals in their own personal quest for achievement. The stories I have chosen to tell are about those with whom I have spent the most time and therefore know the best. The stories are from my point of view and with their permission.

The first time I saw Robert, he was walking around with his baby daughter's pacifier. He is an NFL defensive end, which means he is big. A big young man with a pacifier was a sight to see. When I first met Robert, he was at the peak of his career, going to the Pro Bowl more than once. He is one of the most polite and respectful persons I have ever met. He has played his entire football career with one NFL team. This is a rare occurrence these days. Because of this he has established a strong and enduring influence on the local community and plans to continue living in the Detroit area.

Robert is a man of family values. He loves his wife and kids. During the time I have worked with him, two more babies have been born. I have had the opportunity to be part of the pregnancy experience with his wife. I continue to work with her and with Robert.

Being a professional athlete's wife is not easy. I truly admire what it takes to maintain the infrastructure of a relatively normal family experience. Kim has been able to pull this off.

As of this writing, Robert is in his thirteenth year of professional football. He has been the rookie, the star, and now for the last 2 years the mentor for the young players coming up. I most admire his commitment to the mentoring aspect of his career.

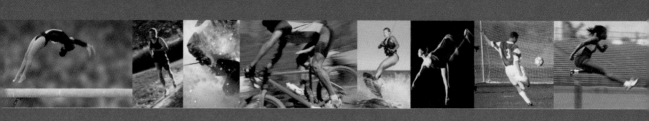

Being involved in professional sports is demanding on the emotional, spiritual, and physical being. No one remains at peak performance forever. Many do not make the transition easily. I have watched Robert work though many different stages during the years I have been his massage therapist. Right now he is at the end of his career. He has managed to remain relatively injury free partly because he does yoga, gets regular massage, and partly because he is strong and physically able to withstand the ongoing trauma.

He has done very well in preparing for the next stage of his life so that as he makes this transition from football player to businessman and community leader, all the pieces are in place. One of his future goals is to help other football players make this transition. Most football players only play 3 or 4 years before injury or other circumstances end their careers, and many do not transition well.

Even though Robert has endured his years of football without major injory, there are lingering physical issues. I have agreed to continue to work with him and his wife even after he retires from football. Even though he will leave football, his years as a professional athlete will continue to affect him his entire life.

Working with Robert all these years has been more about maintenance than injury rehabilitation. Week after week during the season I would massage out the aches and pains. Now this is a big job because Robert is a big man. Week after week I have observed him evolve from a kid to a man.

The year that most stands out in my mind was the year that the family was separated during the season. Kim and the kids needed to live elsewhere during the football season that year. This period was hard on the whole family, but since I spent the most time with him, that is the perspective I got.

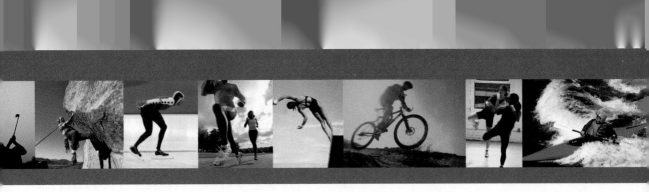

He was lonely. I do not think I have ever seen someone as lonely as Robert was that year. One of the benefits of massage is an increase in the neurochemicals that make one feel less alone. I would show up for the massage, he would put in a movie, and I would time the massage to be over when the movie was over. We seldom talked, but he was not alone and he did not feel so lonely for a while. The massage helped him endure the separation. We talked about it—later—like several years later. Sometimes it is best just to do the job without making a big deal of it. Recently, he shared with me that he does not want to be separated from his family ever again.

I remember that Kim became ill just after the last baby girl was born. I happened to be there for massage, and because of circumstances, Robert and I had the baby with us. There we were, this great big football player, this week-old baby, and me. The baby was on his chest for most of the massage. For a while he was on his side while he fed her and then she was back on his chest. She spit up on him. I wiped it off, and eventually they both went to sleep.

Over the years, I have watched Robert and Kim be very involved with community charities. One of their focuses has been cancer research and treatment. It has been a privilege to observe this family travel though the demands of living in the public eye and achieve and sustain a sort of normalcy. The last time I was at their home just before writing this story, I observed Robert vacuuming the floor, Kim handing her oldest daughter supplies to clean the bathroom, their son running around in a Batman costume, and their youngest running around in nothing. A family. ■

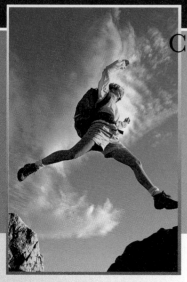

CHAPTER

9 PHYSIOLOGIC MECHANISMS OF MASSAGE BENEFITS

OBJECTIVES

Upon completion of this chapter the reader will have the information necessary to:

1 Understand and describe massage outcomes based on known and theoretical physiologic mechanisms.

2 List and describe the four general outcomes for the athlete/fitness and physical rehabilitation population.

3 Incorporate the reflexive and mechanical application of massage to the four general outcomes.

Typically the application of massage and bodywork is described in terms of methods and modalities instead of physiologic response. To better understand the relationship of massage application to the synergistic interface with sport performance it is necessary to move beyond the classic description of massage in terms such as effleurage or gliding strokes, petrissage or kneading, compression, friction, vibration, rocking, shaking (oscillation), tapotement or percussion, and joint movement. Modalities such as reflexology, shiatsu, Rolfing, Trager, and so forth also do not describe mechanisms of benefits and outcomes. Instead, massage application needs to be described by the stimulus that is being applied to a specific receptor or the force that is being applied to affect a specific tissue type or physiologic function. Variations in depth of pressure, drag on the tissue, speed of application, direction of movement, frequency of application, duration of application, and rhythm allow for extensive application options based on treatment plan outcomes.

OVERVIEW AND REVIEW

Massage and **bodywork** can be described as a manual application to the body that influences multiple body responses. Research has shown that massage has validity in influencing body structure and

Autonomic nervous system (ANS)
Bodywork
Bending loading
Combined loading
Compression loading
Condition management
Cortisol
Counterirritation
Dopamine
Energy systems
Entrainment

Epinephrine/adrenaline
Fluid movement
Growth hormone
Hyperstimulation analgesia
Massage
Mechanical methods
Motor tone
Muscle tome
Myofascial dysfunction
Nerve impingement
Norepinephrine/noradrenaline

Neuroendocrine regulation
Oxytocin
Palliative care
Performance enhancement
Recovery
Reflex response
Serotonin
Shear loading
Tension loading
Vestibular apparatus

function. It is the body's ability to respond, and to adapt to the stimuli and forces applied to it, that achieves the outcomes.

This chapter reviews and expands on the concept of massage benefits based on outcomes related to the structure and function of the body. This is important information if the massage therapist is going to make intelligent decisions regarding massage application for the target population. Research data are beginning to identify patterns of the underlying physiologic mechanisms that massage addresses. Research results identify a pattern of physiologic effects regardless of the philosophy of the system used and indicate that soft tissue method benefits seem to be attributable to a cluster of physiologic effects. It is important to remember that ongoing research will change how the effects of massage are understood. Future research findings will either confirm or conflict those to-date. Either is fine, as the evolution continues to clarify what makes therapeutic massage beneficial.

Current understanding indicates that the effects of massage occur through the interrelationships of the central nervous system (CNS) and the peripheral nervous system (and their reflex patterns and multiple pathways), the **autonomic nervous system (ANS)**, and neuroendocrine control. The current consensus is that massage produces effects due to a combination of neural, chemical, mechanical, and psychological factors that are important in supporting athletic performance and a fitness lifestyle.

In general terms, the total sensory input to the CNS affects overall tension throughout the body. This is why nonphysical emotional and mental stress can lead to physical symptoms such as headaches, digestive problems, and muscular discomfort. Massage works on many levels, which aim to reduce the symptoms that cause negative sensory input and to increase the positive sensory input. This accounts for the general well-being that clients usually feel after treatment.

Massage can affect the nervous system in several ways. It stimulates the nerve receptors in the tissues that control tissue tension. On a sensory level, the mechanoreceptors' response to touch, pressure, warmth, and so on are stimulated. Generally, a reflex effect leads to further relaxation of the tissues and a reduction in pain.

Tension in the soft tissues can cause overactivity in the sympathetic nervous system. By releasing this tension, massage can restore the balance and stimulate the parasympathetic system, resulting in a positive effect on both minor and sometimes quite major medical conditions, such as high blood pressure, migraine, insomnia, and digestive disorders.

SPORT/FITNESS AND REHABILITATION OUTCOMES

The main outcomes of massage for sport and fitness are increased body stamina, stability,

123

mobility, flexibility, agility, reduced soft tissue tension and binding, normalized fluid (blood and lymph) movement, management of pain, reduction of suffering, support of healing mechanisms, alteration of mood, improved physical and mental performance, and experiences of pleasure. All of these outcomes can be appropriately applied to athlete care or rehabilitation of pathology, especially within the context of a multidisciplinary system.

These outcomes can be classified as four goal patterns for sport and fitness:

1. Performance enhancement/recovery
2. Condition management
3. Rehabilitation/therapeutic change
4. Palliative care

PERFORMANCE ENHANCEMENT/RECOVERY

As previously discussed, fitness and performance are not the same. Optimal performance is most often achieved when fitness is attended to first. Performance motivation and activity exceed fitness requirements by pushing the body to achieve activities that are outside the fitness parameters. Performance therefore becomes a strain on the system. Balancing fitness and performance is tricky with athletes. It is important for those whose goals are fitness-oriented to not exceed the beneficial physical outcomes by being caught up in performance demands that lead to increased strain on adaptive capacity.

Continual performance demand interferes with fitness and compromises health. Normal function and performance are not the same. A person learning to walk again after an accident exerts effort and has similar physical manifestations and demands on the body as an athlete seeking to decrease his or her 40-yard dash time. However, one is seeking to regain normal function and the other is striving for peak performance. Performance is more than normal function.

The sports massage therapist needs to consider how the massage application supports the following client goals

- Achieve normal function through rehabilitation and conditioning.
- Maintain fitness.
- Reduce the negative effects that performance demand places on the body in excess of normal function.

All people who engage in exercise may strive for excellence at some performance level. The elderly person beginning a cardiac rehabilitation program, the professional athlete striving for success in com-petition, the child learning to walk—anyone who uses the body in a precise way—are all concerned about the ability to carry out an action with skill. Their motivations may vary but the desired outcome is the same—increased proficiency when performing the activity. Physical performance involves training, practice, and demand on the body. When desired performance levels are achieved and practiced, they become automatic.

Performance enhancement requires increasing demand on the body through practice. Maintaining performance involves attention to demand on the body and reinforcement. Each individual has a range of peak performance where the triad of body/mind/spirit function in their optimal range. As discussed in Chapter 8, this is called "the zone." Peak performance is difficult to maintain for extended periods of time. **Recovery** is necessary to restore depleted energy and regenerate damaged soft tissue. Most athletes train at levels below peak performance with the desired outcome of reaching that peak during competition. This process is com-promised if ongoing competition is extended over periods of time. This is common in professional athletes, especially in team sports such as baseball, basketball, football, hockey, and soccer.

Massage application can support performance by facilitating recovery and removing impediments to training. The general massage protocol described in Chapter 14 targets performance and enhancing recovery. Obviously the protocol needs to be altered to fit each individual client, but it is a reliable pattern from which to work.

CONDITION MANAGEMENT

The goal of condition management is used to manage ongoing strain that is not going to change. Examples of such strain are inherent joint laxity, previous injury, emotional demands, and playing schedule. Maintaining the status quo is a common outcome for competing athletes, especially toward the end of a playing season. The general massage protocol in Chapter 14 is appropriate as long as the massage therapist understands that the goal is to maintain, not improve.

REHABILITATION/THERAPEUTIC CHANGE

Injury is a common consequence of physical activity. Anyone who has worked with competing athletes knows the importance of injury prevention and of effective, accelerated injury recovery. Most athletes practice or compete when injured at one time or another. When injury is involved, performance is compromised. It takes more energy, accommodation, and compensation to perform when injured. Specifically, rehabilitation is the return to normal function, and for the athlete this means return to peak performance (that is, to function above normal).

Massage in this area is complex and requires the most training. Unit Three of this text deals specifically with injury. The specific massage application for injury is integrated into the general massage protocol described in Chapter 14.

PALLIATIVE CARE

Palliative care includes comfort, support, nurturance, and pleasure, which are essential in the care of the athlete. Attention to warm environment, atmosphere, and ambience is part of the caring experience. Patience, flexibility, and commitment are part of the process. Competing athletes are tired, disappointed, and in pain much of the time. Periods of exhilaration and disappointment occur within complex life experiences. The losing athlete needs more support than the winning one. The older athlete needs more care than the young one. When exercising for fitness, weight loss, and rehabilitation, similar stresses occur. Reducing suffering and offering pleasurable sensation are invaluable to reduce the psychological and physical responses to these stresses.

In both training and rehabilitation, plateaus are reached. The satisfaction of seeing ongoing changes is diminished, and palliative care may be able to support the athlete during these periods. Diminished performance because of fatigue and other pressures can be comforted temporarily by nurturing touch. Sometimes there is just too much aching and pain to endure any longer; in this case, palliative massage is the most beneficial.

An example is rookie football players in the second week of training camp. They are tired, stressed, sore, and a bit difficult. Their adaptive capacity is maxed out at the moment, and yet they are driven to perform. The best massage approach is palliative care, not performance enhancement.

UNDERSTANDING THE EFFECTS OF THERAPEUTIC MASSAGE

For an effective understanding of the overlap of massage/bodywork in the context of sport and fitness, a very mechanistic approach is presented in this text. However, it is important to remember that touch is a multidimensional experience, encompassing both client's and therapist's body/mind/spirit experience and the interplay of these three realms in the therapeutic relationship. Just because massage can be explained in terms of stimuli and forces does not change the fact that it is an integrated experience that is difficult to describe, with important intentions of nurturance, compassion, and respect. Although research has identified most of the physiologic mechanisms of massage effects, the mystery of the unknown remains and must be honored.

The terms *bodywork* and *massage* encompass a huge array of methods and philosophies. This chapter does not intend to teach the application of these methods and styles because excellent instructional texts already exist (see the recommended reading list at the end of the book). The focus of this chapter is to describe the underlying theme of all of the methods and the relationship to sport and fitness goals, measurable outcomes, and physiologic pleasurable mechanisms, even though research has not totally proven the response correlation.

Massage effects are determined by reflexive and mechanical outcomes or some combination of both. **Reflex response** results from stimulus of the nervous system to activate feedback loops with the therapeutic intent of adjustment in neuromuscular, neurotransmitter, endocrine, or ANS homeostatic mechanisms. For example, light stimulus of the skin usually results in a tickle or itch response and is arousing and stimulating.

Mechanical methods impose various forces such as tension, compression, rotation or torsion, bending, and shearing and the combination of these forces to change body structure or function (Figure 9-1). This is explained more fully in Chapter 13. Thus, the outcome of massage application is to influence the adaptive, restorative, and healing capacity of the body. Anatomic and physiologic outcomes include:

- Local tissue repair, such as a sprain or contusion.
- Connective tissue normalization that affects elasticity, stiffness, and strength, such as increased pliability of scar tissue or overall flexibility.
- Shifts in pressure gradients to influence body fluid movement.
- Neuromuscular function interfacing with the muscle length-tension relationship; force couples; motor tone of muscles; concentric, eccentric, and isometric functions; and con-

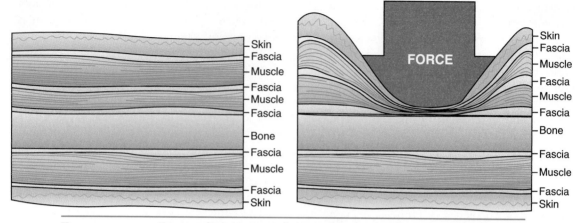

FIGURE 9-1 ■ Massage applications systematically generate force through each tissue layer. This figure provides a graphic representation of force applied, which would begin with light superficial application, progressing with increased pressure to the deepest layer. (From Fritz S: *Mosby's fundamentals of therapeutic massage*, ed 3. St. Louis, 2004, Mosby.)

traction patterns of muscles working together to support efficient movement.

- Mood and pain modulation through shifts in ANS function, yielding neurochemical and neuroendocrine responses.
- Increased immune response to support systemic health and healing.

Each of these common outcomes for massage supports rehabilitation, fitness, and performance recovery.

Structure can be thought of as anatomy and function as physiology. Most massage outcomes influence physiology through both reflexive and mechanical applications. Some massage applications can shift structure, primarily though influence on the connective tissue of the body. Massage always has a physiologic result because of the adaptation required to the presence of the massage practitioner, the sensory stimulation of various touch receptors, and the client's perception of the therapeutic interaction. Therefore, massage can achieve primarily physiologic responses of the body, and we cannot isolate massage results as strictly structural outcomes. This is an important concept in understanding the synergistic and multidisciplinary use of various modalities to support the athlete.

Even though massage can be explained by the following descriptions, it is seldom simple. Mechanical massage application can feel intense and be interpreted as painful, but comforting measures that are more reflexive can support the acceptance of the method. What is considered a reflexive stimulus usually results from a mechanical force applied to the body. A skilled practitioner recognizes the complexity of touch interaction. The following reductive description can simplify the thought processes necessary during clinical reasoning, but the practitioner needs to integrate the experience of the client during analysis of the results achieved.

STRUCTURAL/MECHANICAL EFFECTS

Manual methods of massage that most specifically affect body structure occur as the result of the application of forces to the body to load the tissue. Connective tissue and fluid dynamics are most affected by force.

The forces created by massage are tension loading, compression loading, bending loading, shear loading, rotation or torsion loading, and combined loading.

Tension Loading

9-1 Tissues elongate under **tension loading** with the intent of lengthening shortened tissues (Figure 9-2). Tension force is created by methods such as traction, longitudinal stretching, and stroking with tissue drag. Tension forces also cause an aggregation of collagen, resulting in thicker and denser tissue to improve direction of fiber development, stiffness, and strength. Tension loading is effective during the secondary phase of healing after the acute inflammatory stage has begun to dissipate.

Compression Loading

9-2 During **compression loading** (Figure 9-3), tissue shortens and widens, increasing the pressure within the tissue and affecting fluid flow.

FIGURE 9-2
TENSION LOADING

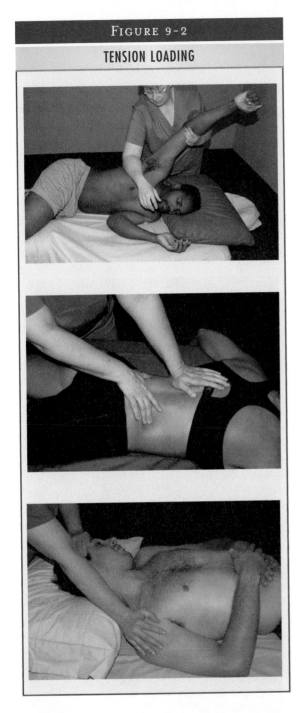

FIGURE 9-3
COMPRESSION LOADING

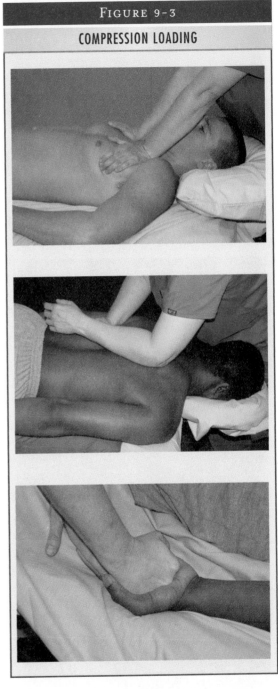

Compression is effective as a rhythmic pumplike method to facilitate fluid dynamics. Sustained compression results in more pliable connective tissue structures and is effective in reducing tissue density and binding.

Bending Loading

9-3

In **bending loading** (Figure 9-4), the therapist applies combined forces of tension on the convex side and compression on the concave side of the tissue. Bending is used when combined effects of lengthening and shortening and an increase in pliability are desired.

Shear Loading

9-4

In **shear loading** (Figure 9-5), the massage therapist moves tissue back and forth, creating a combined pattern of compression and

FIGURE 9-4

BENDING LOADING

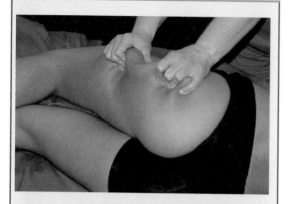

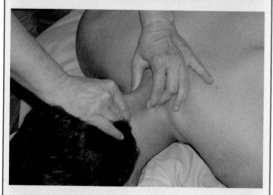

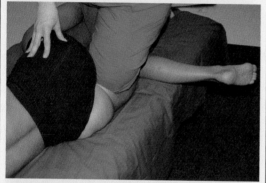

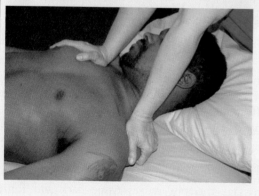

FIGURE 9-5

SHEAR LOADING

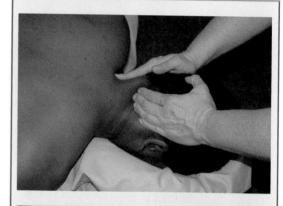

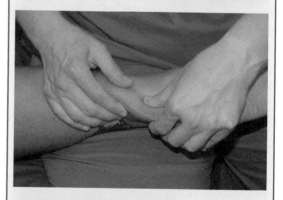

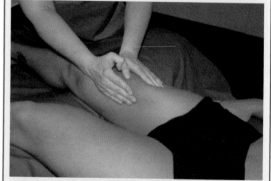

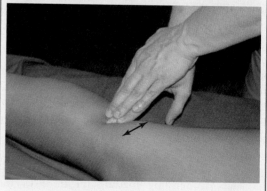

elongation of tissue. This method is particularly effective in creating controlled inflammation and in ensuring that tissue layers slide over one another instead of adhering to underlying layers, creating binding.

9-5 Rotation or Torsion Loading (Figure 9-6)

Rotation or torsion loading (Figure 9-6) is a combined application of compression and wringing resulting in elongation of tissue along the axis of rotation. It is used when a combined effect of both fluid dynamics and connective tissue pliability is desired.

9-6 Combined Loading

In **combined loading** (Figure 9-7) two or more forces are used to load tissue. The more forces applied to tissue, the more intense the response. Tension and compression underlie all the different modes of loading; therefore, any form of manipulation is either tension, compression, or a combination of these. Tension is important in conditions in which tissue needs to be elongated; compression is important when fluid flow needs to be affected. Oscillation of tissue can be considered combined loading.

CONNECTIVE TISSUE INFLUENCES

The mechanical behavior of soft issue in response to tissue loading is related to the property of connective tissue viscoelasticity, as described in the anatomy and physiology review in Unit One. Connective tissue is a biological material that contains a combination of stiff and elastic fibers embedding a gel medium. Connective tissue, the structural component of the body, is the most abundant body tissue. Its functions include support, structure, space, stabilization, and scar formation. It assumes many forms and shapes, from fluid blood to dense bone. The pliability of connective tissue, which is based on its water-binding components, is significantly affected by connective tissue massage. Connective tissue is adaptive and responsive to a variety of influences, such as injury, immobilization, overuse (increased demand), and underuse (decreased demand).

The basic connective tissue massage approach consists of mechanically softening the tissue through introducing various mechanical forces that result in pressure, pulling, movement, and stretch on the tissues, which allow them to rehydrate and become more pliable. The process is similar to softening gelatin by warming it. If you want connec-

FIGURE 9-6

ROTATIONAL/TORSION

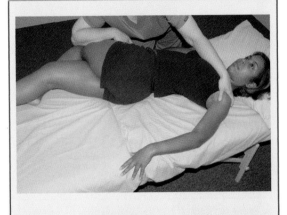
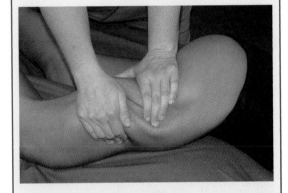
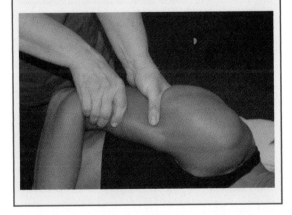

tive tissue to stay soft, water must be added. This is one reason why it is important for the client to drink water before and after the massage.

The stretching, pulling, or pressure on the connective tissue is a little different from that of neuromuscular methods. Neuromuscular techniques usually flow in the direction of the fibers to affect the proprioceptive mechanism and create a quick response. Connective tissue approaches are slow

FIGURE 9-7

COMBINED LOADING

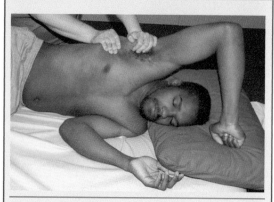

A, Tension and torsion.

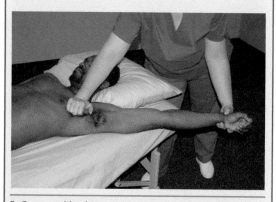

B, Tension and bending.

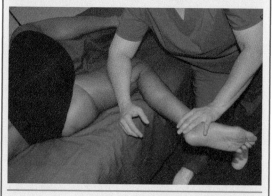

C, Compression and bending

and sustained, usually against or across the fibers. Connective tissue stretching is elongated or telescoped at the point of the tissue movement barrier.

Another aspect of connective tissue massage application is the generation of healing potentials from creating controlled therapeutic inflammation.

The most specific localized example of this type of application is Dr. James Cyriax's cross-fiber friction concept. This method is effective, especially around joints, where the tendons and ligaments become bound down to underlying or adjacent tissue. Deep transverse friction is always a specific rehabilitation intervention. It introduces therapeutic inflammation through the creation of a specific and controlled acute reinjury of the tissues. The frictioning can last as long as 15 minutes to create the controlled reinjury of the tissue, which introduces a small amount of inflammation and traumatic hyperemia to the area. The result is the restructuring of the connective tissue, increased circulation to the area, and temporary analgesia.

Proper rehabilitation after friction massage is essential for the friction technique to be effective and produce a mobile scar or rehealing of the tissue. The frictioned area must be contracted painlessly without any strain put on the frictioned tissue. This is done by fixing the joint in a position in which the muscle is relaxed, and then having the client contract the muscle as far as it will go. This is sometimes called a *broadening contraction* (Figure 9-8). This exercise is repeated 5 to 10 repetitions, three to four time a day.

The Myofascial System

Fascia is loose, irregular connective tissue with a multidirectional network of collagen and elastin fibers. It has a large percentage of ground substance. As previously described, fascia has many thixotropic and colloidal qualities.

Fascia in some form surrounds and separates almost every structure and cell in the body. It forms the interstitial spaces (spaces between individual cells). Fascia is involved in structural and visceral support, as well as separation and protection, and therefore influences respiration, elimination, metabolism, fluid flow, and the immune system. Fascia is stress-responsive, becoming thicker in response to real or perceived threats, as well as any other activation of the sympathetic ANS nervous system. This emotional response of the fascial guarding system is sometimes called *body armoring.* It is an important factor in the

FIGURE 9-8

BROADENING CONTRACTION

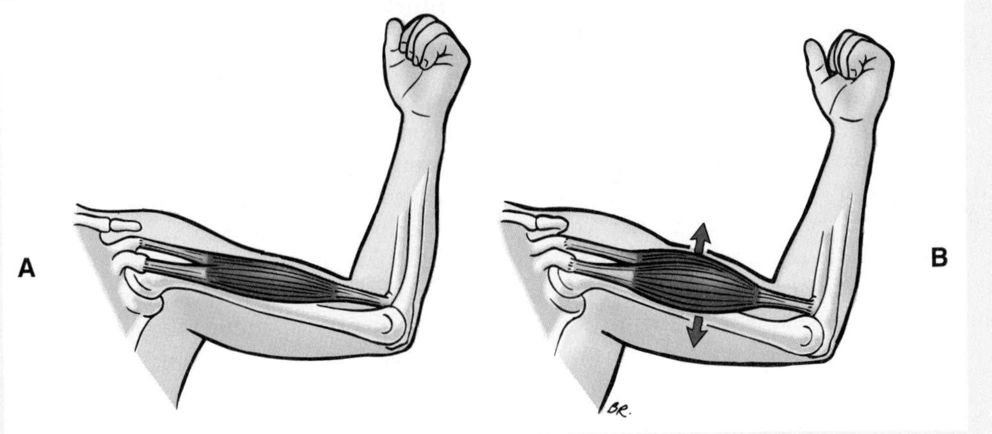

A, Beginning point. **B,** Contract the muscle by flexing the joint. (From Fritz S: *Mosby's fundamentals of therapeutic massage,* ed 3. St. Louis, 2004, Mosby.)

relationship between the body and emotional expression. This factor is often a component of body/mind approaches.

The body has a tensegretic form. Although every structure is ultimately held together by a balance of tension and compression, tensegrity structures are characterized by continuous tension and local compression.

Tension forces naturally transmit over the shortest distance between two points; therefore, these structures offer a maximum amount of strength for a given amount of material.

A tensegrity model of the body combines the tension (muscle or fascia) and compression (bones) factors of a mechanical model of the musculoskeletal display, but the compression members are islands, floating in a sea of continuous tension. The compression members push outward against the tension members, which pull inward. As long as the two sets of forces are balanced, the structure is stable. A tent constructed of canvas, poles, and tension supplied by ropes is a good example of tensegrity.

A tensegrity structure generally is less stiff and more resilient than a continuous compression structure. Load one "corner" of a tensegrity structure, and the whole structure gives a little to accommodate. Load it too much, and the structure ultimately breaks, but not necessarily anywhere

near where the load was placed. Because strain is distributed throughout the structure along the lines of tension, the tensegrity structure may "give" at a weak point remote from the area of applied strain. All the interconnected structural elements of a tensegrity model rearrange themselves in response to a local stress. As the applied stress (load) increases, more of the structures come to lie in the direction of the applied stress, resulting in a linear stiffening of the material. Tensegrity structures, therefore, are resilient, becoming more stable the more they are loaded.

Because the body is a tensegrity structure, an injury at any given site often begins as long-term strain in other parts of the body. The injury manifests where it does because of inherent weakness, or previous injury, not purely or always because of local strain or a direct impact. Discovering these points of tension and easing chronic strain in the body is a natural part of restoring balance in the structure, and tends to prevent future injuries.

As mentioned previously, the bones of the body are compressing structures, and the myofascial tissues are surrounding tension structures. In this model the bones are seen as "spacers" that push out into the soft tissue, and the tone of the tensile myofascia becomes the determinant of balanced structure. To change the relationships among the bones, change the tensional balance through the soft tissue, and the bones will rearrange themselves.

Whenever movement occurs in the body, the extracellular matrix extends, cells distort, and the interconnected molecules that constitute the internal framework of the cell feel the pull. The mechanical restructuring of the cell and cytoskeleton apparently tells the cell what to do. Very flat cells, with their cytoskeletons stretched, sense that more cells are needed to cover the surrounding area, as in wound repair, and that cell division is needed. Rounding indicates that too many cells are competing for space on the matrix and that cells are proliferating too rapidly; some must die to prevent tumor formation. In between those two extremes, normal tissue function is established and maintained.

This research points toward a holistic role for the mechanical distribution of strain in the body that goes far beyond merely dealing with localized tissue pain. Creating an even tone across the bones and myofascial component and, further, across the entire fascial net, can have profound implications for health, both cellular and general. The goal for massage is to support balance in the myofascial systems.

Classifications of fascial layering are artificial, because the tensegric nature of fascia is one large, interconnected, three-dimensional microscopic dynamic grid structure that connects everything with everything. Through the fascial system, if you pull on the little toe you affect the nose, and if the structure of the nose is dysfunctional, it can pull anywhere in the body, including the little toe.

Although fascia generally orients itself vertically in the body, it will orient in any directional stress pattern. For example, scar tissue may redirect fascial structures, as can trauma, repetitive strain patterns, and immobility. This redirection of structural forces occurs as a result of compensation patterns. During physical assessment, the body appears "pulled" out of symmetry or stuck.

There are also three or four transverse fascial planes in the body (depending on the resource you use). They are located at the cranial base, cervical thoracic area, diaphragm, and lumbar and pelvic floor areas. Transverse planes exist for joints as well.

Myofascial/Connective Tissue Dysfunction

Myofascial/connective tissue dysfunction compromises the efficiency of the body, requiring an increase in energy expenditure to achieve functioning ability. Fatigue and pain often result.

Fascial shortening and thickening restrict movement, and the easy undulations of the body rhythms and entrainment mechanisms are disturbed. Twists and torsions of the fascia bind and restrict movement from the cellular level outward to joint mobility. This binding can be likened to ill-fitting clothing or, more graphically, "fascial wedgies." The dysfunctions are difficult to diagnose medically, are not apparent with standard medical testing, and are a factor in many elusive chronic pain and fatigue patterns. They can disrupt athletic performance demands.

Healing of damage to body tissues requires the formation of connective tissue. In the first stages of healing, the inflammatory response is one trigger that generates the healing process. When the inflammatory response does not effectively resolve itself, more new tissue than is needed forms, and adhesions or fibrotic tissue develop. An adhesion is an attachment of connective tissue to structures not directly involved with the area of injury. Fibrosis is abnormal tissue formation, often in response to increased protein content in stagnant edematous tissue. Massage can be used to affect chronic inflammation, adhesion, and fibrotic tissue formation. Forces are applied to the adhesions and fibrotic tissue to create mild inflammation to stimulate connective tissue remodeling.

Connective tissue dysfunction usually is suspected as a factor in disorders older than 12 weeks, especially if the inflammatory response and muscle tone patterns have not effectively resolved during normal healing.

Two basic massage approaches are used to address connective tissue dysfunction, and more importantly, to prevent dysfunction from occurring:

1. Some methods address the ground substance, which is thixotropic, meaning that the substance liquefies on agitation and reverts to a gel when standing. Ground substance is also a colloid. A colloid is a system of solids in a liquid medium that resists abrupt pressure but yields to slow, sustained pressure. (Think silly putty or clay).
2. Other methods address the fibers contained within the ground substance. The fibers are collagenous (ropelike), elastic (rubber band–like), or reticular (meshlike).

Methods that primarily affect the ground substance have a quality of slow, sustained pressure and agitation. Use of shearing, bending, and torsion forces and tension (tensile stretch) applied during massage adds energy to the matrix, softening it and encouraging rehydration. Most massage methods can soften the ground substance as long as the application is not abrupt.

Thermal influences from repeated loading and unloading create hysteresis, which is the process of energy loss due to friction when tissues are loaded and unloaded. On/off application of compression and oscillation methods that are intense enough to load tissues are often used. Heat will be produced during such a sequence, affecting the viscosity of the ground substance. The increase in pliability is due to the thixotropic nature of connective tissue ground substance through the introduction of energy by the application of forces, particularly shear and torsion, which cause a gel to become less viscous, because the tissue is hydrophilic and attracts water. Attention to these methods and outcomes is supportive of athletic massage goals.

Due to the water content of connective tissue, the balance of fluid flow, appropriate hydration, and principles of fluid dynamics in the body is integral to applying effective massage. Thermal or warming modalities support this process.

The fiber component of connective tissue is affected by methods that elongate the fibers past the elastic range (i.e., past the normal give) into the plastic range (i.e., past the bind or point of restriction). For chronic conditions, an acute inflammatory response can be created by using massage to create minor rupture of collagen fibers, leaving free endpoints. These endpoints initiate an inflammatory response and synthesis of collagen by the fibroblasts. The collagen is deposited to reunite the endpoints. The newly formed tissue has a low tensile strength, is more susceptible to forces imposed, and can be encouraged to change structure, including increased or decreased tissue density, direction, and layering. Continued massage applications serve to influence tissue direction, length, and pliability, as well as support effective healing. The positive therapeutic objective is to create therapeutic inflammation to encourage adaptation to controlled damage. The methods used to create the therapeutic inflammatory process are intense and may be interpreted as pain. The method used most often is friction (shear force).

Fascial restrictions can create abnormal strain patterns that can crowd or pull the osseous structures out of proper alignment. This results in compression of joints, producing pain and/or movement dysfunction. Neural and vascular structures can also become entrapped in these restrictions causing neurological or ischemic conditions. Shortening of the myofascial fascicle can limit its functional length, reducing its strength, contractile potential, and deceleration capacity.

Chaitow and DeLany* describe a typical sequence of how dysfunction occurs after an event:

The longer the immobilization, the greater the amount of infiltrate there will be.

If immobilization continues beyond 12 weeks collagen loss is noted; in the early days of any restriction, a significant degree of ground substance loss occurs, particularly glycosaminoglycans and water.

Since one of the primary purposes of ground substance is the lubrication of the tissues it separates (collagen fibers), its loss leads inevitably to the distance between these fibers being reduced.

Loss of interfiber distance impedes the ability of collagen to glide smoothly, encouraging adhesion development.

This allows crosslinkage between collagen fibers and newly formed connective tissue, which reduces the degree of fascial extensibility as adjacent fibers become more and more closely bound.

Because of immobility, these new fiber connections will not have a stress load to guide them into a directional format and they will be laid down randomly.

Similar responses are observed in ligamentous as well as periarticular connective tissues.

Mobilization of the restricted tissues can reverse the effects of immobilization as long as the condition is fairly new.

If, due to injury, inflammatory processes occur as well as immobilization, a more serious evolution occurs, as inflammatory exudate triggers the process of contracture, resulting in shortening of connective tissue.

This means that following injury, two separate processes may be occurring simultaneously: scar tissue development in the traumatized tissues and also fibrosis in the surrounding tissues as a result of the presence of inflammatory exudate.

FLUID MOVEMENT

The movement of fluids in the body is also a mechanical process. Forces applied to the body mimic various pumping mechanisms of the heart,

---

*From Chaitow L, DeLany JW: *Clinical applications of neuromuscular techniques, vol 2, The lower body.* Edinburgh, 2002, Churchill Livingstone.

arteries, veins, lymphatic, muscles, respiratory system, and digestive tract.

PHYSIOLOGIC/REFLEXIVE

Influences of therapeutic massage involve the nervous system. These include CNS processing of cognitive perception of the massage events, and effects on the peripheral somatic and ANS, including fluctuations in neurotransmitters and hormones that influence nervous system response. Physiology for the athlete is discussed in depth elsewhere in this text; this section describes the use of manual methods and their effects on the peripheral nervous system and the neuroendocrine system.

SOMATIC INFLUENCE

The effects of massage can be processed through the somatic division of the peripheral nervous system. The somatic division controls movement and muscle contraction and relaxation patterns, as well as muscle and motor tone. **Muscle tone** is a mixture of tension in the connective tissue elements of the muscle and the intermuscular fluid pressure. An example of muscle tone dysfunction is delayed-onset muscle soreness. Muscle tone is influenced more by mechanical massage applications previously discussed. **Motor tone** is produced by motor neuron excitability and influenced by reflexive massage application that inhibits motor neuron activity. The most common reason for increase in motor tone is increase in sympathetic arousal and sustained sympathetic dominance. Another cause is proactive muscle guarding after injury and nervous system damage. Both situations are common in athletes.

The usual outcome of reflexive massage is inhibitory and anti-arousal. Anti-arousal massage (relaxation massage) may influence motor tone activity in the same way that pharmaceutical muscle relaxers do, because the main reason for motor tone difficulties is sympathetic arousal.

When working with the neuromuscular mechanism in massage, the basic premises are:

- Substitute a different neurologic signal stimulation to support a normal muscle resting length.
- Influence muscle and motor tone by lengthening and stretching of muscles and connective tissue.
- Normalize fluid dynamics.
- Reeducate the muscles involved.

Dysfunction of soft tissue (muscle and connective tissue) without proprioceptive hyperactivity or hypoactivity is uncommon. It is believed that proprioceptive hyperactivity causes tense or spastic muscles and hypoactivity of opposing muscle groups. The main proprioceptors influenced by massage are the spindle cell and the Golgi tendon receptor. The mechanoreceptors of the skin are also influenced by stretching, compression, rubbing, and vibration of the skin. Stimulation of joint mechanoreceptors affects the adjacent muscles, and the stimulation of the skin overlying muscle and joint structures also has beneficial effect, due to shared innervations.

Deep broad-based massage has a minimal and short-term inhibitory effect on motor tone of muscle. It is used primarily to support a muscle reeducation process such as therapeutic exercise or to temporarily reduce motor tone so that muscle activation sequences (firing patterns) can be reset. Inhibiting motor tone allows more mechanical methods to address tissue shortening without causing muscle spasm.

Active movements of the body, using techniques such as active assisted joint movement, and/or the application of active muscle contraction and release used during muscle energy methods of tense and relax, reciprocal inhibition, and combined methods of strain/counterstrain do seem to improve motor function by interaction with proprioceptive function.

Somatic effects are produced by the following means:

- Neuromuscular methods
- Hyperstimulation analgesia
- Vestibular and cerebellum stimulation
- Counterirritation
- Reduction of nerve impingement (entrapment and compression)
- Reduction of muscle inhibition from fluid pressure

Vestibular Apparatus and Cerebellum

The **vestibular apparatus** is a complex system composed of sensors in the inner ear (vestibular labyrinth), upper neck (cervical proprioception), eyes (visual motion and three-dimensional orientation), and body (somatic proprioception) processed in several areas of the brain (brainstem, cerebellum, parietal and temporal cortex). Reflex activity affects the eyes (vestibulo-ocular reflexes), neck (vestibulocollic reflexes), and balance (vestibulospinal reflexes) by sending and receiving information at the same time about how we are oriented to the environment around us. As an example, many amusement park rides create disorienting sensations in the vestibular apparatus that contribute to the effects of the ride.

The vestibular apparatus and the cerebellum are interrelated. The output from the cerebellum goes to the motor cortex and brainstem. Stimulating the cerebellum by altering motor tone of muscles, position of the body, and vestibular balance stimulates the hypothalamus to adjust ANS functions to restore homeostasis. Reflex response time seems to be quicker in athletes than in nonathletes. Most athletes are extremely sensitive in this area.

The massage techniques that most strongly affect the vestibular apparatus and therefore the cerebellum are those that produce rhythmic oscillation, including rocking during the application of massage. Rocking produces movement at the neck and head that influences the sense of equilibrium. Rocking stimulates the inner ear balance mechanisms, including the vestibular nuclear complex and the labyrinthine righting reflexes, to keep the head level. Stimulation of these reflexes produces a body-wide effect involving stimulation of muscle contraction patterns.

Massage can alter body positional sense, and the position of the eyes in response to postural change. It initiates specific movement patterns that change sensory input from the muscles, tendons, joints, and skin and stimulates various vestibular reflexes. This feedback information, which adjusts and coordinates movement, is relayed directly to the motor cortex and the cerebellum, allowing the body to integrate the sensory data and adjust to a more efficient postural balance. If massage application involves vestibular influences, short-term nausea and dizziness can occur while the mechanisms rebalance. Using massage to restore appropriate muscle activation firing pattern sequences and gait reflexes is valuable. Influencing the balance of the various force couples in the body can shift the relationship of the eyes, neck, hips, and so forth and influences positional balance, mobility, and agility.

Hyperstimulation Analgesia

In 1965, Melzack and Wall proposed the gate control theory. Although some aspects of the original theory have been modified over the past 40 years, the basic premise remains viable. According to this theory, a gating mechanism functions at the level of the spinal cord. Pain impulses pass through a "gate" to reach the lateral spinothalamic system.

Pain impulses are transmitted by large-diameter and small-diameter nerve fibers. Stimulation (e.g., rubbing, massaging) of large-diameter fibers prevents the small-diameter fibers from transmitting signals and helps suppress the sensation of pain, especially sharp or visceral pain. Various massage methods, including pressure, positioning, and lengthening, provide this stimulation at sufficient intensity to activate the gating mechanism and produce **hyperstimulation analgesia**. Pain sensation may be reduced by manual analgesia by stimulating the sensory gating achieved when multiple sensations are processed at the same time. The reflexology (foot massage) benefit seems to be mediated by hyperstimulation analgesia.

Tactile stimulation produced by massage travels through the large-diameter fibers. These fibers also carry a faster signal. In essence, massage sensations win the race to the brain, and the pain sensations are blocked because the gate is closed. Stimulating techniques, such as percussion or vibration of painful areas to activate "stimulation-produced analgesia," or hyperstimulation analgesia, also are effective. Pain management for those involved with sport and fitness is essential. Therefore these methods are beneficial.

Counterirritation

Counterirritation is a superficial irritation that masks some irritation of deeper structures. Counterirritation may be explained by the gate control theory. Inhibition in central sensory pathways, produced by rubbing or oscillating (shaking) an area, may explain counterirritation.

All methods of massage can be used to produce counterirritation. Any massage method that introduces a controlled sensory stimulation intense enough to be interpreted by the client as a "good pain" signal will work to create counterirritation.

Massage therapy in many forms stimulates the skin over an area of discomfort. Techniques that friction the skin and underlying tissue to cause reddening of the skin are effective. Many sport therapeutic ointments contain cooling and warming agents and mildly caustic substances (capsicum), which are useful for muscle and joint pain. This is also a form of counterirritation.

Nerve Impingement

A nerve that is compressed or squeezed is a **nerve impingement**. Tissues that can bind include skin, fascia, muscles, ligaments, joint structures, and bones. An increase in fluid in an area can also result in nerve impingement. Shortened muscles and connective tissue (fascia) often impinge on major and minor nerves, causing discomfort. Tissues that are long and taut can also impinge on a nerve.

The specific nerve root, trunk, or division affected determines the condition, such as thoracic outlet syndrome, sciatica, or carpal tunnel syndrome. Therapeutic massage techniques work in many ways to reduce pressure on nerves. The main ways are to:

- Reflexively change the tension pattern and lengthen the short muscles.
- Mechanically stretch and soften connective tissue.
- Reduce localized edema.
- Interrupt the pain-spasm-pain cycle caused by protective muscle spasm that occurs in response to pain.
- Support effectiveness of therapeutic exercise to shift posture and function.
- Support the use of medications such as antispasmodics, analgesics, anti-inflammatories, and circulation enhancers such as vasodilators.

AUTONOMIC NERVOUS SYSTEM EFFECTS

Excessive sympathetic output causes most of the stress-related diseases and dysfunction, including headaches, gastrointestinal difficulties, high blood pressure, anxiety, muscle tension and aches, and sexual dysfunction.

Long-term stress (i.e., stress that can't be resolved by fleeing or fighting) may also trigger the release of **cortisol**, a cortisone manufactured by the body. Long-term high blood levels of cortisol cause side effects similar to those of the drug cortisone, including fluid retention, hypertension, muscle weakness, osteoporosis, breakdown of connective tissue, peptic ulcer, impaired wound healing, vertigo, headache, reduced ability to deal with stress, hypersensitivity, weight gain, nausea, fatigue, and psychological disturbances.

Because of its generalized effect on the ANS and associated functions, massage can cause changes in mood and excitement levels and can induce the relaxation/restorative response. Massage seems to be a gentle modulator, producing feelings of general well-being and comfort. The pleasure aspect of massage supports these outcomes. This is espe-

cially important for sport recovery. The emotional arousal often found in rehabilitation situations is also favorably influenced.

Initially massage stimulates sympathetic functions. The increase in autonomic, sympathetic arousal is followed by a decrease if the massage is slowed and sustained with sufficient pleasurable pressure and lasts about 45 to 50 minutes. The pressure levels must be relatively deep but not painful. Slow repetitive stroking, broad-based compression, rhythmic oscillation, and movement all initiate relaxation responses. Sufficient pressure applied with a compressive force to the tissues supports serotonin functions and vagal nerve tone. Compression and a fast-paced massage style stimulate sympathetic responses and may lift depression temporarily.

Point holding, such as acupressure or reflexology, releases the body's own painkillers and mood-altering chemicals from the entire endorphin class. These chemicals stimulate the parasympathetic responses of relaxation, restoration, and contentment. These methods of massage depend on the creation of moderate, controlled pain to relieve pain. It takes a larger pain or stress stimulus to generate the endorphin response than the perception of the existing pain. When the release of substance P triggers pain, enkephalins are released suppress the pain signal. A negative feedback system activates the release of serotonin and endogenous opiates, which inhibit pain. Therapeutic massage methods can be used to create a controlled, noxious (pain) stimulation that triggers this cycle. Clients often refer to this noxious stimulation as good pain.

Altering the muscles so that they are more or less tense, or changing the consistency of the connective tissue, affects the ANS through the feedback loop, which in turn affects the powerful body/mind phenomenon.

ENTRAINMENT

Entrainment is an important reflexive effect that seems to be processed through the ANS and CNS.

Entrainment is the coordination of or synchronization to a rhythm. Biological oscillators, such as the heart rate/respiratory rate/thalamus synchronization, combine to support the entrainment process, and other, subtler body rhythms follow. There is a synaptic traveling wave that results in neural rhythmic synchronization. The synchronization of the rhythms of our heart, respiration, and digestion promotes this balance, or homeostasis, to support a healthy body.

Athletes are especially sensitive to entrainment mechanisms, and performance is often disrupted if entrainment is disturbed. Athletes often call optimal entrainment "being in the zone." A balance between the sympathetic and parasympathetic divisions of the ANS influences the sinus node of the heart and the vascular system, which in turn modulates heart rate and blood pressure. Our nasal reflexes, stimulated by the movement of air through the nose, rhythmically interact with the heart, lungs, and diaphragm. Thus the entire body is affected, because biological rhythms are interconnected.

The CNS includes a series of rhythms classified by frequency, as alpha, beta, gamma, and theta. The effects of massage on these particular rhythms are the subject of current investigation. Entrainment methods that synchronize the motions and rhythms of the body could provide benefit, because these rhythms are associated with sensory processing and cognitive states. There are also Traube Hering-Mayer (THM) oscillations of 4 to 8 waves per minute, which are rhythmic variations in blood pressure of 6 to 10 cycles per minute. These oscillations can be felt all over the body. Many experts theorize that these oscillations may be the mechanisms of cranial sacral therapy or biofield/energetic modulations. What is known is that the THM oscillations and ANS function are interrelated.

The body also entrains to external rhythms. Any activity that uses a repetitive motion or sound, depending on its rhythmic speed or pace, quiets or excites the nervous system through entrainment and thereby alters the physiologic processes of the body. Sometimes the body rhythms are disrupted. Pounding music and other forms of discord can be disruptive, as can multiple rhythms out of sync in the same environment. This can be seen with visiting teams and the influence of the home field advantage. Athletes become fatigued or "out of sorts" in these disharmonic environments.

When a person experiences positive emotional states, the biologic rhythms naturally tend to begin to oscillate together, or entrain.

To encourage entrainment, massage is provided in a quiet, rhythmic manner. The rhythmic application of massage and the proximity of a centered and compassionate professional's breathing rate and heart rate can support restorative entrainment if the client's body rhythms are out of sync. The focused, centered professional introduces his own ordered rhythms as part of the environment; they serve as an additional external influence that enables the client's the client's body rhythms to become synchronized. Oscillation, in the form of rhythmic rocking affecting the vestibular mechanism, has an anti-arousal effect. When synchronization occurs, homeostatic mechanisms seem to work more efficiently.

NEUROENDOCRINE REGULATION

Neuroendocrine substances carry messages that regulate physiologic functions. **Neuroendocrine regulation** is a continuous, ever-changing chemical mix that fluctuates with each external and internal demand on the body to respond, adapt, or maintain a functional degree of homeostasis. The immune system also produces and responds to these communication substances. The substances that make up this "chemical soup" remain the same, but the proportion and ratio change with each regulating function or message transmission. The "flavor" of the soup, which is determined by the ratio of the chemical mix, affects such factors as mood, attentiveness, arousal, passiveness, vigilance, calm, ability to sleep, receptivity to touch, response to touch, anger, pessimism, optimism, connectedness, loneliness, depression, desire, hunger, love, and commitment.

Research now indicates that most problems in behavior, mood, and perception of stress and pain, as well as other so-called mental/emotional dysfunction, are caused by dysregulation or failure of certain biochemical agents. These behaviors, symptoms, emotional and physical states often are the result of normal chemical mixes that occur at inappropriate times. Athletes are particularly sensitive to neurochemical influences. Highs and lows, wins and losses, pain, and so forth place increased demands on the system.

The effects of neurotransmitters released during massage may explain and validate the use of sensory stimulation methods for treating chronic pain, anxiety, and depression. Much of the research on massage, especially that done at the Touch Research Institute of the University of Miami School of Medicine, revolves around shifts in the proportion and ratio of the composition of the body's "chemical soup" brought about by massage.

NEUROENDOCRINE CHEMICALS

Neuroendocrine chemicals influenced by massage include:

- Dopamine
- Serotonin
- Epinephrine/adrenaline
- Norepinephrine/noradrenaline
- Enkephalins, endorphins, and dynorphins
- Oxytocin
- Cortisol
- Growth hormone

Dopamine

Dopamine influences motor activity that involves movement (especially learned, fine movement such as handwriting), conscious selection (the ability to focus attention), and mood (in terms of inspiration, possibly intuition, joy, and enthusiasm). Dopamine is involved in pleasure states, seeking behavior, and the internal record system. Low levels of dopamine result in opposite effects, such as lack of motor control, clumsiness, inability to focus attention, and boredom. Massage seems to increase the available level of dopamine in the body, which can explain the pleasure and satisfaction experienced during and after massage. The importance of optimal dopamine levels for the athlete is evident.

Serotonin

Serotonin allows a person to maintain context-appropriate behavior; that is, to do the appropriate thing at the appropriate time. It regulates mood in terms of appropriate emotions, attention to thoughts, and calming, quieting, comforting effects; it also subdues irritability and regulates drive states so that the urge to talk, touch, and be involved in power struggles can be suppressed. Serotonin also is involved in satiety; adequate levels reduce the sense of hunger and craving, such as for food or sex. It also modulates the sleep/wake cycle. A low serotonin level has been implicated in depression, eating disorders, pain disorders, and obsessive-compulsive disorders. There is a balancing effect between dopamine and serotonin much like agonist and antagonist muscles. Athletic competition supports dopamine dominance but recovery time is serotonin-dependent. Aggressive and impulsive behavior of athletes may be related to imbalances in this area. Massage seems to increase the available level of serotonin. Massage may support the optimal ratio of serotonin and dopamine, especially when being used to aid

recovery after competition. Care needs to be taken prior to competition to not disrupt the delicate balance of these neurotransmitters.

Epinephrine/Adrenaline and Norepinephrine/Noradrenaline

The terms **epinephrine/adrenaline** and **norepinephrine/noradrenaline** are used interchangeably in scientific texts. Epinephrine activates arousal mechanisms in the body, whereas norepinephrine functions more in the brain. These are the activation, arousal, alertness, and alarm chemicals of the fight-or-flight response and of all sympathetic arousal functions and behaviors. Athletic competition supports the release of these chemicals. If the levels of these chemicals are too high or if they are released at an inappropriate time, a person may feel as if something very important is demanding his or her attention or may react with the basic survival drives of fight or flight (hypervigilance and hyperactivity). The person might have a disturbed sleep pattern, particularly in a lack of rapid eye movement (REM) sleep, which is restorative sleep. The individual with low levels of epinephrine and norepinephrine is sluggish, drowsy, fatigued, and underaroused.

Massage seems to have a regulating effect on epinephrine and norepinephrine through stimulation or inhibition of the sympathetic and parasympathetic nervous systems. This generalized balancing function of massage seems to recalibrate the appropriate adrenaline and noradrenaline levels. Depending on the response of the ANS, massage can just as easily wake a person up and relieve fatigue as it can calm down a person who is anxious and pacing the floor.

It should be noted that initially touch stimulates the sympathetic nervous system, whereas it seems to take 15 minutes or so of sustained stimulation to begin to engage the parasympathetic functions. Therefore it makes sense that a 15-minute chair massage tends to increase production of epinephrine and norepinephrine, which can help athletes become more attentive, whereas a 1-hour slow, rhythmic massage engages the parasympathetic functions, reducing epinephrine and norepinephrine levels and encouraging a good night's sleep necessary for recovery and healing.

Enkephalins, Endorphins, and Dynorphins

Enkephalins, endorphins, and dynorphins are mood-lifters that support satiety and modulate pain. Massage increases the available levels of these chemicals. The massage effect is delayed until chemical levels rise to an inhibitory level. It usually takes about 15 minutes for the blood level of enkephalins, endarphins, and dynorphins to begin to rise. Appropriate availability of these pain-modulating chemicals is essential for athletes.

Oxytocin

The hormone **oxytocin** has been implicated in pair or couple bonding, parental bonding, feelings of attachment, and care-taking, along with its more clinical functions during pregnancy, delivery, and lactation. Massage tends to increase the available level of oxytocin, which could explain the connected and intimate feeling of massage.

Because athletes tend to be single-minded and hyperfocused, the oxytocin influence can support dependence on the therapist. If the massage routine is disrupted, the athlete's performance can be affected. In this sense, commitment and consistency by the therapist working with competing athletes are essential.

Cortisol

Cortisol and other glucocorticoids are stress hormones produced by the adrenal glands during prolonged stress. Elevated levels of these hormones indicate increased sympathetic arousal. Cortisol and other glucocorticoids have been implicated in many stress-related symptoms and diseases, including suppressed immunity states, sleep disturbances, and increases in the level of substance P. Athletes and those in extensive physical rehabilitation programs are particularly susceptible to increased and sustained cortisol levels. Massage has been shown to reduce levels of cortisol.

Growth Hormone

Growth hormone promotes cell division and in adults has been implicated in the functions of tissue repair and regeneration. This hormone is necessary for healing and is most active during sleep. Massage increases the availability of growth hormone indirectly by increased vagal stimulation, predisposing to parasympathetic dominance, encouraging sleep, and reducing the level of cortisol. Again, especially in competing athletes, recovery is a primary goal and optimal levels of growth hormone are necessary.

It can be summarized that therapeutic massage balances the blood levels of serotonin, dopamine, and endorphins, which in turn facilitates the production of natural killer cells in the immune system

and regulates moods. This response indicates that it would be beneficial to include massage as part of the total treatment program for athletes as well as fitness programs. Oxytocin tends to increase supporting feelings of connectedness. At the same time, massage stimulates vagus nerve function, reduces cortisol levels, and regulates epinephrine and norepinephrine levels, which facilitates the action of growth hormone.

ENERGY SYSTEMS

Some methods of massage, especially the more subtle **energy systems**, have not yet been researched enough to be scientifically validated. It is possible that the effectiveness of various kinds of hands-on bodywork can be the result of the entrainment of electrical and magnetic rhythms from therapist to client.

These methods, based on the subtle electrical energy of the body, have been around for eons (Figure 9-9). Most ancient healing practices are based on the interaction with these subtle energy fields. The concept of the vibratory nature of these bodywork approaches is intriguing. It should not be discounted because science has yet to validate eons of experiential evidence. We cannot measure compassion and respect using the scientific method either, but we know they exist. It has been my experience that athletes, especially those that seek the "zone experience," are very sensitive to, and accepting of, these methods as long as they are presented in a nonmystical way and applied matter-of-factly.

SUMMARY

Figure 9-10 presents a brief summary of this chapter.

Generally, therapeutic massage and bodywork stimulate neuroendocrine responses that are antiarousing, which in turn has implications in managing stress-induced difficulties, modulation of pain perception, and increase in effective autoregulation of mood and restorative functions. In addition, mechanical application improves fluid movement and connective tissue structure supporting efficient function. Specifically massage application can be designed to support an existing physiologic process or stimulate a change in structure or function. Physical and tactile measures are necessary to reduce

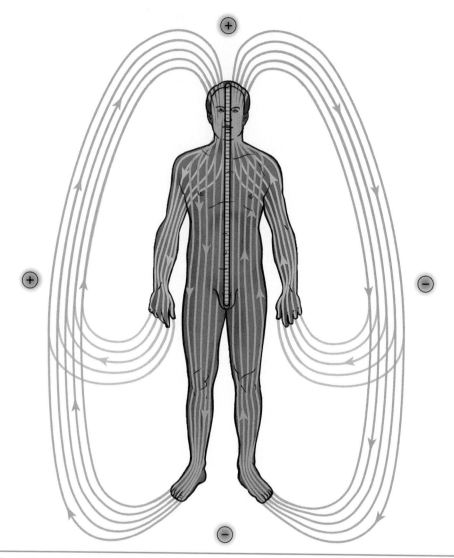

FIGURE 9-9 ■ Electromagnetic currents traveling vertically on the body. (From Fritz S: *Mosby's fundamentals of therapeutic massage*, ed 3. St. Louis, 2004, Mosby.)

arousal and promote self regulation and therefore result in perception of comfort. Pleasure is an important experience in health and healing. Pain causes muscular contraction, withdrawal, abrupt movement, breath holding, increased heart rate, and increased generalized stress response. The perception of pain is dependent on the psychological state, especially anxiety or depression. Low self-esteem and apprehension reduce pain tolerance.

Pleasure can counteract the pain response. Massage provides pleasurable sensation. Pleasurable pain often accompanies massage application. Pain sensation generated by manual techniques needs to result in pleasurable outcomes and should never be sharp, bruising, or tearing in nature.

Emotional states such as apprehension, anxiety, anger, depression, and tension are usually results of increased muscle tone, whereas relaxed states supported by pleasure sensation produce a reduction in muscular tone. These responses are modulated by the limbic system. Applications of touch that are perceived as pleasurable are usually sedative and parasympathetic in nature. Initial adaptation to touch, and touch perceived as uncomfortable, aggressive, and nonproductive, increases sympathetic arousal.

The importance of these pleasurable factors during massage is evident in supporting the athlete for achieving and maintaining performance, as well as recovering from injury. One of the biggest

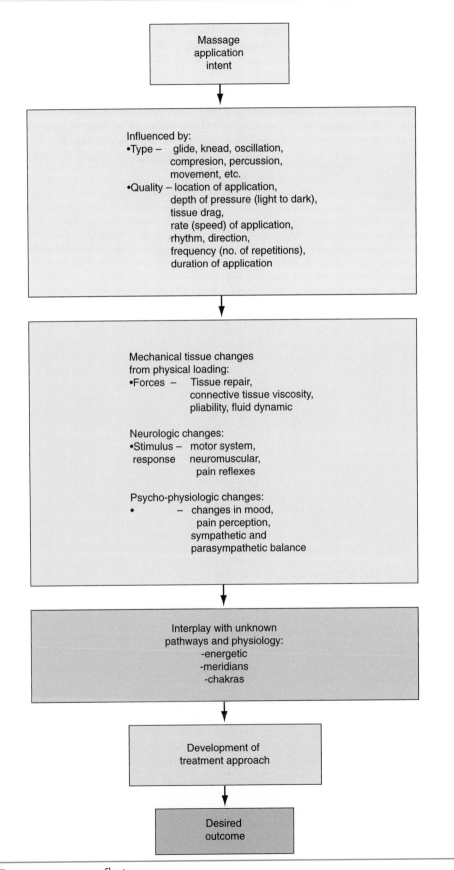

FIGURE 9-10 ■ Chapter summary.

mistakes of those providing sports massage is to undervalue this aspect of massage. The massage application is often too aggressive and painful. There is a misconception that sports massage is "deep tissue" massage (whatever that is). This is not necessarily so. It depends on the outcomes and the individual situation of the athlete.

The general protocol for care of the athlete contains all of these responses to massage application. Those involved in rehabilitation programs are especially sensitive to adaptive strain. Athletes at peak performance are particularly fragile. Appropriate treatment plan development and massage application are necessary. The athlete is ever-changing. That is why sports and fitness massage is a clinical reasoning process and not a protocol application. It is outcome-based, not modality-based. It requires practice and knowledge to make the appropriate choices to benefit and not harm the client.

1 List the four general outcomes discussed in this chapter and provide a case example of each.

Example: Performance/recovery–Athlete is a 22 year old female collegiate volleyball player. The team is poised to win the championship in its division. The coach has indicated everyone has to "step up" performance and wants to see everyone's personal list.

_____

_____

_____

_____

_____

_____

_____

_____

_____

_____

_____

_____

_____

_____

_____

_____

_____

_____

_____

_____

_____

_____

_____

_____

_____

_____

_____

_____

2 Using each of your four case studies, identify the mechanical reflexive approach and list the physiology mechanisms most targeted to achieve the client's outcomes.

Example: To support performance and recovery, the following would be targeted: increase ground substance pliability and fluid movement using compression, torsion, and tension force application; reduce sympathetic dominance and support parasympathetic dominance through entrainment using rhythmic, rocking, and deep compression.

_____

_____

_____

_____

_____

_____

_____

_____

_____

_____

_____

_____

_____

_____

_____

_____

_____

_____

_____

_____

_____

_____

_____

_____

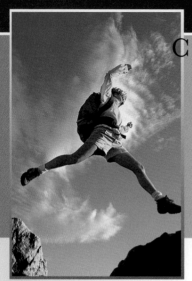

10

INDICATIONS AND CONTRAINDICATIONS FOR MASSAGE

OUTLINE

OBJECTIVES

Upon completion of this chapter the reader will have the information necessary to:

1 List the general indications for massage.

2 Describe illness and injury and how they predispose a client to contraindication or caution for massage application.

3 Evaluate various medications for indication/contraindication for massage.

4 Identify and avoid endangerment sites.

Massage can be very beneficial for athletes and those involved in physical performance activity such as dance, if the professional performing the massage understands the multidimentional aspects of the client's experience. If not, massage can impair optimal function of the performance. Because of the intense physical activity involved in sports, an athlete may be more prone to injury. The massage therapist often works with clients from many different sport or fitness activities. Physical rehabilitation programs are also varied. The author owns just about every sport for dummies and idiot's guide to various sport performance books. I often use these types of books to help me understand various sport activities and determine indications and benefits of massage. Unit I discusses the basic movement functions an athlete uses to accomplish a sport-specific task. Massage is beneficial, is used to allow the body to complete these movements, and can manage compensation patterns that can result from repetitive movement.

Because therapeutic massage has widespread effects on the physiologic functions of the body, it is the massage professional's responsibility, when applying massage techniques, to have knowledge of pathology, contraindications, and endangerment sites. It is difficult to obtain a consensus on such information, however, because not all sources agree.

Acute inflammation
Anxiety and depressive disorders
Deep-vein thrombosis
Diabetes
Endangerment sites
General contraindications
Herpes simplex virus
Inflammation

Lymphangitis
Melanoma
Myositis ossificans
Nerve compression
Nerve entrapment
Pain and fatigue syndromes
Pain threshold
Pain tolerance

Posttraumatic stress disorder
Regional contraindications
Somatic pain
Therapeutic inflammation
Tumors
Varicose veins
Visceral pain

INDICATIONS FOR MASSAGE

Normal physiologic mechanisms inhibit the tendency to function at the body's anatomical and physiologic limits. We usually do not run as fast as we can, work as long as we can, or exert all of our energy to complete a task. Instead the body signals fatigue, pain, or strain before the anatomic or physiologic limits are reached, and we back off. This very important protective mechanism allows us to live within a healthy range of energy expenditure while maintaining functioning energy reserves in case of emergency or extraordinary demand. This is not necessarily the case for athletes, who often strive to exceed normal physical and mental functioning.

Dysfunction occurs when energy reserves run low because restorative mechanisms are not able to function effectively or when the body begins to limit function in an attempt to maintain higher energy reserves.

If a person plays tennis and overstretches the shoulder reaching for the serve, the body senses a danger of harm to the joint. Neurologic sensors may reset muscle patterns, limiting range of motion slightly to prevent this from happening again. Physiologically, protective space has been created even though range of motion has been sacrificed. If this continues, eventually the limited range of motion interferes with the ability to play tennis. Dysfunction occurs. If perpetuated and compensated for over a period of time, pathology usually develops. The person could end up with a frozen shoulder or tendonitis.

Massage intervention just after the first event, coupled with a more conservative playing style or improved playing form, might reverse the process, and dysfunction would not develop. Intervention applied at the point when range of motion limits are first observed would likely still be effective in reversing the dysfunctional process. Interventions introduced after pathology has begun are more complex, sometimes aggressive, and occasionally too late to support repair and restoration of function. Also it may take longer before benefits are noticed.

Massage can support the restorative process to help athletes maintain peak performance for extended periods. The benefits of massage are most effectively focused on assisting people to stay within the healthy range of physical functioning and supporting those who wish to achieve fitness.

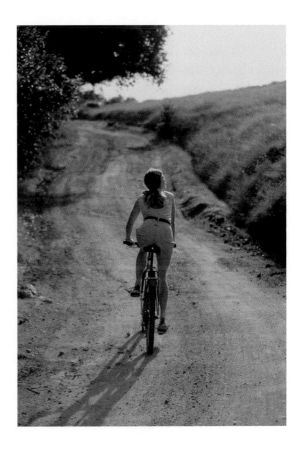

Illness occurs when a body process breaks down. A person whose immune system did not effectively fight off a cold virus becomes ill with a cold. A person with diabetes is ill. Chronic fatigue syndrome, ulcers, cancer, and multiple sclerosis are all examples of illness.

Injury occurs when tissue is damaged. Cuts, bruises, burns, contusions, fractured bones, sprains, and strains are examples of injuries.

Illness tends to indicate general cautions and contraindications, whereas injury more often indicates regional cautions and contraindications.

Therapeutic massage is indicated for both illness and injury. Massage techniques for illness involve very general application of massage to support the body's healing responses (e.g., stress management, pain control, restorative sleep). This approach to massage, sometimes called general constitutional application, is more reflexive in nature and is used to reduce the stress load so that the body can heal. (See Unit Three for specific massage interventions for illness and sport injury.)

Massage for injury incorporates aspects of general constitutional massage, because healing is necessary for tissue repair. The more mechanical application of lymphatic drainage is used to control edema. Gliding methods are used to approximate (bring close together) the ends of some types of injured tissue , such as in minor muscle tears and sprains. Hyperstimulation analgesia and counterirritation reduce acute pain. Methods to increase circulation to the area support tissue formation. Connective tissue applications are used to manage scar tissue formation. Inflammation is a factor in both illness and injury, because healing in both cases involves appropriate activation of the inflammatory response system.

Healing an injury is taxing on the body and strains the restorative mechanism. If an injured person is not in a state of health to begin with, it is common for the stress of the injury to compromise the immune system, and the person then becomes susceptible to illness.

Because many diseases and injuries have similar symptoms, it is difficult to determine the specific underlying causes of pathology. The massage professional must refer clients to qualified, licensed health care providers for a specific diagnosis.

In general, massage is indicated for:
- Relaxation and pleasure
- Anxiety reduction
- Mild depression management
- Effective digestion and elimination
- Efficient circulation of body fluids
- Enhanced growth, development, and regeneration of injured tissue
- Enhanced immune function
- Exercise recovery and performance
- Inflammation management
- Mood management
- Nerve impingement syndrome
- Pain management
- Soft tissue dysfunction

The following areas of effect are especially beneficial for the population targeted in this textbook.

INFLAMMATION

Therapeutic massage seems to be beneficial in cases of prolonged inflammation. Possible theories regarding this include the following:

1. The stimulation from massage activates a release of the body's own antiinflammatory agents.
2. Certain types of massage increase the inflammatory process (**therapeutic inflammation**) to a small degree, triggering the body to complete the process.
3. Massage may facilitate dilution and removal of the irritant by increasing lymphatic flow.

The processes of **inflammation** trigger tissue repair. Tissue repair is the replacement of dead cells with living cells. In the type of tissue repair called *regeneration,* the new cells are similar to those they replace. In another type of tissue repair called *replacement,* the new cells are formed from connective tissue and are different from those they replace, resulting in a scar. Often fibrous connective tissue replaces the damaged tissue. Most tissue repairs are a combination of regeneration and replacement. A goal in the healing process is to promote regeneration and keep replacement to a minimum. Massage has been shown to slow the formation of scar tissue and to keep scar tissue pliable when it does form (Table 10-1).

Because the inflammatory response is part of the healing process, the deliberate creation of inflammation can generate or "jump start" healing mechanisms. Certain methods of massage are used to create a controlled, localized area of therapeutic inflammation. Deep frictioning techniques and connective tissue stretching methods are the most common approaches.

The benefit derived from the use of therapeutic inflammation depends on the body's ability to

TABLE 10-1	STAGES OF TISSUE HEALING AND MASSAGE INTERVENTIONS	
STAGE 1 (3-7 DAYS)—ACUTE: INFLAMMATORY REACTION	**STAGE 2 (14-21 DAYS)— SUBACUTE: REPAIR AND HEALING**	**STAGE 3 (3-12 MO)—CHRONIC: MATURATION AND REMODELING**
Vascular changes	Growth of capillary beds into area	Maturation and remodeling of scar
Inflammatory exudate	Collagen formation	Contracture of scar tissue
Clot formation	Granulation tissue; caution necessary	Collagen aligns along lines of stress force (tensegrity)
Phagocytosis, neutralization of irritants	Fragile, easily injured tissue	Absence of inflammation
Early fibroblastic activity	Decreased inflammation	Pain after tissue resistance
Inflammation	Pain during tissue resistance	Return to function
Pain prior to tissue resistance	Controlled motion	Increase strength and alignment of scar tissue
Protection	Promote development of mobile scar	Cross-fiber friction of scar tissue coupled with
Control and support effects of inflammation:	Cautious and controlled soft tissue mobilization of scar tissue along	directional stroking along the lines of tension away from injury
PRICE (protection, rest, ice, compression, elevation)	fiber direction toward injury	Progressive stretching and active motion; full-range
Promote healing and prevent compensation patterns	Active and passive, open- and closed-chain range of motion, mid-range	Support rehabilitation activities with full-body massage
Passive movement, mid-range	Support healing with full-body massage	
General massage and lymphatic drainage with caution		
Support rest with full-body massage		

From Fritz S: *Mosby's fundamentals of therapeutic massage*, ed 3. St. Louis, 2004, Mosby.

generate healing processes. If healing mechanisms are suppressed, methods that create therapeutic inflammation should not be used. For example, therapeutic inflammation is not used in situations in which sleep disturbance, compromised immune function, a high stress load, or systemic or localized inflammation is already present. This method is also contraindicated if any condition that consists of impaired repair and restorative functions (e.g., fibromyalgia) is present, unless application is carefully supervised as part of a total treatment program. Training and competing athletes may not have enough adaptive capacity to resolve inflammation, so caution is advised when considering using methods to create inflammation.

Client use of antiinflammatory medications is another factor that must be considered. If a person is taking such medication, either steroidal or nonsteroidal, the effectiveness of therapeutic inflammation is negated or reduced, and restoration mechanisms are inhibited. When these medications are used, any methods that create inflammation are to be avoided (Table 10–2).

PAIN

The massage professional especially needs to understand the mechanisms of pain. Pain receptors are found in almost every tissue of the body and may respond to any type of stimulus. When stimuli for other sensations, such as touch, pressure, heat, and cold, reach a certain intensity, they stimulate the sensation of pain as well. Injured tissue may release prostaglandins, making peripheral nociceptors more sensitive to the normal pain response (hyperalgesia). Aspirin and other nonsteroidal antiinflammatory drugs (NSAIDs) inhibit the action of prostaglandins and reduce pain.

Excessive stimulation of a sensory organ causes pain. Additional stimuli for pain receptors include excessive distention or dilation of a structure (typically fluid pressure), prolonged muscular contractions, muscle spasms, inadequate blood flow to tissues, and the presence of certain chemical substances. Because of their sensitivity to all stimuli, pain receptors perform a protective function by identifying changes that may endanger the body.

The point at which a stimulus is perceived as painful is called the **pain threshold.** This varies somewhat from individual to individual. One factor affecting the pain threshold is *perceptual dominance,* in which the pain felt in one area of the body diminishes or obliterates the pain felt in another area. Not until the most severe pain is diminished does the person perceive or acknowledge the other pain. This

TABLE 10-2	DISORDERS RELATED TO CHRONIC INFLAMMATION*

DISORDER	MECHANISM
Allergy	Mediators induce autoimmune reactions
Alzheimer's disease	Chronic inflammation destroys brain cells
Anemia	Mediators attack erythropoietin production
Aortic valve stenosis	Chronic inflammation damages heart valves
Arthritis	Inflammatory mediators destroy joint cartilage and synovial fluid
Asthma	Mediators close the airways
Cancer	Chronic inflammation causes most cancers
Congestive heart failure	Chronic inflammation causes heart muscle wasting
Fibromyalgia	Mediators are elevated in fibromyalgia patients
Fibrosis	Mediators attack traumatized tissue
Heart attack	Chronic inflammation contributes to coronary atherosclerosis
Kidney failure	Mediators restrict circulation and damage nephrons
Lupus	Mediators induce an autoimmune attack
Pancreatitis	Mediators induce pancreatic cell injury
Psoriasis	Mediators induce dermatitis
Stroke	Chronic inflammation promotes thromboembolic events
Surgical complications	Mediators prevent healing

*Seemingly unrelated disorders often have a common link—inflammation. This is a partial list of common medical problems associated with chronic inflammation.
From Fritz S: *Mosby's fundamentals of therapeutic massage*, ed 3. St. Louis, 2004, Mosby.

mechanism is often activated with massage application that produces a "good hurt" and creates hyperstimulation analgesia and counterirritation.

Pain tolerance refers to the length of time or intensity of pain that the person endures before acknowledging the pain and seeking relief. Unlike the pain threshold, pain tolerance is more likely to vary from one individual to another. A person's tolerance to pain is influenced by a variety of factors,

including personality type, psychological state at the onset of pain, previous experiences, sociocultural background, and the meaning of the pain for that person (e.g., the ways in which it affects the person's lifestyle). Factors that decrease pain tolerance include repeated exposure to pain, fatigue, sleep deprivation, and stress. Warmth, cold, distraction, alcohol consumption, hypnosis, and strong religious beliefs or faith all act to increase pain tolerance.

The origins of pain can be divided into two types: somatic and visceral. **Somatic pain** arises from stimulation of receptors in the skin (superficial somatic pain) or from stimulation of receptors in skeletal muscles, joints, tendons, and fascia (deep somatic pain). **Visceral pain** results from stimulation of receptors in the viscera (internal organs).

Pain is usually classified as acute, chronic, intractable, phantom, or referred.

Evaluation and Management of Pain

Because pain is a primary indicator in many disease processes, the massage practitioner must have a basic evaluation protocol for pain to refer his or her clients to the appropriate health care provider. The following guidelines for evaluating pain will help in this process.

Pain has many characteristics. Location, for example, can be divided into four categories:

1. Localized pain is pain confined to the site of origin.
2. Projected pain is typically a result of proximal nerve compression. This pain is perceived in the tissue supplied by the nerve.
3. Radiating pain is diffuse pain, which is not well localized, around the site of origin.
4. Referred pain is felt in an area distant from the site of the painful stimulus.

Pain can be divided into five types:

1. Pricking or bright pain—This type of pain is experienced when the skin is cut or jabbed with a sharp object. It is short-lived but intense and easily localized.
2. Burning pain—This type is slower to develop, lasts longer, and is less accurately localized. It is experienced when the skin is burned or inflammation is present. It often stimulates cardiac and respiratory activity.
3. Aching pain—Aching pain occurs when the visceral organs are stimulated. It is constant, not well localized, and is often referred to areas of the body far from where the damage

is occurring. This type of pain is important because it may be a sign of a life-threatening disorder of a vital organ.

4. Deep pain—The main difference between superficial and deep sensibility is the different nature of the pain evoked by noxious stimuli. Unlike superficial pain, deep pain is poorly localized, nauseating, and frequently associated with sweating and changes in blood pressure. Deep pain can be elicited experimentally in the periosteum and ligaments by injecting them with hypertonic saline. Pain produced in this fashion initiates reflex contraction of nearby skeletal muscles. This reflex contraction is similar to the muscle spasm associated with injuries to bones, tendons, and joints. The steadily contracting muscles become ischemic, and ischemia stimulates the pain receptors in the muscles. The resultant pain, in turn, initiates more spasms, creating a vicious cycle called the *pain-spasm-pain cycle* (Figure 10-1).

5. Muscle pain—If a muscle contracts rhythmically in the presence of an adequate blood supply, pain does not usually result. However, if the blood supply to a muscle is occluded (closed off), contraction soon causes pain. The pain persists after the contraction until blood flow is reestablished. If a muscle with a normal blood supply is made to contract continuously without periods of relaxation, it also begins to ache, because the maintained contraction compresses the blood vessels supplying the muscle.

Nonverbal behaviors such as facial grimacing, flinching, tearing, abnormal gait or posture, muscle tension, and guarding of the body are common indicators of pain. Verbal and emotional signals indicating pain may include crying, moaning, groaning, irritability, sadness, and changes in voice tone.

Pain scales, such as a 1-10 scale, or a mild, moderate, and severe scale, are helpful for measuring pain perception. Only the client can determine the degree of severity. Pain is rarely the same at all times. It is felt (perceived) differently over time and differs with various precipitating and aggravating factors. Pain can range from excruciating to mild and may be difficult for the client to verbalize.

Many ways exist to alleviate pain. The massage professional, as part of a health care team, can contribute valuable manual therapy in various pain conditions using direct tissue manipulation and reflex stimulation of the nervous system and the

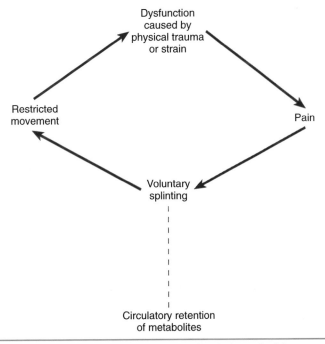

FIGURE 10-1 ■ Pain-spasm-pain cycle. (From Fritz S: *Mosby's fundamentals of therapeutic massage*, ed 3. St. Louis, 2004, Mosby.)

circulation. As a therapeutic intervention, massage may help reduce the need for pain medication, thus reducing the side effects of medication.

All medications, including over-the-counter products available without a prescription, have side effects. Obviously, with clients in extreme pain, the massage therapy must be monitored by a physician or other appropriate health care professional. Most people experience pain in less severe forms occasionally throughout life. Massage may provide temporary symptomatic relief of moderate pain brought on by daily stress, replacing over-the-counter pain medications or reducing their use.

Acute pain and chronic pain are managed somewhat differently; therefore, it is important to make the distinction between the two. Intervention for acute pain is less invasive and focuses on supporting a current healing process. Chronic pain is managed with either symptom relief or a more aggressive rehabilitation approach that incorporates a therapeutic change process.

IMPINGEMENT SYNDROMES

The two types of nerve impingement syndromes are compression and entrapment. **Nerve compression** is pressure on a nerve by a bony structure, and **nerve entrapment** is pressure on a nerve from soft tissue. Massage is beneficial for entrapment and can manage some symptoms of nerve compression, even though the direct causal factor is not addressed.

Cervical Plexus

If the cervical plexus is being impinged, the person experiences headaches, neck pain, and breathing difficulties. The muscles most responsible for pressure on the cervical plexus are the suboccipital and sternocleidomastoid muscles. Shortened connective tissues at the cranial base will also press on these nerves.

The cervical plexus is formed by the ventral rami of the upper four cervical nerves. The phrenic nerve is part of this plexus. It innervates the diaphragm, and any disruption to this nerve affects breathing. Many cutaneous (skin) branches of the cervical plexus transmit sensory impulses from the skin of the neck, ear, and shoulder. The motor branches innervate muscles of the anterior neck.

Brachial Plexus

The brachial plexus, situated partly in the neck and partly in the axilla, provides virtually all the nerves that innervate the upper limbs. Any imbalance that causes pressure on this complex of nerves results in pain in the shoulder, chest, arm, wrist, and hand.

The muscles most often responsible for impingement of the brachial plexus are the scalenes, pectoralis minor, and subclavius. Muscles of the arm occasionally impinge branches of the brachial plexus. Brachial plexus nerve impingement is responsible for thoracic outlet symptoms, which are often misdiagnosed as carpal tunnel syndrome. Whiplash injury involves the brachial plexus.

Lumbar Plexus

Lumbar plexus nerve impingement may give rise to low back discomfort with a belt distribution of pain, as well as pain in the lower abdomen, genitals, thigh, and medial lower leg. The main muscles that impinge on the lumbar plexus are the quadratus lumborum and the psoas. Shortening of the lumbar dorsal fascia exaggerates a lordosis and causes vertebral impingement of the lumbar plexus.

Sacral Plexus

The sacral plexus has approximately a dozen named branches. Almost half of these serve the buttocks and lower limbs; the others innervate pelvic structures. The main branch is the sciatic nerve. Impingement of this nerve by the piriformis muscle gives rise to sciatica.

Ligaments that stabilize the sacroiliac joint can affect the sacral plexus. Pressure on the sacral plexus can cause gluteal pain, leg pain, genital pain, and foot pain.

Massage methods can soften and stretch connective tissues that may impinge nerves, as well as normalize muscle tension patterns, restoring a more normal resting length to shortened muscles and thereby reducing pressure on nerves.

PSYCHOLOGICAL DYSFUNCTIONS

Science has validated the body/mind link in terms of health and disease. Many risk factors for the development of physical (body) pathology are mentally (mind) influenced, such as stress level and lifestyle choices. The same is true for mental health and pathology. The physical state of an individual has a strong influence on mental functioning. Usually when people feel well physically, they also feel well mentally; the reverse, too, is often the case—feeling bad mentally results in physical dysfunctions. Neurochemicals such as serotonin and dopamine exert a strong influence on a person's mental state.

The major mental health dysfunctions affecting Western society are post-traumatic stress disorder and other stress-related illnesses, and pain and fatigue syndromes coupled with anxiety and depression. If a person is involved in athletic competition or a rehabilitation program, it is safe to assume there has been strain on the mind/body connection.

Trauma is defined as:

- Physical injury caused by violent or disruptive action or by a toxic substance
- Psychic injury resulting from a severe emotional shock, either short-term or long-term

Post-traumatic stress disorder, as defined by the Diagnostic and Statistical Manual of Mental Disorders (DSM-IV), includes flashback memory experiences, state-dependent memory, somatization, anxiety, irritability, sleep disturbance, concentration difficulties, times of melancholy or depression, grief, fear, worry, anger, and avoidance behavior. Post-traumatic stress disorder can have long-term effects and often occurs after athletic injury.

Pain and fatigue syndromes are defined as multicausal and often chronic nonproductive patterns that interfere with well-being, activities of daily living, and productivity. Some current conditions in this category are fibromyalgia, chronic fatigue syndrome, Epstein-Barr viral infection, sympathetic reflex dystrophy, headache, arthritis, chronic cancer pain, neuropathy, low back syndrome, idiopathic pain, somatization disorder, and intractable pain syndrome. Acute pain can be a factor, as can acute "episodes" of chronic conditions.

Anxiety and depressive disorders are common. Anxiety is an uneasy feeling usually connected with increased sympathetic arousal responses. Depression is characterized by a decrease of vital functional activity and mood disturbances of exaggerated emptiness, hopelessness, and melancholy, or unbridled periods of high energy with no purpose or outcome.

It is common to see **anxiety and depressive disorders** in conjunction with pain and fatigue syndromes. Panic behavior, phobias, and a sense of impending doom, along with feelings of being overwhelmed and hopelessness, are common with these disorders. Mood swings, breathing pattern disorder, sleep disturbance, concentration difficulties, memory disturbances, outbursts of anger, fatigue, and changes in habits of daily living,

appetite, and activity levels are symptoms of these disorders.

Stress-Related Illness

Stress-related illness is defined as an increased stress load or reduced ability to adapt that depletes the reserve capacity of individuals, increasing their vulnerability to health problems. Stress-related illness can encompass the previously mentioned conditions as the primary cause of dysfunction or as the result of the stress of the dysfunction. Excessive stress sometimes manifests as cardiovascular problems, including hypertension; digestive difficulties, including heartburn, ulcer, and bowel syndromes; respiratory illness and susceptibility to bacterial and viral infection; endocrine dysfunction, particularly adrenal and thyroid dysfunction and delayed or reduced cellular repair; sleep disorders; and breathing pattern disorder, just to mention a few conditions. Clients, especially those with injury, should be carefully monitored for signs of psychological dysfunction (see Chapter 8).

Indications for Massage

Massage intervention has a strong physiologic effect through the comfort of compassionate touch, as well as a physical influence on mental state through its effect on the ANS and neurochemicals.

IN MY EXPERIENCE...

I have worked with many athletes over the years who had the cluster effect of pain and anxiety coupled with depression and fatigue. I remember one player especially who was playing extremely well but with a team that was struggling. As a result, all of his accomplishments were ignored. He became discouraged but continued to perform well. Over time he developed intestinal irritation and headaches. The next year he transferred to a different school whose team performed well. The player's symptoms disappeared, he thrived, and he currently plays in a professional league. Massage for this young man was a method of symptom relief when the situation was unable to be changed.

Those experiencing mental health problems, therefore, may derive benefits from massage. Management of pain is an important factor in the athletic community and for those in rehabilitation programs. Because therapeutic massage often can offer symptomatic relief from chronic pain, the helplessness that accompanies these difficulties may dissipate as the person realizes that management methods exist. Soothing of ANS hyperactivity or hypoactivity provides a sense of inner balance. Normalization of the breathing mechanism allows the client to breathe without restriction and can reduce the tendency toward breathing pattern disorder, which feeds anxiety and panic.

Therapeutic massage can provide intervention on a physical level to restore a more normal function to the body, which supports appropriate interventions by qualified mental health professionals. Certainly strong and appropriate indications exist for the use of massage therapy in the restoration of mental health, but caution is indicated in terms of the establishment of dual roles and boundary difficulties. It is very important to work in conjunction with mental health providers such as sport psychologists in these situations.

SLEEP SUPPORT

There are many causes of sleep interruption, including pain that repeatedly wakes the person, external random noise (such as traffic noise), tending infants and children, varied work schedules, a restless or snoring bed partner, sinus or other respiratory difficulties such as coughing, and urinary frequency. The list is endless. Regardless of the perpetuating factors, sleep is compromised and the stage of deep sleep is seldom achieved.

> ### IN MY EXPERIENCE...
>
> Many athletes love to sleep while on the massage table. Sometimes I feel as if I could bury someone in a blanket on the table—take a picture and it would represent about 90% of my athlete clients over the years. Sleeping during massage is so common that I have included a special section in this book* on how to work effectively while the client is sleeping.
>
> What is important is that athletes need to sleep 8 to 10 hours a day to sustain performance.

Sleep patterns may also be disrupted because of insomnia, snoring, sleep apnea, hormone fluctuations, high cortisol (stress hormone) levels, medications, and stimulants such as caffeine. Stimulant use, especially caffeine, is common in the sports world. Again, quality sleep is sacrificed. Travel across time zones also interferes with sleep.

Light/dark cycles regulate sleep patterns. For effective sleep we need adequate exposure to daylight, which stimulates serotonin. We also need adequate exposure to darkness. With the advent of artificial lighting we spend less and less time in the dark, which disturbs sleep patterns. Absence of light supports release of melatonin, a pineal gland hormone that is involved in the sleep pattern.

During sleep the body renews, repairs, and generally restores itself. Growth hormone is an important factor in this process, with more than half of its daily secretions taking place during sleep. If the deeper stages of sleep are not sustained, the body's restorative mechanisms are compromised. Sleep disturbances are a major factor in many chronic pain and fatigue syndromes, diminished athletic performance, injury predisposition, and delayed recovery. Massage is very effective in supporting restorative sleep.

CONTRAINDICATIONS FOR MASSAGE

When contraindications exist and massage is indicated, adjustment of application may be required to apply methods safely. Massage applications should be monitored by a health care professional such as a physician, nurse, physical therapist, athletic trainer, or other qualified personnel.

In professional team sports, usually there is an athletic training department in charge of maintaining health and injury rehabilitation of athletes. Recommendations by personnel of this department are valuable when determining appropriate massage application. It is most difficult when this type of support is not available, such as occurs with amateur team sports or working with individual athletes such as golfers.

A general recommendation when working with all athletes is to be cautious and to not take risks. The closer to competition, the more important this is.

Conditions that may present contraindications requiring avoidance or alteration in application include:

- Acute injury
- Systemic infection and acute inflammation
- Contagious conditions
- Loss of sensation
- Loss of voluntary movement
- Acute or severe cardiac, liver, and kidney diseases
- Use of sensation-altering substances, both prescribed, such as pain medication, and recreational, such as alcohol.

- Medication that thins blood, both over-the-counter, such as aspirin, and prescribed, such as Coumadin (warfarin)

Contraindications are unique to each client, as well as to each region of the body. The ability to reason clinically is essential to making appropriate decisions about the advisability of, modifications to, or avoidance of massage interventions. It is important to understand when to refer a client for diagnosis and when to obtain assistance in modifying the approach to the massage session so that it will best serve the client. A medical professional must always be consulted if any doubt exists concerning the advisability of therapy. *When in doubt, refer!*

Contraindications can be separated into regional and general types.

Regional contraindications are those that relate to a specific area of the body. For our purposes, a regional (or local) contraindication means that massage may be provided but not to the problematic area. However, the client should be referred to a physician, who can make a diagnosis and rule out underlying conditions.

General contraindications are those that require a physician's evaluation to rule out serious underlying conditions before any massage is applied. If the physician recommends massage, he or she will need to help the massage therapist develop a comprehensive treatment plan with appropriate cautions.

As discussed, massage usually is indicated for musculoskeletal discomfort, circulation enhancement, relaxation, stress reduction, and pain control, as well as in situations in which analgesics, antiinflammatory drugs, muscle relaxants, and blood pressure, antianxiety, and antidepressant medications may be prescribed. Therapeutic massage, appropriately provided, can support the use of these medications and manage some side effects, and in mild cases may be able to replace them.

The general effects of stress and pain reduction and increased circulation, as well as the physical comfort derived from therapeutic massage, complement most other medical and mental health treatment modalities. However, when other therapies, including medication, are being used, the physician must be able to evaluate accurately the effectiveness of each treatment the client is receiving. If the physician, physical therapist, or athletic trainer is unaware that the client is receiving massage, the effects of other therapies may be misinterpreted.

Clients with any vague or unexplainable symptoms of fatigue, muscle weakness, and general aches and pains should be immediately referred to a physician. Many disease processes share these symptoms. This recommendation may seem overly cautious, but in the early stages of some very serious illnesses, the symptoms are not well defined. If the physician is able to detect a disease process early in its development, there is often a more successful outcome. A specific diagnosis is essential for effective treatment. Massage should be avoided in all infectious diseases suggested by fever, nausea, and lethargy until a diagnosis has been made and recommendations from a physician can be followed.

Specific conditions that present contraindications and caution for the athletic and rehabilitation population are discussed here.

ACUTE LOCAL SOFT TISSUE INFLAMMATION

Acute inflammation can occur in any of the soft tissues, including skin, (wounds and blisters), muscles, tendons, ligaments, bursae, synovial capsule, intervertebral discs, and periosteum. Common causal factors are overuse and injury.

Common symptoms of acute inflammation include pain and dysfunction in the affected area, heat and redness, and swelling local to the injury. Frequently there is a history of recent trauma.

Superficial signs and symptoms are usually easy to identify, but less so in inflammation of the deep tissues, when the symptoms may not be visible but only palpable. On palpation, areas of acute inflammation deep in the tissues are harder and more dense than surrounding tissue. Focused pressure may cause a sharp pain. These symptoms may indicate an acute problem that requires caution in massage application, with a focus on lymphatic drain.

To test for acute inflammation, apply enough pressure to the area to cause mild discomfort. Maintain this fixed pressure for up to 10 seconds. If the discomfort increases, this suggests that the tissues are in an acute state; if it decreases, it is safe to apply massage.

BONE AND JOINT INJURIES

These conditions are usually not seen initially by a massage therapist, but if they are, then the histories, as well as the symptoms, normally make them quite obvious. If a fall or impact is involved, a fracture should always be ruled out. (Note: with fractures or dislocations of the wrist, fingers, ankle, or toes, the symptoms may be less obvious.) Fractures tend to be characterized by pain and tenderness around the injury site with any movement or weight-bearing. Stress fractures are very difficult to diagnose. Be especially concerned if the pain persists and is coupled with swelling and bruising in the injured area.

Massage in the acute stage of these conditions is obviously contraindicated, as it would cause further damage.

DIABETES

Diabetes can affect the peripheral circulation, especially in the feet, causing the tissues to become brittle and fragile. Diabetes can also affect the nerves and reduce a person's sensitivity to pressure. Deep massage techniques can damage the brittle tissues, and, with an impaired pain response, which is common in diabetes, feedback mechanisms may be ineffective.

The stimulating effect of massage on the circulation sometimes seems to have the same effect as exercise on a diabetic's blood sugar level. Clients should be made aware of this possibility so that their medication and/or diet can be altered accordingly. Although caution is required, if massage is applied correctly, clients with diabetes can receive much benefit.

FUNGAL INFECTIONS

Ringworm and athlete's foot are the most common fungal infections and can affect warm, moist areas, such as between the toes, in the armpits, or under the breast. The affected area may appear red, with white flaky skin. Although massage does not worsen the problem, it can cause irritation and may be transmitted to the therapist's hands. For these reasons, treatment of the area should be avoided.

BACTERIAL INFECTIONS

Boils are superficial abscesses that appear as localized swellings on the skin, which eventually rupture and discharge pus. Folliculitis is a condition in which the hair follicles become inflamed; it appears as a rash of very small blisters. Massage can break the blisters, leaving the skin open to further infection. These areas are regional contraindications.

Lymphangitis

Bacteria can invade the lymphatic system through open wounds, resulting in inflammation of lym-phatic vessels, or **lymphangitis.** The local area around the wound, which may itself be very minor, will appear red and swollen. A dark line can sometimes be seen running up the limb toward the affected lymph nodes, which may also be swollen and tender. Massage may spread the infection. Medical treatment is required.

VIRAL INFECTIONS

Herpes simplex virus (HSV) infection is a communicable disease and presently has no cure. Cold sores are a common symptom of HSV infection and usually appear on the face and on or near mucous membranes in that area. The cold sores will keep recurring from time to time. Before they erupt, the skin usually feels hypersensitive and tingling. HSV infection is a regional contraindication.

Other viral infections, such as warts and verrucae, should also be considered regional contraindications, because these infections can be transmitted to other parts of the body and to the massage therapist.

MELANOMA (SKIN CANCER)

Skin melanomas are becoming more common, probably because of overexposure of the skin to the sun.

Melanoma appears first as a change in pigmentation of the skin and looks like a large freckle. There is increased concern if there is an increase in size or a change in shape or bleeding, itching, or tingling. If given prompt medical treatment, this is an easily treatable condition, but if left untreated, it can be fatal.

MYOSITIS OSSIFICANS

In **myositis ossificans,** a large hematoma, which can occur with a deep bruise that goes untreated for a long time, ossifies, and forms small pieces of bony deposits within the soft tissues. This is more likely to happen when a fracture has also been involved, because osteoblasts move into the tissues, and can be the catalysts for the calcification. Massage on the area could cause a piece of bone to damage the surrounding soft tissues.

Although this is a rare condition, it should be considered when clients have had a long recovery from a serious fracture or other major impact trauma. Myositis ossificans is a regional contraindication, so avoid the area.

OPEN WOUNDS

The presence of an open wound is the most obvious contraindication and should be a matter of common sense. However, after a large wound has healed, there may be a residual problem due to scar tissue, and this can be treated by massage (see Unit Three).

TUMORS

Undiagnosed **tumors** should be referred to a medical practitioner. Massage, particularly friction massage, of a tumor may stimulate its development and help its spread to other areas. If the tumor is diagnosed as benign, then the tumor area is regionally contraindicated. If the area is malignant, then massage application should follow the physician's recommendation.

BLEEDING DISORDERS

Hemophilia is a hereditary disease that prevents the ability of the blood to clot. There are several different types and severity of the disease. Males are primarily affected. Many people also take medication that thins the blood and predisposes them to bleeding.

Anything that could cause trauma to the tissues, on any level, should be avoided. The client's physician will be able to advise on what is safe and possible for massage application.

DEEP-VEIN THROMBOSIS

A *thrombus* (blood clot) can form in a vein and be dislodged, or a fragment (embolus) may break off, during the application of massage. When this occurs in one of the deep veins of the lower limbs, the condition is known as **deep-vein thrombosis** (DVT). Because the veins get larger as they travel toward the heart, the clot can pass through the chambers of the heart and into the pulmonary circulation. The vessels become smaller as they divide and enter the lungs, and the clot may eventually block the vessels and may occlude an area of the lung. If the clot is large enough, it may block the circulation to a major part of the lung (pulmonary embolism), which can lead to death within minutes.

Factors that may lead to DVT include long periods of immobility or bed rest, which reduces circulation and can compress the veins; recent major surgery; varicose veins, heart disease, and diabetes; use of contraceptive pills; and impact trauma, which may cause damage inside the vein. Although very rare, DVT can occur in seemingly healthy people as the result of other predisposing factors.

Acute pain and hard swelling may be felt when minimal pressure is applied and may be confused with an acute muscle strain. There may be general swelling and discoloration in the distal part of the limb due to restricted circulation. The client may feel more pain and aching in the area when resting than would be expected if it were a muscle strain. There would be no history to suggest such an injury.

If a DVT is suspected, the client should be referred to a physician or hospital immediately.

VARICOSE VEINS

Varicose veins usually occur at the back of the leg. The valves within the veins, which prevent a back flow in the circulation, break down, and stop functioning.

In minor cases, light superficial stroking over the area should do no harm and may in fact ease the pressure on the vein and aid repair. Deep pressure and drag should not be applied because further damage to the walls of the blood vessels can occur. In advanced cases, even superficial stroking should be avoided because there is the added risk of DVT.

This contraindication relates only to the actual location of the vein. The tissues adjacent to the area can be massaged. This will improve circulation away from the varicose vein and relieve some of the pressure.

MEDICATIONS

The massage professional needs to be aware of any medications the client is taking. Massage therapists should have a current *Mosby's Drug Consult* or similar drug reference book so that all medications listed on the client information form can be researched. Internet search programs for researching medications are available as well. Also, the client may be able to provide information about each medication being taken.

In general, a medication is prescribed to do one of the following:
- Stimulate a body process
- Inhibit a body process
- Replace a chemical in the body

Therapeutic massage can also stimulate and inhibit body processes. When the medication and massage stimulate the same process, the effects are synergistic and the result can be too much stimulation. If the medication and massage inhibit the same process, the result is again synergistic, but this time there is too much inhibition. If the medication stimulates an effect and massage inhibits the same effect, massage can be antagonistic to the medication.

Although massage seldom interacts substantially with a medication that replaces a body chemical, it is important to be aware of possible synergistic or inhibitory effects.

Massage often can be used to manage undesirable side effects of medications. In particular, medications that stimulate sympathetic ANS function can cause uncomfortable side effects such as digestive upset, anxiety and restlessness, and sleep disruption. The mild inhibitory effects of massage resulting from stimulation of parasympathetic activity can sometimes provide short-term relief from the undesirable effects of a medication without interfering with its desired action. Caution is required, and close monitoring by the primary care physician is necessary.

The massage professional should be able to assess the effects of medications and should be aware of the ways massage may influence these effects. Massage practitioners need to be specifically knowledgeable about antiinflammatory drugs, muscle relaxants, anticoagulants (blood thinners), analgesics (pain modulators), and other medications that alter sensation, muscle tone, standard reflex reactions, cardiovascular function, kidney and liver function, and personality. They also should be aware of the effects of over-the-counter medications, herbs, and vitamins as well. If a client is taking medication, it is important to have the client's physician confirm the advisability of therapeutic massage.

evolve Refer to the Evolve website accompanying this book for a list of common medications and possible interactions with massage.

ENDANGERMENT SITES

Endangerment sites are areas in which nerves and blood vessels surface are close to the skin and are not well protected by muscle or connective tissue. Consequently, deep, sustained pressure into these areas could damage the vessels and nerves. Areas containing fragile bony projections that could be broken off are also considered endangerment sites. The kidney area is considered an endangerment site because the kidneys are loosely suspended in fat and connective tissue. Heavy pounding is contraindicated in that area.

When the massage therapist is working over an endangerment site, avoidance or light pressure is indicated to prevent damage. The areas shown in Figure 10-2 show commonly considered endangerment sites.

Other endangerment sites include the following:
- Eyes
- Inferior to the ear—fascial nerve, styloid process, external carotid artery
- Posterior cervical area (spinous processes, cervical plexus)
- Lymph nodes
- Medial brachium—between the biceps and triceps
- Musculocutaneous, median, and ulnar nerves
- Brachial artery
- Basilic vein
- Cubital (anterior) area of the median nerve, radial and ulnar arteries, and median cubital vein
- Area of application of lateral pressure to the knees

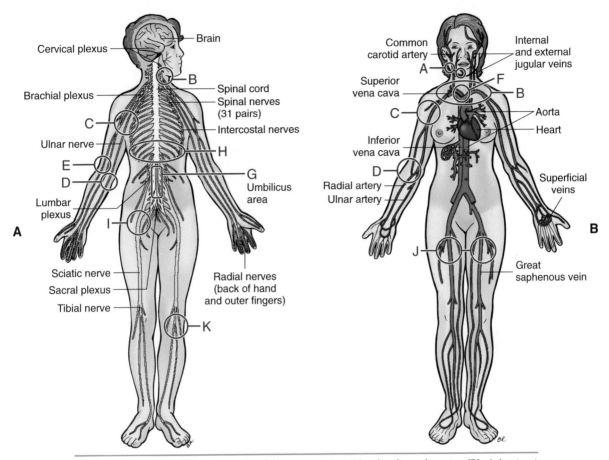

FIGURE 10-2 ■ Endangerment sites of the nervous system **(A)** and cardiovascular system **(B)**. *A,* Anterior triangle of the neck (carotid artery, jugular vein, and vagus nerve), which are located deep to the sternocleidomastoid. *B,* Posterior triangle of the neck—specifically the nerves of the brachial plexus, the brachiocephalic artery and vein superior to the clavicle, and the subclavian arteries and vein. *C,* Axillary area—the brachial artery, axillary vein and artery, cephalic vein, and nerves of the brachial plexus. *D,* Medial epicondyle of the humerus—the ulnar nerve; also the radial and ulnar arteries. *E,* Lateral epicondyle—the radial nerve. *F,* Area of the sternal notch and anterior throat—nerves and vessels to the thyroid gland and the vagus nerve. *G,* Umbilicus area—to either side; descending aorta and abdominal aorta. *H,* Twelfth rib, dorsal body—location of the kidney. *I,* Sciatic notch—sciatic nerve (the sciatic nerve passes out of the pelvis through the greater sciatic foramen, under cover of the piriformis muscle). *J,* Inguinal triangle located lateral and inferior to the pubis—medial to the sartorius, external iliac artery, femoral artery, great saphenous vein, femoral vein, and femoral nerve. *K,* Popliteal fossa—popliteal artery and vein and tibial nerve. (From Fritz S: *Mosby's fundamentals of therapeutic massage,* ed 3. St. Louis, 2004, Mosby.)

SUMMARY

Massage is a valuable treatment for most conditions, ranging from stress to severe illness and injury. However, it must be applied intelligently, based on the current condition of the client. Competing athletes usually seem to have a bang, bruise, blister, sprain, strain, or wound, and regional avoidance or altered massage application is necessary. Persons in physical rehabilitation are there because of some illness or injury, so contraindications and cautions are part of working with this population.

It is important to not assume that minor symptoms equate to minor causes. Nothing is lost by being cautious. Just make sure that during referral the communication approach does not scare the client, and do not overstep the scope of practice by diagnosing.

The statement I often use is, "I need to have these things ruled out by the doctor or trainer so the massage can be given without undue restriction. If I don't know what it is, I have to be extra cautious, so let's just eliminate these possibilities and proceed from there."

1 List the situation(s) that you feel you will most often encounter in which massage is indicated. Refer back to Chapter 9 and describe the physiologic mechanism of benefit for massage application.

_____

_____

_____

_____

_____

_____

_____

_____

_____

_____

2 Develop a position statement on the value of massage for performance fitness and rehabilitation based on the indications discussed in this chapter.

_____

_____

_____

_____

_____

_____

_____

_____

_____

_____

3 Develop a checklist for screening for contraindications.

_____

_____

_____

_____

_____

_____

_____

_____

_____

_____

_____

_____

_____

_____

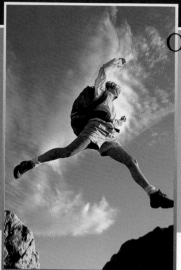

CHAPTER

11

ASSESSMENT FOR SPORTS MASSAGE AND PHYSICAL REHABILITATION APPLICATION

OBJECTIVES

Upon completion of this chapter the reader will have the information necessary to:

1 Apply a clinical reasoning process to treatment plan development.

2 Complete a comprehensive history.

3 Complete a comprehensive physical assessment.

4 Relate assessment data to first-degree, second-degree, and third-degree dysfunction and categorize the adaptation response to stage 1, 2, or 3 pathology.

5 Integrate ongoing assessment data channeled into appropriate massage treatment strategies.

ASSESSMENT

The massage therapist working with athletes, physical rehabilitation, and those involved with fitness has an expanded assessment responsibility. **Assessment** identifies the structures that need to be worked with, creates a clear intention about the treatment goals, provides a baseline of objective information to measure the effectiveness of the treatment, and helps identify conditions that are contraindicated. When working with a client who is striving for optimal performance or has pain, dysfunction, or disability, the massage therapist needs to gather information about both long-term and short-term treatment goals, and relevant data about activities and training activity, as well as pain or decreased function.

Information from the athletic trainer, coaches, or other professionals is important. The massage therapist must understand and apply assessment information provided by the trainer. If at any time you do not understand, ask clarifying questions. Information gathered by the massage therapist should be shared with the athletic trainer or other appropriate member of the sport and/or medical team in a concise and intelligent manner.

Active movements
Assessment
Charting
Clinical reasoning
Connective tissue changes
End-feel
First-degree, second-degree, and third-degree distortion in functioning

Functional stress
Functional tension
Gait assessment
History
Kinetic chain
Micro-trauma
Muscle firing pattern
Muscle strength testing

Outcome goals
Palpation assessment
Phasic (mover) muscles
Physical assessment
Postural (stabilizer) muscles
Posture
Range of motion (ROM)

A massage treatment plan based on efficient biomechanical movement should focus on reestablishing or supporting effective movement patterns. Biomechanically efficient movement is smooth, bilaterally symmetric, and coordinated, with easy, effortless use of the body. Functional assessment measures the efficiency of coordinated movement. During assessment, noticeable variations need to be considered.

A general protocol is presented in Chapter 14, which includes suggestions for assessment and the treatment process.

Once the treatment plan is determined, the massage therapist needs to develop strategies for achieving the goals pertaining to the therapeutic massage. Teamwork is essential, with cooperation and consensus among the various professionals attending to the client. It is important for the massage therapist to maintain an appropriate scope of practice and not infringe on the professional responsibilities and expertise of others.

CLINICAL REASONING PROCESS

As the volume of knowledge pertaining to massage increases, and as soft tissue modalities such as massage are integrated into the areas of sport fitness and physical rehabilitation, it is becoming increasingly important to be able to think or reason through an intervention process and justify its effectiveness. Therapeutic massage practitioners must be able to gather information effectively, analyze that information to make decisions about the type and appropriateness of an intervention,

and evaluate and justify the benefits derived from the intervention.

Effective assessment, analysis, and decision making are essential to meet the needs of each client. Routine or a recipe-type application of therapeutic massage does not work for this population because each person's set of presenting circumstances and outcome goals is different. An experienced sports massage professional possesses effective clinical reasoning skills targeted to this complex population.

Fact gathering is an initial part of the **clinical reasoning** process. Each unique client situation needs to be thoroughly researched. This text provides only a portion of the information needed. Additional research is almost always necessary.

Every massage professional who works with athletes needs to have a medical dictionary and comprehensive texts on athletic training, kinesiology, and pathology, as well as resources on the particular sport and references on medication and nutritional supplements. See the resource list in this text for recommendations. The internet is also a vast resource.

Each sport has its ideal performance requirement and common injuries; however, a sprain in a football player, soccer player, and skate boarder is still a sprain. The sprain should be addressed according to the recommendations in this text. Understanding the demands of the sport is important. However, it is not necessary for the massage professional to be an expert in the sport activity. The sport activity is the context that the massage outcomes support.

Subjective and objective assessment is also a fact source and is the major topic of this chapter. Analysis of the factual data in the assessment leads to treatment plan development.

OUTCOME GOALS AND CARE OR TREATMENT PLAN

Outcome goals need to be *quantified*. This means that they are measured in terms of objective criteria such as time, frequency, 1-10 scales, measurable increase or decrease in the ability to perform an activity, and/or measurable increase or decrease in sensation, such as relaxation or pain.

Outcome goals also need to be *qualified*. How will we know when the goal is achieved? What will the client be able to do after the goal has been reached that he or she is not able to do now? For example: How fast will the client be able to run? What performance skills will the client be able to perform?

After the analysis of the history and assessment data is complete and problems and goals have been identified, a decision needs to be made about the care or treatment plan. Depending on the situation, the massage treatment plan may need to be approved by the appropriate supervising personnel.

Short-term goals typically support a session-by-session process and are dependent on the current status of the client. Long-term goals typically support recovery, performance, or rehabilitation. Long-term goals focus on what is being worked toward. Short-term goals focus on what currently is being worked on, as well as incremental steps toward achieving long-term goals. Short-term goals should not be in conflict with long-term goals.

For example, a golfer is involved in a conditioning program in preparation for going on tour. She has been working on core strength and cardiovascular fitness with a strength and conditioning coach. She has also been working on swing mechanics with the golf coach. The long-term goals for this client are to maintain range of motion (ROM) and manage a chronic tendency for low back pain. In this particular session, the client has indicated that she has a headache and delayed onset muscle soreness. The focus of the current massage must consider both short-term and long-term goals. Short-term goals are to reduce headache pain and fluid retention as part of the existing long-term treatment plan.

How much time is allocated to each goal set depends on the adaptive capacity of the client. For example, massage targeting connective tissue application as part of the long-term goals plan may be reduced or eliminated in the areas where delayed-onset muscle soreness exists. Muscle energy

application may require more effort than the client is willing to expend because of the headache.

It is this ever-changing dynamic of past history, current conditions, and future outcomes that makes any sort of massage routine useless. Each and every session is uniquely developed and applied based on multiple factors. There are many influencing factors to consider when treating athletes or those in physical rehabilitation of any type. Assessment is the identification of all of these influences. Clinical reasoning is the sorting and developing of an appropriate treatment session.

CHARTING

As the treatment plan is implemented, it is recorded sequentially, session by session, in some form of **charting** process such as SOAP (*s*ubjective, *o*bjective, *a*ssessment [*a*nalysis], and *p*lan). The plan is reevaluated and adjusted as necessary. This process should have been learned in entry-level massage training.

Various charting methods are used in the sport and fitness realm. Regardless of the particular style, the basic SOAP plan is easily modified to other charting styles. *Be very clear with the supervisory personnel, usually the trainer, about the type and depth of information included on the client's charts.*

Good record keeping provides the therapist with the information necessary to communicate with health care and other personnel and furnishes an accurate record about what treatment goals are specified, the methods of massage, and the effectiveness of treatment.

ASSESSMENT DETAILS

How extensive the assessment is depends on whether you are working under the direction of a doctor, a trainer, or another health care provider or are working independently. It is the responsibility of the primary care provider to take a thorough history, perform a complete examination, and inform the massage therapist regarding the client's condition and desired outcomes for the massage. If you are working independently, it is your responsibility to perform the appropriate comprehensive assessment, especially to note contraindications and clarify treatment goals.

This text assumes that the reader already has completed a comprehensive therapeutic massage course of study that included assessment procedures such as history taking, physical assessment, treatment plan development, and charting.*

The following procedures are recommended for targeting this specific population.

HISTORY

The **history** interview provides subjective information pertaining to the client's health history, the reasons for massage, a history of the current condition, a history of past illness and health, and a history of any family illnesses that may be pertinent. It also contains an account of the client's current health practices.

Targeting this information to the athlete or person in physical rehabilitation is the focus of this text. In addition to the general history, anyone who is working with an athlete or a person in physical rehabilitation needs to explore the following for each client.

- Surgery or medical procedures
- Medications and supplements
- Use of hydrotherapy
- Use of electrostimulation
- Therapeutic exercise activities
- Physical therapy intervention
- Nutrition
- Training protocols
- Training types such as strength and conditioning and agility.
- Sleep patterns
- Breathing patterns
- Mood
- Cognitive load (how much mental training required)
- Competition schedule
- Practice and training schedules
- Previous massage experience
- Use of alternative therapies (essential oils, magnets)

The client's history may vary depending on whether the problem is the result of sudden trauma or chronic. The following questions should be addressed if the athlete has an acute injury. Usually it is the doctor or trainer who performs the initial injury assessment.

Has the client hurt the area before?
How did the client hurt the area?

---

*For more in-depth information, see Fritz S: *Mosby's fundamentals of therapeutic massage*, ed 3, St. Louis, 2004, Mosby; and Fritz S: *Mosby's essential sciences for therapeutic massage*, ed 2, St. Louis, 2004, Mosby.

What was heard when the injury occurred—a crack, snap, or pop?
How bad was the pain and how long did it last?
Is there any sense of muscle weakness?
How disabling was the injury?
Could the client move the area right away?
Was the client able to bear weight for a period of time?
Has a similar injury occurred before?
Was there immediate swelling, or did the swelling occur later (or at all)?
Where did the swelling occur?

For an athlete with a chronic condition ask the following:

What was the nature of the injury (trauma or repetitive use)?
How much does it hurt?
Where does it hurt?
What is the nature of the pain—hot, pokey, sharp?
Does it hurt to the touch?
Does it hurt when you move?
When does the pain occur—when bearing weight or after activity?
What injuries have occurred in the past?
What first aid and therapy, if any, were given for these previous injuries?

Additional questions address when the client first noticed this condition to help to identify any previous incident or injury prior to the current condition.

What are the details of onset?
Did the condition arise suddenly or gradually?
Was there a specific injury?

Typically, a gradual onset suggests an overuse syndrome, postural stresses, or somatic manifestations of emotional or psychological stresses common in athletes.

Where is the location of the area? Show me.

Ask the client to point as well as explain the area of complaint.

What were the prior treatments—medication, surgery?
What was the outcome?

It is also important to know whether the client has had massage therapy before, whether it was helpful, and the type of massage application.

What medications are being taken?

If the client has taken pain medication within 4 hours of assessment and treatment, the medication may be giving the client a false sense of comfort during assessment and during massage. Be aware of anti-inflammatories, muscle relaxers, and so forth.

What diagnostic studies have been performed—radiography, magnetic resonance imaging?
What were the results?
What is the nature of the progress?
Is the client getting better, worse, or in need of a referral?

GESTURES

Pay attention to gestures used by the client. The general guidelines for gestures listed are not written in stone. Professional experience indicates that those listed here are fairly dependable starting points when interpreting an individual's body language.

It is the professional's responsibility to understand what a gesture means for a particular individual.

The following are common gestures:

- A finger pointing to a specific area suggests an acupressure or motor point hyperactivity or a joint problem. What the pointing means depends on the area indicated.
- If the finger is pointed to a specific area and then the hand swipes in a certain direction, it may be a trigger point problem.
- If the area is grabbed, pulled, or held and moved as if being stretched, this often indicates muscle or fascial shortening.
- If movement is needed to show the area of concern, the area may need muscle lengthening combined with muscle energy work to prepare for the stretch and reset of neuromuscular patterns.
- If the client moves into a position and then acts as if stuck, the area may need connective tissue stretching.
- If the client draws lines on his body, it may indicate nerve entrapment in the fascial planes or grooves.

SYMPTOMS

What is the frequency of the discomfort?

It is important to determine how often the client notices the dysfunction or disability. Is it once a day, two or three days a week, once a week, or constant? Grade 1 and 2 sprains and strains to the muscles, tendons, and ligaments usually hurt when they are being used, and are relieved with rest. Constant pain may be associated with a severe injury or underlying pathology. A client with constant pain should be referred to a physician.

How long is the duration?

The more serious the condition, the longer it will last.

What is the nature of the symptoms?

Typical words used by the client to describe the symptoms are stiff, achy, tight, stuck, and heavy. These words are associated with muscles, tendons, ligaments, and joint capsules and their associated connective tissue and usually describe simple tension or mild overuse of the soft tissue or edema. If an ache is more than mild, is frequent, and lasts a long time, it is more serious and represents inflammation. A referral is required to rule out a more serious condition.

Typically, *tight* means an increase in neuromuscular activity. *Achy* and *fat* often indicates fluid retention or swelling. *Stiff* sensations often indicate a connective tissue pliability issue. *Heavy* sensation of the limbs indicates a firing pattern or gait reflex problem. *Stuck* sensations often mean a joint problem.

Other terms used to describe symptoms include:

Sharp stabbing, tearing describes a more severe injury to the musculoskeletal system or a nerve root condition. This is the type of sensation experienced with muscle or ligament tears, especially when the muscle or ligament is being used. The sensation is usually relieved at rest. A nerve root inflammation can elicit a sharp or stabbing pain, independent of movement.

Tingling, numbing, picky describes a nerve compression, either near the spine or in the extremities, or a circulation impairment.

Throbbing, hot is associated with acute injury inflammation and swelling, such as an abrasion puncture wound or an acute bursitis. Severe throbbing is a contraindication to massage.

Gripping, cramping is typically used to describe a serious condition, often a nerve root injury or visceral condition. Gripping and cramping pain is a contraindication to massage and requires referral to a doctor.

The client can choose from the following descriptors:

- Sore
- Tight
- Stiff
- Weak
- Stuck
- Knot
- Balled up
- Fat, cold
- More pain in the morning or night
- Heavy
- Tired
- Burning
- Cramp
- Poking
- Twisted
- Hurt to touch
- Hurt during movement
- Pinching

Does the symptom radiate?

Irritation or injury to the soft tissue can refer to the extremities, with diffuse pain and aching. Nerve entrapment and trigger point pain can radiate. Sharp well-localized pain in the extremities felt even at rest typically indicates a nerve root problem and requires a referral.

How severe are the symptoms?

Ask the client to rate his or her pain on a 0 to 10 scale, with 10 being the worst pain ever experienced (incapacitating pain) and 0 being no pain. Moderate pain (5 to 9) interferes with a person's ability to perform sport-related activities. Mild pain (1 to 4) does not interfere with a person's activities of daily living but may interfere with sport performance.

What activities make the condition worse—moving, sitting, standing, walking, or resting?
What sport movement is affected—running, jumping, cutting, swinging, acceleration, or deceleration?

The most simple strains and sprains of the musculoskeletal system are irritated by too much movement and relieved by rest. When a condition hurts more with rest, it indicates either inflammation or pathology.

What activities make the condition better—resting, moving, or applying ice or heat?

As the soft tissue heals, it feels good to move the injured area. Stretching tight muscles, shortened ligaments, and joint capsules feels good, despite some mild discomfort. Acute injuries involving the soft tissue are painful with large movements

and are relieved with rest. Muscle guarding makes stretching painful.

When does the pain occur?

Pain caused by inflammation and tumors is worse at night. Constant, gripping pain that is worse at night requires immediate referral to a doctor. An area that hurts at night but is relieved with movement usually indicates inflammation. Joint pain and stiffness with fascial shortening is usually worse in the morning.

Clarifying assessment questions to ask:

What can you do? Show me.
What can't you do? Show me.
What do you want to improve? Show me.
What does the pain feel like?

If you could fix it yourself, what would you do?

The client should demonstrate for the massage therapist. Trust the client's impressions. They usually are right. Then translate what the client is saying into a massage application.

The client should draw a picture of his or her condition. When the client draws the picture, give as few directions as possible. Evaluate the drawing for location and intensity of the symptom. Does the client use hard zigzag lines or small or large circles? Then ask the client to explain.

evolve See the Evolve site to accompany this book for an example.

All the history information should be consolidated and considered when developing treatment plans and session outcomes.

PHYSICAL ASSESSMENT

After the history is complete, the physical assessment is performed. The objective date is obtained during physical assessment.

Accurate assessment is best achieved using a sequence to ensure that all the relevant information has been gathered. A major aspect of a massage session is palpation assessment.

In general, physical assessment includes:
- Visual (blisters, bruises, rash) assessment
- Palpation
- Stability
- Firing patterns
- Gait
- Range of motion (ROM)
- Tissue pliability
- Mobility

- Agility
- Stamina
- Strength
- Performance skills

Identify any scars or muscle atrophy. Scars indicate either prior surgery or prior injury and reveal that the area is compromised. Ask the client to describe how he or she received the scar.

An area of atrophy has either been deconditioned owing to lack of use or indicates neurologic involvement. Simple atrophy can be a result of immobilization caused by prior fracture or lack of use due to pain.

PHYSICAL ASSESSMENT OF POSTURE

Notice the **posture** of the client in both standing and seated positions, and the posture or position of the area of complaint. Look for areas of asymmetry. Asymmetry usually results when overly tense muscles or shortened connective tissue pulls the body out of alignment.

Direct trauma pushes joints out of alignment. Weak stabilizing mechanisms, such as overstretched ligaments or inhibited antagonist muscles, contribute to the problem. In these situations a chiropractor, an osteopath, or another trained medical professional skilled in skeletal manipulation is needed. Often a multidisciplinary approach to client care is necessary.

First observe the client during general movement as opposed to formal assessment to identify natural function. Then perform the following structured standing assessment and compare the findings.

Standard Posture Front View:
- Head: Neutral position neither tilted nor rotated
- Shoulders: Level, not elevated or depressed
- Pelvis: Level with both anterior superior iliac spines in same transverse plane
- Hip joints: Neutral position neither adducted nor abducted nor internally or externally rotated
- Lower extremities: Straight
- Feet: Parallel

Standard Posture Back View:
- Head: Neutral position neither tilted nor rotated
- Shoulders: Level, not elevated or depressed
- Scapulae: Neutral position, medial borders essentially parallel and approximately three to four inches apart

- Thoracic and lumbar spines: Straight
- Pelvis: Level with both posterior superior iliac spines in same transverse plane
- Hip joints: Neutral position neither adducted nor abducted or rotated (internal or external)
- Lower extremities: Straight
- Feet: Parallel

Standard Posture Side View:
- Head: Neutral position, not tilted forward or backward
- Cervical spine: Normal curve, slightly convex to anterior
- Scapulae: Flat against upper back
- Thoracic spine: Normal curve, slightly convex to posterior
- Lumbar spine: Normal curve, slightly convex to anterior
- Pelvis: Neutral position, anterior superior iliac spine in same vertical plane as symphysis pubis
- Hip joints: Neutral position, leg vertical at right angle in sole of foot

Note: An imaginary line should run slightly behind the lateral malleolus, through the middle of the femur, the center of the shoulder, and the middle of the ear.

Chart the findings and relate them to the client's history (Figure 11-1).

For the physical assessment, the main considerations are body balance, efficient function, and basic symmetry (Box 11-1).

IN MY EXPERIENCE...

The big and the small of it. These things tickle me . . .

A great big body builder carrying a little pink bag with a kitten on it. It was a present for his girlfriend.

A really short head coach scolding a big tall basketball player.

A great big football lineman walking around with his baby's pacifier.

A tiny figure skater driving a great big truck.

A beat up old hockey player helping his young daughter dress her Barbie doll.

. . . After all, athletes are just people and observation can be fun.

The body is not perfectly symmetric, but the right and left halves of the body should be similar in shape, ROM, and ability to function. The greater the discrepancy in symmetry, the greater the potential for soft tissue dysfunction.

MASSAGE ASSESSMENT/PHYSICAL PALPATION AND GAIT

PRE
POST ⊘

Client Name: _____   Date: _____

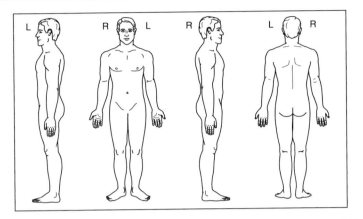

OBSERVATION & PALPATION	OBSERVATION & PALPATION	GAIT ASSESSMENT
ALIGNMENT	**RIBS**	
Chin in line with nose, sternal notch, navel	Even	**HEAD**
Other:	Springy	Remains steady/eyes forward
HEAD	Other:	Other:
Tilted (L)	**ABDOMEN**	**TRUNK**
Tilted (R)	Firm and pliable	Remains vertical
Rotated (L)	Hard areas	Other:
Rotated (R)	Other:	**SHOULDERS**
EYES	**WAIST**	Remain level
Level	Level	Rotate during walking
Equally set in sockets	Other:	Other:
Other:	**SPINE CURVES**	**ARMS**
EARS	Normal	Motion is opposite leg swing
Level	Other:	Motion is even (L) and (R)
Other:	**GLUTEAL MUSCLE MASS**	Other:
SHOULDERS	Even	(L) swings freely
Level	Other:	(R) swings freely
(R) high / (L) low	**ILIAC CREST**	Other:
(L) high / (R) low	Level	**HIPS**
(L) rounded forward	Other:	Remain level
(R) rounded forward	**KNEES**	Other:
Muscle development even	Even/symmetrical	Rotate during walking
Other:	Other:	Other:

FIGURE 11-1 ■ Physical assessment form. (Feel free to copy this form to use as an assessment tool.) (From Fritz S: *Mosby's fundamentals of therapeutic massage*, ed 3. St. Louis, 2004, Mosby.)

Continued

SCAPULA	PATELLA		LEGS
Even	(L) ☐ movable ☐ rigid		Swing freely at hip
Move freely	(R) ☐ movable ☐ rigid		Other:
Other:	**ANKLES**		**KNEES**
CLAVICLES	Even		Flex and extend freely through stance and swing phase
Level	Other:		Other:
Other:	**FEET**		**FEET**
ARMS	Mobile		Heel strikes first at start of stance
Hang evenly (internal) (external)	Other:		Plantar flexed at push-off
(L) rotated ☐ medial ☐ lateral	**ARCHES**		Foot clears floor during swing phase
(R) rotated ☐ medial ☐ lateral	Even		Other:
ELBOWS	Other:		**STEP**
Even	**TOES**		Length is even
Other:	Straight		Timing is even
WRISTS	Other:		Other:
Even	**SKIN**		**OVERALL**
Other:	Moves freely and resilient		Rhythmic
FINGERTIPS	Pulls/restricted		Other:
Even	Puffy/baggy		
Other:	Other:		

FIGURE II-I CONT'D ■ Physical assessment form.

BOX II-I   LANDMARKS THAT HELP IDENTIFY LACK OF SYMMETRY

The following landmarks can be used for comparison. Be sure to observe the client from the back, the front, the left and right sides.

- The middle of the chin should sit directly under the tip of the nose. Check the chin alignment with the sternal notch. These two landmarks should be a direct line.
- The shoulders and clavicles should be level with each other.
- The shoulders should not roll forward or backward or be rotated with one forward and one backward.
- The arms should hang freely and at the same rotation out of the glenohumeral (shoulder) joint.
- The elbows, wrists, and fingertips should be in the same plane.
- The skin of the thorax (chest and back) should be even and should not look as if it is pulled or is puffy.
- The naval, located on the same line as the nose, chin, and sternal notch, should not look pulled.
- The ribs should be even and springy.
- The abdomen should be firm but relaxed and slightly rounded.
- The curves at the waist should be even on both sides.

- The spine should be in a direct line from the base of the skull and on the same plane as the line connecting the nose and the navel. The curves of the spine should not be exaggerated.
- The scapulae should appear even and should move freely. You should be able to draw an imaginary straight line between the tips of the scapulae.
- The gluteal muscle mass should be even.
- The tops of the iliac crests should be even.
- The greater trochanter, knees, and ankles should be level.
- The circumferences of the thigh and calf should be similar on the left and right sides.
- The legs should rotate out of the acetabulum (hip joint) evenly in a slightly external rotation.
- The knees should be locked in the standing position but should not be hyperextended. The patellae (kneecaps) should be level and pointed slightly laterally.
- A line dropped from the nose should fall through the sternum and the navel and should be spaced evenly in between.

From Fritz S: *Mosby's fundamentals of therapeutic massage*, ed 3. St. Louis, 2004, Mosby.

Three major factors influence posture: *heredity*, *disease*, and *habit*. These factors must be considered when evaluating posture. The easiest influence to adjust is habit. By normalizing the soft tissue and teaching balancing exercises, the massage practitioner can play a beneficial role in helping clients overcome habitual postural distortion. Effects may arise from occupational habits (e.g., a shoulder rotation from golf) and recreational habits (e.g., a forward-shoulder position in a bike rider), or they may be sleep-related (long-term use of high pillows).

Clothing, sport equipment, shoes, and furniture affect the way a person uses his or her body. Tight clothing or equipment around the neck restricts breathing and contributes to neck and shoulder problems. Restrictive belts or tight pants also limit breathing and affect the neck, shoulders, and midback. Shoes with high heels or those that do not fit the feet comfortably interfere with postural muscles. Shoes with worn soles imprint the old postural pattern, and the client's body assumes the dysfunctional pattern if he or she puts them back on after the massage. If postural changes are to be maintained, it is important to wear shoes that do not have worn soles.

Sleep positions can contribute to a wide range of problems. Furniture that does not support the back or that is too high or too low perpetuates muscular tension. Competing athletes travel and therefore change beds often. The seats in airplanes are seldom comfortable for athletes.

When assessing posture, it is important for the massage therapist to notice the complete postural pattern. Most compensatory patterns are in response to external forces imposed on the body. However, if the client has had an injury, maintains a certain position for a prolonged period, or overuses a body area, the body may not be able to return to a normal dynamic balance efficiently. The balance of the body against the force of gravity is the fundamental determining factor in a person's posture or upright position. Even subtle shifts in posture demand a whole-body compensatory pattern (Figure 11-2).

The cervical, thoracic, lumbar, and sacral curves develop because of the need to maintain an upright position against gravity (Figure 11-3).

Standing posture requires various segments of the body to cooperate mechanically as a whole. Passive tension of ligaments, fascia, and the connective tissue elements of the muscles supports the skeleton. Muscle activity plays a small but impor-

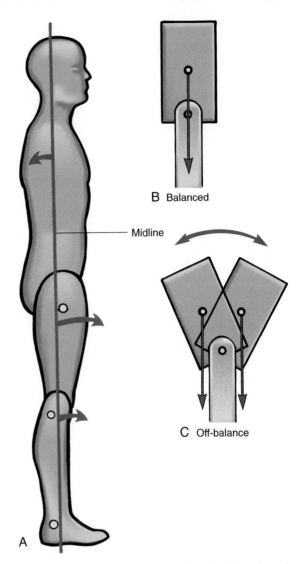

FIGURE 11-2 ■ In normal relaxed standing (**A**), the leg and trunk tend to rotate slightly off the midline of the body but maintain a counterbalance force. Balance is achieved in **B**, but not in **C**. Whenever the trunk moves off this midline balance point, the body must compensate. (From Fritz S: *Mosby's fundamentals of therapeutic massage*, ed 3. St. Louis, 2004, Mosby.)

tant role. Postural muscles maintain small amounts of contraction that stabilize the body upright in gravity by continually repositioning the body's weight over the mechanical balance point.

In relaxed symmetric standing, both the hip and the knee joints assume a position of full extension to provide the most efficient weight-bearing position. The knee joint has an additional stabilizing element in its "screw home" mechanism. The femur rides backward on its medial condyle and rotates medially about its vertical axis to lock the

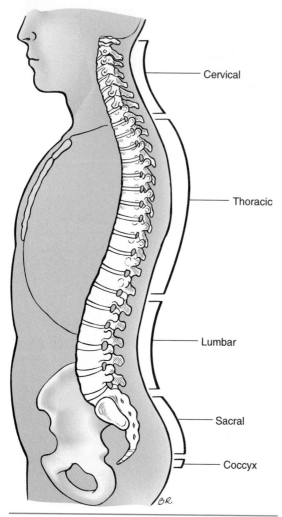

FIGURE 11-3 ■ Normal spinal curves. (From Fritz S: *Mosby's fundamentals of therapeutic massage*, ed 3. St. Louis, 2004, Mosby.)

joint for weight bearing. This happens only in the final phase of extension. The hamstrings are the major muscles that resist the force of gravity at the knees.

At the ankle joint, bones and ligaments do little to limit motion. Passive tension of the two-joint gastrocnemius muscle (i.e., the muscle crosses two joints) becomes an important factor. This stabilizing force is diminished if high-heeled shoes are worn. For example, rodeo riders wear cowboy boots. The heel of the shoe puts the gastrocnemius on a slack. If these heels are worn constantly, the muscle and the Achilles tendon shorten.

Posture is primarily determined by hereditary factors, such as bone structure and muscle type, and even by habitual movement patterns. These can create natural imbalances, but these alone do not normally lead to painful conditions until later in life. They can, however, combine with other stresses such as athletic activity, and together can lead to injury. Little can be done to change these hereditary factors, and regular exercise and soft tissue treatment are often the only way of avoiding such symptoms.

Upright posture is maintained by a series of muscles running down the body. These need to balance each other, in terms of strength and tension, and together resist the forces of gravity. Any postural change will nearly always be in a downward and forward direction, as fatigue or injury reduces the ability of the postural muscles to combat gravity. This creates increased curvature in particular sections of the spine, which can be seen by the therapist when observing the client's standing posture.

Postural dysfunction occurs in the three planes of movement (sagittal, frontal, and transverse) as well as supination and pronation (Figures 11-4 and 11-5).

ASSESSMENT OF JOINT AND MUSCLE FUNCTION

Although the muscular system looks highly complicated, it is important to realize that the actual mechanics involved in movement is simple. A muscle can do only two things; it can contract and shorten and it can relax and lengthen. The system is a complex pattern of movement composed of many simple levers and pulleys. Movement is created by a muscle shortening, which pulls bones together that are connected at the joint.

Many muscles working in functional units provide the widest variety of movements and the ability to do them with stability, control, and efficiency. For example, the knee is basically a hinge joint capable of moving on only one plane, and so theoretically it should need only one pulley (muscle) to flex it and one to extend it. But for extension there are the four quadriceps muscles, each of which pulls across the joint in a slightly different direction. During flexion three hamstrings accomplish the same thing. This muscle interaction stabilizes the joint and enables it to adapt to variations in movement and to the random direction of forces from the outside environment. The whole of the muscular system works in unison to enable the body to cope with the stresses caused by gravity when movement takes place. It is important to see move-

FIGURE 11-4

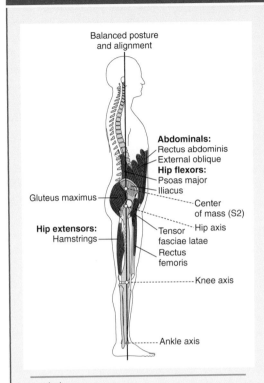

A Ideal posture.

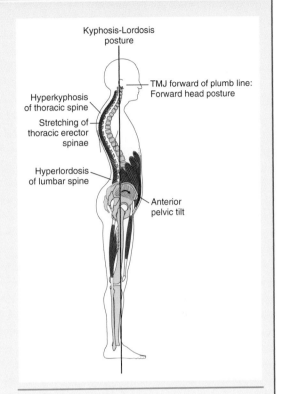

C Kypholordotic posture.

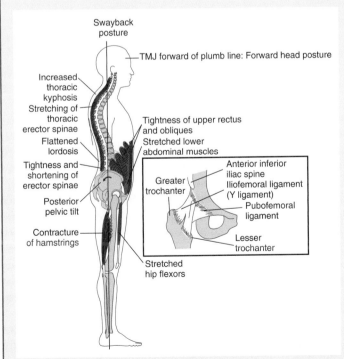

B Swayback posture.

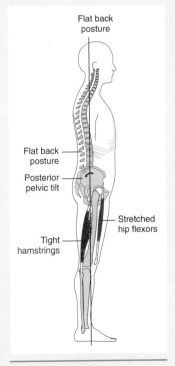

D Flat back posture.

Effects of postural imbalance. (Modified from Saidoff DC, McDonough AL: *Critical pathways in therapeutic intervention: extremities and spine.* St. Louis, 2002, Mosby.)

FIGURE 11-5

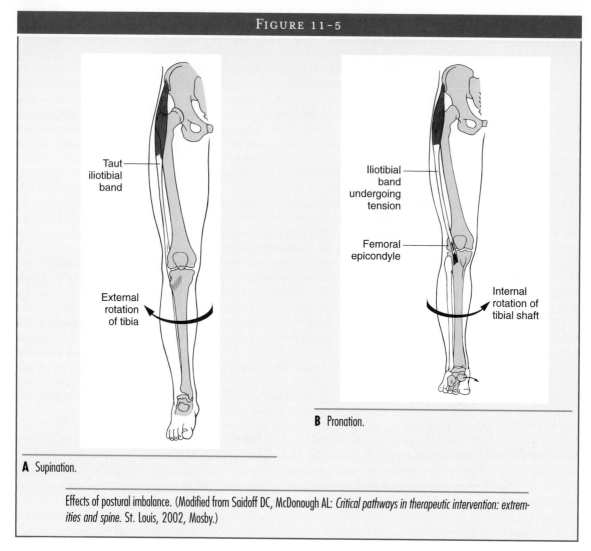

A Supination.

B Pronation.

Effects of postural imbalance. (Modified from Saidoff DC, McDonough AL: *Critical pathways in therapeutic intervention: extremities and spine*. St. Louis, 2002, Mosby.)

ment in terms of patterns of activity (movement strategies) taking place within a system rather than as the action of individual muscles. Almost all movement strategies involve the gait (walking) process.

Overuse problems develop in parts of a system that are put under greater stress, or repetitive use, compared to the rest of the system. The running action, for instance, does not just involve the leg muscles. Many muscles work to create a complicated pattern of rotation and spiral movements throughout the entire body. If this did not happen, and movement was confined just to the legs, then all the stress of impact and push-off would be absorbed by the ankle, knee, and hip joints, and the forces on these joints would cause damage. The spiraling movement up the body absorbs the stress and distributes the impact through many joints. Because no individual structure absorbs too much stress, the human body is therefore able to function for many years.

Coordinated movement involves many muscles working together in a pattern to create the power and control needed to accomplish a task. Each muscle has a preferred function within a movement pattern; therefore, a particular movement will involve greater effort from certain individual muscles. For example, kicking a soccer ball involves a strong effort from the quadriceps muscles. Each of the four muscles within the group acts on the joint from a different angle; therefore, depending on the degree of rotation in the lower leg and the angle of the force, one muscle may have to keep working slightly more than the rest.

The muscular system develops based on how the body is used. Each individual has a unique pattern of muscle function adaptation, many of which are beneficial and in harmony with the person's activities and lifestyle, and some will be negative or excessive. Assessment provides information about beneficial or detrimental function.

For example, a mid-field soccer player who often has to pass the ball with the inside of the foot will tend to use the vastus medialis, and the adductors may be involved. Therefore, the soccer player would naturally develop increased strength in the vastus medialis and adductors while training. Although this may appear to create an imbalance within the other quadriceps muscles, it could be natural for the individual, and therefore this may not be a situation requiring remedial treatment. The same imbalance found in a distance runner complaining of patellofemoral syndrome or groin pain would be a treatment priority.

MICRO-TRAUMA

A muscle can suffer acute strain, with its fibers being torn, if overused or overloaded. The same can also occur on a microscopic level, even if just a few fibers are overused. When this breakdown occurs on a microscopic level, the pathologic changes that take place are just the same as with any soft tissue tear: bleeding, swelling, muscle tension, guarding in the surrounding tissues, and scar tissue formation. The delayed-onset muscle soreness experienced in muscles after hard exercise in part is due to this type of trauma (**micro-trauma**).

Scar tissue can continue to build up gradually with repetitive activity. Adhesions can form and affect the elasticity within that particular area of the muscle, making muscles vulnerable to further micro-trauma. This process results in fibrotic changes in the muscle.

As function deteriorates in a small part of the muscle, it can create imbalance within a functional muscle unit (a group of muscles working together). As the condition builds up gradually, in the early stages it may develop unnoticed. The increased tension can then put excessive stress on adjoining structures such as the tendons, which can become more vulnerable to acute trauma. Biomechanical alterations develop as natural movement patterns compensate. In the long run, the overuse syndrome can lead to many problems, both locally as well as in other parts of the body. Several muscle dysfunctions can develop.

Massage is possibly the most effective way of identifying this type of problem. Palpation assessment identifies fibrotic changes in a muscle. This is the most important benefit in general preventive massage.

These areas should be treated in much the same way as any chronic muscle injury. Mechanical force is applied to break down the scar tissue to improve flexibility and to realign tangled fibers.

Static positions, such as standing at attention in the military for long periods of time, put stress on specific tissues, causing micro-trauma in a similar way to the active type of overuse, but from isometric overload instead of eccentric or concentric function. Lack of movement in the muscles also slows the blood and lymph flow through the area, which can increase congestion and add to the problem.

ACTIVE MOVEMENTS

General understanding of biomechanics is especially important to the massage professional who works with athletes. The assessment question "What do you want your body to do?" will result in answers such as run, ride, throw, catch, jump, bend, rotate, lift, and press. The massage professional needs to break down the movements of the activity, assess for soft tissue changes that interfere with these movements, and then identify massage applications that can support these movements. For example, in response to an assessment question, "What do you need to do that you are having problems with?" I will often hear something like run backwards or swing. Then I will ask the athlete to show me, and while I observe the movements, I can begin to target the specific outcomes.

Perhaps the athlete says, "I can't stand on my left foot with the same balance as my right foot" (which is important for many sport activities). I ask the athlete to stand on the right foot, and I observe and palpate to determine the "normal" activity they can perform. This is a general assessment and treatment principle. The least affected movement pattern or structure becomes the "normal" for evaluation and comparison purposes. Regardless of the situation, in practical application this works. I then ask the athlete to stand on the left foot, where the problem exists, and I compare it to the more normal function. Then I assess for the difference between the two—tissue texture and pliability, ROM, and firing patterns. Choices about what treatments to use are based on the assessment information.

The next part of the examination is divided into two sections. In active movement assessment, the massage therapist asks the client to perform movements in specific directions in all planes of movement. ment. The squat assessment is particularly beneficial. In passive movement assessment, the massage therapist moves the client.

Injuries and dysfunctions of the musculoskeletal system are symptomatic when the injured area is actively moved. More complex conditions such as inflammation of the nervous system, systemic conditions such as heart disease, and pathologies such as tumors are not significantly affected by movement. If an area does not hurt at rest, but it does with movement, then soft tissue dysfunctions are indicated.

Remember that each individual joint movement pattern is part of an interconnected aspect of the neurologic coordination pattern of muscle movement called the **kinetic chain.** The support system involves the tensegric nature of the body's connective design. Both posture and movement dysfunctions identified in an individual joint pattern must be assessed and treated in broader terms of kinetic chain interactions, muscle tension/length relationships, and the effects of stress and strain on the entire system.

When active ROM is performed, the client moves the joint through the planes of motion that are normal for that joint. Any pain, crepitus, or limitation that is present during the action should be reported. This assessment identifies what the client is willing or able to do.

11-2

Passive ROM is performed when the massage therapist moves the joint passively through the planes of motion that are normal for the joint. The assessment identifies limitation (hypomobility) or excess movement (hypermobility) of the joint.

Passive ROM is done carefully and gently to allow the client to fully relax the muscles while the assessment is performed. The client reports the point at which pain or bind, if present, occurs. The massage therapist stops the motion at the point of pain or bind, unless assessing for joint end feel. Then a tiny increase in resistance is used to assess the quality of movement just past the bind. Passive ROM gives information about the joint capsule and ligaments and other restricting mechanisms, such as muscles.

ROM is measured in degrees. Joint movement is measured from the neutral line of anatomic position. Movement of a joint in the sagittal, frontal, or transverse plane is described as the number of degrees of flexion, extension, adduction, abduction, and internal and external rotation (Figure 11-6). For example, the elbow has approximately 150 degrees of flexion at the end range and 180 degrees of extension. Anything less than this is hypomobility, and anything more is considered hypermobility. Massage therapists typically estimate degrees of movement, while other professionals will use specific equipment to obtain precise information. The normal ROM of joints is found in anatomy texts such as *Mosby's Essential Sciences for Therapeutic Massage.*

Each movement pattern (e.g., flexion and extension of the elbow and knee, circumduction and rotation of the shoulder and hip, movement of the trunk and neck) is assessed in sequential positioning in each area of all available movement patterns, testing for strength, range, and ease of movement. Functional assessment is the combination of all previously described assessments.

Muscle strength assessment is performed by applying resistance to a specific group of muscles. Resistance (pressure against) applied to the muscles is focused at the end of the lever system (Figure 11-7).

For example, when assessing the function of the shoulder, resistance is focused at the distal end of the humerus, not at the wrist. When assessing extension of the hip, resistance is applied at the end of the femur. When assessing flexion of the knee, resistance is applied at the distal end of the tibia.

Resistance is applied slowly, smoothly, and firmly at an appropriate intensity as determined by the size of the muscle mass. Stabilization is essential to assess movement patterns accurately. Only the area assessed is allowed to move. Movement in any other part of the body must be stabilized. A stabilizing force is usually applied by the massage therapist. As one hand applies resistance, the other provides the stabilization. Sometimes the client can provide the stabilization by holding onto the masssage table. Some methods use straps to provide stabilization. The easiest way to identify the area to be stabilized is to move the area to be assessed through the ROM. At the end of the range, some other part of the body begins to move; this is the area of stabilization. Return the body to a neutral position. Provide the appropriate stabilization to the area identified and begin the assessment procedure (Figure 11-8).

During assessments, muscles should be able to hold against appropriate resistance without strain or pain from the pressure and without recruiting or using other muscles. Appropriate resistance is applied slowly and steadily and with just enough force to induce the muscles to respond to the stimulus. Large muscle groups require more force than small ones. The position should be easy to assume and comfortable to maintain for 10 to 30 seconds. Contraindications to this type of assessment include joint and disk dysfunction, acute pain, recent trauma, and inflammation.

When a movement pattern is evaluated, two types of information are obtained in one functional assessment.

FIGURE 11-6

EXAMPLES OF APPROXIMATE DEGREES OF MOVEMENT

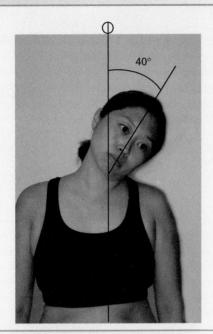

A 40 degrees of lateral flexion.

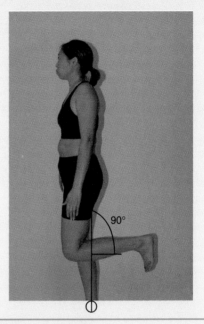

B 90 degrees of knee flexion.

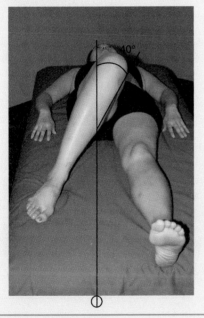

C 40 degrees of internal hip rotation.

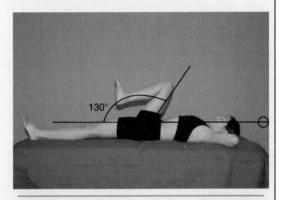

D 130 degrees of hip flexion.

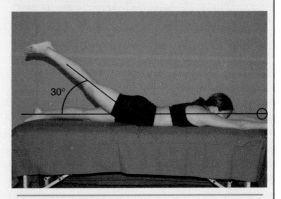

E 30 degrees of hip extension.

Continued

FIGURE 11-6 CONT'D

EXAMPLES OF APPROXIMATE DEGREES OF MOVEMENT

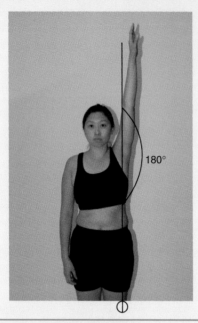

F 180 degrees of shoulder abduction.

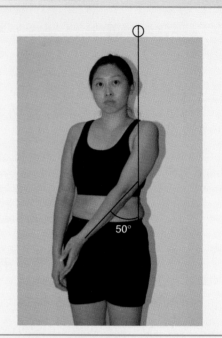

G 50 degrees of shoulder adduction.

FIGURE 11-7

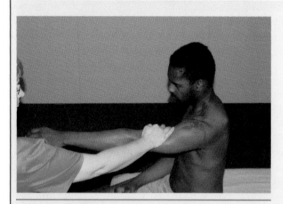

A Resistance at end of lever.

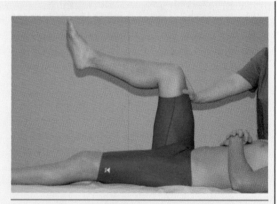

B Resistance at end of lever.

First, when a jointed area moves into flexion and the joint angle is decreased, the prime mover and synergists concentrically contract, antagonists eccentrically function while lengthening, and the fixators isometrically contract and stabilize. Bodywide stabilization patterns also come into play to assist in allowing the motion. During assessment, resistance can be applied to load the prime mover groups and synergists to assess for neurologic function of strength and, to a lesser degree, endurance, as the contraction is held for a period of time. At the same time, the antagonist pattern or the tissues that are lengthened when positioning for the functional assessment can be assessed for increased tension patterns or connective tissue shortening. Dysfunction shows itself in limited ROM by restricting the

FIGURE 11-8

EXAMPLES OF MUSCLE TESTING

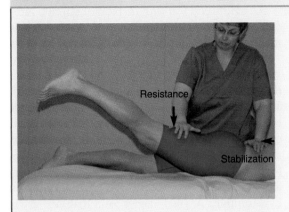

A Hip extension.

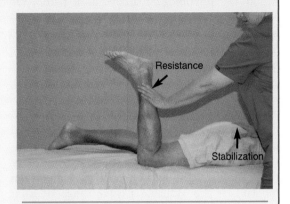

B Knee flexion.

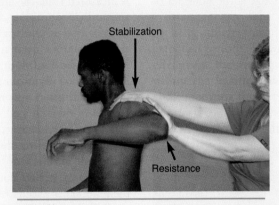

C Shoulder retraction.

movement pattern. Therefore, when placing a jointed area into flexion, the extensors are assessed for increased tension or shortening. When the jointed area moves into extension, the opposite becomes the case. The same holds for adduction and abduction, internal and external rotation, plantar and dorsiflexion, and so on.

During actual movement assessment, the following categories are noted by the massage therapist:

Range of motion (ROM). Is the motion normal, decreased, increased? Determining normal ROM is more complex than it might seem. You need to consider the client's age and sex, sport type, and muscle texture. There is less ROM as we age. Women typically have greater ROM than men. If the complaint is in the extremities, then begin with the non-involved side, and always compare both sides. The less involved side becomes the "normal side" for comparison.

Limits to joint movement. Joints have various degrees of ROM. Anatomic, physiologic, and pathologic barriers to motion exist. Anatomic barriers are determined by the shape and fit of the bones at the joint. The anatomic barrier is seldom reached because the possibility of injury is greatest in this position. Instead the body protects the joint by establishing physiologic barriers.

For a comprehensive strength testing sequence, see the Evolve site. **evolve**

Physiologic barriers are the result of the limits in ROM imposed by protective nerve and sensory function to support optimal function. An adaptation in the physiologic barrier so that the protective function limits instead of supports optimal functioning is called a *pathologic barrier*. Pathologic barriers often are manifested as stiffness, pain, or a "catch."

When using joint movement techniques, remain within the physiologic barriers. If a pathologic barrier exists that limits motion, use massage techniques to gently and slowly encourage the joint to increase the limits of the ROM to the physiologic barrier.

The stretch on the soft tissues, such as muscles, tendons, fascia, and ligaments, and the arrangement of the joint surfaces determine the ROM of the joint and therefore the joint's normal end-feel.

Overpressure is the term used when the massage therapist gradually applies more pressure when the end of the available passive range of joint motion has been reached. The sensation transmitted to the therapist's hands by the tissue resistance at the end of the available range is the **end-feel** of a joint.

Types of End-Feel

Normal End-Feel. Soft tissue approximation end-feel occurs when the full ROM of the joint is restricted by the normal muscle bulk; it is painless and has a feeling of soft compression. Muscular, or tissue stretch, end-feel occurs at the extremes of muscle stretch, such as in the hamstrings during a straight leg raise; it has a feeling of increasing tension, springiness, or elasticity. Capsular stretch, or leathery, end-feel occurs when the joint capsule is stretched at the end of its normal range, such as with external rotation of the glenohumeral joint; it is painless and has the sensation of stretching a piece of leather. Bony, or hard, end-feel occurs when bone contacts bone at the end of normal range, as in extension of the elbow; it is abrupt and hard.

Abnormal End-Feel. There are many types of abnormal end-feel. Empty end-feel occurs when there is no physical restriction to movement except the pain expressed by the client. Muscle spasm end-feel occurs when passive movement stops abruptly because of pain; there may be a springy rebound from reflexive muscle spasm. Boggy end-feel occurs when edema is present; it has a mushy, soft quality. Springy block, or internal derangement, end-feel is a springy or rebounding sensation in a noncapsular pattern; this indicates loose cartilage or meniscal tissue within the joint. Capsular stretch (leathery) end-feel that occurs before normal range indicates capsular fibrosis with no inflammation. Bony (hard) end-feel that occurs before

normal range indicates bony changes or degenerative joint disease or malunion of a joint after a fracture.

An empty end feel with no bind or stability indicates a seriously damaged joint, and referral is required.

Interpreting Range of Motion Assessment Findings

The ROM of a joint is measured in degrees. A full circle is 360 degrees. A flat horizontal line is 180 degrees. Two perpendicular lines (as in the shape of a capital L) create a 90-degree angle. When the ROM of a joint allows 0 to 90 degrees of flexion, anything less is hypomobile and anything more is hypermobile. A great degree of variability exists among individuals as to the actual normal ROM. The degrees provided are general guidelines. ROM is measured from the anatomic position. Anatomic position is considered 0 degrees of motion, regardless whether the client is standing, supine, or side-lying.

Decreased ROM is caused by either pain or changes in the joint position, or soft tissue bind. If the loss of motion is not a result of pain, more information is needed to determine whether the lack of motion is caused by adhesions in the joint capsule, muscle guarding, joint degeneration, or other factors.

Increased ROM that is significantly different from the other side indicates a moderate to severe injury to the ligaments, joint capsule, or both. Increased ROM on both sides compared with normal anatomic ROM suggests a generalized hypermobility syndrome and potential instability in the joints.

If active movement is painful, ask the client to describe its location, quality, and severity. The three stages of healing that elicit pain at different ranges of the movement are as follows:

1. Acute conditions yield pain before the normal ROM.
2. Subacute conditions give pain at the end of the normal range.
3. Chronic conditions may elicit pain with slight overpressure at the end of active or passive motion.

Pain with passive motion at different ranges of the movement indicates a stage of healing that is the same as for active motion.

Active and passive ROM can identify limits of movement. If an empty capsular or hard end-feel is identified, the joint is damaged. Referral is needed for acute conditions. ROM limited by muscle contraction may indicate an underlying problem with joint laxity, and caution is indicated before reducing the muscle guarding. Proceed slowly until a balance between increased ROM and maintaining joint stability is achieved. If joint stability is reduced, the client usually experiences pain in the joint for a day or two after the massage. Simple edema around a joint is managed with lymphatic drain. Any unexplained edema should be referred for diagnosis.

ROM should improve as the client's tissues normalize with general massage. Progressive mobilization in ROM is an indication of improved function. Never force an increase in ROM. Instead, allow it to be a natural outcome of effective massage application.

Interpreting Muscle-Specific Testing Findings

Muscle strength testing determines a muscle's force of concentric contraction. The preferred method is to isolate the muscle or muscle group by positioning the muscle with its attachment points as close together as possible. The muscle or muscle group being tested should be isolated as specifically as possible.

The client holds or maintains the contracted position of the muscle isolation while the therapist slowly and evenly applies a counterpressure to pull or push the muscle out of its isolated position. The massage therapist must use sufficient force to recruit a full response by the muscles being tested but not enough to recruit other muscles in the body. The client should not hold his or her breath during assessment. If strength testing is done this way, there is little chance that the therapist will injure the client. As with all assessment, it is necessary to compare the muscle test with a similar area—usually the same muscle group on the opposite side.

Another muscle testing method is to compare a muscle group's strength with its antagonist pattern. The body is designed so that the flexor, internal rotator, and adductor muscles are about 25% to 30% stronger than the extensor, external rotator, and abductor muscles. It is also designed so that flexors and adductors usually work against gravity to move a joint. The main purposes of extensors and abductors are to restrain and control the movement of the flexor and adductor muscles and to return the joint to a neutral position. Less strength is required because gravity is assisting the function. A third form is strength testing to assess for facilitator and inhibitor patterns during gait function (see Box 11-2).

Strength testing should reveal a difference in the pattern between the flexors, internal rotators, and adductors, and the extensors, external rotators, and abductors in an agonist/antagonist pattern. These groups should not be equally strong. Flexors, internal rotators, and adductors should show more muscle strength than extensors, external rotators, and abductors.

Muscle strength testing indicates the following possible findings:
- A strong and painless contraction indicates a normal structure.
- A painful but strong contraction indicates an injury or dysfunction in the tested muscle-tendon-periosteal unit.

A weak and painless contraction may be caused by one or more of the following situations:
- The muscle is inhibited due to a hypertonic antagonist pattern.
- The muscle is inhibited due to dysfunction or injury to adjacent joint structures.
- A spinal nerve condition is causing impingement on or irritation of the motor nerve and weakness in the muscles innervated by that nerve.
- A nerve is injured.
- The muscle is deconditioned due to disuse as a result of previous injury or disease.
- The length-tension relationship is long.
- The length-tension relationship is short.
- The gait pattern is dysfunctional.

See Box 11-2 for a complete muscle test.

POSTURAL AND PHASIC MUSCLES

Postural (stabilizer) and phasic (mover) muscles are made up of different kinds of muscle fibers. Postural muscles have a higher percentage of slow-twitch red fibers, which can hold a contraction for a long time before fatiguing. Phasic muscles have a higher percentage of fast-twitch white fibers, which contract quickly but tire easily. These two types of muscle develop different types of dysfunction and are tested differently.

Postural Muscles

Postural (stabilizer) muscles are relatively slow to respond compared with phasic muscles. They do not produce bursts of strength if asked to respond quickly, and they may cramp. They are the deliberate, slow, steady muscles that require time to respond. Using the analogy of the tortoise and the hare, these muscles are the tortoise. Inefficient neurologic patterns, muscle tension, reorganization of

Text continued on p. 189.

BOX 11-2   GAIT TESTING

Kinetic Chain Protocol Testing

Control group: Serves as standard or reference for comparison with a test group and is the group of muscles that initiates the reflex response.

Test group: The muscle group that responds to the stimulus from the control group.

Many gait-related kinetic chain patterns exist. We will concentrate on the main patterns involved in flexion, extension, abduction, and adduction at the shoulder and pelvic girdle. For testing the arm flexors/extensors, one should stabilize the humerus superior to the elbow joint and the femur above the knee.

The control group is activated first, the test group is next, and then both contractions are held simultaneously. Both groups should hold strong and steady during the test. One should chart the data to show any inhibitions.

The antagonist pattern should be inhibited during the test. The antagonists should let go. If they do not let go, the contraction maintained is concentric instead of eccentric. One should chart the data.

I. Contralateral Patterns

A. Left Arm Flexor Test

1. Isolate and stabilize left arm and right leg in supine flexion.
2. Control group: Use right leg as control and have client hold right leg position against therapist's inferior/caudal pressure.
3. Test group: Test left arm flexors by having client hold left arm position against practitioner's inferior/caudal pressure.
4. Both groups should hold equally strong and steady. If test group is inhibited, chart the data.

Antagonist Test: Test left arm extensors by having client hold against practitioner's superior/cranial pressure. These muscles should inhibit (let go). If test group remains concentrically contracted and holds, one should chart data.

B. Right Arm Flexor Test

1. Isolate and stabilize left leg and right arm in supine flexion.
2. Control group: Use left leg as control and have client hold left leg position against practitioner's inferior/caudal pressure.
3. Test group: Test right arm flexors by having client hold right arm position against practitioner's inferior/caudal pressure.
4. Both groups should hold equally strong and steady. If test group is inhibited, chart data.

Antagonist test: Test right arm extensors by having client hold right arm position against practitioner's superior/cranial pressure. These muscles should inhibit (let go). If test group remains concentrically contracted and holds, chart data.

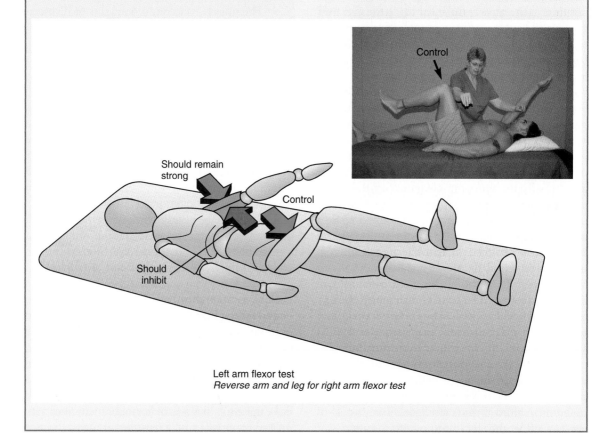

Left arm flexor test
Reverse arm and leg for right arm flexor test

Box 11-2   GAIT TESTING—cont'd

C. *Left Leg Flexor Test*
   1. Isolate and support/stabilize left leg and right arm in supine flexion.
   2. Control group: Use right arm as control and have client hold right arm position against therapist's inferior/caudal pressure.
   3. Test group: Test left leg flexors by having client hold left leg position against practitioner's inferior/caudal pressure.
   4. Both groups should hold equally strong and steady. If test group is inhibited, chart data.

   Antagonist Test: Test left leg extensors by having client hold against practitioner's superior/cranial pressure. These muscles should inhibit (let go). If test group remains concentrically contracted and holds, chart data.

D. *Right Leg Flexor Test*
   1. Isolate and stabilize left arm and right leg in supine flexion.
   2. Control group: Use left arm as control and have client hold left arm position against practitioner's inferior/caudal pressure.
   3. Test group: Test right leg flexors by having client hold right leg position against practitioner's inferior/caudal pressure.
   4. Both groups should hold equally strong and steady. If test group is inhibited (let go), chart data.

   Antagonist test: Test right leg extensors by having client hold right leg position against practitioner's superior/cranial pressure. These muscles should inhibit (let go). If test group remains concentrically contracted and holds, chart data.

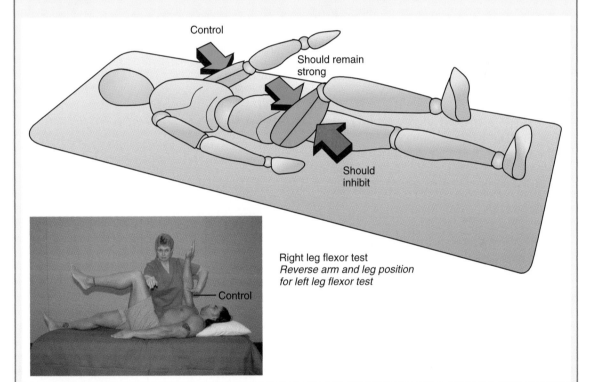

Control

Should remain strong

Should inhibit

Right leg flexor test
Reverse arm and leg position for left leg flexor test

Control

II. *Contralateral Extensors*
A. *Left Arm Extensor Test*
   1. Isolate and stabilize left arm and right leg in supine flexion.
   2. Control group: Right leg is control. Have client hold leg position against practitioner's superior/cephalad pressure.
   3. Test group: Test left arm extensors by having client hold arm position against practitioner's superior/cephalad pressure.
   4. Both groups should stay equally strong and steady. If test group is inhibited, chart data.

   Antagonist test: Test left arm flexors by having client hold left arm position against practitioner's inferior/caudal pressure. These muscles

should inhibit (let go). If test group remains concentrically contracted and holds, chart data.

B. *Right Arm Extensor Test*
   1. Isolate and stabilize left leg and right arm in supine flexion.
   2. Control group: Left leg is control. Have client hold leg position against practitioner's superior/cephalad pressure.
   3. Test group: Test right arm extensors by having client hold arm position against practitioner's superior/cephalad pressure.
   4. Both groups should stay equally strong and steady. If test group is inhibited, chart data.

Continued

Box 11-2   GAIT TESTING—cont'd

Antagonist test: Test right arm flexors by having client hold right arm position against practitioner's inferior/caudal pressure. These muscles should inhibit (let go). If test group remains concentrically contracted and holds, chart data.

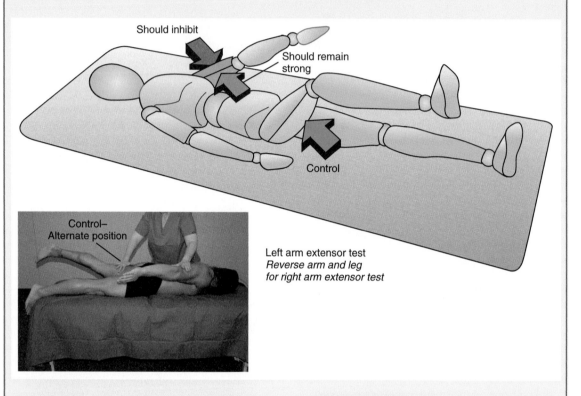

Left arm extensor test
*Reverse arm and leg
for right arm extensor test*

C. *Left Leg Extensor Test*
  1. Isolate and stabilize left leg and right arm in supine flexion.
  2. Control group: Right arm is control. Have client hold arm position against practitioner's superior/cephalad pressure.
  3. Test group: Test left leg extensors, have client hold leg position against practitioner's superior/cephalad pressure.
  4. Both groups should stay equally strong and steady. If test group is inhibited, chart data.

Antagonist test: Test left leg flexor by having client hold left leg position against practitioner's inferior/caudal pressure. These muscles should inhibit (let go). If test group remains concentrically contracted and holds, chart data.

D. *Right Leg Extensor Test*
  1. Isolate and stabilize left arm and right leg in supine flexion.
  2. Control group: Left arm is control. Have client hold arm position against practitioner's superior/cephalad pressure.
  3. Test group: Test right leg extensors by having client hold leg position against practitioner's superior/cephalad pressure.
  4. Both groups should stay equally strong and steady. If test group is inhibited, chart data.

Antagonist test: Test right leg flexors by having client hold right leg position against practitioner's inferior/caudal pressure. These muscles should inhibit (let go). If test group remains in a concentrically contracted pattern and holds, chart data.

BOX 11-2 GAIT TESTING—cont'd

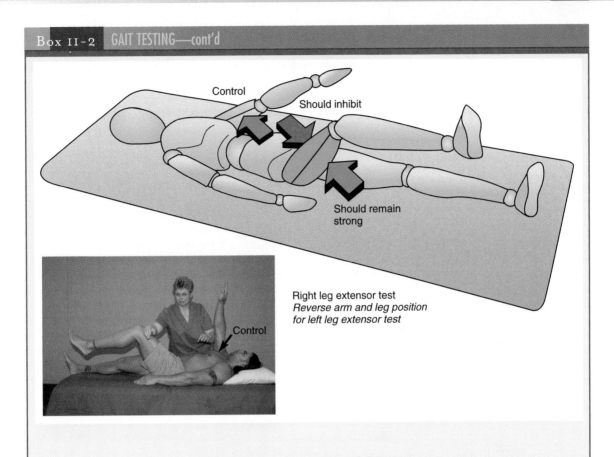

Right leg extensor test
*Reverse arm and leg position
for left leg extensor test*

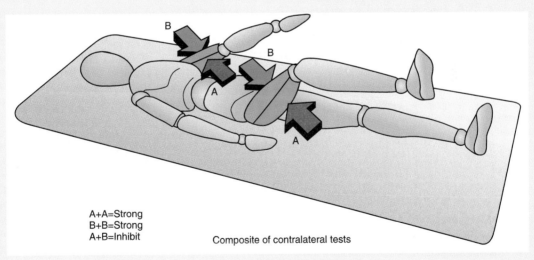

A+A=Strong
B+B=Strong
A+B=Inhibit

Composite of contralateral tests

Continued

BOX 11-2   GAIT TESTING—cont'd

III. Unilateral Flexors

A. Left Arm Flexor Test

1. Isolate and stabilize left arm and left leg in supine flexion.
2. Control group: Left leg is control. Have client hold leg position against practitioner's superior/cephalad pressure (contracting extensors).
3. Test group: Test left arm flexors by having client hold arm position against practitioner's inferior/caudal pressure (testing flexors).
4. Both groups should stay equally strong and steady. If test group is inhibited, chart data.

Antagonist test: Test left arm extensors by having client hold left arm position against practitioner's superior/cranial pressure. These muscles should inhibit (let go). If test group remains concentrically contracted and holds, chart data.

B. Right Arm Flexor Test

1. Isolate and stabilize right arm and right leg in supine flexion.
2. Control group: Right leg is control. Have client hold leg position against practitioner's superior/cephalad pressure (contracting extensors).
3. Test group: Test right arm flexors by having client hold arm position against practitioner's inferior/caudal pressure (testing flexors).
4. Both groups should stay equally strong and steady. If test group is inhibited, chart data.

Antagonist test: Test right arm extensors by having client hold right arm position against practitioner's superior/cranial position. These muscles should inhibit (let go). If test group remains concentrically contracted and holds, chart data.

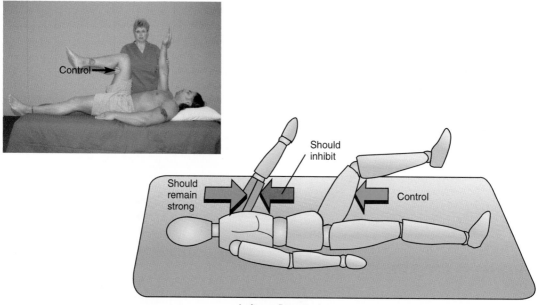

Left arm flexor test
Reverse arm and leg position for right arm flexor test

C. Left Leg Flexor Test

1. Isolate and stabilize left arm and left leg in supine flexion.
2. Control group: Left arm is control. Have client hold arm position against practitioner's superior/cephalad pressure (contracting extensors).
3. Test group: Test left leg flexors by having client hold leg position against practitioner's inferior/caudal pressure (testing flexors).
4. Both groups should stay equally strong and steady. If test group is inhibited, chart data.

Antagonist test: Test left leg flexors by having client hold left leg position against practitioner's inferior/caudal pressure. These muscles should inhibit (let go). If test group remains concentrically contracted and holds, chart data.

D. Right Leg Flexor Test

1. Isolate and stabilize right arm and right leg in supine flexion.
2. Control group: Right arm is control. Have client hold arm position against practitioner's superior/cephalad pressure (contracting extensors).

BOX 11-2 GAIT TESTING—cont'd

3. Test group: Test right leg flexors by having client hold leg position against practitioner's inferior/caudal pressure (testing flexors).
4. Both groups should stay equally strong and steady. If test group is inhibited, chart data.

Antagonist test: Test right leg extensors by having client hold leg position against practitioner's superior/cranial position. These muscles should inhibit (let go). If test group remains concentrically contracted and holds, chart data.

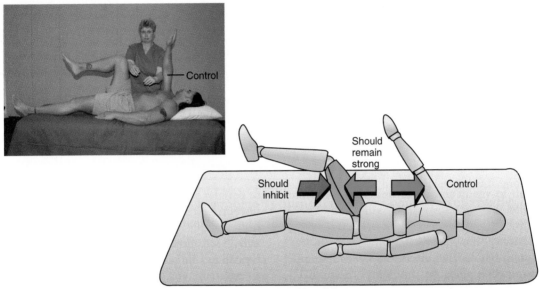

Right leg flexor test
Reverse arm and leg position for left leg flexor test

IV. Unilateral Extensors

A. Left Arm Extensor Test
1. Isolate and stabilize left arm and left leg in supine flexion.
2. Control group: Left leg is control. Have client hold leg position against practitioner's inferior/caudal pressure (contracting flexors).
3. Test group: Test left arm extensors by having client hold arm position against practitioner's superior/cephalad pressure (testing extensors).
4. Both groups should stay equally strong and steady. If test group is inhibited, chart data.

Antagonist test: Test left arm flexors by applying inferior/caudal pressure. These muscles should inhibit (let go). If test group remains concentrically contracted and holds, chart data.

B. Right Arm Extensor Test
1. Isolate and stabilize right arm and right leg in supine flexion.
2. Control group: Right leg is control. Have client hold leg position against practitioner's inferior/caudal pressure (contracting flexors).
3. Test group: Test right arm extensors by having client hold arm position against practitioner's superior/cephalad pressure (testing extensors).
4. Both groups should stay equally strong and steady. If test group is inhibited, chart data.

Antagonist test: Test right arm flexors by applying inferior/caudal pressure. These muscles should inhibit (let go). If test group remains concentrically contracted and holds, chart data.

Continued

BOX 11-2   GAIT TESTING—cont'd

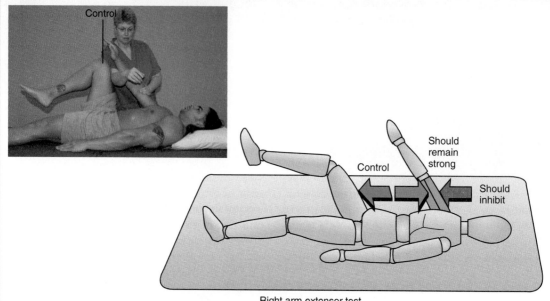

Right arm extensor test
Reverse arm and leg position for left arm extensor test

C. Left Leg Extensor Test

1. Isolate and stabilize left arm and left leg in supine flexion.
2. Control group: Left arm is control. Have client hold arm position against practitioner's inferior/caudal pressure (contracting flexors).
3. Test group: Test left leg extensors by having client hold leg position against practitioner's superior/cephalad pressure (testing extensors).
4. Both groups should stay equally strong and steady. If test group is inhibited, chart data.

Antagonist Test: Test left leg flexors by applying inferior/caudal pressure. These muscles should inhibit (let go). If test group remains in concentric contraction and holds, chart data.

D. Right Leg Extensor Test

1. Isolate and stabilize right arm and right leg in supine flexion.
2. Control group: Right arm is control. Have client hold arm position against practitioner's inferior/caudal pressure (contracting flexors).
3. Test group: Test right leg extensors by having client hold leg position against practitioner's superior/cephalad pressure (testing extensors).
4. Both groups should stay equally strong and steady. If test group is inhibited, chart data.

Box 11-2 GAIT TESTING—cont'd

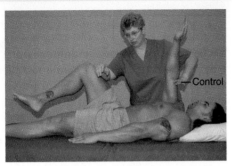

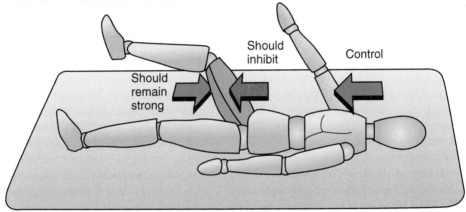

Right leg extensor test
Reverse arm and leg position for left leg extensor test

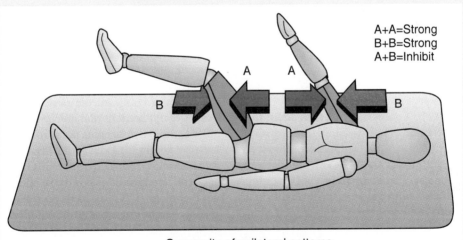

A+A=Strong
B+B=Strong
A+B=Inhibit

Composite of unilateral patterns

Antagonist test: Test right leg flexors by applying inferior/caudal pressure. These muscles should inhibit (let go). If test group remains concentrically contracted, chart data.

Continued

BOX 11-2   GAIT TESTING—cont'd

V. Medial/Lateral Symmetry

A. Bilateral Arm Adductor Test

1. Isolate and stabilize arms bilaterally in supine 90% flexion and legs bilaterally in flexion.
2. Control group: Bilateral legs are control. Have client hold position against practitioner's lateral pressure or squeeze a ball (contracting adductors).
3. Test group: Test bilateral arm adductors by having client hold position against practitioner's lateral pressure (testing adductors).
4. Both groups should be equally strong and steady. If test group is inhibited, chart data.

Antagonist test: Test bilateral arm abduction by having client hold arm position against medial pressure. These muscles should inhibit (let go). If test group remains concentrically contracted, chart data.

B. Bilateral Leg Adductor Test

1. Isolate and stabilize arms bilaterally in supine 90% flexion and legs bilaterally in flexion.
2. Control group: Bilateral arms are controls. Have client hold position against practitioner's lateral pressure or have client press palms together (contracting adductors).
3. Test group: Test bilateral leg adductors by having client hold position against practitioner (testing adductors).
4. Both groups should be equally strong and steady. If test group is inhibited, chart data.

Antagonist test: Test bilateral leg abductors by having client hold against practitioner's medial pressure. These muscles should inhibit (let go). If test group remains concentrically contracted, chart data.

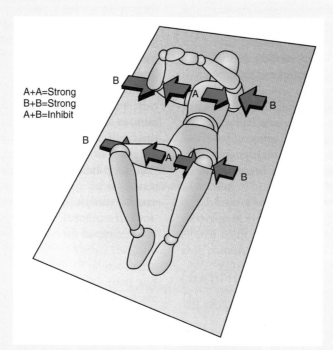

A+A=Strong
B+B=Strong
A+B=Inhibit

Intervention: Use any massage method to inhibit muscles that test too strong by remaining in concentric contraction patterns. Appropriate methods are slow compression, kneading, gliding, and shaking. Strengthen muscles that inhibit when they should hold strong. Appropriate methods are tapotment and rhythmic tensing of inhibited muscles. Then retest pattern; it should be normal.

connective tissue with fibrotic changes, and trigger points are common in postural muscles.

If posture is not balanced, postural muscles must function more like ligaments and bones. When this happens, additional connective tissue develops in the muscle to provide the ability to stabilize the body in gravity. The problem is that the connective tissue freezes the body in the position because, unlike muscle, which can actively contract and lengthen, connective tissue is static.

Postural muscles tend to shorten and increase in tension when under a strain-tension-length relationship. This information is important when attempting to assess which muscles are tense and short, and therefore in need of lengthening, and which groups of muscle are apt to develop connective tissue changes and require stretching. Connective tissue shortening is dealt with mechanically through forms of stretch. Hypertension of concentric contraction muscles is dealt with through muscle energy methods and reflexive lengthening procedures.

Phasic Muscles

Phasic (mover) muscles jump into action quickly and tire quickly. It is more common to find musculotendinous junction problems in phasic muscles. The four most common problems are microtearing of the muscle fibers at the tendon, inflamed tendons (tendonitis), tendons adhering to underlying tissue, and bursitis.

Phasic muscles usually weaken in response to postural muscle shortening. Sometimes the weakened muscles also shorten. This shortening allows the weak muscle to retain the same contraction power on the joint. It is important not to confuse this condition with hypertense muscles. These muscles are inhibited and weak.

Phasic muscles occasionally become overly tense and short. This almost always results from some sort of repetitive behavior and is a common problem in athletes. Phasic muscles also become short in response to a sudden posture change that causes the muscles to assist the postural muscles in maintaining balance. These common, inappropriate muscle patterns often result from an unexpected fall or near-fall, an automobile accident, or some other trauma. Basic massage methods discussed in this text can be used to reset and retrain out-of-sync muscles.

KINETIC CHAIN ASSESSMENT OF POSTURE

Consider the body as a circular form divided into four quadrants: a front, a back, a right side, and a left side with divisions on the sagittal and frontal planes, the body must be balanced in three dimensions to withstand the forces of gravity.

The body moves and is balanced in gravity in the following transverse plane areas that easily allow movement: the atlas; the C6 and C7 vertebrae; the T12 and L1 vertebrae (the thoracolumbar junction); the L4, L5, and S1 vertebrae (the sacrolumbar junction); and at the hips, knees, and ankles (Figure 11-9). If a postural distortion exists in any of the four quadrants or within one of the jointed areas, the entire balance mechanism must be adjusted. This occurs as a pinball-like effect that jumps front to back and side to side in the soft tissue between the movement lines (see Figure 11-9).

To gain an understanding of postural balance, use a pole of some type (a broom handle without the broom portion will work). Tie a string around the pole. Now, try to balance the pole on its end with the string. Note that you work opposite the pattern when trying to counter the fall pattern of the pole. If the pole tends to fall forward and to the left, you apply a counterforce back and to the right.

This is also what the body does if part of it moves off the balance line. The body is made up of many different poles stacked on top of one another. The poles stack at each of the movement segments. Muscles between the movement segments must be three-dimensionally balanced in all four quadrants to support the pole in that area. Each area needs to be balanced. If one pole area tips a bit to the right, the body compensates by tipping the adjacent pole areas (above and/or below) to the left. If a pole area is tipped forward, adjacent poles are tipped back. A chain reaction occurs, such that when compensating poles tip back, their adjacent areas must counterbalance the action by tipping forward. This is how the body-wide compensation patterns occur.

Whether the pole areas sit nicely on top of each other with evenly distributed muscle action or whether they are tipped in various positions and counterbalanced by compensatory muscle actions, the body remains balanced in gravity. However, the "tippy pole" pattern is much more inefficient than the "balanced pole pattern" (Figure 11-10).

Intervention plans attempt to normalize the balance process by relaxing the tension pattern in overly tight and short areas, strengthening muscles in corresponding taut and long but weak areas, and allowing the poles to straighten out. If a pole is per-

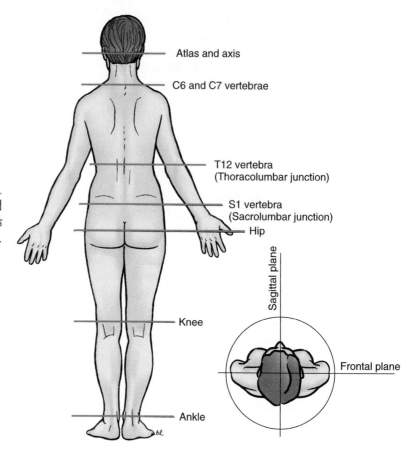

FIGURE II-9 ■ Quadrants and movement segments. (From Fritz S: *Mosby's fundamentals of therapeutic massage,* ed 3. St. Louis, 2004, Mosby.)

manently tippy, such as with scoliosis or kyphosis, intervention plans attempt to support the appropriate compensation patterns and prevent them from increasing beyond what is necessary for postural balance.

Muscle imbalance, discovered by observation, palpation, and through muscle testing procedures, often indicates how the body is compensating for postural and movement imbalances. Muscle testing also can locate the main muscle problems. When the primary dysfunctional group of muscles is concentrically contracted against resistance, the main compensatory patterns are activated, and the other body compensation patterns are activated and exaggerated. The massage professional must then become a detective, looking for clues to unwind the pattern by concentrating on methods that restore symmetry of function.

A major muscle problem is overly tense muscles. If these muscles can be relaxed, lengthened, and, if necessary, stretched to activate connective tissue changes, the rest of the dysfunctional pattern often resolves.

If the extensors and abductors are stronger than the flexors and adductors, major postural imbalance and postural distortion result. Similarly, if the extensors and abductors are too weak to balance the other movement patterns, the body curls into itself, and nothing works properly.

If gait and kinetic chain patterns are inefficient, more energy is required for movement, and fatigue and pain can result.

Shortened postural (stabilizer) muscles must be lengthened and then stretched. This takes time and uses all the massage practitioner's technical skills. Because of the fiber configuration of the muscle tissue (slow-twitch red fibers or fast-twitch white fibers), techniques must be sufficiently intense and must be applied long enough to allow the muscle to respond.

Shortened and weak phasic muscles must first be lengthened and stretched. Eventually, strengthening techniques and exercises will be needed. Long and weak muscles need therapeutic exercise. If the hypertense phasic muscle pattern is caused by repetitive use, the muscles can be normalized

FIGURE 11-10

POSTURE BALANCE AND IMBALANCE

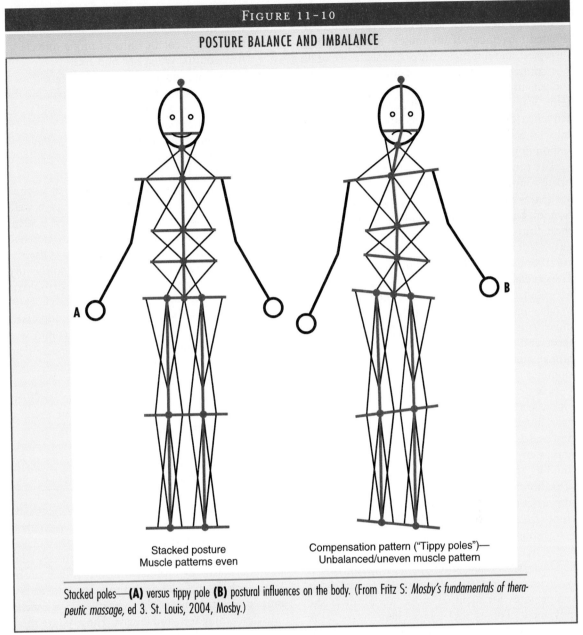

Stacked posture
Muscle patterns even

Compensation pattern ("Tippy poles")—
Unbalanced/uneven muscle pattern

Stacked poles—**(A)** versus tippy pole **(B)** postural influences on the body. (From Fritz S: *Mosby's fundamentals of therapeutic massage*, ed 3. St. Louis, 2004, Mosby.)

with muscle energy techniques and then lengthened. Overly tense muscles often increase in size (hypertrophy). Muscle tissue that has undergone hypertrophy begins to return to normal if it is not used for the activity. The client must reduce the activity of that muscle group until balance is restored, which usually takes about 4 weeks. Athletes often display this pattern and very likely will resist complete inactivity. A reduced activity level and a more balanced exercise program, combined with flexibility training, can be beneficial for them. Refer these individuals to appropriate training and coaching professionals, if indicated.

People usually complain of problems in the tight but long eccentrically functioning and inhibited muscle areas. Massage in these areas makes the symptoms worse because massage further lengthens the area. Instead, identify the shortened tissues and apply massage to lengthen and stretch tense areas. Assessment must identify the concentrically contracted shortened areas so that correction can be applied.

MUSCLE FIRING PATTERNS

11-3   A **muscle firing pattern** (or muscle activation sequence) is the sequence of muscle contraction involvement with agonist and synergist to best produce joint motion. Muscles also contract, or fire, in a neurologic sequence to produce coordinated movement. If the muscle firing pattern is disrupted, and if muscles fire out of sequence or do not contract when they are supposed to, labored movement and postural strain result. Firing patterns can be assessed by initiating a particular sequence of joint movements and palpating for muscle activity to determine which muscle is responding to the movement.

The central nervous system recruits the appropriate muscles in specific muscle activation sequences to generate the appropriate muscle function of acceleration, deceleration, or stability. If these firing patterns are abnormal, with the synergist becoming dominant, efficient movement is compromised and the joint position is strained. The general activation sequence is (1) prime mover, (2) stabilizer, and (3) synergist. If the stabilizer has to also move the area (acceleration) or control movement (deceleration), it typically becomes short and tight. If the synergist fires before the prime mover, the movement is awkward and labored.

If one muscle is tight and short, reciprocal inhibition occurs. *Reciprocal inhibition* exists when a tight muscle decreases nervous stimulation of its functional antagonist, causing it to reduce activity. For example, a tight and short psoas decreases (inhibits) the function of the gluteus maximus. The activation and force production of the prime mover (gluteus maximus) is decreased, leading to compensation and substitution by the synergists (hamstrings) and stabilizers (erector spinae), creating an altered firing pattern.

The most common firing pattern dysfunction is synergistic dominance, in which a synergist compensates for a prime mover to produce the movement. For example, if a client has a weak gluteus medius, then synergists (the tensor fascia lata, adductor complex, and quadratus lumborum) become dominant to compensate for the weakness. This alters normal joint alignment, which further alters the normal length-tension relationships of the muscles around the joint. See Box 11-3 for the most commonly used assessment procedures and interventions for altered firing patterns.

Each jointed area has a movement muscle activation sqeuence. The movement is a product of the entire mechanism, including the following:

- Bones, joints, and ligaments
- Capsular components and design
- Tendons, muscle shapes, and fiber types
- Interlinked fascial networks, nerve distribution, and myotatic units of prime movers
- Antagonists, synergists, and fixators
- Neurologic kinetic chain interactions
- Bodywide influence of reflexes, including the positional and righting reflexes of vision and the inner ear and gait reflex
- Circulatory distribution
- General systemic balance
- Nutritional influences

Assessment of a movement pattern as normal indicates that all parts are functioning in a well-orchestrated manner. When a dysfunction is identified, the causal factors can arise from any one or a combination of these elements. Often a multidisciplinary diagnosis is necessary to identify clearly the interconnected nature of the pathologic condition.

Inappropriate firing patterns can be addressed by inhibiting the muscles that are contracting out of sequence and stimulating the appropriate muscles to fire. Compression to the muscle belly effective inhibits a muscle. Tapotement is a good technique to stimulate muscles. If the problem does not normalize easily, referral to an exercise professional may be indicated (Box 11-4).

 GAIT ASSESSMENT

11-4

Understanding the basic body movements of walking helps the massage therapist recognize dysfunctional and inefficient gait patterns.

Disruption of the gait reflexes creates the potential for many problems. Common gait problems include a functional short leg caused by muscle shortening, tight neck and shoulder muscles, aching feet, and fatigue. The massage therapist must understand biomechanics, including posture, interaction of joint functions, and gait, and expand the knowledge to the demands of sport performance.

This is especially important in rehabilitation progress in which walking is either the goal or part of the program. It is important to observe the client from the front, back, and both sides. To begin, the massage practitioner should watch the client walk, noticing the heel-to-toe foot placement. The toes should point directly forward with each step (Figure 11-11).

Text continued on p. 197.

Box 11-3   COMMON MUSCLE FIRING PATTERNS

Trunk Flexion

1. Normal firing pattern
   a. Transverse abdominus
   b. Abdominal obliques
   c. Rectus abdominus
2. Assessment

a. Client is supine with knees and hips at 90 degrees.
b. The client is instructed to perform a normal curl up.
c. The massage practitioner assesses the ability of the abdominal muscles functionally to stabilize the lumbo-pelvic-hip complex by having the client draw the abdominal muscle in as when bringing the umbilicus toward the back and then doing a curl just lifting the scapula off the table while keeping both feet flat.

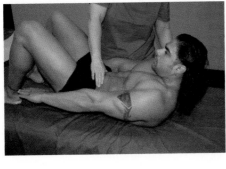

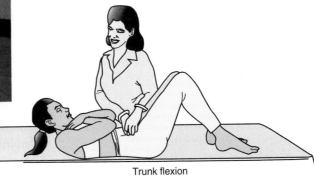

Trunk flexion

The inability to maintain the drawing in position or to activate the rectus demonstrates altered firing of the abdominal stabilization mechanism.

3. Altered firing pattern
   a. Weak agonist: Abdominal complex
   b. Overactive antagonist: Erector spinae
   c. Overactive synergist: Psoas or rectus abdominus
4. Symptoms
   a. Low back pain
   b. Buttock pain
   c. Hamstring shortening

Hip Extension

1. Normal firing pattern
   a. Gluteus maximus
   b. Opposite erector spinae
   c. Same-side erector spinae and hamstring

Or
   a. Gluteus maximus
   b. Hamstring
   c. Opposite erector spinae
   d. Same-side erector spinae
2. Assessment
   a. With the client prone the massage practitioner palpates the erector spinae with the thumb and index finger of one hand and palpates the muscle belly of the gluteus maximus and hamstring with the little finger and the thumb of the opposite hand.
   b. The practitioner instructs the client to extend the hip more than 15 degrees from the table.

Continued

BOX 11-3   COMMON MUSCLE FIRING PATTERNS—cont'd

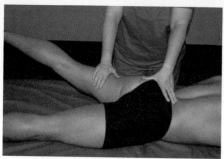

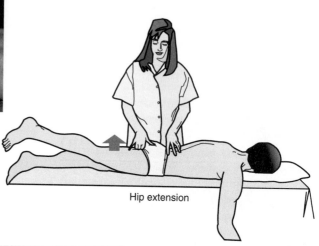

Hip extension

3. Altered firing pattern
   a. Weak agonist: Gluteus maximus
   b. Overactive antagonist: Psoas
   c. Overactive stabilizer: Erector spinae
   d. Overactive synergist: Hamstring
4. Symptoms
   a. Low back pain
   b. Buttock pain
   c. Recurrent hamstring strains

Hip Abduction
1. Normal firing pattern
   a. Gluteus medius
   b. Tensor fasciae latae
   c. Quadratus lumborum
2. Assessment
   a. With the client side-lying the massage practitioner stands behind the client and palpates the client's quadratus lumborum with one hand and the tensor fasciae latae and gluteus medius with the other hand.
   b. The practitioner instructs the client to abduct the leg from the table.

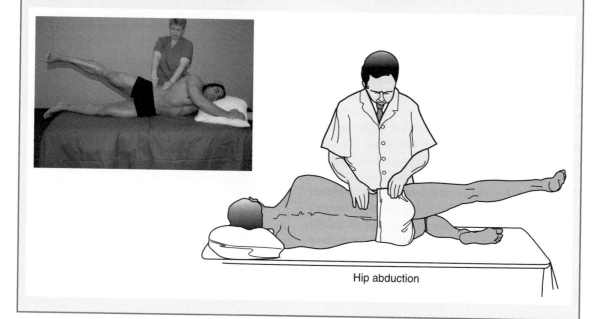

Hip abduction

Box 11-3   COMMON MUSCLE FIRING PATTERNS—cont'd

3. Altered firing pattern
   a. Weak agonist: Gluteus medius
   b. Overactive antagonist: Adductors
   c. Overactive synergist: Tensor fasciae latae
   d. Overactive stabilizer: Quadratus lumborum
4. Symptoms
   a. Low back pain
   b. Sacroiliac joint pain
   c. Buttock pain
   d. Lateral knee pain
   e. Anterior knee pain

Knee Flexion
1. Normal firing pattern
   a. Hamstrings
   b. Gastrocnemius
2. Assessment
   a. With client lying prone the massage practitioner places fingers on the hamstring and gastrocnemius.
   b. The client flexes the knee.

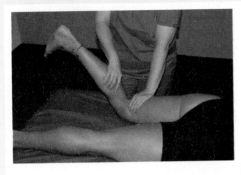 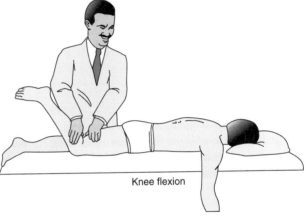

Knee flexion

3. Altered firing pattern
   a. Weak agonist: Hamstrings
   b. Overactive synergist: Gastrocnemius
4. Symptoms
   a. Pain behind the knee
   b. Achilles' tendonitis

Knee Extension
1. Normal firing pattern
   a. Vastus medialis
   b. Vastus intermedialis and vastus lateralis
   c. Rectus femoris

2. Assessment
   a. Client lies supine with leg extended. The practitioner asks the client to pull the patella cranially (up). The massage practitioner places finger on vastus medialis oblique, vastus lateralis, and rectus femoris.

Continued

Box II-3   COMMON MUSCLE FIRING PATTERNS—cont'd

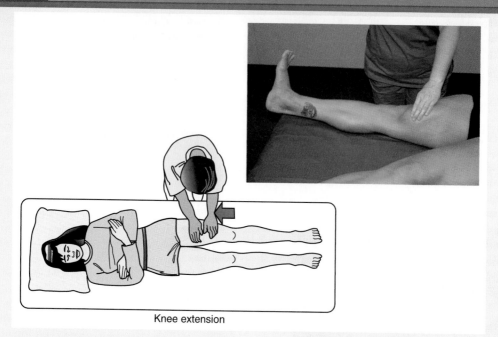

Knee extension

3. Altered firing pattern
   a. Weak agonist: Vastus medius, primarily the oblique portion
   b. Overactive synergist: Vastus lateralis
4. Symptoms
   a. Knee pain under patella
   b. Patellar tendonitis
5. Intervention for altered firing patterns
   a. Use appropriate massage application to inhibit dominant muscle and then strengthen the weak muscles.

Shoulder Flexion
1. Normal firing pattern
   a. Supraspinatus
   b. Deltoid
   c. Infraspinatus
   d. Middle and lower trapezius
   e. Contralateral quadratus lumborum
2. Assessment
   a. Massage practitioner stands behind seated client with one hand on shoulder and the other on the contralateral quadratus area.
   b. The practitioner asks the client to abduct shoulder to 90 degrees.

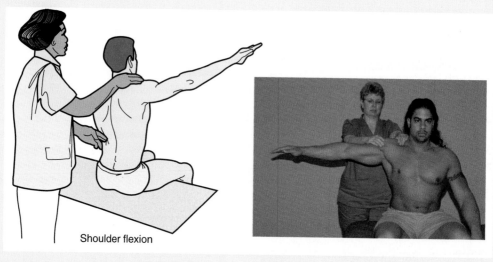

Shoulder flexion

Box 11-3	COMMON MUSCLE FIRING PATTERNS—cont'd

3. Altered Firing Pattern
   a. Weak agonist: Levator scapula
   b. Overactive antagonist: Upper trapezius
   c. Overactive stabilizer: Ipsilateral quadratus lumborum

4. Symptoms
   a. Shoulder tension
   b. Headache at base of skull
   c. Upper chest breathing
   d. Low back pain

FIGURE 11-11

FOOT POSITION DURING WALKING

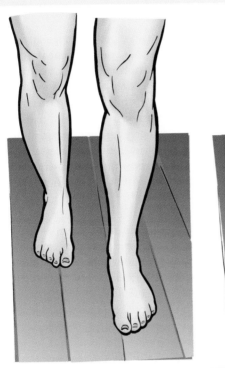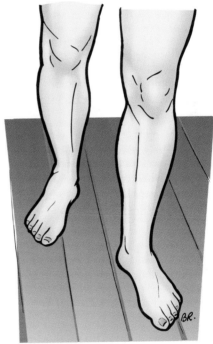

Proper—**(A)** and improper **(B)** foot position in walking. (From Fritz S: *Mosby's fundamentals of therapeutic massage,* ed 3. St. Louis, 2004, Mosby.)

Observe the upper body. It should be relaxed and fairly symmetric. The head should face forward with the eyes level with the horizontal plane. There is a natural arm swing that is opposite to the leg swing. The arm swing begins at the shoulder joint. On each step the left arm moves forward as the right leg moves forward and then vice versa. This pattern provides balance. The rhythm and pace of the arm and leg swing should be similar. Increased walking speed increases the speed of the arm swing. The length of the stride determines the arc of the arm swing (Figure 11-12).

Observe the client walking, and note his or her general appearance. The optimal walking pattern is as follows:

1. The head and trunk are vertical, with the eyes easily maintaining forward position and level with the horizontal plane; the shoulders are level.
2. The arms swing freely opposite the leg swing, allowing the shoulder girdle to rotate opposite the pelvic girdle.
3. Step length and step timing are even.
4. The body oscillates vertically with each step.

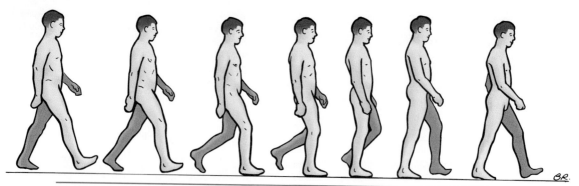

FIGURE 11-12 ■ Efficient gait position. (From Fritz S: *Mosby's fundamentals of therapeutic massage*, ed 3. St. Louis, 2004, Mosby.)

5. The entire body moves rhythmically with each step.
6. At the heel strike, the foot is approximately at a right angle to the leg.
7. The knee is extended but not locked.
8. The body weight is shifted forward into the stance phase.
9. At push-off, the foot is strongly plantar-flexed, with defined hyperextension of the metatarsophalangeal joints of the toes.
10. During the leg swing, the foot easily clears the floor with good alignment and the rhythm of movement remains unchanged.
11. The heel contacts the floor first.
12. The weight then rolls to the outside of the arch.
13. The arch flattens slightly in response to the weight load.
14. The weight then is shifted to the ball of the foot in preparation for the spring-off from the toes and the shifting of the weight to the other foot.

During walking the pelvis moves slightly in a side-lying figure-of-eight pattern. The movements that make up this sequence are transverse, medial, and lateral rotation. The stability and mobility of the sacroiliac joints play very important roles in this alternating side figure-of eight movement. If these joints are not functioning properly, the entire gait is disrupted. The sacroiliac joint is one of the few joints in the body that is not directly affected by muscles that cross the joint. It is a large joint, and the bony contact between the sacrum and ilium is broad. It is common for the rocking of this joint to be disrupted (Figure 11-13).

The hips rotate in a slightly oval pattern, beginning with a medial rotation during the leg swing and heel strike, followed by a lateral rotation through the push-off. The knees move in a flexion and extension pattern opposite each other. The extension phase never reaches enough extension to initiate the normal knee lock pattern that is used in standing. The ankles rotate in an arc around the heel at heel strike and around a center in the forefoot at push-off. Maximal dorsiflexion at the end of the stance phase and maximal plantar flexion at the end of push-off are necessary.

When assessing gait, observing for areas of the body that do not move efficiently during walking is a good means of detecting dysfunctional areas. Pain causes the body to tighten and alters the normal relaxed flow of walking. Muscle weakness and shortening interfere with the neurologic control of the agonist (prime mover) and antagonist muscle action. Hypomobility (limitation of joint movement) and hypermobility (laxity) both result in protective muscle contraction.

If the situation becomes chronic, both muscle shortening and muscle weakness result. Changes in the soft tissue, including all the connective tissue elements of the tendons, ligaments, and fascial sheaths, restrict the normal action of muscles. Connective tissue usually shortens and becomes less pliable.

Amputation disrupts the body's normal diagonal balance. Obviously, any amputation of the lower limb disturbs the walking pattern. What is not so obvious is that amputation of any part of the upper limb affects the counterbalance movement of the arm swing during walking. The rest of the body must compensate for the loss. Loss of any of the toes greatly affects the postural information sent to the brain from the feet.

It is possible to have soft tissue dysfunction without joint involvement. Any change in the tissue around a joint has a direct effect on the joint function. Changes in joint function eventually cause problems with the joint. Any dysfunction of

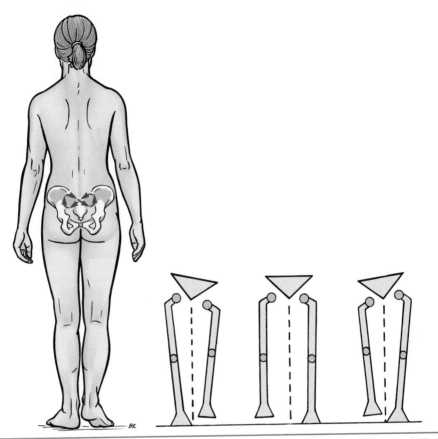

FIGURE 11-13 ■ The mechanism of the slight rocking movement of the sacroiliac joint. (From Fritz S: *Mosby's fundamentals of therapeutic massage*, ed 3. St. Louis, 2004, Mosby.)

the joint immediately involves the surrounding muscles and other soft tissue.

Disruption of the gait demands that the body compensate by shifting movement patterns and posture. Because of this, all dysfunctional patterns are whole-body phenomena. Working only on the symptomatic area is ineffective and offers only limited relief. Therapeutic massage with a whole-body focus is extremely valuable in dealing with gait dysfunction Corrective measures include normalizing muscle firing patterns and gait reflex patterns (See Box 11-2 and Box 11-3).

Interpreting Gait Assessment Findings

When interpreting the information gathered from gait assessment, the massage practitioner should focus on areas that do not move easily when the client walks and areas that move too much. Areas that do not move are restricted; areas that move too much are compensating for inefficient function. By releasing the restrictions through massage and reeducating the reflexes through neuromuscular work and exercise, the practitioner can help the client improve the gait pattern.

The techniques followed are similar to those for postural corrections. The shortened and restricted areas are softened with massage and then the neuromuscular mechanism is reset with muscle energy techniques, muscle lengthening, stretching, and normalizing firing patterns.

The client should be taught slow lengthening and stretching procedures. After stimulating the muscles in weakened areas, the practitioner can refer the client for strengthening exercises. The therapist must be sure the adaptation methods are built into the context of a complete massage rather than spot work on isolated parts of the body. Suggestions can be made to the client to evaluate factors that may contribute to these adaptations, such as posture, footwear, chairs, tables, beds, clothing, work stations, physical tasks (e.g., shoveling), and repetitive exercise patterns.

SACROILIAC JOINT FUNCTION

11-5 Proper functioning of the sacroiliac (SI) joint is an important factor in walking patterns. Because sacroiliac joint movement has no direct muscular component, it is difficult to use any kind of muscle energy lengthening when working with this joint. The SI joint is embedded deep in supporting ligaments. To keep the surrounding ligaments pliable, direct and specific connective tissue techniques are indicated unless the joint is hypermobile. If that is the case, external bracing combined with rehabilitative movement may be indicated. Sometimes the ligaments restabilize the area. Stabilization of the jointed area should be interspersed with massage and gentle stretching to ensure that the ligaments remain pliable and do not adhere to each other. This process takes time.

To assess for possible SI joint involvement, apply deep broad-based compression over the joint (Figure 11-14). If symptoms increase, SI joint dysfunction is indicated. Another assessment is to have the client stand on one foot and then extend the trunk. This loads the SI joint and would increase symptoms of SI joint dysfunction. Have the client lie prone and extend the hip. Then apply resistance to the opposite arm and have the client push against the resistance by extending the shoulder and arm (Figure 11-15), and then, while doing this, also extend the contralateral hip. If it is easier to lift and symptoms are relieved, then SI joint function can be improved by exercise and massage, because force closure mechanisms are able to be addressed. If there is no improvement, then external bracing may help.

The diagnosis of specific joint problems and fitting for external bracing is outside the scope of practice for therapeutic massage, and the client must be referred to the appropriate professional.

ANALYSIS OF MUSCLE TESTING AND GAIT PATTERNS

11-6

It is important to consider the pattern of muscle interactions that occurs with walking. Remember that gait has a certain pattern for efficient movement. For example, if the left leg is extended for the heel strike, the right arm also is extended. This results in activation of the flexors of both the arm and leg and inhibition of the extensors. It is common to find a strength imbalance in this gait pattern. One muscle out of sequence with the others can set up tense (too strong) or inhibited (weak) muscle imbalances. Whenever a muscle contracts with too much force, it overpowers the antagonist group, resulting in inhibited muscle function. The imbalances can occur anywhere in the pattern.

evolve Strength muscle testing should reveal that the flexor and adductor muscles of the right arm activate, facilitate, and coordinate with the flexors and adductors of the left leg. The opposite is also true: left arm flexors and adductors activate, facilitate, and coordinate with the right leg flexors and adductors. Extensors and abductors in the limbs coordinate in a similar fashion.

If the flexors of the left leg are activated, as occurs during strength testing, the flexors and adductors of the right arm should be facilitated and should be strong in strength testing. The flexors and adductors of the right leg and left arm should be inhibited and should be weak in strength testing. Also, the extensors and abductors in the right arm and left leg should be inhibited. All associated patterns follow suit (i.e., activation of the right arm flexor pattern facilitates the left leg flexor pattern and inhibits left arm and right leg flexor muscles while facilitating extensors and abductors). In a similar way, activation of the adductors of the right

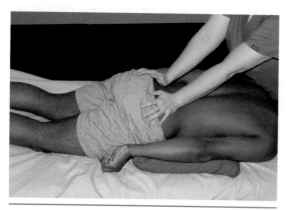

FIGURE 11-14 ■ Broad-based compression over the sacroiliac joint. Form closure assessment.

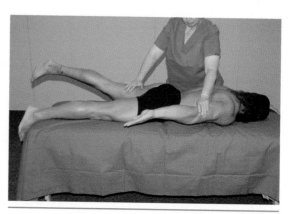

FIGURE 11-15 ■ Sacroiliac joint assessment—force closure.

leg facilitates the adductors of the left arm and inhibits the abductors of the left leg and right arm. The other adductor/abductor patterns follow the same interaction pattern.

All these patterns are associated with gait mechanisms and reflexes. If any pattern is out of sync, gait, posture, and efficient function are disrupted (See Box 11-2).

GAIT MUSCLE TESTING AS AN INTERVENTION TOOL

An understanding of gait provides a powerful intervention tool. For example, a person trips and strains the left hip extensor muscles. Gait muscle testing reveals an imbalanced pattern by showing that the left hip extensor muscles are weak, whereas the flexors in the left hip and right arm/shoulder are overly tense. The hip and leg are sore and cannot be used for work, but the arm muscles are fine. By activating the extensors in the right shoulder and arm, movement of the left hip extensor muscles can be facilitated. By activating the flexors of the left arm, the flexors of the left hip are inhibited. This process may restore balance in the gait pattern. Many combinations are possible based on the gait pattern and reflexes. Gait muscle testing provides the means of identifying these interactions.

PALPATION ASSESSMENT

Identifying changes in texture, tension, or actual damage in the soft tissues is a very important part of massage assessment. The massage therapist must understand the anatomy and physiology of the whole body to such an extent that the palpation methods actually form the area like a hologram in the practitioner's kinesthetic senses. You simply cannot study anatomy and physiology enough.*

All assessment is comparison of and contrast with the normal to identify deviations from the norm. It is necessary to identify very localized areas that feel irregular or different compared to the adjacent tissues. As mentioned previously, the least affected area is the norm for comparison. The client's pain perception is important in helping in this assessment process. Nonverbal clues such as

facial expression, clenching the fist, or curling the toes are helpful. While applying deep palpation with one hand, the therapist's other hand should be in gentle contact with the client. In this way it is often possible to sense a pain response.

Pain alone does not necessarily mean that there is a problem. There are areas in the body that are naturally a little painful when deeply palpated. There are certain tissues, such as the iliotibial band, that naturally need a fairly high degree of tension for normal function, and these areas can feel painful when pressed deeply. If the tissues feel normal to the massage therapist but cause pain when palpated, compare them with the same areas on the other side of the body. If there is a difference, then there may be a problem; if they feel the same, there is no problem and the feeling is normal.

There is no benefit in applying deep pressure to a small area, because this only shows what those particular tissues feel like and gives no information about how they compare with the surrounding tissues. Instead, it is necessary to palpate all the tissues in the area, using the to plasticity of the skin and subcutaneous layers to glide in all directions throughout the area to feel any textural changes.

Damage can occur in soft tissue at any level. One mistake sometimes made during palpation assessment is to explore deeper and deeper into the tissues in an effort to find the problem, only to miss it because it is located more superficially. It is therefore necessary to vary the degree of pressure used, from fairly light to very deep, to assess all the different tissue layers.

It also is necessary to feel the surfaces of the bony structures where fibrosis or scar tissue may occur. When palpating around a joint it is good to move it into different positions, as this gives access to different surfaces of the bones and soft tissues.

Pressing into tissue and removing all the slack puts the tissue in tension. Normally, there is no pain with pressing into the soft tissue, only a sense of pressure. However, if there is injury, the following sensations may occur:

Acute: The client feels pain before tissue is in tension.

Subacute: The client feels pain when tissue is in tension.

Chronic: The client may feel pain with overpressure.

Palpation assessment is a major aspect of the massage. In any given massage, about 90% of the

---

*This text assumes that the therapist has been trained in the fundamentals of palpation. To review palpation skills, see Fritz S: *Mosby's fundamentals of therapeutic massage*, ed 3, St. Louis, 2004, Mosby.

touching is also assessment developed as part of glidng, kneading, or joint movement. Palpation assessment makes contact with tissue but does not override it or encourage it to change. This type of work generally relaxes or stimulates the client, depending on the type of strokes used.

Palpation findings of soft tissue include the following:

Normal: The soft tissue feels resilient, homogeneous, relaxed, and pliable.

Chronic: The soft tissue feels fibrous, thickened, stiff, and tight.

Acute: The soft tissue feels boggy, warm, or hot.

Atrophy: The soft tissue feels mushy and flaccid because of loss of tone.

Normal fluid dynamics: Normal soft tissue is hydrated without feeling boggy or swollen; warm without feeling hot or sweaty; blanches when compressed and then quickly returns to normal color.

Temperature: Heat is an indication of inflammation. Cold is often a circulation impairment.

It is important not to limit a palpation sense only to the hand. Body layers, differences in tissue, movement, heat, sensitivity, texture, and other sensations can be felt with the entire body. It is essential that the massage therapist's entire self becomes sensitive to subtle differences in the client's body.

The recommended sequence of applications of palpation is as follows:

1. Near-touch palpation
2. Palpation of the skin surface
3. Palpation of the skin itself
4. Palpation of the skin and superficial connective tissue
5. Palpation of the superficial connective tissue only
6. Palpation of vessels and lymph nodes
7. Palpation of muscles
8. Palpation of tendons
9. Palpation of fascial sheaths
10. Palpation of ligaments
11. Palpation of bones
12. Palpation of abdominal viscera
13. Palpation of body rhythms

NEAR-TOUCH PALPATION

The first application of palpation does not involve touching the body. Near-touch palpation detects hot and cold areas and is best performed just off the skin using the back of the hand, because the back of the hand is very sensitive to heat. The general temperature of the area and any variations should be noted. Very sensitive cutaneous (skin) sensory receptors detect changes in air pressure and currents and movement of the air. Being able to consciously detect these subtle sensations is an invaluable assessment tool.

Hot areas may be caused by inflammation, muscle spasm, hyperactivity, or increased surface circulation. When the focus of intervention is to cool down hot areas, one method is application of ice (see section on hydrotherapy). Another way to cool an area is to reduce the muscle spasm and encourage more efficient blood flow in the surrounding areas.

Cold areas often are areas of diminished blood flow, increased connective tissue formation, or muscle flaccidity. Cold areas may have heat applied to them. Stimulation massage techniques increase muscle activity, thus heating up the area. Connective tissue approaches soften connective tissue, help restore space around the capillaries, and release histamine, a vasodilator, to increase circulation. These approaches can warm a cold area.

PALPATION OF THE SKIN SURFACE

The second application of palpation is very light stroking of the skin surface (Figure 11-16). First, determine whether the skin is dry or damp. Damp areas feel a little sticky, or the fingers drag. This light stroking causes the root hair plexus that senses light touch to respond. It is important to notice whether an area reacts with more "goose bumps" than other areas (pilomotor reflex). This is a good time to observe for color, especially blue or yellow coloration. The practitioner also should note and keep track of all moles and surface skin growths, pay attention to the quality and texture of the hair, and observe the shape and condition of the nails.

PALPATION OF THE SKIN ITSELF

Palpation of the skin itself is done through gentle, slight stretching of the skin in all directions, comparing the elasticity of these areas (Figure 11-17 and 11-18). The skin also can be palpated for surface texture. By applying light pressure to the skin surface, roughness or smoothness can be felt.

Skin should be contained, hydrated, resilient, elastic, and have even and rich coloration. Skin that does not spring back into its original position after a slight pinch may be a sign of dehydration. The skin should have no blue, yellow, or red tinges.

FIGURE 11-16

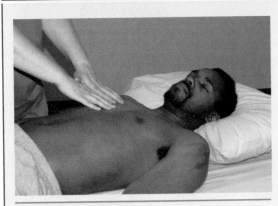

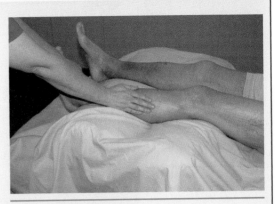

A Palpation of skin surface.

B Surface stroking of the skin.

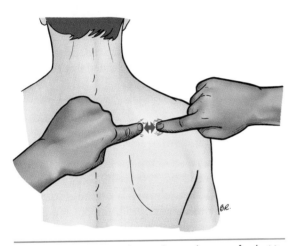

FIGURE 11-17 ■ Skin stretching used to assess for elasticity. Skin that seems tight compared with surrounding skin may indicate dysfunctional areas. (From Fritz S: *Mosby's fundamentals of therapeutic massage*, ed 3. St. Louis, 2004, Mosby.)

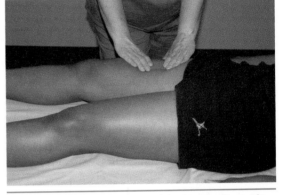

FIGURE 11-18 ■ Palpation of the skin using skin stretching.

Blue coloration suggests lack of oxygen; yellow indicates liver problems, such as jaundice; and redness suggests fever, alcohol intake, trauma, or inflammation. Color changes are most noticeable in the lips, around the eyes, and under the nails.

Bruises must be noted and avoided during massage. If a client displays any hot red areas or red streaking, he or she should be referred to a physician immediately. This is especially important when symptoms are present in the lower leg because of the possibility of deep-vein thrombosis (blood clot).

The skin should be watched carefully for changes in any moles or lumps. As massage

professionals, we often spend more time touching and observing a person's skin than anyone else, including the person being massaged. If we keep a keen eye out for changes and refer clients to physicians early, many skin problems can be treated before they become serious.

Depending on the area, the skin may be thick or thin. The skin of the face is thinner than the skin of the lower back. The appearance of the skin in each particular area, however, should be consistent. The skin loses its resilience and elasticity over areas of dysfunction. It is important to be able to recognize visceral referred pain areas in the skin (Figure 11-19). If changes occur to the skin in these areas, refer the client to a physician.

The skin is a blood reservoir. At any given time it can hold 10% of the available blood in the body. The connective tissue in the skin must be soft to allow the capillary system to expand to hold the

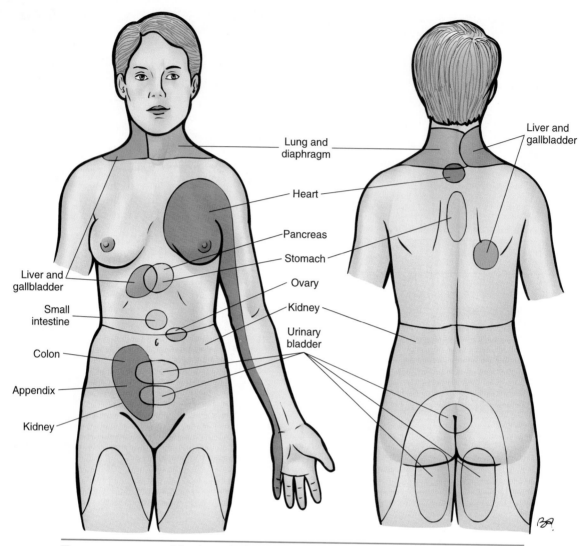

FIGURE 11-19 ■ Referred pain. The diagram indicates cutaneous areas to which visceral pains may be referred. The massage professional encountering pain in these areas needs to refer the client to a physician for diagnosis to rule out visceral dysfunction. (From Fritz S: *Mosby's fundamentals of therapeutic massage*, ed. 3. St. Louis, 2004, Mosby.)

blood. Histamine, which is released from mast cells found in the connective tissue of the superficial fascial layer, dilates the blood vessels. Histamine is also responsible for the sense of "warming and itching" in an area that has been massaged.

Damp areas on the skin are indications that the nervous system has been activated in that area. This small amount of perspiration is part of a sympathetic activation called a *facilitated segment.* Surface stroking with enough pressure to drag over the skin elicits a red response over the area of a hyperactive muscle. Deeper palpation of the area usually elicits a tender response. The small erector pili muscles attached to each hair are under the control of the sympathetic autonomic nervous system. Light

fingertip stroking produces goose bumps over areas of nerve hyperactivity. All of these responses can indicate potential activity, such as trigger points in the layers of muscle under the indicated area.

The hair and nails are part of the integumentary system and reflect health conditions. The hair should be resilient and secure; hair loss should not be excessive when the scalp is massaged.

The nails should be smooth. Vertical ridges may indicate nutritional difficulties, and horizontal ridges may be signs of stress caused by changes in circulation that affect nail growth. Clubbed nails may also indicate circulation problems. The skin around the nails should be soft and free of hangnails.

It is important to continuously monitor the skin and associated structures. During times of stress, the epithelial tissues are affected first. Signs of prolonged stress, medication side effects, and pathologic conditions include hangnails, split skin around the lips and nails, mouth sores, hair loss, dry scaly skin, and excessively oily skin. This area is one of the best for assessing adaptive capacity. For example, slow wound healing would indicate strain in the system.

PALPATION OF THE SKIN AND SUPERFICIAL CONNECTIVE TISSUE

In palpation of both the skin and superficial connective tissue, a method such as skin rolling is used to further assess the texture of the skin by lifting it from the underlying fascial sheath (Figure 11-20) and measuring the skin fold or comparing the two sides for symmetry (Figure 11-21). The skin should move evenly and glide on the underlying tissues. Areas that are stuck, restricted, or too loose should be noted, as should any areas of the skin that become redder than surrounding areas.

PALPATION OF THE SUPERFICIAL CONNECTIVE TISSUE ONLY

The fifth application of palpation is the superficial connective tissue, which separates and connects the skin and muscle tissue. It allows the skin to glide over the muscles during movement. This layer of tissue is found by applying compression until the fibers of the underlying muscle are felt. The pressure then should be lightened so that the muscle cannot be felt, but if the hand is moved, the skin also moves. This area feels a little like a very thin water balloon. The tissue should feel resilient and springy, like gelatin. Superficial fascia holds fluid. If surface edema is present, it is in the superficial fascia. This water-binding quality gives this area the feel of a water balloon, but it should not feel boggy or soggy or show pitting edema (i.e., the dent from the pressure remains in the skin).

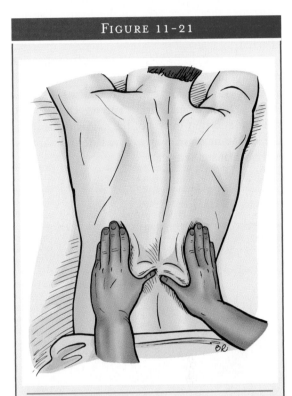

FIGURE 11-21

A Use of kneading to assess the skin and superficial connective tissues by lifting of the tissues.

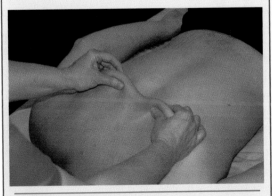

B Measuring skin fold for symmetry. (**A** from Fritz S: *Mosby's fundamentals of therapeutic massage*, ed 3. St. Louis, 2004, Mosby.)

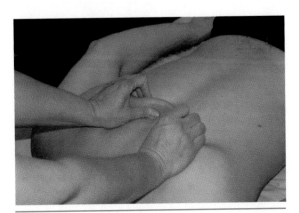

FIGURE 11-20 ■ Skin roll.

Methods of palpation that lift the skin, such as kneading and skin rolling, provide much information. Depending on the area of the body and the concentration of underlying connective tissue, the skin should lift and roll easily (Figure 11-22). Loosening of these areas is very beneficial, and the practitioner can achieve this by applying the assessment methods (kneading and skin rolling) slowly and deliberately, allowing a shift in the tissues. A constant drag should be kept on the tissues, because both the skin and superficial connective tissue are affected.

Any area that becomes redder than the surrounding tissue or that stays red longer than other areas is suspect for connective tissue changes (Figure 11-23). Usually, lifting and stretching (bend, shear, and torsion forces) of the reddened tissue or use of the myofascial approaches (tension forces) will normalize these areas.

PALPATION OF VESSELS AND LYMPH NODES

The sixth application of palpation involves circulatory vessels and lymph nodes. Just above the muscle and still in the superficial connective tissue lie the more superficial blood vessels. The vessels are distinct and feel like soft tubes. Pulses can be palpated, but if pressure is too intense, the feel of the pulse is lost (Figure 11-24). Palpating for pulses helps detect this layer of tissue.

In this same area are the more superficial lymph vessels and lymph nodes. Lymph nodes usually are located in joint areas and feel like small, soft "gelcaps." The compression of the joint action assists in lymphatic flow. A client with enlarged lymph nodes should be referred to a medical professional for diagnosis. Very light, gentle palpation of lymph nodes and vessels is indicated in this circumstance.

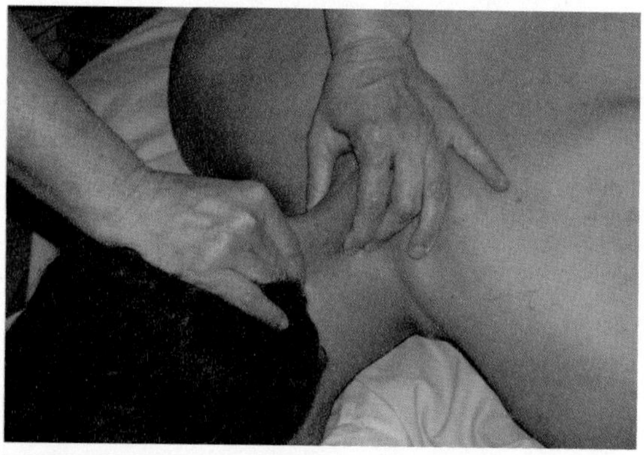

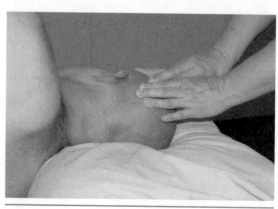

FIGURE 11-22 ■ Skin lift and roll.

FIGURE 11-23 ■ Areas of reddening indicates connective tissue changes.

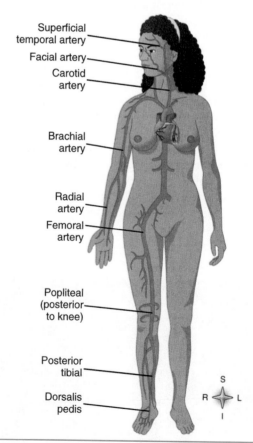

FIGURE 11-24 ■ Pulse points. Each pulse point is named after the artery with which it is associated. (From Thibodeau GA, Patton KT: *Anatomy and physiology*, ed. 5, St. Louis, 2003, Mosby.)

Vessels should feel firm but pliable and supported. If bulging, mushiness, or constriction is noted in any areas, the massage therapist should refer the client to a physician.

Pulses should be compared by feeling for a strong, even, full-pumping action on both sides of the body. If differences are perceived, the massage practitioner should refer the client to a physician. Sometimes the differences in the pulses can be attributed to soft tissue restriction of the artery or to a more serious condition that can be diagnosed by the physician. Refill of capillaries in nail beds after compression of the nail should take approximately 3 to 5 seconds and be equal in all fingers.

Enlarged lymph nodes may indicate local or systemic infection or a more serious condition. The client should be referred to a physician immediately.

PALPATION OF SKELETAL MUSCLES

The seventh application of palpation is skeletal muscle. Muscle is made up of contractile fibers embedded in connective tissue. Muscle has a distinct fiber direction. Its texture feels somewhat like corded fabric or fine rope. The area of the muscle that becomes the largest when the muscle is concentrically contracted is in the belly of the muscle. Where the muscle fibers end and the connective tissue continues, the tendon develops; this is called the *musculotendinous junction*.

It is a good practice activity to locate both of these areas for all surface muscles and as many underlying ones as possible. Almost all muscular dysfunctions, such as trigger points or microscarring from minute muscle tears, are found at the musculotendinous junction or in the belly of the muscle. Most acupressure points, often classified as *motor points,* also are located in these areas.

Often three or more layers of muscle are present in an area. These layers are separated by fascia, and each muscle layer should slide over the one beneath it (Figure 11-25).

In palpation of the muscles, compressing systematically through each layer until the bone is felt is important (Figure 11-26). Pressure used to reach and palpate the deeper layers of muscle must travel from the superficial layers down to the deeper layers. To accomplish this, the compressive force must be even, broad-based, and slow. There should be no "poking" quality to the touch, or abrupt pressure pushing through muscle layers, because the surface layers of muscle will tense up and guard,

FIGURE 11-25

SLIDING OF MUSCLE LAYERS

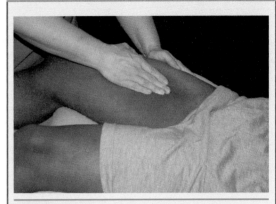

A First layer.

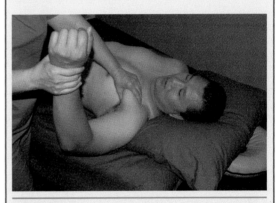

B Second layer.

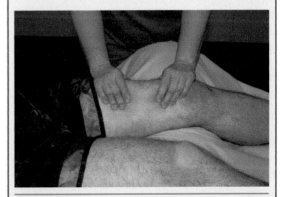

C Third layer.

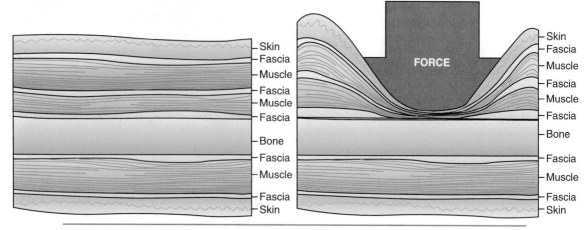

FIGURE 11-26 ■ Massage applications systematically generate force through each tissue layer. This figure provides a graphic representation of force applied, which would begin with light superficial applications, progressing with increased pressure to the deepest layer. (From Fritz S: *Mosby's fundamentals of therapeutic massage*, ed 3. St. Louis, 2004, Mosby.)

preventing access to the deeper layers. Muscle tends to push up against palpating pressure when it is concentrically contracting. Having the client slowly move the joint that is affected can help in identifying the proper location of muscles being assessed (Figure 11-27).

Palpation of each specific muscle area involves sliding each layer of muscle back and forth over the underlying layer to make sure there is no adherence between the muscle layers and systematic compression through each muscle layer (Figure 11-28).

Muscle layers usually run cross-grain to each other. The best example of this is the abdominal muscle group. Even in the arm and leg, where all the muscles seem to run in the same direction, a diagonal crossing and spiraling of the muscle groups is evident.

Interpreting Skeletal Muscle Assessment Findings

Muscles can feel tense and ropy in both concentric (short) and eccentric (long) patterns. Therefore think of muscle functioning as short and tight and long and tight.

Skeletal muscle is assessed both for texture and for function. It should be firm and pliable. Soft, spongy muscle or hard, dense muscle indicates connective tissue dysfunction. Muscle atrophy results in a muscle that feels smaller than normal. Hypertrophy results in a muscle that feels larger than normal. Application of the appropriate techniques can normalize the connective tissue component of the muscle. Excessively strong or weak muscles can be caused by problems with neuromuscular control or imbalanced work or exercise demand. Weak

muscles can be a result of wasting (atrophy) of the muscle fibers.

Tension can be felt in muscles that are either concentrically short or eccentrically long. Tension that manifests in short muscles that are concentrically contracted results in tissue that feels hard and bunched. When muscles are tense from being pulled into an extension pattern, they feel like long, taut bundles with some contraction and shortened muscle fiber groups. Usually, flexors, adductors, and internal rotators become short, whereas extensors, abductors, and external rotators palpate tense but are long and have eccentric contraction patterns. Massage treatment most often first addresses the short concentrically contracted muscles, in order to lengthen them, rather than the long muscles, because massage methods usually result in longer tissues, which would ultimately worsen the problem. Therapeutic exercise is necessary to restore normal tone to the "long muscles."

Spot work on isolated areas is seldom effective. Neurologic muscle imbalances are kinetic chain interactions linked by reflex patterns, most notably the gait reflexes and the interaction between postural and phasic muscles.

Important areas are the musculotendinous junction and the muscle belly, where the nerve usually enters the muscle. As was pointed out earlier, motor points cause a muscle contraction with a small stimulus. Disruption of sensory signals at the motor point causes many problems, including trigger points and referred pain, hypersensitive acupressure points, and restricted movement patterns

FIGURE 11-27

EXAMPLES OF PALPATION OF CONTRACTING MUSCLES

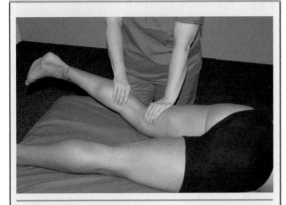

A Gastrocnemius and hamstring.

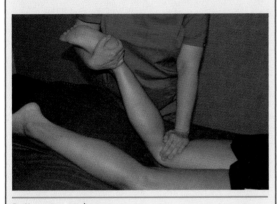

B Hamstring attachment.

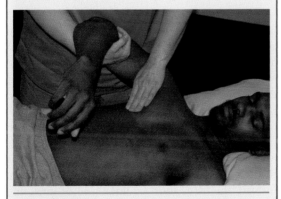

C Pectoralis major.

caused by the increase in the physiologic barrier and the development of pathologic barriers.

PALPATION OF TENDONS

The eighth application of palpation is the tendons. Tendons have a higher concentration of collagen fibers and feel more pliable and less ribbed than muscle. Tendons feel like duct tape. Under many tendons is a cushion of fluid-filled bursae that assists the movement of the bone under the tendon.

Tendons should feel elastic and mobile. If a tendon has been torn, it may adhere to the underlying bone during the healing process. Some tendons, such as those of the fingers and toes, are enclosed in a sheath and must be able to glide within the sheath. If they cannot glide, inflammation builds up, and the result is *tenosynovitis*. Overuse also can cause inflammation. Inflammation signals the formation of connective tissue, which can interfere with movement and cause the tendons to adhere to surrounding tissue. In tendons without a sheath, this condition is called *tendonitis*. Frictioning techniques help these conditions. Usually, tight tendon structures are normalized when the muscle's resting length is normalized.

PALPATION OF FASCIAL SHEATHS

The ninth application of palpation is fascial sheaths. Fascial sheaths feel like sheets of plastic wrap. They separate muscles and expand the connective tissue area of bone for muscular attachment. Some, such as the lumbodorsal fascia, the abdominal fascia, and the iliotibial band, run on the surface of the body and are thick, like a tarp. Others, such as the linea alba and the nuchal ligament, run perpendicular to the surfaces of the body and the bone like a rope. Still others run horizontally through the body. The horizontal pattern occurs at joints (see Figure 11-9), the diaphragm muscle (which is mostly connective tissue), and the pelvic floor. Fascial sheaths separate muscle groups. They provide a continuous, interconnected framework for the body that follows the principles of tensegrity. Fascial sheaths are kept taut by the design of the cross-pattern and the action of muscles that lie between the sheaths, such as the gluteus maximus, which lies between the iliotibial band and the lumbodorsal fascia (Figure 11-29).

The larger nerves and blood vessels lie in grooves created by the fascial separations. Careful comparison reveals that the location of the tradi-

FIGURE 11-28

EXAMPLE OF PALPATION OF A SPECIFIC MUSCLE AREA

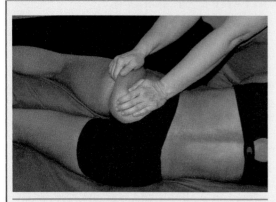

A Muscle layer should slide over the one under it.

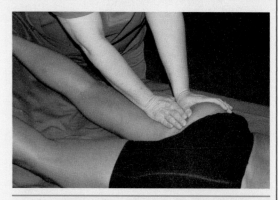

B Layer 1. Compress systematically through the tissue layers.

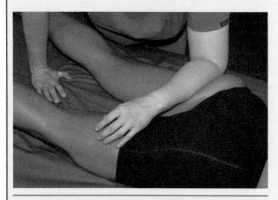

C Layer 2. Maintain broad-based compression.

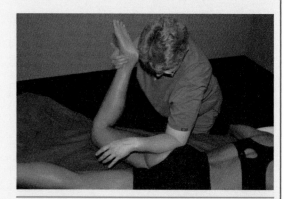

D Layer 3. Position superficial layers so that deep layers are easily accessed.

tional acupuncture meridians corresponds to these nerve and blood vessel tracts. The fascial separations can be made more distinct and more pliable by palpating with the fingers. With sufficient pressure, the fingers tend to fall into these grooves, which can then be followed. These areas need to be resilient and pliable but distinct, because they serve both as stabilizers and separators.

Fascial sheaths should be pliable, but because they are stabilizers, they may be more dense than tendons in some areas. Problems arise if the tissues these sheaths separate or stabilize become stuck to the sheath or if the fascial sheath becomes less pliable.

Myofascial approaches are best suited to dealing with the fascial sheaths. Mechanical work, such as slow, sustained stretching, and methods that pull and drag on the tissue are used to soften the sheaths. Because it often is uncomfortable, creating a burning, pulling sensation, the work should not

be done unless the client is committed to regular appointments until the area is normalized. This may take 6 months to 1 year.

Chronic health conditions almost always show dysfunction of the connective tissue and fascial sheaths. Any techniques categorized as connective tissue approaches are effective as long as the practitioner proceeds slowly and follows the tissue pattern. The massage therapist should not override the tissue or force the tissue into a corrective pattern. Instead, the tissue must be untangled or unwound gradually following ease and bend directions.

Fascial separations between muscles create pathways for the nerves and blood vessels. When palpated, these pathways feel like grooves running between muscles. If these areas become narrow or restricted, blood vessels may be constricted and nerves impinged. A slow, specific, stripping gliding along these pathways can be beneficial (Figure 11-

FIGURE 11-29

FASCIAL SHEATHS

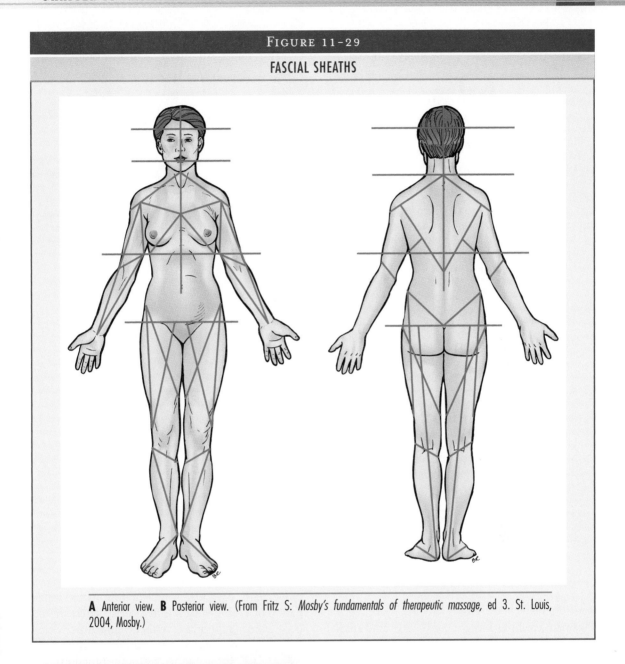

A Anterior view. **B** Posterior view. (From Fritz S: *Mosby's fundamentals of therapeutic massage,* ed 3. St. Louis, 2004, Mosby.)

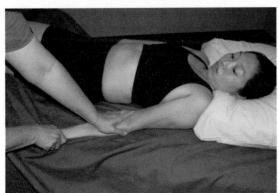

FIGURE II-30 ■ Gliding in fascial grooves.

30). The nerves run in these fascial pathways, and the nerve trunks correlate with the traditional meridian system. Therefore most meridian and acupressure work takes place along these fascial grooves (Figure 11-31). Muscle layers are also separated by fascia, and because muscles must be able to slide over each other, it is necessary to make sure that there is no adherence between muscles. This situation often occurs in the legs. If assessment indicates that the muscles are stuck to each other, kneading and gliding can be used to slide one muscle layer over the other.

Water is an important element of connective tissue. To keep connective tissue soft, the client must rehydrate.

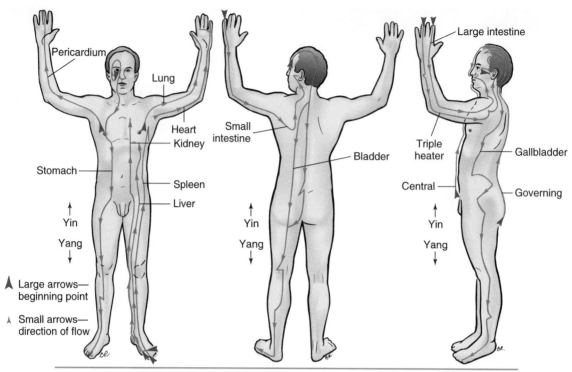

FIGURE 11-31 ■ Typical location of meridians. Meridians tend to follow fascial nerves and grooves. Yin and yang meridians are paired as follows:

Yin Meridian	Yang Meridian
Pericardium	Triple heater
Liver	Gallbladder
Kidney	Bladder
Heart	Small intestine
Spleen	Stomach
Lung	Large intestine

(From Fritz S: *Mosby's fundamentals of therapeutic massage*, ed. 3. St. Louis, 2004, Mosby.)

PALPATION OF LIGAMENTS

Ligaments feel like bungee cords and some are flat when palpated. Ligaments should be flexible enough to allow the joint to move, yet stable enough to restrict movement. It is important to be able to recognize a ligament and not mistake it for a tendon. With the joint in a neutral position, if muscles are isometrically contracted, the tendon moves but the ligament does not. If ligaments are not pliable or are tender, shear force is used to normalize the tissue.

PALPATION OF JOINTS

The eleventh application of palpation is the joints. Careful palpation should reveal the space between the synovial joint ends. Joints often feel like hinges. Most assessment is of active and passive joint movements. An added source of information is palpation of a joint while it is in motion. There should be a stable, supported, resilient, and unrestricted range of motion. (Refer to the Evolve site *evolve* for a summary of joint function).

When palpating joints, it is important to assess for end-feel, as previously discussed Simply put, end-feel is the perception of the joint at the limit of its ROM, and it is either soft or hard. In most joints it should feel soft. This means that the body is unable to move any more through muscular contraction, but a small additional move by the therapist still produces some give. A hard end-feel is what the bony stabilization of the elbow feels like on extension. No more active movement is possible, and passive movement is restricted by bone.

For the massage practitioner, it is important to be able to palpate the bony landmarks that indicate the tendinous attachment points of the muscles and to trace the bone's shape.

Movement of the joints through a comfortable ROM can be used as an evaluation method. Comparison of the symmetry of ROM (e.g., comparing the circumduction pattern of one arm with that of the other) is effective for detecting limitations of a particular movement. Muscle energy methods, as well as all massage manipulations, can be used to support symmetric ROM functions.

All these tissues and structures are supported by general massage applications, which result in increased circulation, increased pliability of soft tissue, and normalized neuromuscular patterns.

Massage can positively affect the normal limits of the physiologic barrier. When joints are traumatized, the surrounding tissue becomes "scared," almost as if saying, "This joint will never get in that position again." When this happens, all the proprioceptive mechanisms reset to limit the ROM, setting up a pathologic barrier. Massage and appropriate muscle lengthening and general stretching, combined with muscle energy techniques and self-help, can have a beneficial effect on ligaments and joint function. Ligaments are relatively slow to regenerate, and it takes time to notice improvement.

PALPATION OF BONES

The twelfth application of palpation is the bones. Those who have developed their palpation skills find a firm, but detectable pliability when palpating bone. Bones feel like young sapling tree trunks and branches.

PALPATION OF ABDOMINAL VISCERA

The thirteenth application of palpation is the viscera. The abdomen contains the viscera, or internal organs of the body. It is important for the massage professional to be able to locate and to know the positioning of the organs in the abdominal cavity (Figure 11-32). The massage therapist

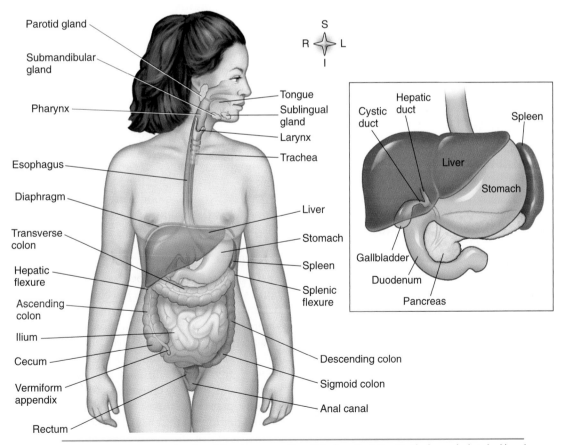

FIGURE 11-32 ■ Location of digestive organs. (From Thibodeau GA, Patton KT: *The human body in health and disease,* ed 3. St. Louis, 2002, Mosby.)

should be able to palpate the distinct firmness of the liver and location of the large intestine.

Refer the client to a physician if any hard, rigid, stiff, or tense areas are noted in the abdomen or if pain increases when palpation pressure ceases. Close attention must be paid to the visceral referred pain areas. If tissue changes are noted in these areas, the practitioner must refer the client to a physician.

The skin often is tighter in areas of visceral referred pain. As a result of cutaneous/visceral reflexes, benefit may be obtained by stretching the skin in these areas. There is some indication that normalizing the skin over these areas has a positive effect on the functioning of the organ. If nothing else, circulation is increased and peristalsis (intestinal movement) may be stimulated.

In accordance with the recommendations for colon massage, repetitive stroking in the proper directions may stimulate smooth muscle contraction and can improve elimination problems and intestinal gas (Figure 11-33). Psoas work is often done through the abdomen.

PALPATION OF BODY RHYTHMS

The fourteenth application of palpation is the body rhythms. Body rhythms are felt as even pulsations or undulations. Body rhythms are designed to operate in a coordinated, balanced, and synchronized manner. In the body, all the rhythms are entrained. When palpating body rhythms, the practitioner should get a sense of this harmony. Although the trained hand can pick out some of the individual rhythms, just as one can hear individual notes in a song, it is the whole connected effect that is important. When a person feels "off" or "out of sync," often he or she is speaking of disruption in the entrainment process of body rhythms.

Respiration

The breathing rhythm is easy to feel. It should be even and should follow good principles of inhalation and exhalation. To palpate the breath, while the client goes through three or more breathing cycles the practitioner places his or her hands over the client's ribs and evaluates the evenness and fullness of the breaths. Relaxed breathing should result in a slight rounding of the upper abdomen and lateral movement of the lower ribs during inhalation. Movement in the shoulders or upper chest indicates potential difficulties with the breathing mechanism.

Improved breathing function helps the entire body. The muscular mechanism for inhalation and exhalation of air is like a simple bellows system and depends on unrestricted movement of the musculoskeletal components of the thorax. The muscles of respiration include the scalenes, intercostals, anterior serratus, diaphragm, abdominals, and pelvic floor muscles. If a breathing pattern disorder is a factor and the person is prone to anxiety, intervention softens and normalizes the upper body and supports the mechanism of breathing.

Because of the whole-body interplay between muscle groups in all actions, including breathing, it is not uncommon to find tight lower leg and foot muscles interfering with breathing. Disruption of function in any of these muscle groups inhibits full and easy breathing.

General relaxation massage and stress reduction methods seem to help breathing the most. The client can be taught slow lengthening and stretching methods and the breathing retraining pattern. The client also can be advised not to wear restrictive clothing or hold in the stomach. (See specific protocol for breathing dysfunction.)

Circulation

The movement, or circulation, of the blood is felt at the major pulse points. The pulses should be balanced on both sides of the body. Basic palpation of the movement of the blood is done by placing the fingertips over pulse points on both sides of the body and comparing for evenness.

The vascular refill rate is another means of assessing the efficiency and rhythm of the circulation. To assess this rate, press the nail beds until they blanch (push blood out), then let go and count the seconds until color returns. A normal rate is 3 to 5 seconds.

Assessment of Subtle Body Rhythms

There are many other biologic oscillators that function in a rhythmic pattern, but they are more difficult to palpate. The body rhythms are assessed before and after massage. An improvement in rate and evenness should be noticed after the massage. Massage offered by a centered practitioner with a focused, rhythmic intent provides patterns for the client's body to use to entrain its own rhythms. The massage practitioner must remain focused on the natural rhythms of the client. Although the entrainment pattern of the practitioner and the massage provides a pattern for the client, it should not superimpose an unnatural rhythm on the client.

FIGURE 11-33

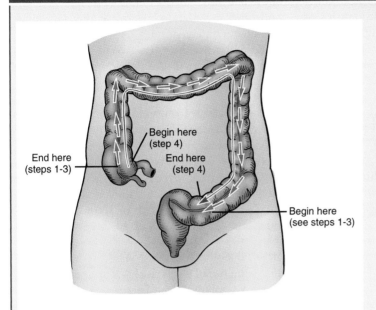

End here
(steps 1-3)

Begin here
(step 4)

End here
(step 4)

Begin here
(see steps 1-3)

A Colon with flow pattern arrows. All massage manipulations are directed in a clockwise fashion. The manipulations begin in the lower left-hand quadrant (on the left side as one views the illustration) at the sigmoid colon. The methods progressively contact all of the large intestine as they eventually end up encompassing the entire colon area.

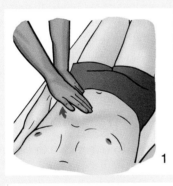

1

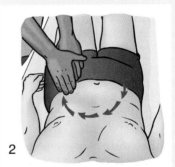

2

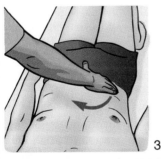

3

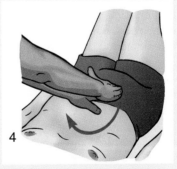

4

B Abdominal sequence. The direction of flow for emptying of the large intestine and colon is as follows: *1,* Massage down the left side of the descending colon using short strokes directed to the sigmoid colon. *2,* Massage across the transverse colon to the left side using short strokes directed to the sigmoid colon. *3,* Massage up the ascending colon on the right side of the body using short strokes directed to the sigmoid colon. End at the right side of the ileocecal valve located in the lower right-hand quadrant of the abdomen. *4,* Massage entire flow pattern using long, light to moderate strokes from the ileocecal valve to the sigmoid colon. Repeat sequence. (Modified from Fritz S: *Mosby's fundamentals of therapeutic massage,* ed. 3. St. Louis, 2004, Mosby.)

Any foreign patterns ultimately will be rejected by the client's body. Instead, the practitioner should support the client in reestablishing his or her innate entrainment rhythm. Supported by rocking methods and a rhythmic approach to the massage and the appropriate use of music, the body can reestablish synchronized rhythmic function.

UNDERSTANDING ASSESSMENT FINDINGS

The results of an assessment identify either appropriate function or dysfunction of each area. When all assessments have been completed, the overall result is described as normal or as stage 1, stage 2, or stage 3 dysfunction. Typical dysfunction includes local functional block, local hypermobility or hypomobility, altered firing patterns, and postural imbalance, all of which lead to changes in motor function and are accompanied by temporary or chronic disorders of the joints, muscles, and nervous system.

Functional assessment defines mobility through active and passive movements of the body as well as palpation and observation of distortion in these movements. Muscle testing and definition of the functional relationships of muscles are also performed.

Distortions in functioning are often measured and categorized in the following manner:

First-degree distortion–Shortening or weakening of some muscles or the formation of local changes in tension or connective tissue in these muscles. For usual and simple movements, a person has to use additional muscles from different parts of the body. As a result, movement becomes uneconomical and labored.

Second-degree distortion–Moderately expressed shortening of postural muscles and weakening of antagonist muscles. Moderately peculiar postures and movements of some parts of the body are present. Postural and movement distortions, such as altered firing patterns, begin to occur.

Third-degree distortion–Clearly expressed shortening of postural muscles and weakening of antagonist muscles, with the appearance of specific, nonoptimal movement. Significantly expressed peculiarity in postures and movement occurs. Increased postural and movement distortions result.

It is important to define which muscles are shortened and which are inhibited and likely long and taut, in order to determine the appropriate therapeutic intervention.

Based on the three levels of distorted function, three stages exist in the development of postural and movement pathology:

Stage 1 Dysfunction (Functional Tension). At stage 1 dysfunction (functional tension), a person tires more quickly than normal. This fatigue is accompanied in the first- or second-degree limitation of mobility, painless local myodystonia (changes in muscle length-tension relationship and motor tone), postural imbalance of the first or second degree, and nonoptimal motor function of the first degree.

Stage 2 Dysfunction (Functional Stress). Stage 2 dysfunction (functional stress) is characterized by a feeling of fatigue following moderate activity, discomfort, slight pain, and the appearance of one or more degrees of limited mobility that is painless or that results in first-degree pain. It may be accompanied by local hypermobility or hypomobility. Functional stress is also characterized by reflex vertebral-sensory dysfunction, fascial/connective tissue changes, and regional postural imbalance. It is accompanied by distortion of motor function of the first or second degree increase in motor tone and firing pattern alterations.

Stage 3 Dysfunction (Connective Tissue Changes in the Musculoskeletal System). The reasons for connective tissue changes are overloading, disturbances of tissue nutrition, microtrauma, microhemorrhage, unresolved edema, and other endogenous (inside the body) and exogenous (outside the body) factors. Hereditary predisposition is also a consideration. In stage 3 dysfunction, changes in the spine and weight-bearing joints may appear, with areas of local hypermobility and instability of several vertebral motion segments, hypomobility, widespread painful muscle tension, fascial and connective tissue changes in the muscles, regional postural imbalance of the second or third degree in many joints, and temporary nonoptimal motor function with second- or third-degree distortion. Visceral disturbances may be present.

Implications for Massage Treatment
(functional tension) can often be managed effectively by massage methods applied by practitioners with training equivalent to 500 to 1000 hours that

includes an understanding of the information presented in this text and technical training in the chosen method. Working with stages 2 and 3 (functional stress and connective tissue changes) usually requires more training and proper supervision within a multidisciplinary approach.

Assessment also identifies areas of resourceful and successful compensation. These compensation patterns occur when the body has been required to adapt to some sort of trauma or repetitive use pattern. Permanent adaptive changes, although not as efficient as optimal functioning, are the best pattern that the body can develop in response to an irreversible change in the system. Resourceful compensation is not to be eliminated but supported.

Years of clinical experience have taught many therapists that most symptoms and dysfunctional patterns are compensatory patterns. Some problems are recent, and some qualify for archaeologic exploration, having developed in early life and having been compounded through time. Compensatory patterns often are complex, but the client's body frequently can show us the way if we can listen to the story it tells.

There are many instances of **resourceful compensation,** a term used for the adjustments the body makes to manage a permanent or chronic dysfunction. Protective muscle spasm (guarding) around a compressed disc is an example. The splinting action of the spasms protects the nerves and provides additional stability in the area.

Decisions must be made regarding how and to what degree the compensatory pattern should be altered. It seems prudent to assume that the body knows what it is doing. The wise therapist spends time learning to understand the reasons for the compensatory patterns presented by the body. When resourceful compensation is present, therapeutic massage methods are used to support the altered pattern and prevent any further increase in postural distortion than is necessary to support the body change.

Some compensatory patterns are also set up for short-term situations that do not require permanent adaptation. Having a leg in a cast and walking on crutches for a period of time is a classic example. The body catching itself during an "almost" fall is another classic set-up pattern. Unfortunately, the body often habituates these patterns and maintains them well beyond their usefulness. As a result, over time the body begins to show symptoms of pain or inefficient function, or both.

Many compensatory patterns develop to maintain a balanced posture, and even though the posture becomes distorted during compensation, the overall result is a balanced body in a gravitational line. It also is important to consider the pattern of muscle interactions, such as the ones that occur when walking, and to recognize that gait has a certain pattern for the most efficient movement that the body can manage.

There is no set system for figuring out the compensatory patterns. All these factors must be considered in devising a plan that best serves the client.

Remember, as indicated above, first-degree and stage 1 dysfunction can usually be managed by general massage application. Stage 2 and stage 3 dysfunction should be referred to the appropriate health care professional, and cooperative multidisciplinary treatment plans should be developed. Keeping this in mind, the massage therapist honors the limits of their scope of practice.

If the massage therapist is working in a sports team environment, the athletic trainer in conjunction with the team doctor and the physical therapist would do a majority of the assessment. They would also provide the treatment plan and outcome goals to be carried out by the massage therapist. This does not mean that the massage therapist does not also do an assessment to identify the focus for massage application. Findings are submitted to the trainer.

ORGANIZING ASSESSMENT INFORMATION INTO TREATMENT STRATEGIES

The body is an interrelated, relatively symmetric functional form. Both for assessment purposes and treatment approaches, it is helpful to consider these interrelationships. Science does not totally understand how our molecules stay together, let alone how the body constantly adapts second by second to internal and external environmental demands. Yet natural design is usually very simple and set up in repeating patterns that function together for efficiency.

SYMPATHETIC/PARASYMPATHETIC BALANCE

In general, excessive sympathetic activation should be balanced by a relaxing massage, and excessive parasympathetic activation should be balanced by a stimulating massage. However, it is not quite that easy. In order to establish rapport and ultimately entrainment, it is recommended that the practitioner work with a client by addressing the client's current state. This is also very true when deciding whether the general massage approach will be stimulation or relaxation.

If the client is functioning from sympathetic nervous system dominance, and relaxation methods such as rocking and slow gliding are used initially, the work often seems irritating to the client. If the session is begun with a more stimulating approach, using such strokes as rapid compression, muscle energy methods, lengthening, and tapotement, the design of the massage fits the physiologic level of the client. After some of the nervous energy has been discharged, the client is ready for the more relaxing methods.

The same is true with parasympathetic dominance patterns. If the client is feeling "down," beginning with a stimulating approach may feel like an attack. It is better to begin with more subtle relaxation methods and progress slowly into the stimulating approaches to encourage balance.

If the client seems "out of sorts," operating more as a collection of parts than the sum of the parts, entrainment processes may be off. The centered, coordinated presence of the professional providing a harmonized approach to the massage is beneficial.

BODY SYMMETRY

Body symmetry interrelationships exist in the nervous system, especially various reflexes—oculopelvic, crossed extensor, withdrawal, gait, and other such patterns. Observation of the body reveals structural similarity in the design of the shoulder and pelvic girdles and the upper and lower limbs. It is logical to assume that similarly shaped areas function in similar ways.

The axial skeleton does not seem to show a design similar to that of the appendicular skeleton; however, with a bit of imagination, one can see that it is there. Consider the rib cage as the central point: above it you have the cervical vertebrae and the head; below it, the lumbar vertebrae, sacrum, and coccyx (what is left of a tail). Most biologic forms have a head at one end and a tail at the other. Imagine if we removed the head or added a tail, and there you go—symmetry (Figure 11-34).

The principles of postural balance and mobility factor in. The axial skeleton displays a mirror image

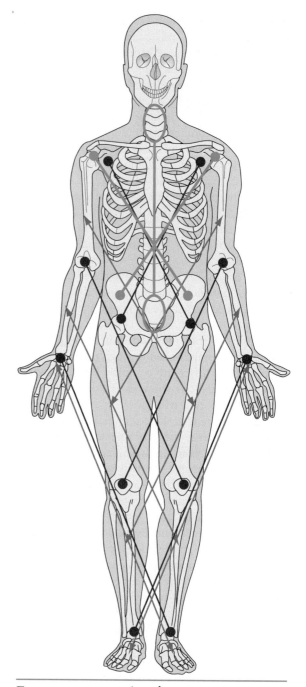

FIGURE II-34 ■ Areas of symmetry.
Arm—Thigh; Forearm—Leg; Hand—Foot; Shoulder—Hip; Elbow—Knee; Wrist—Ankle; Cervical-Sacrum; Shoulder Girdle—Pelvic Girdle.

as a top/bottom with the midpoint about the navel. Therefore, the imaginary tail pairs with the real head, the coccyx pairs with the atlas, the axis with the sacrum, and the lumbar and cervical areas pair together. This mirror image can be considered functional for posture and stability. The muscles pair as follows: Occipital base and suprahyoids with pelvic floor, sternocleidomastoid and longus coli with the psoas and rectus abdominis, scalenes with quadratus lumborum, internal and external intercostals with internal and external obliques, and transversus thoracis with transversus abdominis. On the dorsal aspect of the thorax, you find the posterior serratus superior and inferior paired. Muscles that are oriented more vertically, such as the rectus abdominis and erector spinae group, pair on the dorsal and ventral aspects. If the pairs are also agonist/antagonists, then either a reciprocal inhibition pattern can occur or there can be a co-contraction situation.

Therefore, if a client has a short psoas, the sternocleidomastoid and longus coli may also be short. If the scalenes are short, the quadratus lumborum may show reflex shortening. Dysfunction in the occipital base may also involve pelvic floor dysfunction.

The girdles and limbs that attach to the axial skeleton move in contralateral patterns, the left lower with right upper, and so forth. The scapula and clavicle pair with the pelvis. The sacroiliac joints pair with both sternoclavicular joints. Other pairs are the humerus and femur, the tibia/fibula and radius/ulna, the carpals and tarsals, the metacarpals and metatarsals, the phalanges and the corresponding phalanges, the hip and shoulder joints, the elbow and knee, the ankle and wrist, and the foot and hand.

There is a corresponding symmetry in the functional aspects of the axial soft tissue: the rotator cuff muscles with the deep lateral hip rotators, the deltoid with the gluteal group, the pectoralis minor and coracobrachialis with the pectineus, the pectoralis major and latissimus dorsi with the adductors, the quadriceps with the triceps and aconeus, the hamstrings with the biceps brachii, the brachialis with the popliteus, the wrist and finger flexors with the ankle plantar flexors, the wrist and finger extensors with the dorsiflexors, the supinators with the inverters, the pronators with the everters, and finally, the palm of the hand with the sole of the foot. These relationships should be easy to conceptualize (see Figure 11-34).

Remember that in the appendicular skeleton, a counterbalancing crossed pattern exists, so again the left arm pairs with the right leg and the right arm with the left leg. Thus, if a client has a short hamstring on the left then he or she may also have a short biceps brachii on the right. A bruise on the right quadriceps may result in reflex guarding in the

left triceps. A sprain of the great toe on the right foot may result in reflexive guarding in the left thumb. A short gastrocnemius bilateral may also reflexively include short wrist flexors bilaterally. Guarding patterns for a knee injury may also occur reflexively around the opposite elbow. Right sacroiliac pain may be paired with left sternoclavicular joint dysfunction. Short deep lateral hip rotators on the left may also involve reflexive guarding in the right rotator cuff, with changes in movement of the shoulder. Restricted shoulder/arm movement on the right may be a lingering response to a previous adductor/groin injury on the left. The possible interactions are countless.

One way to use these potential patterns is in analysis of assessment and developing massage application.

For example, if a baseball pitcher has a restricted ROM in the pitching arm (right arm) that has appeared over time and seems unrelated to the common strain in the arm, ask if there was a previous groin injury or increase in groin tightness on the left. For treatment, first address the adductors of the leg and the deep lateral hip rotators on the left while the client moves the right arm slowly through an ROM. Continually palpate for areas in the thigh and hip muscles that seem to overrespond to the arm movement and focus inhibition methods (usually compression in the muscle belly but sometimes in the attachments) in these areas. Then reassess the shoulder and arm for change. Finally, address the remaining arm symptoms.

Another example: A client has quadratus/psoas shortening related low back pain. Ask if he or she is also experiencing any symptoms in the neck. Assess the ROM of the neck and palpate for especially tender areas. Before addressing the low back pain, make sure that the scalenes and sternocleidomastoid muscles are normal and treat dysfunction with muscle energy methods or direct inhibition while the client rotates the pelvis in various directions. As in the previous example, continue to assess for areas that overrespond to the activations of the quadratus lumborum and psoas movement. Focus on those areas and reassess the low back pain. Treat the remaining symptoms of low back pain. While addressing the quadratus lumborum and the psoas, have the client rotate the head in slow large circles to activate the pattern and facilitate the release.

Another example: A soccer player has a thigh bruise and it cannot be directly massaged other than by lymphatic drain. To create a reduction in reflexive guarding and pain, massage is applied to the opposite triceps group. There may be a surprisingly sore area corresponding to the location of the bruise.

When working with these patterns, remember the focus of the massage. If the goal of the massage is to increase mobility of the left ankle, it may be helpful for the client to slowly move the right wrist in circles; the intent is not to treat the wrist, but to influence the dysfunctional ankle. If the goal of the massage is to manage short hamstrings, the biceps muscle of the arm will be part of the treatment approach. While the client may notice changes in the arm when massage is being applied, the client should be moving the knees back and forth so that the hamstrings are affected, since this is the goal of the massage. A client with a groin pull will likely benefit from massage of the arm adductors and abductors, but the intent of the massage of this area is to influence the groin.

The general protocol and many of the other specific recommendations for massage incorporate these concepts. It is prudent for the massage therapist to become proficient with this strategy for organizing and understanding injury and training adaptation. Seemly unrelated symptoms are indeed part of the same process.

Additional guidelines for analyzing problems found through the functional biomechanical assessment include the following:

- If an area is hypomobile, consider tension or shortening in the antagonist pattern as a possible cause.
- If an area is hypermobile, consider instability of the joint structure or muscle weakness in the fixation pattern or problems with antagonist/agonist co-contraction function.
- If an area cannot hold against resistance, consider weakness from reciprocal inhibition of the muscles of the prime mover and synergist pattern, and tension in the antagonist pattern as possible causes.
- If pain or heaviness occurs on passive movement, consider joint capsule dysfunction and nerve entrapment syndromes as possible causes.
- If pain occurs on active movement, consider muscle firing patterns and fascial involvement as a possible cause.
- Always consider bodywide reflexive patterns, as discussed in the sections on posture, gait

assessment, and kinetic chain assessment, as possible causes.

The following guidelines also are important:

- During muscle testing, the ability to easily resist the applied force should be the same or very similar bilaterally.
- Opposite movement patterns should be easy to assume.
- Bilateral asymmetry, pain, weakness, inability to assume the isolation position or to move into the opposite position, fatigue, or a heavy sensation may indicate dysfunction.
- Intervention or referral depends on the severity of the condition (stage 1, 2, or 3) and whether the dysfunction is joint-related, neuromuscular-related, or myofascial-related.

SUMMARY

The main purpose of intervention is to help the body regain symmetry and ease of movement. Therefore, when observing gait or posture, the practitioner notes areas that seem pulled, twisted, or dropped. The massage practitioner's job is to use massage methods to lengthen shortened areas, untwist twisted areas, raise dropped areas, drop raised areas, soften hard areas, harden soft areas, warm cold areas, and cool hot areas.

During assessment, careful attention should be paid to the order of priority in which the client relays the information. If the headache is mentioned first, the knee ache second, and the tight elbow last, the areas should be dealt with in that order, if possible, in the massage flow.

The importance of listening to understand is paramount. Many experienced professionals have learned that if we listen to our clients, they will tell us what is wrong and how to help them restore balance. Athletes are especially attuned to their body function. Slow down, do not jump to conclusions, pay attention, and let the information unfold. Realize that each client is the expert about himself or herself. Clients are your teachers about themselves, and in teaching you they often begin to understand themselves better. In every session, approach each client with fascination about what you will learn from him or her. No textbook, class, or instructor can equal the teaching provided by careful attention to the client.

Note: This chapter does not adapt well to written question responses. The information is skill-based; therefore, the following exercises are recommended. Write a summary in the space provided.

1 Develop a checklist of all history components covered.

_____

_____

_____

_____

_____

_____

2 Develop a checklist of all physical assessment components covered.

_____

_____

_____

_____

_____

_____

3 Complete ten comprehensive assessments using all methods covered in this chapter and your checklists.

_____

_____

_____

_____

4 Develop a treatment plan based on each assessment.

_____

_____

_____

_____

_____

_____

5 Implement the treatment plan and reassess after ten sessions. Chart each.

_____

_____

_____

_____

_____

6 Write a post-assessment narrative describing the outcomes achieved or not achieved by the client.

_____

_____

_____

_____

_____

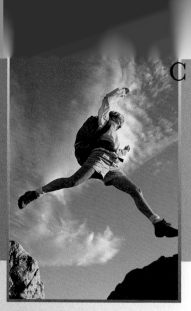

CHAPTER

12

REVIEW OF MASSAGE METHODS

OBJECTIVES

Upon completion of this chapter, the reader will have the information necessary to do the following:

1 Apply all massage applications.

2 Use efficient body mechanics during massage application.

3 Achieve determined outcomes by adjusting depth of pressure, drag, duration, frequency, direction, speed, and rhythm of all massage application.

4 Choose appropriate methods to achieve results.

5 Explain all massage methods in terms of physiologic mechanism.

6 Perform all massage applications using proper body mechanics.

Massage is the application of stimulus and force to create beneficial and physiologic changes in the body. The premise of this textbook is that you already have a solid foundation of therapeutic massage skills. Therefore this chapter presents only a brief review and overview of massage application. I strongly suggest that you reread or read for the first time the following books: *Mosby's Fundamentals of Therapeutic Massage* and *Mosby's Essential Sciences for Therapeutic Massage.*

COMPONENTS OF MASSAGE APPLICATION

All massage consists of a combination of the following qualities of touch:

- **Depth of pressure** (compressive force), which can be light, moderate, deep, or variable. Depth of pressure is important. Most soft tissue areas of the body consist of three to five layers of tissue, including the skin; the superficial fascia; the superficial, middle, and deep layers of muscle; and the various fascial sheaths and connective tissue structures. Pressure

Active assisted movement
Active joint movement
Active range of motion
Active resistive movement
Bending
Bind
Body mechanics
Compression
Counterpressure
Cross-directional stretching
Depth of pressure
Direction
Direction of ease
Drag
Duration
Frequency
Friction

Gliding
Integrated approach
Isometric contraction
Isotonic contraction
Joint movement methods
Joint oscillation
Joint stacking
Kneading
Lengthening and stretching
Longitudinal stretching
Mechanical forces
Methods
Multiple isotonic contractions
Muscle energy techniques
Oscillation
Passive joint movement
Percussion

Perpendicularity
Positional release
Postisometric relaxation
Pulsed muscle energy
Reciprocal inhibition
Resting position
Rhythm
Shear
Skin rolling
Speed
Strain-counterstrain
Stretching
Tension
Torsion
Weight transfer

must be delivered through each successive layer to reach the deeper layers without damage and discomfort to the more superficial tissues. The deeper the pressure, the broader the base of contact required with the surface of the body. It takes more pressure to address thick, dense tissue than delicate tissue (Figure 12-1).

- **Drag** is the amount of pull (stretch) on the tissue (tensile force) (Figure 12-2).

- **Direction** can move from the center of the body out (centrifugal) or in from the extremities toward the center of the body (centripetal). Direction can proceed from origin to insertion (or vice versa) of the muscle following the muscle fibers, transverse to the tissue fibers, or in circular motions (Figure 12-3).

- **Speed** of manipulations can be fast, slow, or variable (Figure 12-4).

- **Rhythm** refers to the regularity of application of the technique. If the method is applied at regular intervals, it is considered even, or rhythmic. If the method is disjointed or irregular, it is considered uneven, or nonrhythmic.

- **Frequency** is the rate at which the method repeats itself in a given time frame. In general, the massage practitioner repeats each method about 3 times before moving or switching to a different approach. The first application is assessment, second is treatment, and third is postassessment. If the postassessment indicates remaining dysfunction, then the frequency is increased to repeat the treatment/postassessment several more times.

- **Duration** is the length of time that the method lasts or that the manipulation stays in the same location. Typically, duration should not be more than 30 to 60 seconds.

Through these varied qualities of touch, the practitioner adapts simple massage **methods** to the desired outcomes of the client. These qualities of touch provide the therapeutic benefit. The mode of application (e.g., **gliding** or **kneading**) provides the most efficient application. Each method can be varied, depending on the desired outcome, by adjusting depth, drag, direction, speed, rhythm, frequency, and duration. In perfecting massage application, the quality of touch is important, more so than the method. The practitioner alters quality of touch when there is a

FIGURE 12-1

DEPTH OF PRESSURE

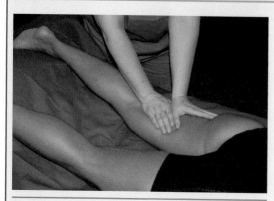

A Light.

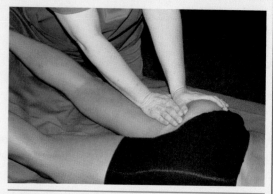

B Medium.

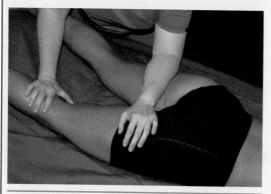

C Deep.

FIGURE 12-2

DRAG

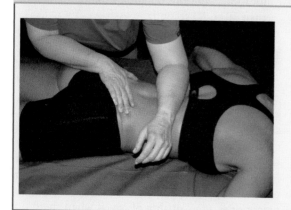

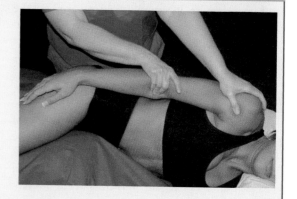

FIGURE 12-3

DIRECTION

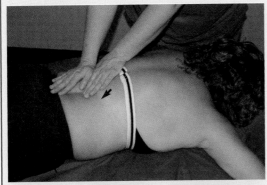

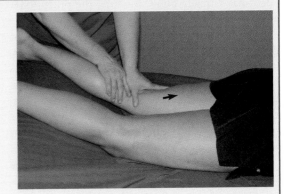

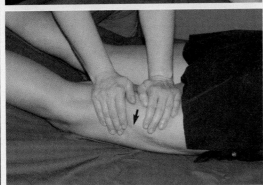

FIGURE 12-4

SPEED

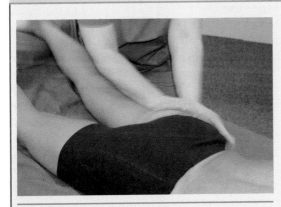

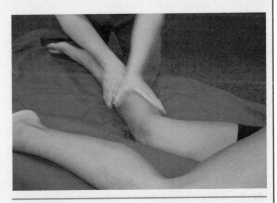

A Speed-fast.

B Speed-slow.

contraindication or caution for massage. For example, when a person is fatigued, the practitioner often reduces the duration of the application; if a client has a fragile bone structure, the practitioner alters depth of pressure.

All massage manipulations introduce forces into the soft tissues. These forces stimulate various physiologic responses. Force may be perceived as mechanical, which we are going to discuss in this chapter, or as field forces, such as gravity or magnetism. Examples of **mechanical forces** are actions that involve pushing, pulling, friction, or sudden loading, such as a direct blow. Mechanical forces can act on the body in a variety of ways. It is helpful to identify the different types of mechanical forces and to understand the ways in which mechanical forces applied during massage act therapeutically on the body.

The five kinds of force that can affect the tissues of the body are **compression, tension, bending, shear,** and **torsion.** Not all tissue is affected the same way by each type of force. We will look at each of the five types of force, the different ways they can produce tissue injuries, and more importantly, the ways in which they produce therapeutic benefits when applied by a skilled massage therapist.

COMPRESSION

Compressive forces occur when two structures are pressed together (Figure 12-5). Compressive force is a component of massage application and is described as depth of pressure. This kind of force may be sudden and strong, as with a direct blow (tapotement), or it may be slow and gradual, as with gliding strokes. The magnitude and duration of the force are important in determining the outcome of the application of compression. Some tissues are resilient to compressive forces, whereas others are more susceptible. Nerve tissue is an interesting example. Nerve tissue is capable of withstanding moderately strong compressive forces if they do not last long (such as a sudden blow to the back of your elbow that hits your "funny bone"). However, even slight force applied for a long time (as occurs with carpal tunnel syndrome) can cause severe nerve damage. The practitioner needs to consider this when determining the duration of a massage application using compression.

Ligaments and tendons are sturdy and resistant to strong compressive loads. Muscle tissue, however, with its extensive vascular structure, is not as resistant to compressive forces. Excess

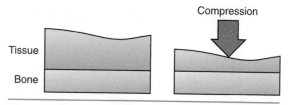

FIGURE 12-5 ■ Compression. (From Fritz S: *Mosby's fundamentals of therapeutic massage*, ed. 3. St. Louis, 2004, Mosby.)

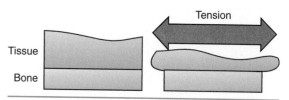

FIGURE 12-6 ■ Tension. (From Fritz S: *Mosby's fundamentals of therapeutic massage*, ed. 3. St. Louis, 2004, Mosby.)

compressive force will rupture or tear muscle tissue, causing bruising and connective tissue damage. This is a concern when pressure is applied to deeper layers of tissue. To avoid tissue damage, the massage therapist must distribute the compressive force of massage over a broad contact area on the body. The more compressive force being used, therefore, the broader the base of contact with the tissue. Compressive force is used therapeutically to affect circulation, nerve stimulation, and connective tissue pliability.

TENSION

Tension forces (also called tensile force) occur when two ends of a structure are pulled apart from one another (Figure 12-6). This is different from muscle tension. Muscular tension is created by excess amounts of muscular contraction and not by strong levels of pulling force applied to the tissue. Muscles that are long from being pulled apart are affected by tensile force. Certain tissues, such as bone, are highly resistant to tensile forces. It would take an extreme amount of force to break or damage a bone by pulling its two ends apart. However, soft tissues are susceptible to tension injuries. In fact, tensile stress injuries are the most common injuries to soft tissues. Examples of such injuries include muscle strains, ligament sprains, tendonitis, fascial pulling or tearing, and nerve traction injuries (i.e., sudden nerve stretching such as occurs in whiplash).

Tension force is used during massage with applications that drag, glide, lengthen, and stretch tissue

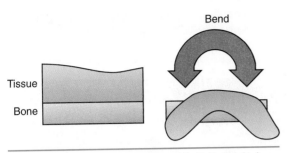

FIGURE 12-7 ■ Bending. (From Fritz S: *Mosby's fundamentals of therapeutic massage*, ed. 3. St. Louis, 2004, Mosby.)

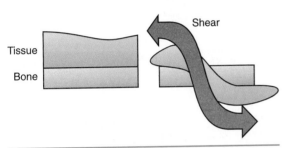

FIGURE 12-8 ■ Shear. (From Fritz S: *Mosby's fundamentals of therapeutic massage*, ed. 3. St. Louis, 2004, Mosby.)

to elongate connective tissues and lengthen short muscles.

BENDING

Bending forces are a combination of compression and tension (Figure 12-7). One side of a structure is exposed to compressive forces while the other side is exposed to tensile forces. Bending occurs during many massage applications. Pressure is applied to the tissue, or force is applied across the fiber or across the direction of the muscles, tendons or ligaments, and fascial sheaths. Bending forces rarely damage soft tissues; however, they are a common cause of bone fractures. Bending force is effective in increasing connective tissue pliability and affecting proprioceptors in the tendons and belly of the muscles.

SHEAR

Shear is a sliding force (Figure 12-8). As a result, significant friction often is created between the structures that are sliding against each other. The massage method of friction uses shear force to generate physiologic change by increasing connective tissue pliability and creating therapeutic inflammation.

Excess friction (shearing force) may result in an inflammatory irritation that causes many soft tissue problems.

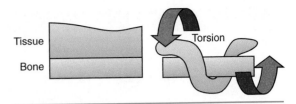

FIGURE 12-9 ■ Torsion. (From Fritz S: *Mosby's fundamentals of therapeutic massage*, ed. 3. St. Louis, 2004, Mosby.)

TORSION

Torsion forces are best thought of as twisting forces (Figure 12-9). Massage methods that use kneading introduce torsion forces.

Torsion force to a single soft tissue structure is not common and is rarely the cause of significant tissue injury. However, torsion force applied to a group of structures (e.g., a joint) is much more likely to be the cause of significant injury. For example, when the foot is on the floor and the individual turns the body, the knee as a whole is exposed to significant torsion force. Torsion force is a major therapeutic force that affects connective tissue in the body.

The methods of massage described next introduce one or a combination of these forces to the body for therapeutic benefit. This process is influenced by the qualities of application: depth of pressure, drag, direction, duration, speed, rhythm, and frequency. Appropriate use of force is necessary. If insufficient force is used, the application will not be effective; conversely, excessive use of force can cause tissue damage.

THE METHODS

 12-7

RESTING POSITION

The practitioner must make initial contact with respect and a client-centered focus. The body needs time to process all the sensory information it receives during massage. Stopping the motions and simply resting the hands on the body provides moments of integration (Figure 12-10).

GLIDING

12-7 The distinguishing characteristic of gliding strokes is that they are applied horizontally in relation to the tissues, generating a tensile force (Figure 12-11).

During gliding stroke, light pressure remains on the skin and moderate pressure extends through the

FIGURE 12-10

EXAMPLES OF RESTING POSITION

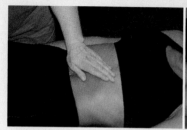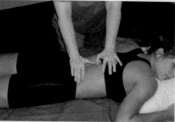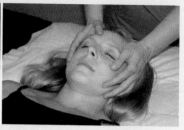

FIGURE 12-11

EXAMPLES OF GLIDING

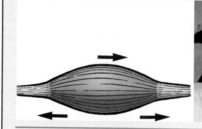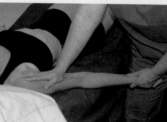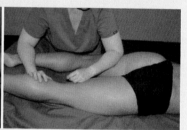

The focus of gliding is horizontal.

subcutaneous layer of the skin to reach muscle tissue but not so deep as to compress the tissue against the underlying bony structure. Moderate to heavy pressure that puts sufficient drag on the tissue mechanically affects the connective tissue and the proprioceptors (spindle cells and Golgi tendon organs) found in the muscle. Heavy pressure produces a distinctive compressive force of the soft tissue against the bone.

Depth of pressure is a result of leverage and leaning on the body. Pressure increases as the angle of the lean increases. Increases in pressure are not achieved by pushing with muscle strength.

Strokes that use moderate pressure from the fingers and toes toward the heart following the muscle fiber direction are excellent for mechanical and reflexive stimulation of blood flow, particularly venous return and lymphatics. Light to moderate pressure with short, repetitive gliding following the patterns for the lymph vessels is the basis for manual lymph drainage.

KNEADING

12-7   Soft tissue is lifted, rolled, and squeezed. The main purpose of this manipulation is to lift tissue, applying bend, shear, and torsion forces.

Kneading is good for reducing muscle tension. The lifting, rolling, and squeezing action affects the spindle cell proprioceptors in the muscle belly. As the belly of the muscle is squeezed (thus squeezing the spindle cells), the muscle feels less tense. When lifted, the tendons are stretched, thus increasing tension in the tendons and the Golgi tendon receptors, which have a protective function.

Kneading also is good for mechanically softening the superficial fascia. The kneading methods are effective in supporting circulation by squeezing the capillary beds in tissues and supporting fluid exchange.

Kneading may incorporate a wringing or twisting component (torsion) after the tissue is lifted. Changes in depth of pressure and drag determine whether the client perceives the manipulation as

FIGURE 12-12

EXAMPLES OF KNEADING AND SKIN ROLLING

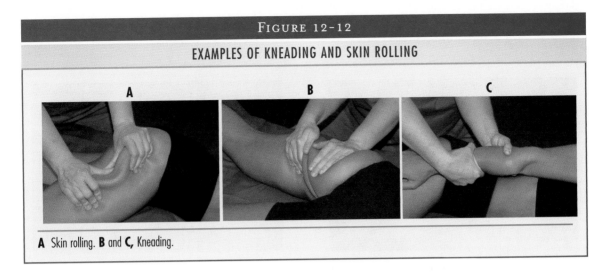

A Skin rolling. **B** and **C**, Kneading.

superficial or deep. By the nature of the manipulation, the pressure and pull peak when the tissue is lifted to its maximum and decrease at the beginning and end of the manipulation (Figure 12-12).

SKIN ROLLING

12-7 A variation of the lifting manipulation is **skin rolling.** Whereas deep kneading attempts to lift the muscular component away from the bone, skin rolling lifts only the skin from the underlying muscle layer. Skin rolling has a warming and softening effect on the superficial fascia, causes reflexive stimulation of the spinal nerves, and is an excellent assessment method. Areas of "stuck" skin often suggest underlying problems. Skin rolling is one of the few massage methods that is safe to use directly over the spine. Because only the skin is accessed and the direction of pull to the skin is up and away from the underlying bones, the spine risks no injury, unlike when any type of downward pressure is used.

Sometimes a client's tissue will not lift. This may be a result of excessive edema (swollen tissue), a heavy fat layer, scarring that extends into the deeper body layers, or thickened areas of connective tissue, especially over aponeuroses (flat sheets of superficial connective tissue). If these conditions exist, applications of kneading or skin rolling will be uncomfortable for the client. Shifting to gliding and compression may soften the tissue enough that kneading can be used more effectively if applied later in the massage session.

COMPRESSION

12-7 Compression moves down into the tissues, with varying depths of pressure adding bending and compressive forces (Figure 12-

13). The manipulations of compression usually penetrate the subcutaneous layer, whereas in the resting position they stay on the skin surface. Much of the effect of compression results from pressing tissue against the underlying bone, causing it to spread.

Compression used in the belly of the muscle spreads the spindle cells, causing the muscle to sense that it is stretching. To protect the muscle from overstretching, the spindle cell signals for the muscle to contract. The lift-press application stimulates the muscle and nerve tissue. These two effects combine to make compression a good method for stimulating muscles and the nervous system. Because of this stimulation, compression is a little less desirable for a relaxation or soothing massage.

Compression is an excellent method for enhancing circulation. The pressure against the capillary beds changes the pressure inside the vessels and encourages fluid exchange. Compression appropriately applied to arteries allows back pressure to build, and when the compression is released, it encourages increased arterial flow.

Compression can be done with the point of the thumb or stabilized finger, palm and heel of the hand, fist, knuckles, forearm, and in some systems, the leg and heel of the foot (Figure 12-14). Even though the compressive pressure is perpendicular to the tissue, the position of the forearm in relation to the wrist is about 120 to 130 degrees. Application against a 45-degree angle of the body (hill) plus the 45-degree angle of the practitioner's hand and forearm results in the 90-degree contact on the tissue. If you are using your knuckles or fist, make sure the forearm is in a direct line with the wrist (Figure 12-15). Avoid use of the thumb if possible,

FIGURE 12-13

EXAMPLES OF COMPRESSION

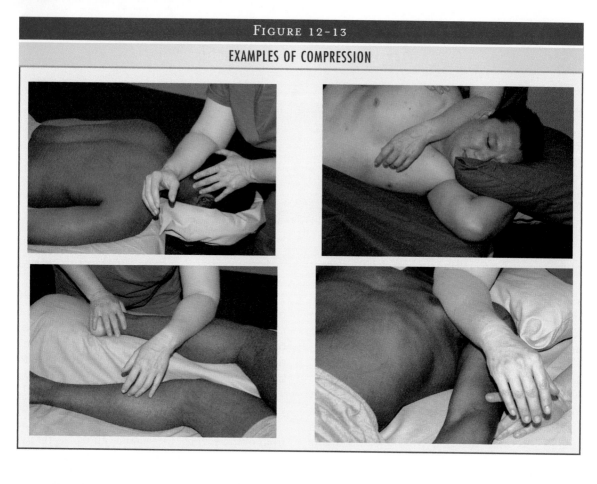

FIGURE 12-14

FOOT, LEG, AND FOREARM COMPRESSION

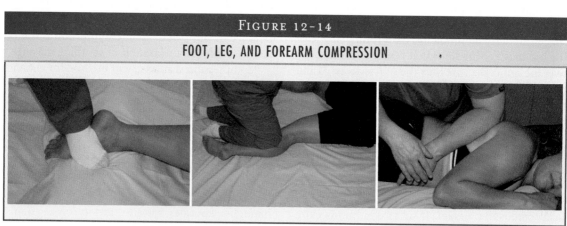

because the thumb can be damaged by extensive use, especially on large muscle masses.

The tip or the radioulnar side of the elbow should not be used for compression. Because the ulnar nerve passes just under the skin and damage can result from extensive compression, use the forearm near the elbow for compression. The massage professional's arm and hand must be relaxed, or neck and shoulder tension will occur. Leverage applied through appropriate **body mechanics** does the work, not muscle strength (Figure 12-16).

Compression proceeds downward into the tissues; the depth is determined by what is to be accomplished, where compression is to be applied, and how broad or specific the contact with the client's body.

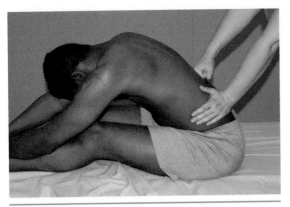

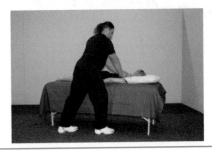

FIGURE 12-16 ■ Body mechanics during compression.

FIGURE 12-15 ■ Position of the hand during compression.

FIGURE 12-17

EXAMPLES OF OSCILLATION

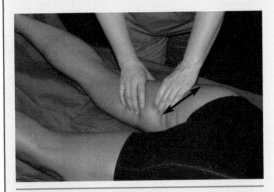

A Shaking, direct.

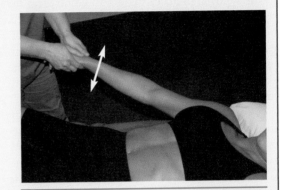

B Shaking.

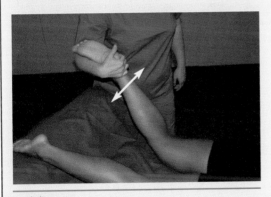

C Shaking.

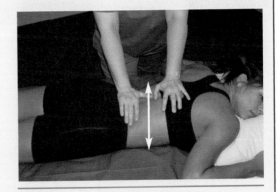

D Rocking.

Deep compression presses tissue against the underlying bone. Because of the diagonal pattern of the muscles, the massage practitioner should stay perpendicular or at a 90-degree angle to the bone, with actual compression somewhere between a 60- and 90-degree angle to the body. Beyond those angles, the stroke may slip and turn into a glide.

12-7 OSCILLATION: SHAKING, ROCKING, VIBRATION

Shaking is a massage method that is effective in relaxing muscle groups or an entire limb (Figure 12-17). Shaking manipulations confuse the positional proprioceptors because the sensory input is too unorganized for the integrating systems of the brain to interpret; muscle relaxation is the natural response in such situations. Athletes respond well to shaking.

Shaking warms and prepares the body for deeper bodywork and addresses the joints in a nonspecific manner. Shaking is effective when the muscles seem extremely tight. This technique is reflexive in effect, but a small mechanical influence may be exerted on the connective tissue as well because of the lift-and-pull component of the method. Shaking begins with a lift-and-pull component. The practitioner grasps, lifts, or shakes a muscle group or a limb (Figure 12-18).

Shaking is not a manipulation to be used on the skin or superficial fascia, nor is it effective to use on the entire body. Rather, shaking is best applied to any large muscle groups that can be grasped and to the synovial joints of the limbs. Good areas for shaking are the upper trapezius and shoulder area, biceps and triceps groups, hamstrings, quadriceps, gastrocnemius, and in some instances, the abdominal muscles and the pectoralis muscles close to the axilla. The joints of the shoulders, hips, and extremities also respond well to shaking.

The larger the muscle or joint, the more intense the method required to be effective. If the movements are performed with all the slack out of the tissue, the focus point of the shake is small and is extremely effective. The more purposeful the approach, the smaller the focus of the shaking applied. You should always stay within the limits of range of motion of a joint and "elastic give" of the tissue.

Vibration is a smaller, more focused **oscillation** that involves very fast, small movements.

Rocking is a soothing, rhythmic method used to calm persons. Rocking is reflexive and chemical in its effects (Figure 12-19).

Rocking also works through the vestibular system of the inner ear and feeds sensory input directly into the cerebellum. Other reflex mechanisms probably are affected as well. Because of this, rocking is one of the most productive massage methods used to achieve entrainment. For rocking to be most effective, the client's body must move so that the fluid in the semicircular canals of the inner ear is affected, initiating parasympathetic mechanisms.

Rocking is rhythmic and should be applied with a deliberate full-body movement.

This attunement to the client's rhythm is a powerful interface point to synchronize entrainment. The easiest way to do this is to take the client's pulse and match the rhythm to that of the pulse. The massage therapist works within the rhythm to maintain and amplify it by attempting gently to extend the limits of movement or by slowing the rhythm. Incorporation of a rocking movement that supports this entrainment process into all massage

FIGURE 12-18

PERFORMING OSCILLATION METHODS

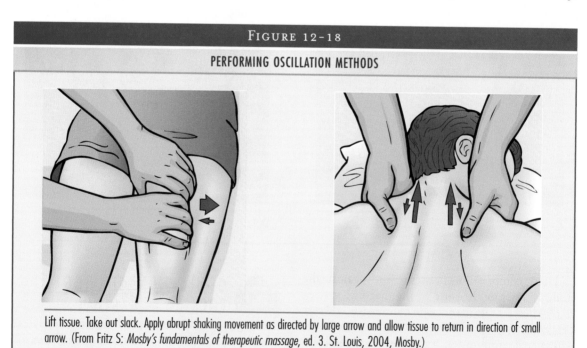

Lift tissue. Take out slack. Apply abrupt shaking movement as directed by large arrow and allow tissue to return in direction of small arrow. (From Fritz S: *Mosby's fundamentals of therapeutic massage*, ed. 3. St. Louis, 2004, Mosby.)

FIGURE 12-19

PERFORMING ROCKING METHOD

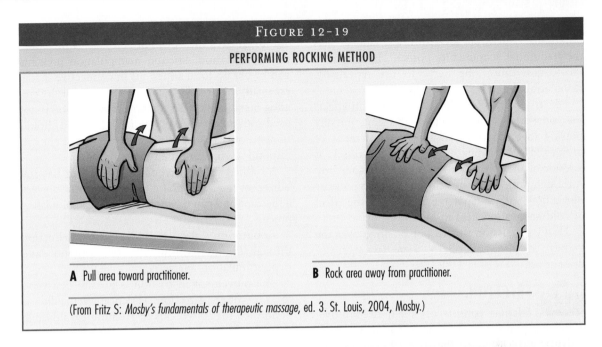

A Pull area toward practitioner.

B Rock area away from practitioner.

(From Fritz S: *Mosby's fundamentals of therapeutic massage*, ed. 3. St. Louis, 2004, Mosby.)

applications effectively individualizes the application and speed of the method. The client seems to relax more easily when a subtle rocking movement, matching his or her innate rhythm pattern, is incorporated as part of the generalized massage approach, along with techniques such as gliding, kneading, compression, joint movement, and especially passive movements.

PERCUSSION, OR TAPOTEMENT

12-7

Percussion is divided into two classifications: light and heavy (Figure 12-20). The difference between light and heavy tapotement is whether the compressive force of the blows penetrates only to the superficial tissue of the skin and subcutaneous layers (light) or deeper into the muscles, tendons, and visceral (organ) structures, such as the pleura in the chest cavity (heavy).

Tapotement is a stimulating manipulation that operates through the response of the nerves. Because of its intense stimulating effect on the nervous system, tapotement initiates or enhances sympathetic activity of the autonomic nervous system. The effects of the manipulations are reflexive except for the mechanical results of percussion in loosening and moving mucus in the chest.

When applied to the joints, percussion affects the joint kinesthetic receptors responsible for determining the position and movement of the body. The quick blows confuse the system, similar to the effect of joint-focused rocking and shaking, but the body muscles tense instead of relax. This method

FIGURE 12-20

EXAMPLES OF PERCUSSION

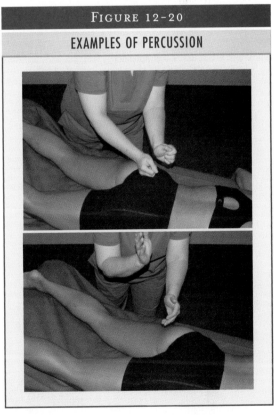

is useful for stimulating weak muscles. The force used must move the joint but should not be strong enough to damage the joint. For example, one finger may be used over the carpal joints, whereas the fist may be used over the sacroiliac joint.

Percussion is effective when used at motor points that usually are located in the same area as the traditional acupuncture points. The repetitive stimulation causes the nerve to fire repeatedly, stimulating the nerve tract (Figure 12-21).

Percussion focused primarily on the skin affects the superficial blood vessels of the skin, initially causing them to contract. Heavy tapotement or prolonged lighter application dilates the vessels as a result of the release of histamine, a vasodilator. Although prolonged tapotement seems to increase blood flow, surface tapotement enhances the effect of cold application used in hydrotherapy.

Heavy percussion should not be done over the kidney area or anywhere there is pain or discomfort.

FRICTION

12-7 Friction consists of small, deep movements performed on a local area (Figure 12-22). It provides shear force to the tissue. Friction burns

may result if the fingers are allowed to slide back and forth over the skin. Friction creates therapeutic inflammation. Friction manipulation prevents and breaks up local adhesions in connective tissue, especially over tendons, ligaments, and scars by creating therapeutic inflammation. This method is not used over an acute injury or fresh scar and should be used only if adaptive capacity of the client can respond to superimposed tissue trauma.

Modified use of friction, after the scar has stabilized or the acute phase has passed, may prevent adhesions and can promote a more normal healing process.

Application also provides pain reduction through the mechanisms of counterirritation and hyperstimulation analgesia.

The movement in friction is usually transverse to the fiber direction. Friction generally is performed for 30 seconds to 10 minutes, although some authorities have suggested a duration of 20 minutes. The result of this type of friction is

FIGURE 12-21

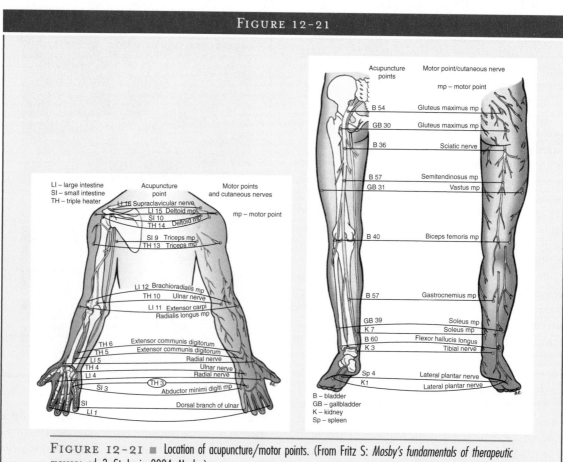

FIGURE 12-21 ■ Location of acupuncture/motor points. (From Fritz S: *Mosby's fundamentals of therapeutic massage*, ed. 3. St. Louis, 2004, Mosby.)

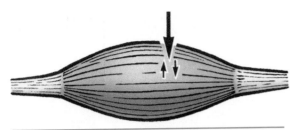

FIGURE 12-22 ■ The focus of friction is a vertical pressing down, applying movement to underlying tissues. (From Fritz S: *Mosby's fundamentals of therapeutic massage*, ed. 3. St. Louis, 2004, Mosby.)

initiation of a small, controlled inflammatory response. Experts disagree on whether an area that is to receive friction should be stretched or relaxed. Because both ways have merit, the practitioner should include both positions when frictioning.

The chemicals released during inflammation result in activation of tissue repair mechanisms with reorganization of connective tissue. This type of work, coupled with proper rehabilitation, is valuable.

Friction is a mechanical approach best applied to areas of high connective tissue concentration such as the musculotendinous junction. Microtrauma from repetitive movement and overstretching are common in this area. Microtrauma predisposes the musculotendinous junction to inflammatory problems, connective tissue changes, and adhesion.

Another use for friction is to combine it with compression. The combination adds a small stretch component. The movement includes no slide. This application has mechanical, chemical, and reflexive effects and is the most common approach today for the use of friction (Figure 12-23).

The main focus when using friction is to move tissue under the skin. No lubricant is used because the tissues must not slide. The practitioner should place the area to be frictioned in a soft or slack position. The movement is produced by beginning with a specific and moderate to deep compression using the fingers, palm, or flat part of the forearm near the elbow. After the pressure required to contact the tissue has been reached, the practitioner moves the upper tissue back and forth across the grain or fiber of the underlying tissue for transverse or cross-fiber friction or around in a circle for circular friction (Figure 12-24).

As the tissue responds to the friction, gradually begin to stretch the area and increase the pressure. The feeling for the client may be intense, but if it

FIGURE 12-23

FRICTION = COMPRESSION + MOVEMENT

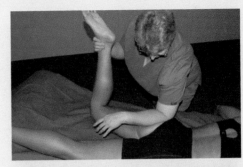

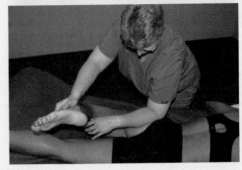

is painful, modify the application to a tolerable level so that the client reports the sensation as a "good hurt." The recommended way to work within the client's comfort zone is to use pressure sufficient for him or her to feel the specific area but not complain of pain. The practitioner should continue friction until the sensation diminishes. Gradually increase the pressure until the client again feels the specific area. Begin friction again and repeat the sequence for up to 10 minutes.

The area being frictioned may be tender to the touch for 48 hours after use of the technique. The sensation should be similar to a mild after-exercise soreness. Because the focus of friction is the controlled application of a small inflammatory response, heat and redness are caused by the release of histamine. Also, increased circulation results in a small amount of puffiness as more water binds with the connective tissue. The area should not bruise.

APPLICATION OF DEEP TRANSVERSE FRICTION

Use the following procedure to apply deep transverse friction:

1. Identify the exact location.

FIGURE 12-24

DIRECTION OF FRICTION

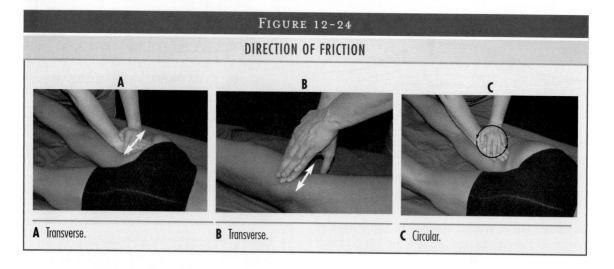

A Transverse.   **B** Transverse.   **C** Circular.

2. The therapist's fingers and the client's skin must move as one. Take care not to cause a blister. The client must understand that deep friction massage can be painful during application and for a few days after treatment.

3. The friction must be given across the fibers composing the affected structure.

4. The friction must be given with sufficient sweep. Pressure only accesses the tender area; it does not replace the friction. Circular friction is not recommended. Only a back-and-forth friction is effective.

5. The friction must reach deep enough. If friction does not reach the lesion, it is of no value.

6. The client must be placed in a suitable position that ensures the appropriate degree of tension or relaxation of the tissues to be frictioned.

7. Muscles must be kept relaxed while being frictioned. Because the connective tissue of the muscle is affected, the massage must penetrate into the muscle and not stay on the surface.

8. Tendons with a sheath must be kept taut during friction massage.

9. Broadening contractions are used between sessions to promote circulation and mobilize scar development during the healing process.

Another effective way to produce friction is a combination of compression and **passive joint movement,** with the bone under the compression used to perform the friction (Figure 12-25). The process begins with a compression as just described, but instead of the massage practitioner moving the tissue back and forth, the massage practitioner moves the client's body under the compression. This automatically adds the slack and stretch positions for the friction methods. The result is the same. This method is much easier for the massage

FIGURE 12-25

DEEP TRANSVERSE FRICTION USING COMPRESSION + MOVEMENT METHOD

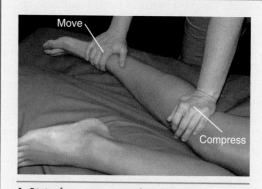

A Friction from compression with movement.

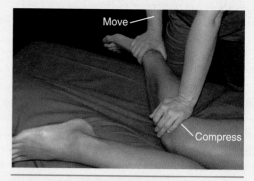

B Move back and forth between positions.

professional to perform and may be more comfortable for the client as well. The movement of the joint provides a distraction from the specific application of the pressure and generalizes the sensation. Broad general methods can be used with a

FIGURE 12-26

COMPARISON OF BROAD-BASED CONTACT AND PINPOINT CONTACT

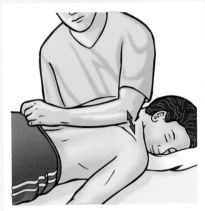

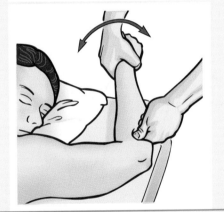

(From Fritz S: *Mosby's fundamentals of therapeutic massage,* ed. 3. St. Louis, 2004, Mosby.)

higher degree of intensity than a pinpointed specific focus (Figure 12-26).

12-8 JOINT MOVEMENT METHODS

Joint movement methods are effective because they provide a means of controlled stimulation to the joint mechanoreceptors (Figure 12-27). Movement initiates muscle tension readjustment through the reflex center of the spinal cord and lower brain centers. As positions change, the supported movement gives the nervous system an entirely different set of signals to process. It is possible for the joint sensory receptors to learn not to be so hypersensitive. As a result, the protective spasm and movement restriction may lessen.

Joint movement also encourages lubrication of the joint and contributes an important enhancement to the lymphatic and venous circulation systems. Much of the pumping action that moves these fluids in the vessels results from compression against the lymph and blood vessels during joint movement and muscle contraction. The tendons, ligaments, and joint capsule are warmed from the movement. This mechanical effect helps keep these tissues pliable.

TYPES OF JOINT MOVEMENT METHODS

Joint movement involves moving the jointed areas within the physiologic limits of range of motion of the client. The two types of joint movement are active and passive.

Active joint movement means that the client moves the joint by active contraction of muscle groups. The two variations of active joint movement are as follows:

1. **Active assisted movement,** which occurs when the client and the massage practitioner move the area (Figure 12-28)
2. **Active resistive movement,** which occurs when the client actively moves the joint against a resistance provided by the massage practitioner (Figure 12-29)

Passive joint movement occurs when the client's muscles stay relaxed and the massage practitioner moves the joint with no assistance from the client. When doing passive joint movement, feel for the soft or hard end-feel of the joint range of motion. This is an important evaluation. **Joint oscillation** is a passive joint movement (Figure 12-30).

Whether active or passive, joint movements are always done within the comfortable limits of the range of motion of the client.

The client's body must always be stabilized, allowing only the joint being worked on to move. Occasionally the entire limb is moved to allow for coordinated interaction among all the joints of the area, but the rest of the body is stabilized. Slow movement is essential, because quick changes or abrupt moves may cause the muscles to initiate protective contractions.

Working within the physiologic ranges of motion for the particular client is within the scope of practice of the massage professional. Let the trainer, physical therapist, or chiropractor deal with joint pathology. The specific method section describes a simple joint play method based on indirect functional techniques, which means identifying the ease position and then having the client move the joint.

Text continued on p. 242.

FIGURE 12-27

JOINT MOVEMENTS

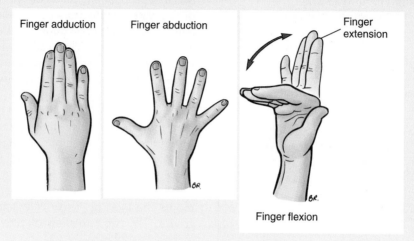

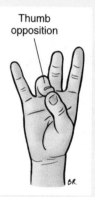

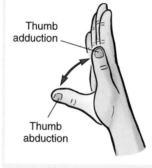

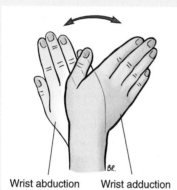

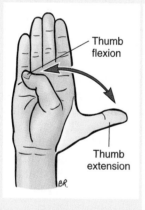

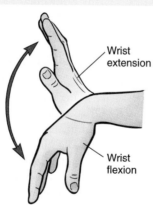

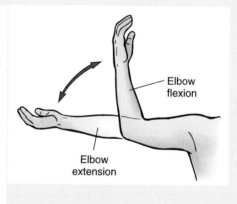

(From Fritz S: *Mosby's fundamentals of therapeutic massage*, ed. 3. St. Louis, 2004, Mosby.)

Figure 12-27 cont'd

JOINT MOVEMENTS

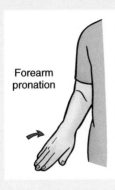

Forearm pronation

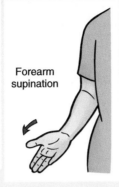

Forearm supination

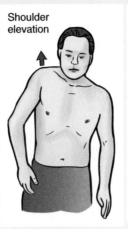

Shoulder elevation

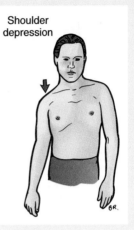

Shoulder depression

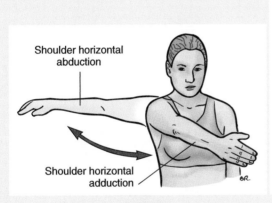

Shoulder horizontal abduction

Shoulder horizontal adduction

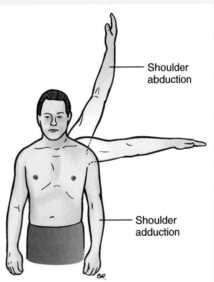

Shoulder abduction

Shoulder adduction

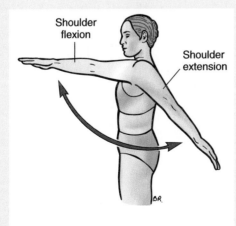

Shoulder flexion

Shoulder extension

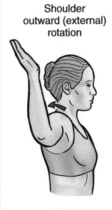

Shoulder outward (external) rotation

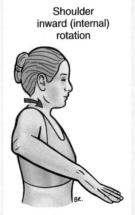

Shoulder inward (internal) rotation

Continued

FIGURE 12-27 CONT'D

JOINT MOVEMENTS

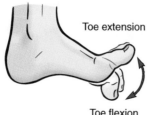

Toe extension

Toe flexion

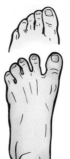

Toe adduction

Toe abduction

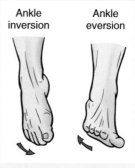

Ankle inversion

Ankle eversion

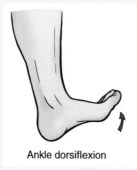

Ankle dorsiflexion

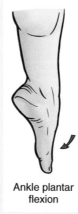

Ankle plantar flexion

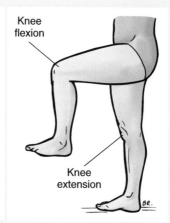

Knee flexion

Knee extension

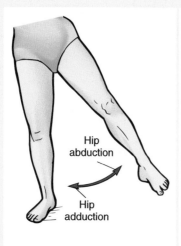

Hip abduction

Hip adduction

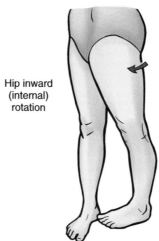

Hip inward (internal) rotation

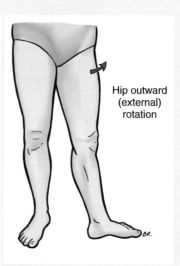

Hip outward (external) rotation

FIGURE 12-27 CONT'D

JOINT MOVEMENTS

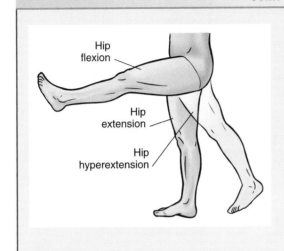

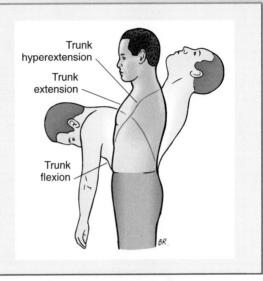

FIGURE 12-28

ACTIVE ASSISTED MOVEMENT

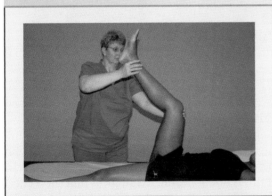

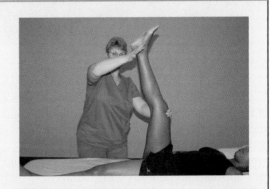

FIGURE 12-29

EXAMPLES OF ACTIVE RESISTED JOINT MOVEMENT

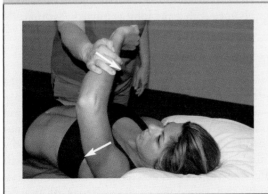

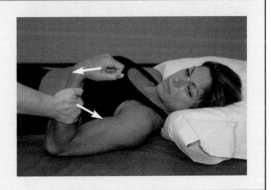

FIGURE 12-30

EXAMPLES OF PASSIVE JOINT MOVEMENT

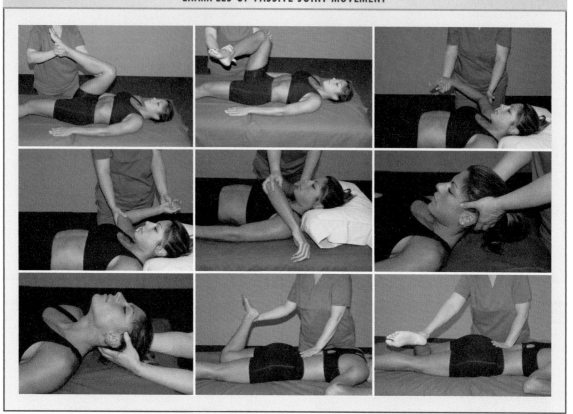

Joint movement becomes part of the application of **muscle energy techniques** to lengthen muscles and of stretching methods to elongate connective tissues. Because of this the massage professional should concentrate on developing the ability to use joint movement efficiently and effectively.

Hand placement with joint movement is important. Make sure that the area is not squeezed, pinched, or restricted in its movement pattern. The practitioner should place one hand close to the joint to be moved to act as a stabilizer and for evaluation. The practitioner places the other hand at the distal end of the bone, and that hand actually provides the movement. Proper use of body mechanics is essential when using joint movement. The stabilizing hand must remain in contact with the client and must be placed near the joint being affected (Figure 12-31).

Another method of placement of the stabilizing hand is to move the jointed area without stabilization and observe where the client's body moves most in response to the range of motion action. Place the stabilizing hand at this point.

Avoid working cross-body. Usually, the hand closest to the joint is the stabilizing hand.

Before joint movement begins, the moving hand lifts and leans back to produce the slight traction necessary to put a small stretch on the joint capsule. If this is not done, the technique is much less effective. When tractioning has been mastered and the joint is moved simultaneously, the size of the movement becomes smaller and the effectiveness increases. Having the client's limbs flailing about in the air is not necessary or desirable. Joint oscillation simply means that the joint is moved rhythmically in small, controlled movement (Figure 12-32).

Active Range of Motion

In **active range of motion** the client moves the area without any type of interaction by the massage practitioner. This is a good assessment method and should be used before and after any type of joint work because it provides information about the limits of range of motion and the improvement after the work is complete. As mentioned previously, two variations of active range of motion

FIGURE 12-31

STABILIZATION AND HAND PLACEMENT DURING JOINT MOVEMENT

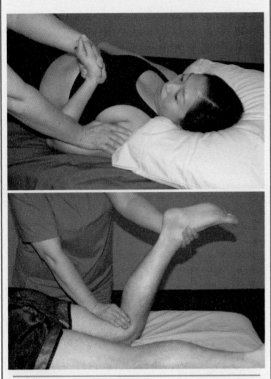

Effective joint movement requires that the body be stabilized.

FIGURE 12-32

STABILIZATION WITH TRACTION

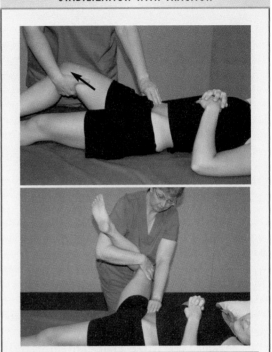

Before joint movement begins, the moving hand lifts and leans back to produce the slight traction necessary to put a small stretch on the joint capsule. If this is not done, the technique is much less effective.

methods exist: active assisted range of motion and active resistive range of motion.

Active Assisted Range of Motion. Active assisted range of motion involves the client moving the joint through the range of motion and the massage practitioner helping or assisting the movement. This approach is useful in cases of weakness or pain with movement. The action remains within the comfortable limits of movement for the client. The focus is to create movement within the joint capsule, encouraging synovial fluid movement to warm and soften connective tissue and support muscle function.

Active Resistive Range of Motion. In active resistive range of motion the massage practitioner firmly grasps and holds the end of the bone just distal to the joint being addressed. The massage therapist places

a small traction to take up the slack in the tissue. Then the practitioner instructs the client to push slowly against a stabilizing hand or arm while moving the joint through its entire range. A tap or light slap against the area to begin the movement works well to focus the client's attention.

Another method is to stabilize the entire circumference of the limb and instruct the client to pull gently or move the area. The job of the massage practitioner is to maintain a gentle traction to prevent slack in the tissue, keep the movement slow, and give the client something to push or pull against, discharging the nervous system so that the area can relax.

The counterforce applied by the massage therapist does not exceed the pushing or pulling action of the client but rather matches it and then allows movement (Figure 12-33).

FIGURE 12-33

EXAMPLE OF ACTIVE RESISTED RANGE OF MOTION

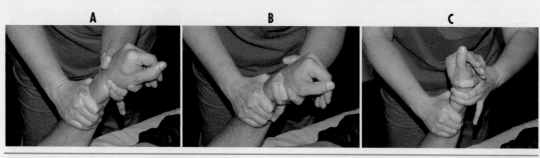

A   **B**   **C**

A, Traction. **B** and **C**, Movement against resistance.

After a form of active range of motion has been completed, the client's body is more apt to accept passive range of motion.

SUGGESTED SEQUENCE FOR JOINT MOVEMENT METHODS

When incorporating joint movement into the massage, follow these basic suggestions:

- If possible, do active joint movement first. Assess range of motion by having the client move the area without participation by the practitioner.
- Have the client move the area against a stabilizing force supplied by the practitioner to increase the intensity of the signals from the contracting muscles, which discharges the nervous system.
- Incorporate any or all of the previously discussed massage methods.
- After the tissue is warm and the nervous system normalized, do the passive range of motion/ joint movement.
- During a massage session, strive to move every joint about 3 times. Each time, take up any slack in the tissues and gently encourage an increase in the range of motion.

MUSCLE ENERGY TECHNIQUES

Muscle energy techniques involve a voluntary contraction of the client's muscles in a specific and controlled direction, at varying levels of intensity, against a specific counterforce applied by the massage therapist (Figure 12-34). Movement of the eyes enhances the effect. Muscle energy procedures have a variety of applications and are considered active techniques in which the client contributes the corrective force. The amount of effort may vary

FIGURE 12-34

USE OF EYES DURING MUSCLE ENERGY TECHNIQUE

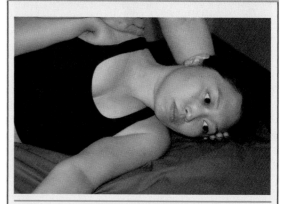

A Looking toward the direction causes target muscle to contract. In this example, target muscles are left lateral neck flexors.

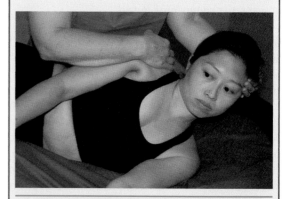

B Looking away inhibits the target muscles supporting stretching.

from a small muscle twitch to a maximal muscle contraction. The duration may be a fraction of a second to several seconds. All contractions begin and end slowly, gradually building to the desired intensity.

The focus of muscle energy techniques is to stimulate the nervous system to allow a more normal muscle resting length. To describe what happens, the term *lengthening* is used because lengthening is more of a neurologic response that allows the muscles to stop contracting and to relax. *Stretching* is defined more correctly as a mechanical force applied to elongate connective tissue. Muscle energy methods are used with both lengthening and stretching.

Muscle energy techniques are focused on specific muscles or muscle groups. It is important for the practitioner to be able to position muscles so that the muscle attachments are close together or in a lengthening phase with the attachments separated. Study muscle charts until you understand the configuration of the muscle patterns, and practice isolating as many muscles as possible, keeping in mind that proper positioning is important. When practicing, make sure that the muscles can be isolated regardless of whether the client is in a supine, prone, side-lying, or seated position.

Types of Muscle Contractions

The massage practitioner uses three types of muscle contraction to activate muscle energy techniques:

Counterpressure is the force applied to an area that is designed to match the effort or force exactly **(isometric contraction)** or partially **(isotonic contraction)** and multiple isotonic contractions.

In an isometric contraction the distance between the proximal and distal (origin and insertion) attachment of the target muscle(s) is maintained at a constant length. A fixed tension develops in the target muscle(s) as the client contracts the muscle against an equal counterforce applied by the massage therapist, preventing shortening of the muscle. In this contraction the effort of the muscle, or group of muscles, is matched exactly by a counterpressure so that no movement occurs, only effort.

An isotonic contraction is one in which the effort of the target muscle or muscles is not matched by the counterpressure, allowing a degree of resisted movement to occur. With a concentric isotonic contraction, the massage practitioner applies a counterforce but allows the client to move

the proximal and distal (origin and insertion) attachment of the target muscle(s) together against the pressure. In an eccentric isotonic movement, the massage practitioner applies a counterforce but allows the client to move the jointed area so that the proximal and distal (origin and insertion) attachment of the target muscle separate as the muscle lengthens against the pressure.

Multiple isotonic contractions require the client to move the joint through a full range of motion against partial resistance applied by the massage practitioner.

Muscle energy techniques usually do not use the full contraction strength of the client. With most isometric work, the contraction should start at about 25% of the strength of the muscle. Subsequent contractions can involve progressively greater degrees of effort but never more than 50% of the available strength.

Many experts use only about 10% of the available strength in muscles being treated in this way and find that they can increase effectiveness by using longer periods of contraction. Pulsed contractions (a rapid series of repetitions) using minimal strength are also effective.

The use of coordinated breathing to enhance particular directions of muscular effort is helpful. During muscle energy applications, all muscular effort is enhanced by inhaling as the effort is made and exhaling on the lengthening phase. Eye position is also effective. Looking toward the direction of the contraction causes or facilitates the target muscles to contract. Looking away from the direction of contraction inhibits the target muscles. Use of eye movement is valuable with athletes who are prone to cramping or are having difficulty using only a small contraction force. It is recommended that eye movement be used first before active target muscle contraction. The following are common examples:

- To increase tension in neck flexors (tense and then relax), have clients look toward their belly, rolling eyes down.
- To decrease tension in neck flexion, have clients look up over their head, rolling eyes up.
- To increase tension in left neck rotation or lateral flexors, have the client look left.
- To decrease tension in left neck rotators or lateral flexors, have client look right.
- Reverse for right rotation or lateral flexor patterns.

Almost all flexor patterns—trunk, hip, knee, ankle, shoulder, arm, and wrist—are increased in tension (facilitated) when the client looks toward the abdomen and are inhibited when the eyes roll up.

Extensor patterns–for example, trunk, hip, knee, and ankle–are facilitated when the client looks up and are inhibited when the client rolls eyes down.

When in doubt about the position, just instruct clients to roll their eyes in big circles slowly and deliberately. The result will be a contract/relax antagonist contract pattern.

The eye movement replaces the contraction of the target muscles, or it can enhance the contraction being used with muscle energy techniques.

A successful application is to lengthen the target area to bind and hold it there. Then begin the eye movement (usually big circles) as the facilitation (contraction) and inhibition (relaxation) takes place, slowly increasing the lengthening force on the target muscles until a more normal resting length is achieved.

12-9 Post-isometric Relaxation

Post-isometric relaxation (PIR, tense-and-relax, contact relax), which occurs after iso-metric contraction of a muscle or when you direct client's eye movement as described previously, results from the activity of the Golgi tendon bodies. Post-isometric relaxation is in the brief latent period of 10 seconds or so after such a contraction that the muscle can be lengthened painlessly, further than it could be before the con-traction. The comfort barrier is the first point of resistance short of the client perceiving any dis-comfort at the physiologic or pathologic barrier.

The isometric contraction involves minimal effort lasting 7 to 10 seconds. Repetitions continue until no further gain is noted.

The following is the procedure for PIR (Figure 12-35):
1. Lengthen the target muscle to the comfort barrier. Back off slightly.
2. Tense the target muscle for 7 to 10 seconds, or use eye position, or use both.
3. Stop the contraction and lengthen the target muscle. Repeat steps 1 to 3 until normal full resting length is obtained.

12-9 Reciprocal Inhibition

Reciprocal inhibition takes place when a muscle contracts, causing its antagonist to relax to allow for more normal movement. Generally, isometric contraction of the antagonist of a shortened target muscle allows the muscle to relax and be taken to a new resting length. Such con-tractions usually begin in the midrange, rather than near the barrier of resistance, and last 7 to 10 seconds. Reciprocal inhibition relaxes a target muscle as the tension increases in its antagonist. This response works through the central nervous system, which cannot allow the prime movers and the antagonists to tighten at the same time in this reflex arc pattern.

The following is the procedure for reciprocal inhibition (Figure 12-36):
1. Lengthen the target muscle to comfort barrier and back off slightly.
2. Contract the antagonist muscle group, or acti-vate eye movement, or both (the muscle in extension).

FIGURE 12-35

POST-ISOMETRIC RELAXATION SEQUENCE

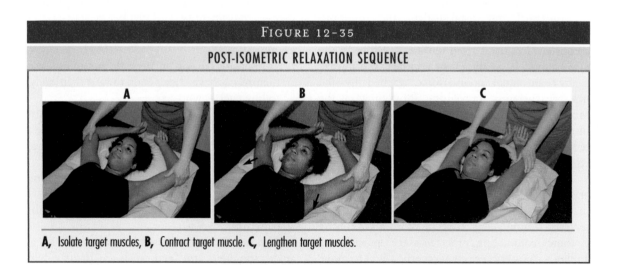

A, Isolate target muscles, **B,** Contract target muscle. **C,** Lengthen target muscles.

FIGURE 12-36

EXAMPLE OF A RECIPROCAL INHIBITION SEQUENCE

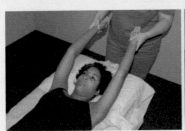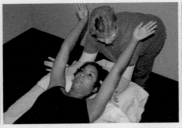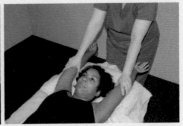

A, Isolate target muscle. **B,** Contract antagonist. **C,** Lengthen target muscle.

FIGURE 12-37

EXAMPLE OF A CONTRACT-RELAX-ANTAGONIST-CONTRACT (CRAC) SEQUENCE (QUADRICEPS)

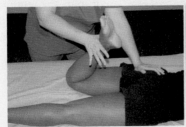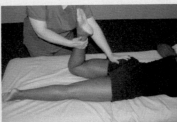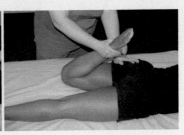

A, Position quadriceps and contract. **B,** Contract hamstrings. **C,** Lengthen quadriceps.

3. Stop the contraction and slowly bring the target muscle into a lengthened state, stopping at resistance.

Repeat steps 2 and 3 until normal full resting length is obtained.

The methods of post-isometric relaxation and reciprocal inhibition can be combined to enhance the lengthening effects. This method can be called contract-relax-antagonist-contract.

The following is the procedure for contract-relax-antagonist-contract (Figure 12-37):

1. Position the target muscles as in the post-isometric sequence.
2. Lengthen the target muscle to the barrier. Back off slightly.
3. Tense the target muscle for 7 to 10 seconds, or have client roll his or her eyes in a big circle, or both.

4. Contract the antagonist as in reciprocal inhibition, or have client roll his or her eyes in a big circle, or both.
5. Stop the contraction of the antagonist.
6. Lengthen the muscle to a more normal resting length.

 Pulsed Muscle Energy

12-9 **Pulsed muscle energy** procedures involve engaging the comfort barrier and using small, resisted contractions (usually 20 in 10 seconds); this introduces mechanical pumping and PIR or resting inhibition, depending on the muscles used.

The following is the procedure for pulsed muscle energy (Figure 12-38):

1. Isolate the target muscle by putting it into a passive contraction.

2. Apply counterpressure for the contraction.
3. Instruct the client to contract the target muscle rapidly in small movements for about 20 repetitions. Go to step 4 or use this variation: maintain the position, but switch the counterpressure location to the opposite side and have the client contract the antagonist muscles for 20 repetitions. Rapid eye movement can replace the pulses or enhance the action.
4. Slowly lengthen the target muscle. Repeat steps 2 to 4 until normal full resting length is obtained.

Note: All contracting and resisting efforts should start and finish gently.

Direct Applications

In some circumstances the client does not wish to or cannot participate actively in the massage (Figure 12-39). This muscle energy technique of direct application is beneficial when the client is sleeping. The principles of muscle energy techniques still can be used by direct manipulation of the spindle cells or Golgi tendons. Pushing muscle fibers together in the direction of the fibers in the belly of a muscle weakens the muscle by working with the spindle cells. As the fibers of the muscle are pushed together, the spindle cells (which sense muscle length) determine that the muscle is too short. The proprioceptive response is to relax the muscle fibers so that the muscle can be comfortable in its chosen position. Pushing muscle fibers together in the belly of the muscle is a way to relieve a muscle cramp. This sometimes is called approximation.

Separating the muscle fibers in the belly of the muscle in the direction of the fibers strengthens the muscle. When this occurs, the spindle cells determine that the muscle is too long; they signal the proprioceptive intelligence of the brain to shorten the muscle so that the muscle can do the job it is supposed to do.

The same responses can be obtained by using the Golgi tendon organs, except that the manipulation of the proprioception signal cells is reversed. Manipulation of the Golgi tendon organs occurs at the ends of the muscle where it joins the tendons. To weaken the muscle, pull apart on the tendon attachments of the target muscle. This tells the pro-

FIGURE 12-38

EXAMPLE OF A PULSED MUSCLE ENERGY SEQUENCE—UPPER TRAPEZIUS

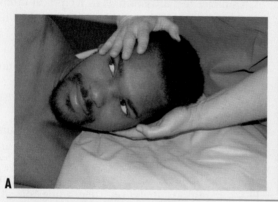
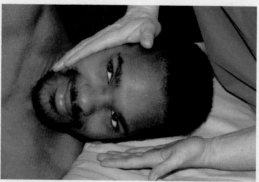

A, Isolate target muscle and position for counterpressure. **B,** Pulse muscle back and forth and then lengthen the muscle. Pulsed muscle energy methods can be difficult for the client to perform. The pulsing contractions are small and precise. The eyes can move back and forth to facilitate the pulsing movement.

FIGURE 12-39

DIRECT MANIPULATION

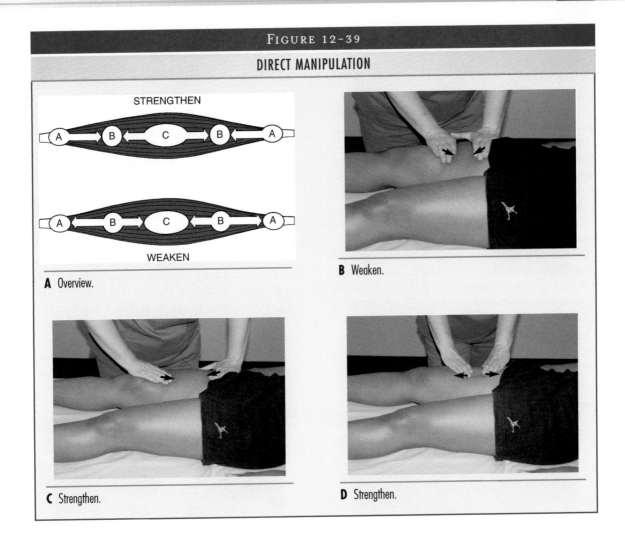

A Overview.

B Weaken.

C Strengthen.

D Strengthen.

prioception center of the body that tension on the tendon is excessive and the muscle should loosen to be in balance. To strengthen the muscle, push the tendon attachments together. This signals the body that too little tension is on the tendon (in relation to the tension within the muscle belly). The muscle, in turn, contracts.

The pressure levels used to elicit the response need to be sufficient to contact the muscle fibers. Pressure that is too light does not access the proprioceptors. Excessive pressure negates the response by activating protective reflexes. Moderate pressure where the muscle itself can be palpated is most effective.

The following is the procedure for direct manipulation of the spindle cells to initiate the relaxation and lengthening response:

1. Place the target muscle in comfortable passive extension.
2. Press the spindle cells together on the target muscle.
3. Pull the spindle cells apart on the antagonist muscle.
4. Lengthen the target muscle.

Repeat steps 2 to 4 until normal full resting length is obtained.

The following is the procedure for directmanipulation of the Golgi tendon organsto initiate the PIR response:

1. Place the target muscle in comfortable passive extension.
2. Pull apart on the tendon attachments of the target muscle.
3. Push the tendon attachments together on the antagonist muscle.
4. Lengthen the target muscle.

Repeat steps 2 to 4 until normal full resting length is obtained.

Positional Release/Strain-Counterstrain

According to Dr. Chaitow, during **positional release** techniques, the spindles of a muscle fiber are influenced by methods that take them into an "ease" state and that theoretically allow them an opportunity to "reset" and reduce hypertonic status. **Strain-counterstrain** and other positional release methods use the slow, controlled return of distressed tissues to the position of strain as a means of offering spindles a chance to reset and so normalize function. This is particularly effective if the spindles have inappropriately held an area in just such protective splinting.

Positional release is a more generic term to describe these methods. Positional release methods are used on painful areas, especially recent strains, before, after, or instead of muscle energy methods. The tender points often are located in the antagonist of the tight muscle because of the diagonal balancing process the body uses to maintain an upright posture in gravity.

Repositioning of the body into the original strain (often the position of a prior injury) allows proprioceptors to reset and stop firing protective signals. By moving the body into the **direction of ease** (i.e., the way the body wants to go and out of the position that causes the pain), the proprioception is taken into a state of safety. Remaining in this state for a time allows the neuromuscular mechanism to reset itself. The massage practitioner then gently and slowly repositions the area into neutral.

The positioning used during positional release is a full-body process. Remember, an injury or loss of balance is a full-body experience. For this reason, the practitioner must consider areas distant to the tender point during the positioning process. Very possibly the position of the feet will have an effect on a tender point in the neck. The eye position is almost always a factor. Often the ease position can be found just with eye movement.

The following is the procedure for positional release (Figure 12-40):

FIGURE 12-40

EXAMPLE OF A POSITIONAL RELEASE SEQUENCE—INTERCOSTAL AND PECTORALIS MAJOR

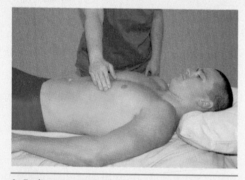

A Tender point, intercostals.

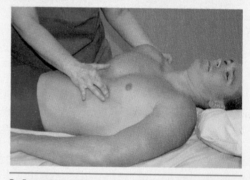

B Ease position.

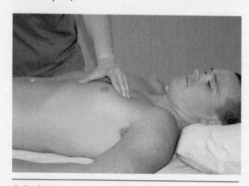

C Tender point, pectoralis major.

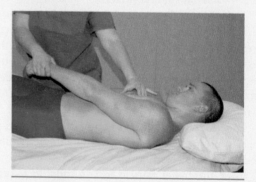

D Ease position.

1. Locate the tender point.
2. Gently initiate the pain response with direct pressure. Remember, the sensation of pain is a guide.
3. Slowly position the body until the pain subsides. Include eye position.
4. Wait at least 30 seconds or longer until the client feels the release, lightly monitoring the tender point.
5. Slowly lengthen the muscle.

Repeat steps 1 to 5 until normal full resting length is obtained.

Positional release techniques are important because they gently allow the body to reposition and restore balance. They are also highly effective ways of dealing with tender areas regardless of the pathologic cause. Sometimes it is impossible to know why the point is tender to the touch. However, if tenderness is present, a protective muscle spasm surrounds it. Positional release is an excellent way to release these small areas of muscle spasm without inducing additional pain.

Integrated Approach

Muscle energy methods can be used together or in sequence to enhance their effects. Muscle tension in one area of the body often indicates imbalance and compensation patterns in other areas of the body. Tension patterns can be self-perpetuating. Often, using an **integrated approach** introduces the type of information the nervous system needs to self-correct. The procedure outlined next relies on the innate knowledge of the body of what is out of balance and how to restore a more normal functioning pattern.

The following is the procedure for an integrated approach. (Use the position from Option A, steps 1 and 2, or Option B, steps 1 and 2, as the starting point for the rest of the process that begins at step 3.)

Option A (Figure 12-41)
1. Identify the most obvious of the postural distortion symptoms.
2. Exaggerate the pattern by increasing the distortion, moving the body into ease. This position becomes the pattern of isolation of various muscles to address in the next part of the procedure. Continue with step 3.

Option B (Figure 12-42)
1. Identify a painful point.
2. Use positional release to move the body into ease until the point is substantially less tender to pressure. The position of ease found becomes the pattern of isolation of various

FIGURE 12-41

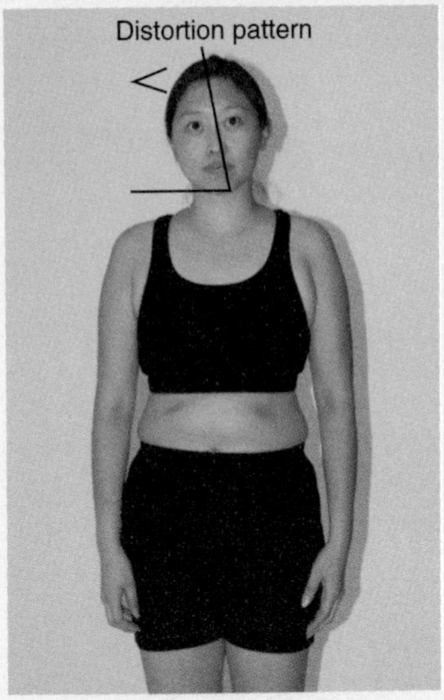

A Distortion pattern.

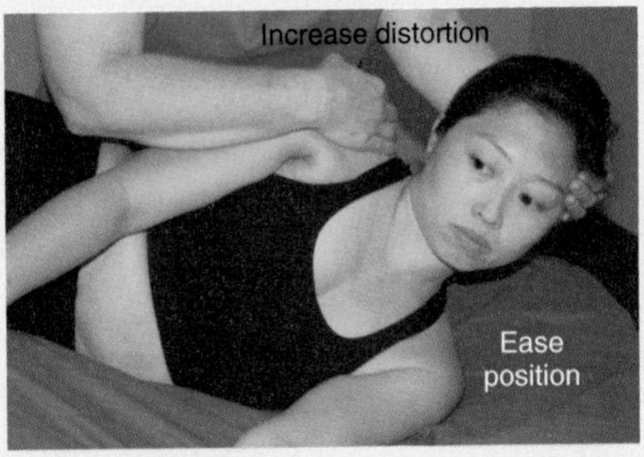

B Increase distortion in ease position.

muscles to address in the next part of the procedure. Continue with step 3.

After choosing from Option A or Option B, continue the procedure as follows:
3. Stabilize the client in as many different directions as possible.
4. Instruct the client to move out of the pattern. Be as vague as possible and do not guide the client because it is important for the client to identify the resistance pattern.
5. Provide resistance for the client to push or pull against (Figure 12-43).
6. Modify the resistance angle as necessary to achieve the most solid resistance pattern for the client (Figure 12-44).

FIGURE 12-42

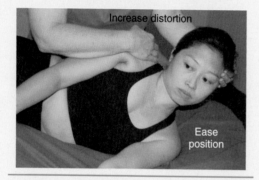

A Pain point.

B Increase distortion in ease position.

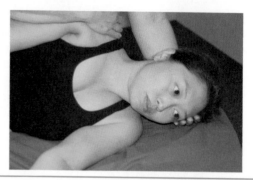

FIGURE 12-43 ■ Stabilization and resistance.

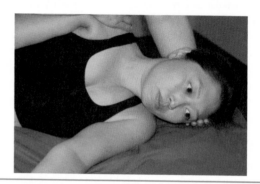

FIGURE 12-44 ■ Modified resistance angle.

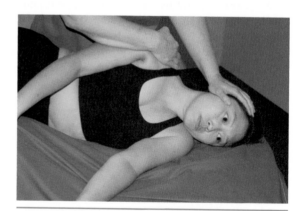

FIGURE 12-45 ■ Lengthening and stretching.

7. Spend a few moments noticing when the client's breathing changes; then, while still providing modified resistance, allow the client to move through the pattern slowly.

8. When the client has achieved as much extension as he or she can, recognize that what the client has achieved is the lengthening pattern.

9. Gently increase the lengthening. If additional elongation in this position is desired, connective tissue stretching can be achieved (Figure 12-45).

10. Pay attention to what body areas become involved besides the one addressed. This is your guide to the next position.

Stretching

Stretching is a mechanical method of introducing various forces into connective tissue to elongate areas of connective tissue shortening (Figure 12-46). Stretching affects the fiber component of connective tissue by elongating the fibers past their normal give so that they can enter the plastic range past the existing **bind.** This creates freeing and unraveling

FIGURE 12-46

STRETCHING

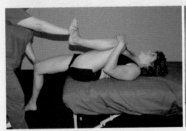

A Longitudinal joint.

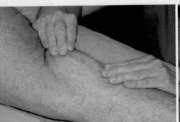

B Direct—longitudinal.

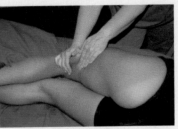

C Direct—cross directional.

of fibers or a small therapeutic inflammatory response that signals for change in the fibers. Stretching also affects the ground substance, warming and softening it and thereby increasing pliability.

Because fascial sheaths provide structural support, it is important to work with a sense of three-dimensional awareness, realizing that shifts in structure have more than a localized effect. Because the body supports stability before mobility and compensation patterns are bodywide, changes in structure need to be balanced with lengthening or strengthening activities that allow the body to maintain a sense of perpendicular orientation in gravity.

If the stability/mobility factor is not considered, the body's method of reacting to changes in structure is to increase muscle spasm and acute pain. This results in a decreased ability to adapt effectively to the changes introduced; it reduces the effectiveness of the methods. Stretching introduces forces of bend, torsion, and tension that mechanically affect connective tissue.

As explained previously, stretching and lengthening are different. Before stretching, usually lengthening of muscles must be done or the muscles of the area may develop protective spasms, because stretching often moves into pathologic barriers formed by connective tissue changes. The connective tissue component cannot be accessed until the muscle has been lengthened. Without stretching, any neuromuscular lengthening may be restricted by shortened connective tissue. Although lengthening without stretching is possible and often desirable, lengthening before stretching is always necessary. During stretching, the two methods work in conjunction. Muscle

energy techniques are used to prepare muscles to stretch by activating lengthening responses.

Longitudinal stretching pulls connective tissue in the direction of the fiber configuration. **Cross-directional stretching** pulls the connective tissue against the fiber direction. Both accomplish the same thing, but longitudinal stretching is done with movement at the joint or direct application to tissue. If longitudinal stretching is not advisable, if it is ineffective in situations of hypermobility of a joint, or if the area to be stretched is not effectively stretched longitudinally, cross-directional stretching is a better choice. Cross-directional stretching focuses on the tissue itself and does not depend on joint movement.

The direction of ease is the way the body allows for postural changes and muscle shortening or weakening compensation patterns, depending on its balance in gravity. Although compensation patterns may be inefficient, the patterns developed serve a purpose and need to be respected. It may seem logical to locate a shortened muscle group or a rotated movement pattern and use direct methods to reverse the pattern. However, this may not be the best approach. Protective sensory receptors prevent any forced stretch out of a compensation pattern. Instead, the practitioner respects the pattern of compensation and exaggerates and coaxes the body into a more efficient position.

For example, a client has shortened pectoralis muscles that pull the shoulders forward, giving a gorilla-like appearance. Instead of pulling the pectoralis muscles into a stretch by forcing the arms back, curl the shoulders and arms more into adduction, providing slack and space to the receptors in the pectoralis muscles. Begin corrective action from this point (Figure 12-47).

FIGURE 12-47

EXAMPLE OF USING DIRECTION OF EASE DURING STRETCHING PROCEDURE

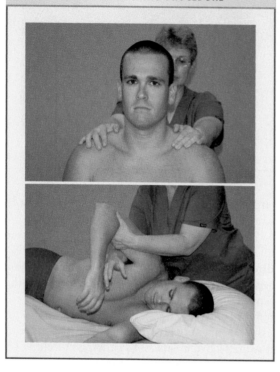

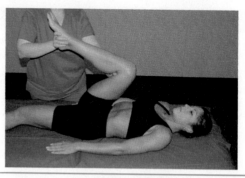

FIGURE 12-48 ■ Position for stretch.

Developing good stretching techniques is perhaps as much an art as it is a science, for there are so many variables involved. An individual muscle needs to be isolated carefully by positioning and stabilizing so that the stretch is focused (Figure 12-48). With the muscles that work one joint only, this is usually simple, but with two-joint muscles it becomes more complicated. One joint needs to be fixed so that it prestretches the muscle while the other joint is moved to increase the stretch. This means that there may be two different techniques for the same muscle to focus the stretch at either end (Figure 12-49).

Within each stretch there needs to be some fine tuning by careful adjustments in the position to try to focus the stretch into the target area. The muscle must be relaxed fully and non–weight bearing; otherwise, it will not stretch fully, even though the client still may feel a sensation of stretch.

When stretching a muscle, the practitioner first should take it slowly to the point where the client feels a mild discomfort and then hold it firmly but comfortably in that position. No client should feel

a sensation of pain, tearing, or burning, for this would suggest that the fibers are being over-stretched and torn. After a period of time the tissues may begin to ease, and the stretch can be increased gently. Many differing opinions exist as to how long to hold a stretch, but it is generally accepted that the length of time is more significant than the intensity of the stretch. Short ballistic-type stretches or using too much force can increase tension through a reflex action. Long, sustained and progressive stretching seems to produce the best results.

The following is the procedure for longitudinal stretching (Figure 12-50):

1. Position the target muscle in the direction of ease. Stabilize and isolate a muscle group.
2. Choose a method to prepare the target muscle to stretch (e.g., gliding, kneading, PIR, resting inhibition, pulsed muscle energy, or direct application).
3. After preparing the target muscle, stretch the muscle to its physiologic or pathologic barrier or to wherever protective contraction is engaged. Back off slightly to avoid muscle spasm. Stay in line with the muscle fibers. Exert effort or movement with the inhalation. Stretch on the exhalation.

The following two approaches are used for the actual stretch phase:

1. Hold the position just off the physiologic or pathologic barrier for at least 10 seconds and up to 30 to 60 seconds to allow for the neurologic reset. This is the lengthening phase. Feel for secondary response (a small give in the muscle).
2. Take up slack and hold for 20 to 30 seconds to create longitudinal pull (tension force) on the connective tissue. You must hold the muscle stretch as instructed to allow for changes in the

FIGURE 12-49

STRETCHING TWO JOINTED MUSCLES

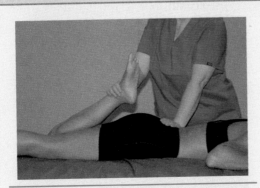

A Stretch position 1.

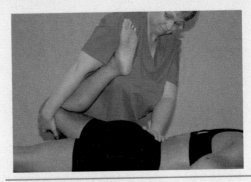

B Stretch position 2.

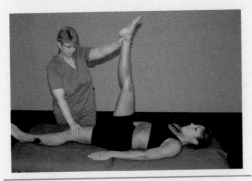

C Stretch position 1.

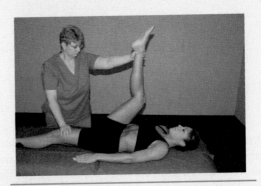

D Stretch position 2.

FIGURE 12-50

LONGITUDINAL STRETCHING

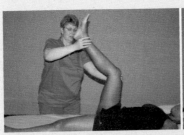

A Position target muscle.

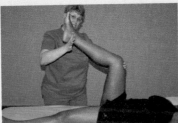

B Use muscle energy method to prepare for stretch.

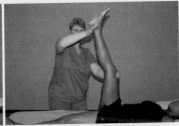

C Lengthening phase. The muscle is ready for stretching.

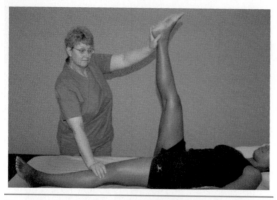

FIGURE 12-51 ■ For actual stretch phase: Take up slack and hold for 20 to 30 seconds to create longitudinal pull (tension force) on the connective tissue. You must hold the muscle stretch as instructed to allow for changes in the connective tissue component of the muscle.

connective tissue component of the muscle (Figure 12-51).

Alternate Procedure for Longitudinal Stretching

If only a small section of muscle needs to be stretched, if the muscle does not lend itself to stretching with joint movement, or if the joints are so flexible that not enough pull is put on the muscles to achieve an effective stretch to the tissues, the practitioner should use the following alternate procedure for longitudinal stretching (Figure 12-52):

1. Locate the fibers or muscle to be stretched.
2. Place the hands, fingers, or forearms in the belly of the muscle or directly over the area to be stretched.
3. Contract the muscle with sufficient pressure to reset the neuromuscular mechanism by having the client push the area into their fingers.
4. Separate the fingers, hands, or forearms (tension force) or lift the tissue with pressure sufficient to stretch the muscle (bending or torsion force). Take up all slack from lengthening and then increase the intensity slightly and wait for the connective tissue component to respond (this may take as long as 30 seconds).

Note: All requirements for preparation of muscle and direction of stretch are the same as described for the previous longitudinal stretching procedure.

The following is the procedure for active assisted longitudinal stretching:

1. Identify and isolate the muscle, making sure it is not working against gravity in this position. Remind the client to exhale during the stretching phase of this technique.

FIGURE 12-52

ALTERNATE PROCEDURE FOR LONGITUDINAL STRETCHING

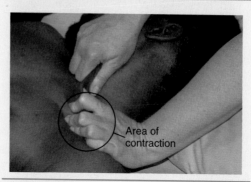

Area of contraction

A Place the hands, fingers, or forearms in the belly of the muscle or directly over the area to be stretched.

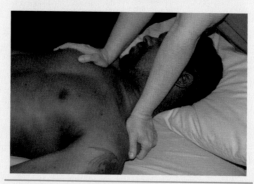

B Lift the tissue with pressure sufficient to stretch the muscle (bending or torsion force).

2. Then lengthen the muscle to its physiologic or pathologic barrier, move it slightly beyond this point, and stretch it gently for 1 to 2 seconds.
3. Return the muscle to its starting position, and repeat this action in a rhythmic, pulse-like fashion for 5 to 20 repetitions.
4. The client will benefit from doing a contraction with the antagonist while lengthening and then stretching the target muscle. As in all proper lengthening and stretching movements, the practitioner must pay attention to the stretch reflex; bouncing is never done because it initiates this reflex.

Cross-Directional Stretching

Cross-directional tissue stretching uses a pull-and-twist component, introducing torsion and

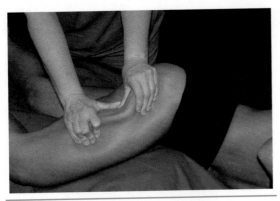

FIGURE 12-53 ■ Cross-directional stretching.

bend forces. The following is the procedure for cross-directional stretching (Figure 12-53):

1. Access the area to be stretched by moving against the fiber direction.
2. Lift or deform the area slightly and hold for 30 to 60 seconds until the area gets warm or seems to soften.

Use the following procedure for skin and superficial connective tissue:

1. Locate the area of restriction.
2. Lift and pull (like taffy), first moving into the restriction and then pulling and twisting out of it, keeping a constant tension on the tissue (think plastic wrap).

 ## 12-10 BODY MECHANICS

Effective body mechanics are essential for working with the sport and fitness population. In general, the therapeutic massage community does a poor job in teaching and practicing proper body mechanics. The concepts of massage as a fluid movement, with flexed knees and arms, are not effective. Concepts of yoga, martial arts, and tai chi do not translate to effective body mechanics. Contrary to common perception, massage is *not* a dynamic movement system. Massage is a repeated series of static activities. If you are going to be successful with the sport and fitness population, effective and ergonomically correct body mechanics are essential. These clients have toned, bulked muscles and often request deep pressure. However, the client does not want to be poked and prodded and dug into. Instead, the client wants all layers of soft tissue from superficial to deep to be addressed. Because of the tissue density, more compressive

force may be required to move sequentially through the tissue layers.

The massage therapist needs to provide a sustained, restrained, and somewhat static movement with pressure focused downward and forward to deliver the various levels of compressive force. Use of forearms, wrists, hands, fingers, thumbs, knees, and feet is effective to deliver the compressive force. Four basic concepts pertaining to body mechanics are common to all techniques used to apply compressive force against the body tissues during massage application. These concepts are as follows:

- **Weight transfer**
- **Perpendicularity**
- Stacking of the joints in close-packed position
- Keeping the back straight (Figure 12-54)

Weight transfer allows the massage practitioner to transfer body weight by shifting the center of gravity forward to achieve a pressure that is comfortable to the client. To transfer weight, the practitioner stands (or kneels) with one foot forward and the other foot (or knee) back in an asymmetric stance (Figure 12-55). In the standing position, the front leg is in a relaxed knee flexion with the foot forward enough to be in front of the knee. The back leg is straight, and the hips and shoulders are aligned so that the back is straight. The transfer happens by taking the weight off the front leg and moving it to the heels of the hands, thumbs, or whichever part of the arm is being used to apply pressure. Pressure is increased or decreased by moving the back leg further away from, or closer to, the client. The weight of the body is distributed to the heel of the weight-bearing leg, not the toes.

Perpendicularity is an important concept that ensures that the pressure is sinking straight into the tissues. The line from the shoulders to the point of contact (e.g., forearm or heel of the hand) must be 90 degrees to the plane of the contact point on the client's body. The client needs to be positioned so that the pressure is applied against a 45-degree incline whenever possible (Figure 12-56).

Stacking the joints one on top of another is essential to the concepts of perpendicularity and weight transfer. The practitioner's body must be a straight line from the heel of the weight-bearing rear foot through the knee, hip, and shoulder, and then from the shoulder to the forearm, or through the elbow acting as an extension of the shoulder, to the heels of the hands. The ankle, knee, hip of the back leg, and spine are stacked and stable in a close-packed joint position. The pelvic girdle and

FIGURE 12-54

PROPER POSITIONING FOR BODY MECHANICS

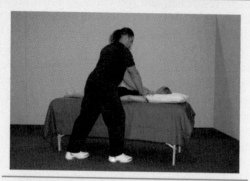

A Perpendicularity: stacking the joints. Keep the back straight.

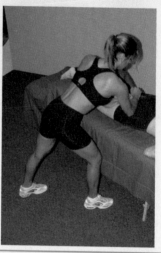

B Alternate view, standing.

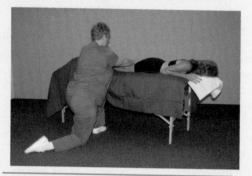

C Alternate view, kneeling.

FIGURE 12-55

TO TRANSFER WEIGHT, THE PRACTITIONER STANDS (OR KNEELS) WITH ONE FOOT FORWARD AND THE OTHER FOOT (OR KNEE) BACK IN AN ASYMMETRIC STANCE

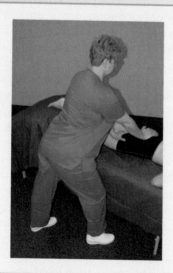

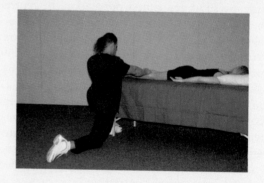

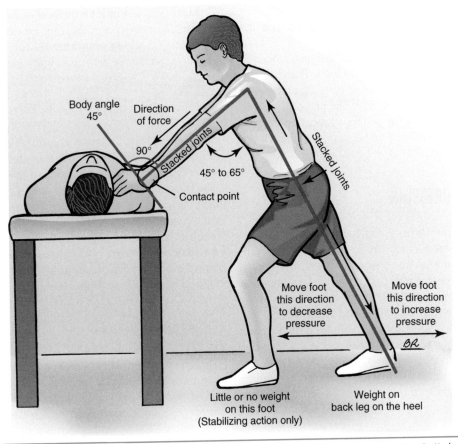

FIGURE 12-56 ■ Correct body mechanics for compressive force required for massage. (From Fritz S: *Mosby's fundamentals of therapeutic massage*, ed. 3. St. Louis, 2004, Mosby.)

shoulder girdle are lined up. The shoulder is stacked over the elbow, which in turn is stacked over the wrist. **Joint stacking** in this way allows the pressure to go straight into the client's body effortlessly as the therapist's center of gravity moves forward.

A straight back and a pressure-bearing leg are other essential components of body mechanics. If the back is not straight, the practitioner often ends up pushing with the upper body instead of using the more effortless feeling of transferred weight. The muscles of the torso, especially the abdomen, are considered the core. Core stability is necessary for back stability.

Most massage therapists will need to develop core stability. The practitioner's weight should be borne on the back leg and on the heel of the foot (Figure 12-56). At first this may feel uncomfortable; however, some of the biggest muscles in the body are in the legs. At least 15 degrees of dorsiflexion in the ankles needs to occur to do this well. Most massage therapists will need to increase their ankle flexibility.

Massage uses primarily a force generated forward and downward with a 90-degree contact against the body. The combination of a 45-degree slant from the contours of the client's body plus the 45-degree angle of force used during appropriate body mechanics results in the 90-degree contact (Figure 12-56). Therefore redistribution of the center of gravity and the weight force is necessary by keeping the weight on the back foot (heels and not toes), the knee and back straight, the weight distribution coming from the abdomen, and the balance point at the object-contact point. The joints of the wrist, arm, shoulder, back, hip, weight-bearing knee, and ankle are stacked for effective delivery of force. As the stance of the body widens, the base of support enlarges. The arm generating the pressure is opposite the weight-bearing leg, which allows proper counterbalance and prevents twisting of the body at the shoulder and pelvic girdle. The shoulder girdle must stay in line with the pelvic girdle, with the head held up and the eyes forward.

Creative use of the massage therapist's body is essential when working with athletes. The ability to use the knee/leg and foot during massage is helpful.

The thumb is seldom used. The braced hand and supported fingers is the proper application because hinge joints effectively move into a stable, closed packed position.

COUNTERPRESSURE

Because of the density and bulk of some athletes' muscle structure, it may be necessary to use a body mechanics strategy to allow you to apply deep compressive force (Figure 12-57). By using counterpressure the massage therapist can reach the deep tissue layers safely without poking the client.

The principle is simple. Combining the forward weight transfer with a pullback motion squeezes the forces together.

1. Apply compressive force as presented by leaning and weight transfer.

FIGURE 12-57

COUNTERPRESSURE

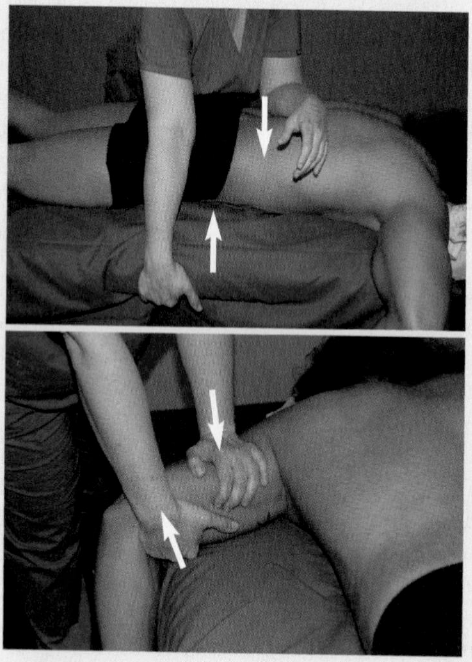

2. Make sure weight is on the heel of the back foot.
3. Use the nonpressure bearing arm to hold the table and pull up to squeeze the forces together. The practitioner may use a body part as well.

12–10 MAT

Some clients will be more comfortable on a mat (Figure 12-58). This is especially true of large athletes who really do not fit on a standard massage table. The body mechanics principles do not change. The only difference is that the weight-bearing contacts on the floor most often are the back knee and shin, whereas the forward upper limb (hand or forearm, for example) used to apply massage becomes the point of contact. The practitioner can easily use the leg and foot when working on a mat.

SUMMARY

This chapter provides a review and detailed population focus of massage methods. The general protocol found in Chapter 14 of this unit and focused massage application as described in Chapter 13 of this unit are based on the methods in this chapter, which then are applied intelligently based on assessment findings to achieve determined outcome. Almost all of the methods described in the chapter are also assessment methods. Indeed, most massage is a form of assessment.

The actual massage is a weaving of palpation and movement assessment with treatment and then post-assessment. Gliding is palpation that first can discern surface edema. Gliding then becomes a method to move the fluid. Kneading is assessment to identify connective tissue bind and then is the method to introduce forces into the tissue to reduce bind. Active and passive joint movement is range of motion assessment that then can become some type of application of muscle energy technique to lengthen and then stretch an area of restricted movement. Post-assessment is again active and passive joint movement. One thing becomes the other and then back again in the assessment, treatment, post-assessment continuum.

You should be able to work a solid 7 to 9 hours per day at least 5 days per week. If you cannot do this, your body mechanics are incorrect. Possibly, you will have to unlearn your current approach and relearn the more effective methods presented in this text.

FIGURE 12-58

EXAMPLES OF MAT WORK

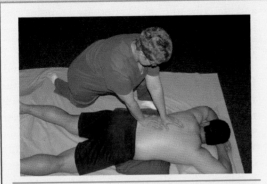

A Basic position 1.

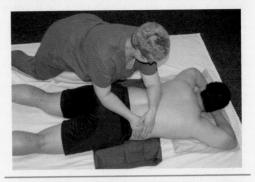

B Basic position 2.

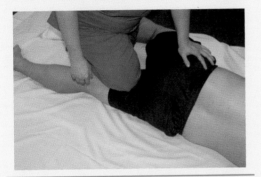

C Using leg.

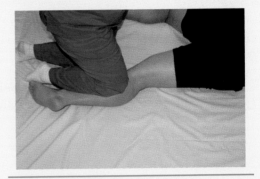

D Using leg.

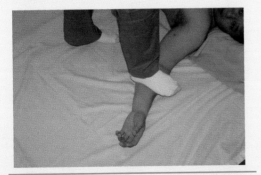

E Using foot/arch.

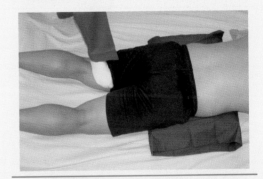

F Using foot/arch.

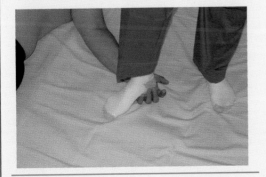

G Using foot/heel.

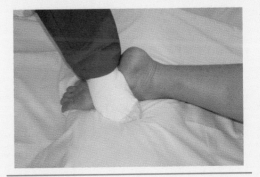

H Using foot/heel.

1 Identify a current bodywork modality with which you are familiar (Swedish, reflexology, shiatsu, deep tissue) and describe it in terms of stimulus and forces.

Examples:

Deep tissue (my own personal pet peeve—there is no such modality, really)
Depth of pressure—moderate to deep
Drag—moderate to intense
Duration—intermediate (45 seconds)
Frequency—two to three repetitions
Speed—slow
Rhythm—even

Consists of mechanical force application to affect connective tissue structures.

Stimulus to deep muscles using inhibiting pressure to the belly or attachment.

Muscle energy methods are appropriate with primary application of localized tissue lengthening and cross-fiber stretching.

_____

_____

_____

_____

_____

_____

_____

2 Watch someone give a massage (can be a video) and describe the application by stimulus and force.

Example: Massage begins with superficial glide to assess for skin temperature, texture, and bind. Glide assessment identified area of bind in the midscapular region. Compressive force was increased to moderate and direction changed, which moved tissue into ease position. Tissue was held for 30 seconds and then moved into bind direction. At bind, drag was increased and sustained for 30 seconds. Then tissue was kneaded . . .

_____

_____

_____

_____

_____

_____

_____

3 Do a massage, providing an ongoing narrative of the process by describing the application, using terminology from this chapter and the previous assessment chapter.

Example: I am beginning the massage with palpation assessment using near touch to identify heat. Now, I am gently touching the skin and using a light pressure with drag to assess for areas of ease and bind. . . .

_____

_____

_____

_____

_____

_____

_____

4 Do a comprehensive evaluation of your body mechanics while giving a massage. Identify areas of strength and weakness and develop a corrective action plan.

_____

_____

_____

_____

_____

_____

_____

_____

_____

_____

_____

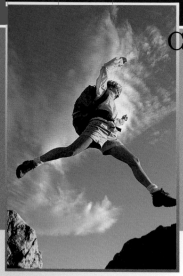

13

FOCUSED MASSAGE APPLICATION

OUTLINE

OBJECTIVES

Upon completion of this chapter, the reader will have the information necessary to correctly perform each of the following:

1 Indirect functional technique

2 Circulation support and lymphatic drain massage

3 Connective tissue application

4 Trigger point therapy

5 Joint play

6 Reflexology

7 Simple acupressure and meridian massage

8 Specific releases

This chapter discusses various massage methods that target specific tissues or body functions. Subjects discussed include indirect functional techniques, fluid dynamics, connective tissue, trigger points, joint play, reflexology, acupressure, and specific releases.

INDIRECT AND DIRECT FUNCTIONAL TECHNIQUES

Indirect functional techniques are usually referred to as indirect techniques or indirect methods of treatment. These methods are very gentle and safe. Rather than being treated as a specific modality, functional indirect methods need to be incorporated into the massage application regardless of whether the focus is soft tissue or joint movement. These methods, rather than engaging and attempting (by whatever means) to overcome resistance **(bind)** do the exact opposite. The soft tissue or joint is taken in all directions from the point of maximum

Active release
Acupressure
Acupuncture points
Anterior rotation
Anterior serratus
Biceps tendon displacement
Bind
Circulation support massage
Connective tissue methods
Deep lateral hip rotators
Diaphragm
Edema
Fluid dynamics
Groin area muscles
Hamstrings

Inflare
Indirect functional techniques
Interspinales
Intertransversarii
Joint play
Lymph nodes
Lymphangions
Lymphatic drain massage
Meridians
Mobilization with movement
Multifidii
Occipitals
Pectoralis minor
Pelvis alignment
Posterior rotation

Psoas
Quadratus lumborum
Rectus abdominis
Reflexology
Rhomboid
Rotatores
Sartorius displacement
Scalenes
Sacroiliac (SI) joint
Sternocleidomastoid
Subscapularis
Trigger points
Yang
Yin

ease. The massage practitioner simply maintains the joint or tissue in this ease position. There is no further treatment at this point, and after a couple of minutes the position is gently released.

A variation is to introduce a mild degree of overpressure at the point of maximum ease, which actually results in taking the soft tissue just into a bit of bind. The result is a reflex release of previously restricted tissues. It is essential that all movements are directed and controlled by the practitioner. A refinement of this application is to add gentle focused oscillation while the tissue or joint is in the ease position. Vibration, tiny shaking movements, and small focused rocking all are effective. In another variation, the client produces the oscillation with tiny pulsed movements against a resistance provided by the massage practitioner (pulsed muscle energy).

Regardless of how the methods are done, the underlying principles are assessment of ease and bind and the natural tendency of the body to seek homeostasis.

Soft tissue or joint mobility is assessed for motion restriction by palpation and/or range of motion and then treated by taking the dysfunctional tissue or joint in the direction of easier movement, which would be away from the restriction or bind and toward the way the tissue or joint wants to go in all planes of movement (sagittal, frontal, transverse). The soft tissue ease position is maintained until a sense of softening is perceived. If the

massage practitioner cannot easily palpate or identify this sensation, then the position should be held in this area 30 to 60 seconds. Breathing can increase the ease position and is assessed by having the client inhale and exhale, typically holding the breath for a few seconds in the direction that further contributes to the ease of tissue tension.

Indirect functional techniques are noninvasive methods and should be the first approach attempted to normalize tissue and joint movement. On the other hand, stretching is considered a direct technique because it engages the bind and moves through it. Stretching is more invasive than indirect methods, increasing the potential for adverse reactions.

A modification that incorporates the indirect method and the more aggressive direct stretching is to move back and forth between the ease position and the bind position. This can be described as indirect/direct. First the ease position is identified and held as previously described. Then the restrictive barrier of a joint or tissue is engaged in each plane of motion and held taut at the barrier until softening occurs. The corrective activating force then moves slightly through the restrictive barrier and again sustains the area in this position for 30 to 60 seconds until the tissue softens. Various forms of oscillation can be added. It is effective to alternate two or three times between direct and indirect application.

Indirect and direct functional methods are also the basis for **connective tissue methods.** Connective tissue methods can be indirect (i.e., a restricted area is placed into a position of little resistance until subsequent relaxation occurs) or direct (i.e., the affected area is placed against a restrictive barrier with constant force [stretched] until fascial release occurs).

Ease/indirect and bind/direct methods can be combined with muscle energy methods. As discussed, during muscle energy application, muscles (contractions) are actively used to support the response. Muscles are placed in a specific direction, which can be either ease or bind, and then the client pushes slowly in a controlled manner against a counterforce usually supplied by the massage therapist.

A sequence of indirect functional techniques is shown in Figure 13-1.

FLUID DYNAMICS

The body is an interconnected network of fluid compartments that contain blood, interstitial fluid, lymph, synovial fluid, and cerebrospinal fluid. Normal flow within the tissue and exchange of fluid between compartments is essential for homeostasis. Any impediment to normal flow leads to fluid stagnation, resulting in impaired tissue nutrition and repair. Stagnant tissue fluid becomes toxic and, as the protein content increases, can lead to fibrotic tissue changes.

Fluid tension in the body is called *hydrostatic pressure*. Body fluid is classified as extracellular (outside the cell) and intercellular (within the cell). About one third of the body fluid is extracellular and is located in two compartments:

1. The blood circulatory system, including the arteries and veins
2. The interstitial or anatomic space around cells and the lymphatic vessels

Fluids also move across compartments by diffusion from areas of high salt concentration to areas of lower salt concentration. The rate and volume of fluid movement are determined by pumping mechanisms such as the heart, muscle contraction and relaxation, rhythmic compression of fascial structure during movement, and respiration. Other factors influencing fluid movement include the viscosity of the fluid, the permeability of the membranes, and the size of the various vessels that the fluid travels through.

Vasodilators and constrictors of the circulatory system therefore influence the movement of body fluid. Massage that addresses the extracellular fluid can mechanically support the movement of fluid within these compartments by stimulating *hydrokinetics* (transport of fluid) along pressure gradients from high pressure to lower pressure. The mechanical pumping and oscillation applications of massage and the reflexive release of vasodilators (primarily histamine) produced during massage, coupled with the vasodilatation or constriction response of hydrotherapy, interplay in various ways to influence the outcome of the application.

INFLAMMATION AND FLUID DYNAMICS

Inflammation results in increased interstitial fluid, which then raises hydrostatic pressure in the area. The tissue swelling produces pain due to pressure on pain receptors. The increase in tissue pressure can serve a protective function by mechanically limiting movement and producing pain. This is important during the first few days after an acute injury, but the process then needs to begin to reverse itself for normal healing to take place.

The inflammatory process heightens the influence of chemical vasodilators affecting the venules and capillaries. There is also greater permeability of blood vessels locally, with a reduced flow velocity. This leads to the formation of local edema and stasis, with reduced exchange of nutrient and waste products. Pressure on vessels, or reduction of tissue space by changes in muscle tone, fascial pliability and length, and bony impingement, can also impede fluid exchange in the tissue. Carpal tunnel syndrome is an example in which the median nerve is impinged by fascial shortening and edema. Restoration of fascial pliability and reduction of edema support normal function. Massage treatment uses tensile forces to elongate shortened connective tissue, compressive forces to support the pumping action encouraging the movement of tissue fluid, and neuromuscular applications to reduce and normalize muscle tone.

Edema

Edema, which is the presence of abnormally large amounts of interstitial fluid, can be caused by a variety of factors, some of which are discussed here.

Lack of Exercise. Exercise, in which muscles alternately contract and relax, stimulates lymph circulation and cleans muscle tissue. If the muscles stay contracted or flaccid, lymph circulation decreases drastically inside muscles, and edema can result.

FIGURE 13-1

EXAMPLES OF DIRECT AND INDIRECT APPLICATION

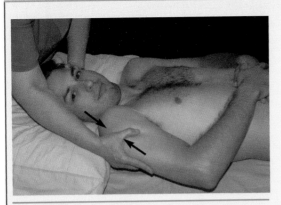

A Ease, indirect.

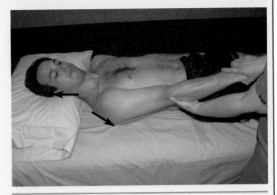

B Bind, direct.

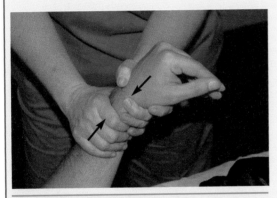

C Ease, indirect.

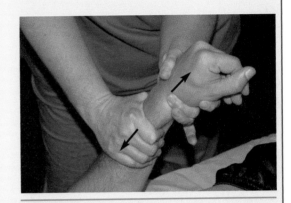

D Bind, direct.

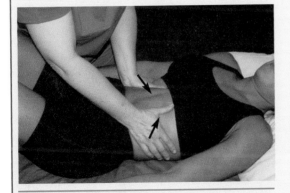

E Ease, indirect.

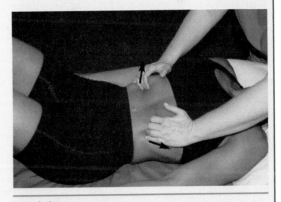

F Bind, direct.

Continued

FIGURE 13-1—CONT'D

EXAMPLES OF DIRECT AND INDIRECT APPLICATION

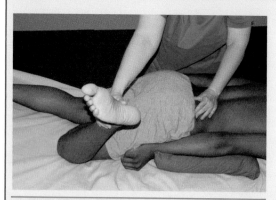

G Ease, indirect.

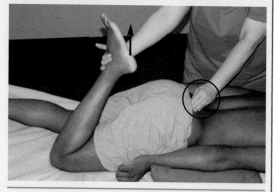

H Bind, direct.

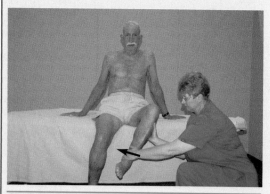

I Ease, indirect.

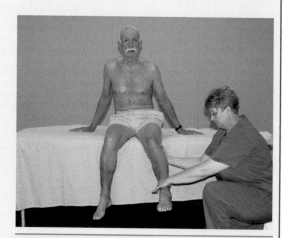

J Bind, direct.

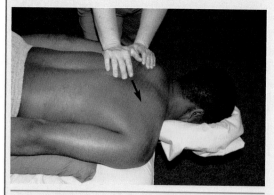

K Ease, indirect.

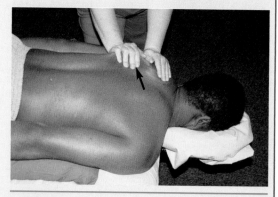

L Bind, direct.

FIGURE 13-1—CONT'D

EXAMPLES OF DIRECT AND INDIRECT APPLICATION

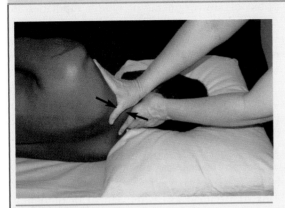

M Ease, indirect.

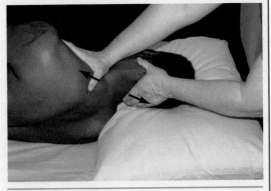

N Bind, direct.

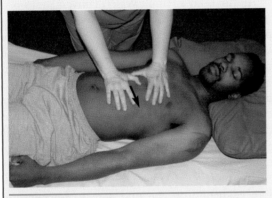

O Ease, indirect.

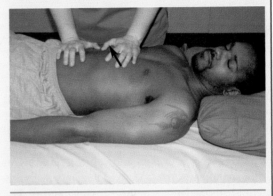

P Bind, direct.

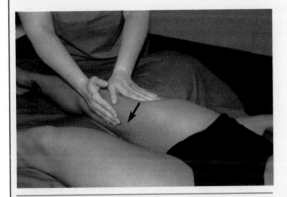

Q Ease, indirect.

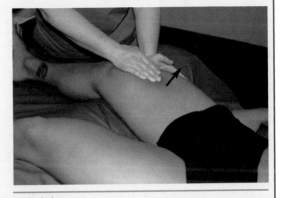

R Bind, direct.

Overexercise. During exercise, blood pressure and capillary permeability both increase, allowing more fluid to seep into the interstitial spaces. If the movement of fluid exceeds the ability of the lymphatic capillaries to drain the areas, the fluid accumulates. This seems to be a contributing factor to delayed-onset muscle soreness.

Salt. The body maintains a specific ratio of salt to fluids. The more salt a person consumes, the more water is retained to balance it, which can result in edema.

Heart and Kidney Disease. These diseases affect blood and lymph circulation. Lymph massage stimulates the circulation of lymph. Caution is indicated, because the increase in fluid volume could possibly overload an already weakened heart and kidneys.

Menstrual Cycle. Water retention and/or a swollen abdomen are common before or during the menstrual cycle.

Lymphedema. Lymphedema is edema of one or both limbs as a result of stasis of lymph secondary to obstruction of lymph vessels or disorders of the lymph nodes. Limbs affected with this condition become very swollen and painful, resulting in difficulty moving the affected limb and disfigurement. Lymphedema can be life-threatening. The interstitial fluid is contaminated and even small wounds can become infected.

Inflammation. Increased blood flow to an injured area and the release of vasodilators, which are part of the inflammatory response, can cause edema in localized areas. This is a common response to injury and surgery.

Other Causes. Medications, including steroids, hormones, and chemotherapy for cancer, may cause edema as a side effect. Scar tissue and muscle tension can cause obstructive edema by restricting lymph vessels.

THE LYMPHATIC SYSTEM

All massage stimulates the circulation and lymph movement. The lymphatic system transports fluid from around the cells through a system of filters. Interstitial fluid becomes lymph fluid once it enters the lymphatic capillaries.

The lymphatic system permeates the entire tissue structure of the body in a one-way drainage network of vessels, ducts, nodes, lacteals, and lymphoid organs. Segments of lymph capillaries are divided by one-way valves and a spiral set of smooth muscles called **lymphangions.** This system moves fluid against gravity in a peristalsis-type undulation.

The lymphatic tubes merge into one another until major channels and vessels are formed. These vessels run from the distal parts of the body toward the neck, usually alongside veins and arteries. Valves in the vessels prevent back flow of lymph.

Lymph nodes are enlarged portions of the lymph vessels that generally cluster at the joints. This arrangement assists movement of the lymph through the nodes by means of the pumping action from joint movement.

All the body's lymph vessels converge into two main channels: the thoracic duct and the right lymphatic duct. Vessels from the entire left side of the body and from the right side of the body below the chest converge in the thoracic duct, which in turn empties into the left subclavian vein, situated beneath the left clavicle. The right lymphatic duct collects lymph from the vessels on the right side of the head, neck, upper chest, and right arm. It empties into the right subclavian vein beneath the right clavicle.

The movement of lymph occurs along a pressure gradient from high-pressure to low-pressure areas. Fluid moves from the interstitial space into the lymph capillaries through a pressure mechanism exerted by respiration, peristalsis of the large intestine, the compression of muscles, and the pull of the skin and fascia during movement. This action is especially prominent at the soles of the feet and palms of the hands, where major lymph plexuses exist. It is likely that the rhythmic pumping of walking and grasping facilitates lymphatic flow.

Lymph circulation involves two steps:
1. Interstitial fluid flows into the lymphatic capillaries. Plasma is forced out of blood capillaries into the spaces around the cell walls. As fluid pressure increases between the cells, cells move apart, pulling on the microfilaments that connect the endothelial cells of the lymph capillaries to tissue cells. The pull on the microfilaments causes the lymph capillaries to open like flaps, allowing tissue fluid to enter the lymph capillaries.
2. Lymph moves through a network of contractile lymphatic vessels. The lymphatic

system does not have a central pump like the heart. Various factors assist in the transport of lymph through the lymph vessels.

The "lymphatic pump" of the body is the spontaneous contraction of lymphatic vessels as a result of the increase in pressure of lymphatic fluid. These contractions usually start in the lymphangions adjacent to the terminal end of the lymph capillaries and spread progressively from one lymphangion to the next, toward the thoracic duct or the right lymphatic duct. The contractions are similar to abdominal peristalsis and are stimulated by increases in pressure inside lymphatic vessels. Contractions of the lymphatic vessels are not coordinated with the heart or breath rate. If the pressure inside the lymphatic vessels exceeds or falls below certain levels, lymphatic contractions cease.

During breath inhalation, the thoracic duct is squeezed, pushing fluid forward and creating a vacuum in the duct. During exhalation, fluid is pulled from the lymphatics into the thoracic duct to fill the partial vacuum.

LYMPHATIC DRAIN MASSAGE

CONTRAINDICATIONS AND CAUTIONS

Edematous tissues have poor oxygenation and reduced function, and they heal slowly after injury. Chronic edema results in chronic inflammation and fibrosis, making the edematous tissue coarse, thicker, and less flexible.

Lymphatic drain massage can lower blood pressure. If the client has low blood pressure, there is the danger that it will fall further and that the client may be dizzy when standing up.

When a person is ill with a viral or bacterial infection and fever, circulation of lymph through the nodes slows, giving the lymphocytes more time to destroy the bacteria or virus. Because massage moves fluid through the lymphatic system more quickly, it can interfere with the body's efforts to defeat the attacking cells and can prolong the illness. During fever, white blood cells multiply rapidly but bacteria and viruses multiply more slowly; fever therefore is part of the body's healing process. Because lymph drain massage lowers the body temperature, do not give such a massage to a client with a fever.

Lymphatic drain massage affects the circulation of fluid in the body and can overwhelm an already weak heart or kidneys. Do not perform lymph drain massage on anyone with congestive heart failure, kidney failure, or undergoing kidney dialysis, unless the massage is specifically ordered by the client's physician.

INDICATIONS

Simple edema, screened for contraindications, responds well to massage focused on the lymphatic system. This approach is helpful for soft tissue injury, which includes surgery (with supervision), because it speeds healing and reduces swelling.

Traveler's edema is the result of enforced inactivity, such as sitting in an airplane or a car for several hours. It can affect anyone who sits for extended periods. Interstitial fluid (tissue fluid) responds to gravity, causing swelling in the feet, hands, and buttocks of a person who has to sit without moving very much for a few hours. Lymph drainage massage can remove the edema and reduce the pain and stiffness caused by the edema. Caution is indicated for the formation of blood clots with prolonged inactivity. Since many professional athletes often travel, this is a concern for massage.

Exercise-induced, delayed-onset muscle soreness is partly the result of increased fluid pressure in the soft tissues. Lymph drain massage is effective in reducing the pain and stiffness of this condition.

Lymph drain massage softens scar tissue and stimulate improved circulation.

PRINCIPLES

The pressure provided by massage mimics the drag and compressive forces of movement and respiration and can move the skin to open the lymph capillaries. The pressure gradient from high pressure to low pressure is supported by creating low-pressure areas in the vessels proximal to the area to be drained.

Depth of pressure, speed and frequency, direction, rhythm, duration, and drag are adjusted to support the lymphatic system. The pressure should be just sufficient to move the skin.

Disagreement exists about the intensity of the pressure used. Some schools of thought recommend very light pressure. Other methods use a deeper pressure and hold that the stronger the compression used, the larger the increase in the flow rate of lymph. This text combines both approaches.

Lymphatics are mostly located in superficial tissues, in the outer 0.3 mm of the skin; surface edema occurs in those superficial tissues, not in the deep tissue. Moving the skin moves the lymphatics. Stretching the lymphatics longitudinally, horizontally, and diagonally stimulates them to contract.

Simple muscle tension puts pressure on the lymph vessels and may block them, interfering with efficient drainage. Massage can normalize this muscle tension. As the muscles relax, the lymph vessels open, and drainage is more efficient.

TREATMENT

In general, massage first drains the surface area using lighter pressure, and then works on the areas of muscle tension using appropriate massage methods and pressure, and then finishes the area with a surface lymph drain again.

The greater the amount of fluid in the tissue, the slower the massage movements. Massage strokes are repeated slowly, at a rate of approximately 10 per minute in an area; this is approximately the rate at which the peripheral lymphatics contract.

Move lymph nodes toward the closest cluster of lymph nodes, which are located in the neck, axilla, and groin for the most part. Massage near nodes first, then move fluid toward them, working proximally from the swollen area toward the nodes. Massage the unaffected side first, and then the obstructed side. For instance, if the right arm is swollen because of scar tissue from a muscle tear, massage the left arm first.

The approach is a rhythmic, slow repetition of the massage movements.

Full-body lymph drain massage lasts about 45 minutes. Focus on local areas for about 5 to 15 minutes.

The methods of lymphatic drain massage are fairly simple, but this is a very powerful technique that elicits bodywide responses. Although disagreement exists about the methodology, all approaches have some validity. Therefore, the technique described in this text combines the various methods used to support lymphatic movement in the body.

The massage session begins with a pumping action on the thorax. Place both hands on the anterior surface of the thoracic cage. While the client exhales completely, passively follow the movements of the thorax with your hands. When the client starts inspiration, resist the movement of the thorax with counterpressure for 5 to 7 seconds. Repeat this procedure four or five times. Pumping action on the thorax increases lymph drainage through the lymphatic ducts by additionally lowering intrapleural pressure and exaggerating the action of inhalation and exhalation of the breath.

The massage application consists of a combination of short, light, pumping, gliding strokes beginning close to the torso at the node cluster and directed toward the torso; the strokes methodically move distally. The phase of applying pressure and drag must be longer than the phase of release. The releasing phase cannot be too short because the lymph needs to drain from the distal segment. Therefore, the optimal duration of the pressure and drag phase is 6 to 7 seconds; for the release phase, it is about 5 seconds. This pattern is followed by long, surface gliding strokes with a bit more pressure to influence deeper lymph vessels. The direction is toward the drainage points (following the arrow on the diagram in Figure 13-2).

The focus of the initial pressure and finishing strokes is on the dermis, just below the surface layer of skin, and on the layer of tissue just beneath the skin and above the muscles. This is the superficial fascial layer, which contains 60% to 70% of the lymphatic circulation in the extremities. It does not take much pressure to contact the area. If too much pressure is applied, the capillaries are pressed closed, which nullifies any effect on the more superficial vessels. Generally, light pressure is indicated initially, which increases to a moderate level (including kneading and compression as well as gliding) during repeated application to the area to reach the deep lymphatic vessels and then returns to lighter pressure over the area.

Drag is necessary to affect the microfilaments and open the flaps at the ends of the capillary vessels. A pumping, rhythmic compression on the soles of the feet and palms of the hands supports lymph movement. Rhythmic, gentle passive and active joint movement reproduces the body's normal means of pumping lymph. The client helps the process by deep, slow breathing, which stimulates lymph flow in the deeper vessels.

When possible, position the area being massaged above the heart so that gravity can assist the lymph flow. See specific protocol, beginning on page 280.

THE CIRCULATORY SYSTEM

The circulatory system is a closed system composed of a series of connected tubes and a pump. The heart pump provides pressure for the blood to move through the body via the arteries and eventually into the small capillaries, where the actual blood gas and nutrient exchange occurs. The blood

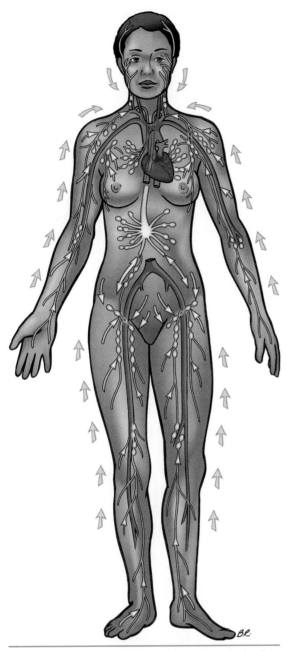

FIGURE 13-2 ■ Direction of strokes for facilitating lymphatic flow. (From Fritz S: *Mosby's fundamentals of therapeutic massage*, ed 3. St. Louis, 2004, Mosby.)

MASSAGE METHODS

The purpose of circulatory massage is to stimulate the efficient flow of blood through the body. This type of massage tends to normalize blood pressure, tone the cardiovascular system, and undo the negative effects of occasional stress. It is an excellent massage approach to use with athletes and anyone else after exercise. Circulatory massage also supports the inactive client by increasing the blood movement mechanically; however, it in no way replaces exercise. Both the circulatory and lymphatic types of massage are beneficial for the client who is unable to walk or exercise aerobically.

Massage to encourage blood flow to the tissues (arterial circulation) is different from massage to encourage blood flow from the tissues back to the heart (venous circulation). Because of the valve system of the veins and lymph vessels, deep, narrow-based stroking over these vessels from proximal to distal (from the heart out) is contraindicated. A small chance exists of breaking down the valves if this is done. However, compression, which does not slide, as does gliding or stripping, is appropriate for stimulating arterial circulation.

TREATMENT

Compression is applied over the main arteries, beginning close to the heart (proximal), and systematically moves distally to the tips of the fingers or toes. The manipulations are applied over the arteries, with a pumping action at a rhythm of approximately 60 beats per minute or whatever the client's resting heart rate is. Compressive force changes the internal pressure in the arteries, stimulates the intrinsic contraction of arteries, and encourages the movement of blood out to the distal areas of the body. Compression also begins to empty venous vessels and forms an arterial-venous pressure gradient, encouraging arterial blood flow (Figure 13-3).

Rhythmic, gentle contraction and relaxation of the muscles powerfully encourage arterial blood flow. Both active and passive joint movements support the transport of arterial blood.

The next step is to assist venous return flow. This process is similar to lymphatic massage in that a combination of short and long gliding strokes is used in conjunction with movement. The difference is that lymphatic massage is done over the entire body and the movements are usually passive. With venous return flow, the gliding strokes move distal to proximal (from the fingers and toes to the

returns to the heart by way of the veins. Venous blood flow is not under pressure from the heart. Rather, it relies on muscle compression against the veins to change the interior venous pressure. As in the lymphatic system, back flow of blood is prevented by a valve system.

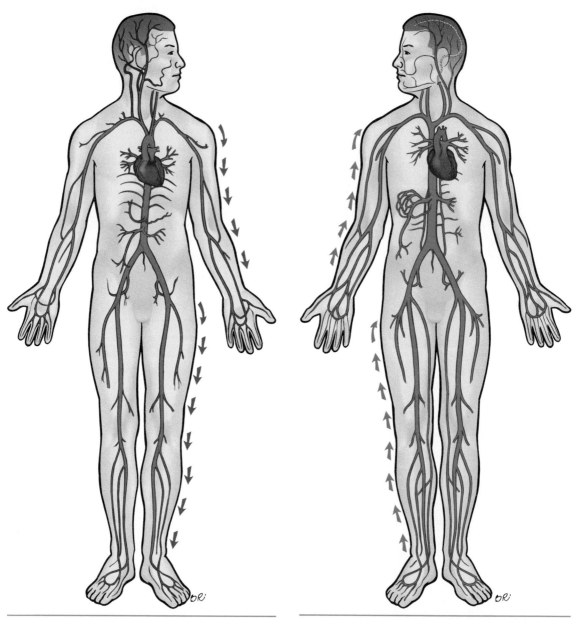

FIGURE 13-3 ■ Direction of compression over arteries to increase arterial flow. (From Fritz S: *Mosby's fundamentals of therapeutic massage,* ed 3. St. Louis, 2004, Mosby.)

FIGURE 13-4 ■ Direction of gliding strokes to facilitate venous flow. (From Fritz S: *Mosby's fundamentals of therapeutic massage,* ed 3. St. Louis, 2004, Mosby.)

heart) over the major veins. The gliding stroke is short, about 3 inches. This enables the blood to move from valve to valve. Long gliding strokes carry the blood through the entire vein. Both passive and active joint movements encourage venous circulation. Placing the limb or other area above the heart brings gravity into assistance (Figure 13-4).

Athletes experience fluid dynamics issues in various ways. Hydration is especially important and

is discussed in Unit One. In terms of methodical application, the massage outcome can target each main fluid area: arterial, venous, and lymphatic function. All of these areas are strained during exercises. Cardiovascular fitness is a major focus of many exercise programs and sport conditioning and training. The application of massage support to influence fluid dynamics is then dependent on whether the massage is applied as part of the "warm up–cool down–recovery," or rehabilitation process.

In general, massage application targeted to increase arterial flow is part of the warm-up process. Venous congestion can occur post exercise, as does an increase in interstitial fluid. Methods to address venous return can also decrease interstitial fluid by moving it into the lymphatic system.

Recovery involves normalizing all fluid movement. Injury rehabilitation involves managing swelling and encouraging effective circulation to the injured area to support healing.

Specific situations involving focused massage applications are injury swelling; sprains, strains, or other contusions; surgery swelling; delayed-onset muscle soreness; and chronic swelling (joint).

Strain, sprains, contusions, and surgery require specific treatment. These local injuries of the first and second degree (mild and moderate) benefit from both local and systemic lymphatic drain massage. It is important to decongest the entire drainage area affecting the injured area—for example, a sprained ankle requires draining of the entire leg into the trunk.

PRICE (*p*rotection, *r*est, *i*ce, *c*ompression, *e*levation) treatment should be used for the first 24 hours. Movement of fluid from superficial tissues can begin after the acute stage begins to diminish—as always, proper medical care needs to be provided and medical team orders followed.

Treatment of delayed-onset muscle soreness can begin as a preventive measure immediately after activity begins. Part of the process of delayed-onset muscle soreness is inflammation with increased capillary permeability. Increased influences of the sympathetic autonomic nervous system on blood pressure also result in more fluid movement from the capillary beds into the tissues. This increases interstitial fluid and hydrostatic pressure in the tissues. The lymph capillaries are unable to effectively drain the area and the congestion increases, which puts pressure on the pain-sensitive receptors.

Chronic swelling usually occurs around the joints, tendons, and bursae. The edema acts as a protective mechanism to attempt to reduce the problem causing the inflammation. A portion of the treatment of this condition involves addressing fluid issues of both blood and lymph. When using massage, the goal is to reduce the fluid enough to increase function but not to interfere with the protective process and increased stability provided by the hydrostatic pressure (Figure 13-5).

With contusions, the entire area around the con-tusion needs to be drained, but caution is necessary because the capillaries have been damaged and the massage must not interfere with the healing process. However, the blood in the interstitial fluid increases the protein content of the fluid, which increases the potential for formation of fibrotic tissue. This is why it is essential that the lymphatic system remove the interstitial fluid containing blood. Appropriate massage application can enhance this process.

The use of massage to increase arterial and venous circulation and lymphatic movement will be recommended throughout the text to serve the athlete and others who are involved in fitness and rehabilitation programs.

The following section is a precise description of the massage application that first affects arterial flow and then venous return; both approaches involve addressing capillary beds. Next, lymphatic drain massage for interstitial (extracapsular) tissue fluid and intracapsular fluid (inside the joint capsule) is described. These three approaches are easily and effectively combined.

The methods of both mechanical and reflexive fluid movement are primarily focused on mechanical force. To understand them, it is necessary to understand both the structure and function of the vascular and lymphatic systems. It is also necessary to appreciate the properties of a fluid, including properties of water, colloids, and viscosity.

Fluids naturally move from high pressure to low pressure with gravity. The more viscous (thick) the fluid, the slower it moves. Fluid moves against gravity only with a pump. The faster and stronger the pump, the more fluid is moved.

Permeability is the rate at which a fluid (water) moves across a membrane. Fluid also moves by *osmosis* and *diffusion*. The application of effective massage is dependent on all of these factors.

Increasing Arterial Circulation

13–2 Various mechanisms can influence arterial circulation (Figure 13-6). The massage application needs to address all these areas. However, the effects of pressure in the vessels and stimulation of vasodilation are especially important. These effects include:

Increased sympathetic arousal, which increases both the stroke volume and heart rate.
Increased build-up of pressure within the vessels.
Vasodilatation of the capillaries.

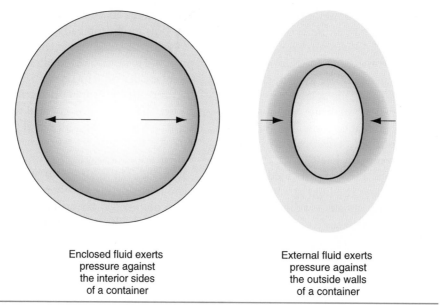

Enclosed fluid exerts
pressure against
the interior sides
of a container

External fluid exerts
pressure against
the outside walls
of a container

FIGURE 13-5 ■ Effect of hydrostatic pressure.

The general massage should be brisk, with a duration of 15 to 30 minutes. Active participation of the client, such as various forms of range of motion and muscle energy methods, is effective both to increase sympathetic arousal and to increase demand for blood as a result of muscle activity.

Deliberate temporary pressure against the arteries results in a build-up of fluid pressure between the heart, and the temporary blockage caused by the therapist's pressure results in an increased flow rate of the blood when the pressure block is released. Compression of the arteries in a rhythmic fashion moves the arterial blood faster toward capillaries to supply the nutritional and oxygen requirements of the tissues. Usually the target areas are the limbs, hands, and feet.

To create temporary pressure:

1. Position the area where increased arterial circulation is desired, below the heart if possible: seated, standing, and semireclined positions are most desirable.

2. A broad-based compression force is used against the tissue over the arteries. Begin close to the torso. If the arms are the target, begin where the arms join the torso (same for the legs).

3. The compression must be deep enough to close off the arteries so that the pressure builds. The rate of the on/off compression of the arteries is timed to the client's heart rate, which is determined by the closest pulse rate in the area. For example, if the pulse rate is 60 beats per minute, then the compression rate would be approximately one second on one second off–it is helpful to count, such as "1–(compress) and (release); 2–(compress) and (release)."

4. The direction systematically moves distal toward the fingers and toes.

5. The athlete can make a fist and release or curl the toes and release at the same rhythm.

Perform three or four repetitions of the area until the distal area increases in temperature.

Next, rhythmically knead and compress the target area to create hyperemia (histamine response and vasodilatation). Squeeze out the capillary beds to allow movement of blood into the venous system, creating space for the arterial blood. This will also facilitate the exchange of nutrients and gases, as well as plasma movement into the interstitial spaces. Pressure and squeezing techniques have a pumping effect on circulation. The pressure forces the blood out of the vessels in one direction only (toward the heart), because of the unidirectional valves. When pressure is released, the vessels refill from the arterial supply.

FIGURE 13-6

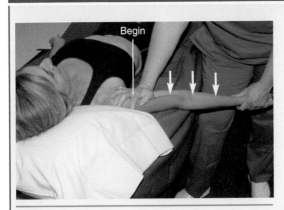

A Begin arterial circulation.

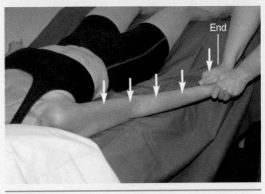

B End arterial circulation.

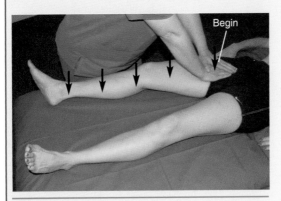

C Begin arterial circulation.

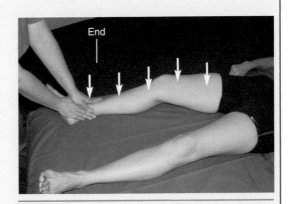

D End arterial circulation.

Microcirculation

The walls of the blood vessels need to be soft and pliable so that they can assist the pumping action and allow filtration and absorption through them. As a massage stroke forces blood through the capillaries and arterioles it has a stretching effect on the vessel walls, which can help increase their size, capacity, and function.

Venous Return

As with all methods, this massage application supports the anatomy and physiology of normal function. To support normal venous circulation, the venous pump is mimicked. A combination of short and long gliding stokes is used over the veins. The depth of pressure is a bit more than that used with lymphatic drain massage, because the intent is to actually pump the blood through a tube. Position the area, usually a limb, somewhat above the heart

to allow gravity to assist the fluid movement (Figure 13-7).

1. As with lymphatic drain, begin close to the torso and glide no more than 3 to 5 inches with the direction toward the heart to take advantage of the valve system in the veins. Systematically move toward the distal end of the limb.

2. Use kneading to move the blood in the capillary beds, dispersing it through the soft tissue.

3. Have the client actively contract and relax the muscles and move the joints in the area. Think of the action as being a pump. Passive joint movement can be used if necessary. It is effective to move the joint through its entire range of motion.

4. Repeat the entire sequence and then shift location a bit to address a different vein.

FIGURE 13-7

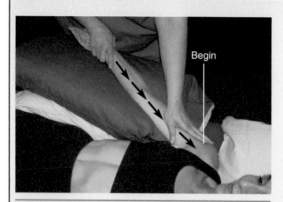

A Begin venous return.

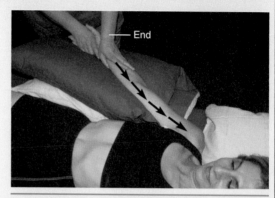

B End venous return.

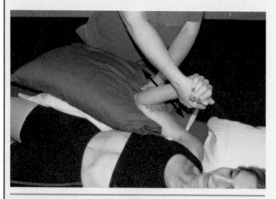

C Joint movement—venous pump.

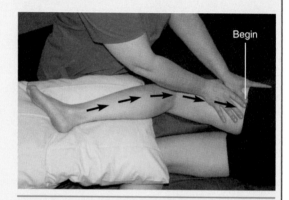

D Begin venous return.

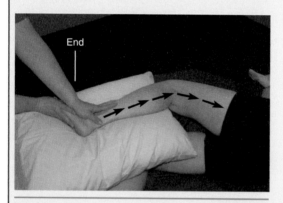

E End venous return.

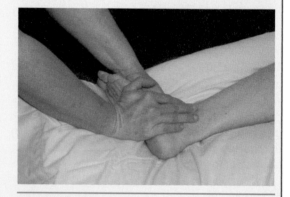

F Pump venous plexus in foot.

5. The calf muscles act as a secondary heart pump, especially influencing venous returning blood flow. The client can move the ankle in slow circles to activate this pumping action. This can also be taught as a self-help method. It is especially effective if the client lies on a slant board with the head slightly lower than the heart. This method is helpful even if the target area is not placed above the heart.

6. The respiratory pump supports venous return by channeling thoracic pressure during breathing. This is primarily caused by diaphragm action. Therefore it is important for the breathing mechanism to be normal.

Lymphatic Drain Massage

The following protocol is meticulous and detailed. It covers all of the current applications for lymphatic drain that are based on physiologic mechanisms. It is presented in the ideal order of application to target lymphatic fluid flow. (Author's note: I personally seldom perform the procedures as written here. Instead I pick, choose, and modify. However, for learning purposes, I strongly suggest you practice the protocols for both full body application and local application until you are comfortable with the procedures, concepts, and outcomes.) The protocol addresses increased movement of interstitial fluid into the lymphatic capillaries without fibrosis. Management of fibrotic tissue is discussed on page 293.

Contraindications for lymphatic drain massage:
- Compromised urinary or cardiovascular function, especially congestive heart or kidney failure.
- Systemic illness with symptoms such as fever, diarrhea, vomiting, and unexplained edema.
- Edema present in the acute phase of an injury (first 24 hours)
- Edema that is contributing to joint stability.

Because surgery, abrasions, and puncture wounds break the protective skin barrier, sanitation around the area of the wound is critical. Lymphatic drain massage around surgical areas and injury can safely be used, but not within the first 24 to 48 hours. Extreme care must be taken not to disturb the tissue healing process. Direct work over an area of surgery needs to be delayed until the incision sites are healed (5 to 7 days, and maybe longer).

Lymphatic drain massage targeted to a specific joint is most effective in the context of a general full body massage application.

Assessment for Increased Interstitial Fluid Volume

Common history components:
- Increased physical activity such as a competition or a game followed by 24- to 48-hour period of relative inactivity.
- Increased physical activity as above, but with insufficient recovery time (common in training camp schedules).
- Increased salt intake
- Increased water intake without appropriate electrolyte balance.
- Decreased fluid intake.
- Water weight gain of 3 to 5 pounds

Common complaints:
- Delayed-onset muscle soreness; sore all over, best described as achy.
- Stiffness that will not stretch out and is not clearly confined to a particular area.
- Sensation of the skin and muscles being "fat or taut."

Visual assessment:
- Loss of muscle and joint definition
- Appearance of being swollen.
- Client appears sluggish

Physical assessment
- Skin and superficial fascia palpated as taut from increased hydrostatic pressure.
- Skin and superficial fascia palpated as boggy, spongy, soggy (increased fluid but not enough to push against skin, as previously described).
- Difficulty palpating muscle fiber structure owing to fluid accumulation overlay.
- Decreased definition of joints.
- Reduced range of motion of joints as a result of edema
- Difficulty in lifting the skin and fascia from the surface layer of muscles.
- Deep, broad-based and narrow, superficial-based compression; both are painful.
- Pitting edema and prolonged blanching of skin after compression.
- Drag on the skin and superficial fascia can create pockets of fluid that feel like small water balloons.

Other observations.
- Reflexive methods are ineffective to resolve complaints.
- Connective tissue applications may make symptoms worse at least temporarily.

Supportive measures:

FIGURE 13-8

LYMPHATIC DRAIN—PHASE I: PREPARING THE TORSO

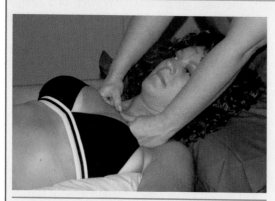

A Lymphatic drain—Phase 1. Prepare the torso.

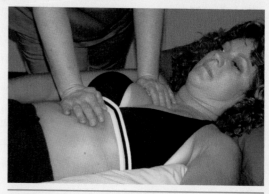

B Prepare torso.

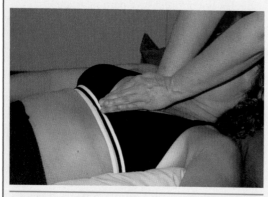

C Prepare torso. Mobilize the ribs.

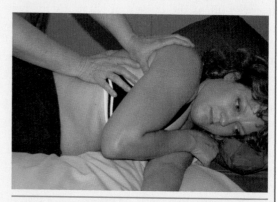

E Prepare torso—side-lying.

1. Epsom salt soak: Use enough salt so that the water has a mineral taste. Too much is better than not enough. This works by diffusion of water from less mineral concentration to more concentration to equalize solutions on either side of a membrane (the skin). The edema close to the skin flows across the skin into the salty water.
2. Increase fluid intake with proper electrolyte balance (50% water-diluted sport drink or pediatric fluid replacement drink such as Pedialight).
3. Eat diuretic-type foods such as pineapple, papaya, berries, cucumbers, radishes, celery.

Full-body lymphatic drain massage takes 45 to 90 minutes depending on the size of the client. Begin working on the least affected areas and then progress to the target area.

STEP-BY-STEP PROTOCOL FOR FULL-BODY LYMPHATIC DRAIN MASSAGE PHASE 1—PREPARING THE TORSO

(FIGURE 13-8)

1. Position the client on back (supine) with arms and legs bolstered above the heart but with no areas of joints in a close-packed position (typically ends of range of motion).
2. Begin on upper thorax and use glide, knead, and compression to prepare the tissue. The goal is to increase skin pliability and connective tissue ground substance pliability and to reduce any areas of muscle tension so that lymph capillaries and vessels are unobstructed. Continue into the abdomen, paying

FIGURE 13-8 CONT'D

LYMPHATIC DRAIN—PHASE I: PREPARING THE TORSO

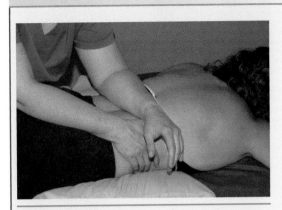

E Prepare torso, prone.

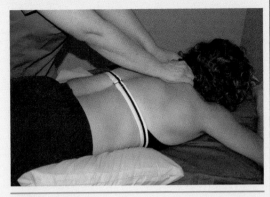

F Prepare torso, prone.

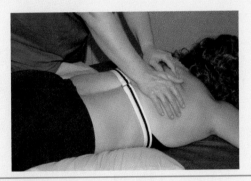

G Mobilize the ribs.

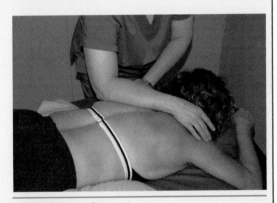

H End preparation of torso.

particular attention to abdominal and diaphragm muscles.

3. Mobilize the ribs by applying gentle but firm broad-based compression beginning at the sternoclavicular joint and work down toward the lower ribs. Make two or three passes, working from the sternum out toward the lateral edge. If an area of restriction is found, various methods can be used to increase mobility in the area. Compressing the restricted area while the client coughs is usually effective. Massage the intercostals.

4. Place client in side-lying position and use glide, knead, and compression to continue to increase tissue pliability and rib mobility. Work from the iliac crests up toward the axilla. Pay particular attention to the anterior serratus. Repeat on other side.

5. Place client in the prone position (face down). Use glide, knead, and compression to increase tissue pliability and rib mobility. Begin at the iliac crest and systematically work toward the shoulder and neck. Do both left and right sides.

Outcome

Torso soft tissue pliability and rib mobility allows effective deep breathing and movement of lymph into the torso.

13-1

PHASE 2—Decongesting and Drain the Torso (Figures 13-9 and 13-10)

1. Reposition client in the supine position with arms and legs bolstered above the heart.

2. Place hand (a flat or loose fist) just below either clavicle and compress and release. Repeat three

FIGURE 13-9

LYMPHATIC DRAIN—PHASE 2: DECONGESTING AND DRAINING THE TORSO

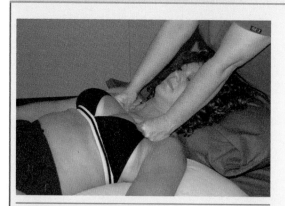

A Decongest and compress the torso.

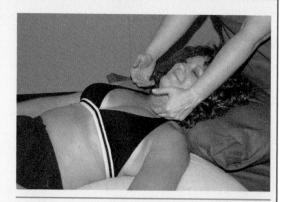

B Release.

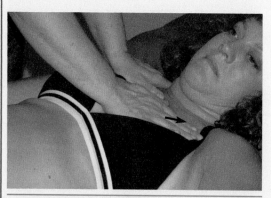

C Drag the skin. Surface drainage.

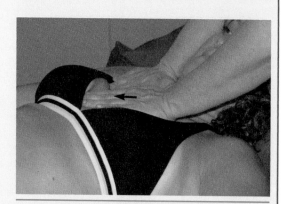

D Drag the skin. Surface drainage.

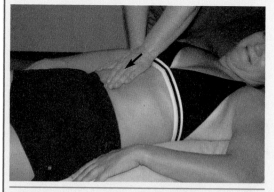

E Skin drag below the diaphragm. Surface drainage.

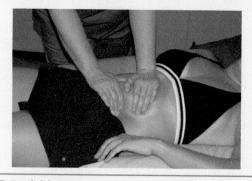

F Knead abdomen.

FIGURE 13-9 CONT'D

LYMPHATIC DRAIN—PHASE 2: DECONGESTING AND DRAINING THE TORSO

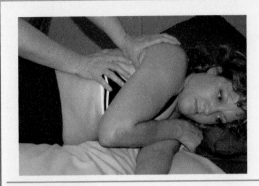

G Drain torso, side-lying.

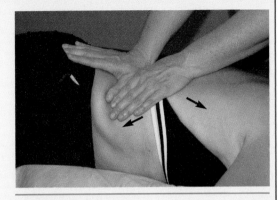

H Side-lying skin drag on torso.

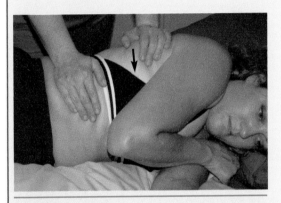

I Side-lying rib compression.

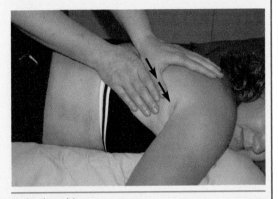

J Skin drag while prone.

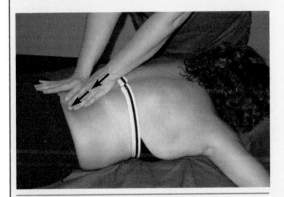

K Skin drag while prone.

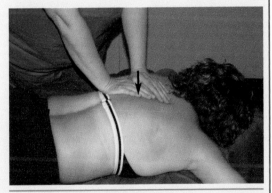

L Compress the ribs. End of Phase 2.

FIGURE 13-10

LYMPHATIC DRAIN—DRAIN THE UPPER LIMB

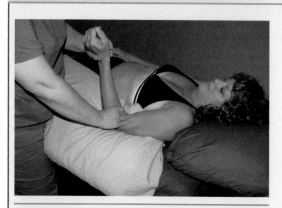

A Active and passive joint movement.

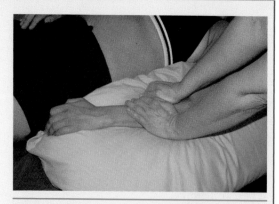

B Prepare the tissues.

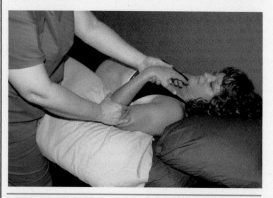

C Repeat joint movements.

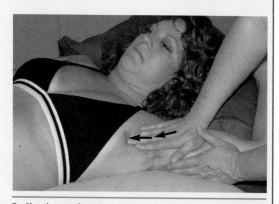

D Skin drag on the arm.

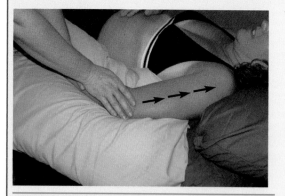

E Skin drag on the arm and continue all the way to hand.

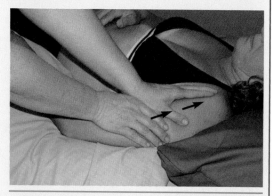

F Gliding, long strokes.

FIGURE 13-10 CONT'D

LYMPHATIC DRAIN—DRAIN THE UPPER LIMB

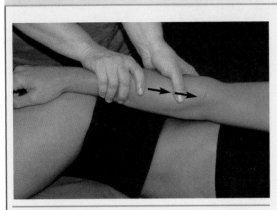

G Skin drag.

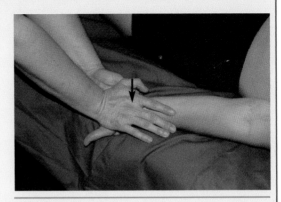

H Rhythmic compression.

or four times. Compress with exhale, release with inhale. This begins to affect the thoracic duct by changing thoracic pressure. Note: Repeat this procedure approximately every 15 minutes during the session.

3. Begin surface draining procedure. This process consists of dragging and sliding of the skin in various directions to pull on the microfilaments, opening the ends of the lymph capillaries, so that the interstitial fluid can move from around the cells into the lower pressure areas of the lymph vessels. This needs to be done in a rhythmic slow manner, like a pump. Drag the skin systematically in each area and then let it return to its original position. Drag skin and let it return, drag skin again, etc. Each skin movement has a slightly different direction vertically, horizontally, diagonally, and circularly. The skin movement phase is a little longer than the release phase. Remember, the massage application is structured to mimic the pull of the skin and fascia that would normally affect the microfilaments attached to the lymphatic capillaries. Begin skin drag at the closest lymph node area and work distal. This decongests and lowers the pressure, allowing fluid to move from high pressure to low pressure.

4. Begin the skin movement at the thorax midline above the diaphragm and work toward the area under the clavicles. (Do both sides.) When this area is thoroughly addressed, repeat chest compression.

5. Continue with the skin movement below the diaphragm, and change direction to drain toward the groin.

6. Have client do deep breathing while you gently but firmly knead the abdomen; then repeat chest compression. Compress on exhale, release on inhale.

7. Position client on side and repeat skin drag method, starting near the axilla, and drain from the waist up toward the axilla; below the waist, drain toward the groin, starting proximal to the region where drainage occurs. Do both sides.

8. While client is in the side-lying position, rhythmically compress the ribs (compress on exhale, release on inhale).

9. Place client in the prone position and drain again: above the waist toward the axilla and below the waist toward the groin. Compress the ribs in rhythm with the breathing.

Outcome

Torso is decongested and able to receive fluid from limbs.

PHASE 3—Limbs (Figures 13-10 and 13-11)

1. With client in the supine, prone, and side-lying position, begin to systematically address the arms and legs. The procedure for both is the same. Address the least congested area first. For example, if the arms have more fluid, begin with the legs. If the right arm is more

FIGURE 13-11

LYMPHATIC DRAIN OF LOWER LIMB—PHASE 3

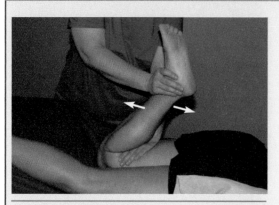

A Passive and active joint movement.

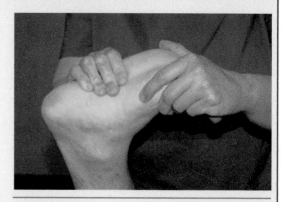

B Passive and active.

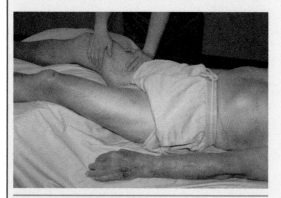

C Prepare tissues, supine.

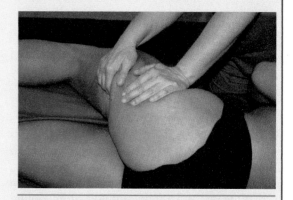

D Prepare tissues, side-lying.

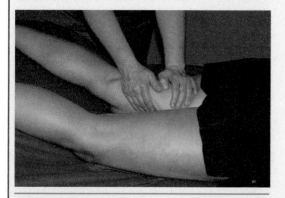

E Prepare tissues, prone.

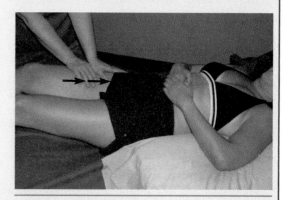

F Skin drag on the leg, supine.

FIGURE 13-11 CONT'D

LYMPHATIC DRAIN OF LOWER LIMB—PHASE 3

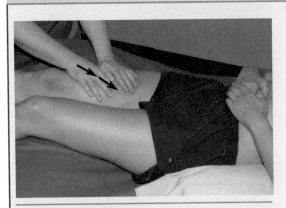

G Continue skin drag down the leg, supine.

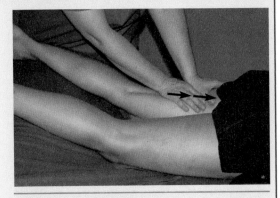

H Skin drag on the leg, prone.

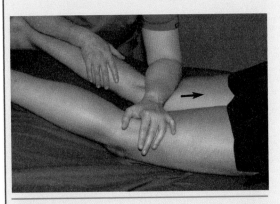

I Gliding, long strokes.

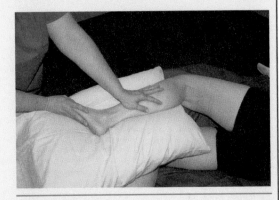

J Knead and compress.

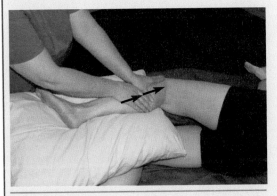

K Skin drag, side-lying.

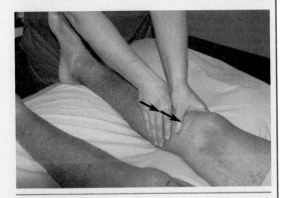

L Skin drag, supine.

FIGURE 13-11 CONT'D

LYMPHATIC DRAIN OF LOWER LIMB—PHASE 3

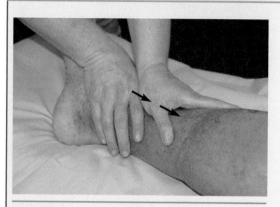

M Skin drag on the leg, supine.

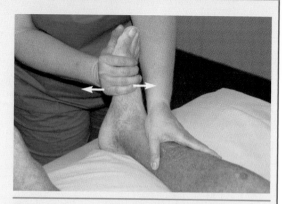

N Active and passive joint movement.

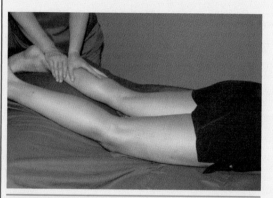

O Complete skin drag.

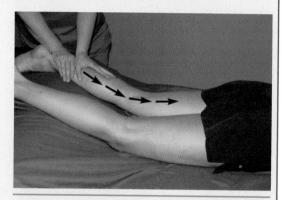

P Long strokes on the leg, prone.

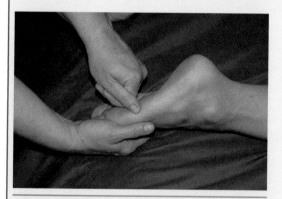

Q Rhythmic compression.

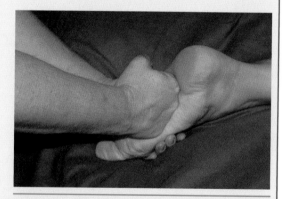

R Rhythmic compression.

FIGURE 13-12

LYMPHATIC DRAIN—PHASE 3 ON THE NECK

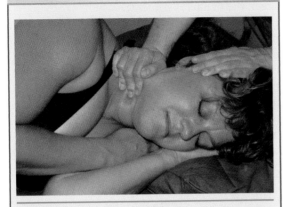

A Knead and compress the neck, side-lying.

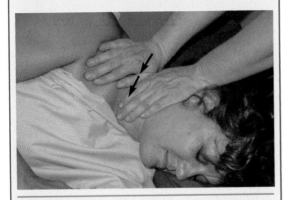

B Skin drag.

closest set of lymph nodes. Work down toward the elbow or knee.

6. Apply moderately deep gliding from the elbow or knee toward the groin or axilla. The intent is to support movement of the fluid once inside the vessels and to activate the lymphangions. Glide with the intent of moving the fluid from valve to valve and increase intravessel pressure. Long, slow, moderately deep gliding from the knee or elbow to the groin or axilla is also appropriate.

7. Apply active and passive joint movements again. The intent is to pump fluid at the nodes located at the joints.

8. Knead and compress the soft tissue of the elbow, knee, axilla, or groin. The intent is to move the interstitial fluid in the deeper tissues to the surface lymphatic capillaries.

9. Repeat steps 3, 4, and 5.

10. Apply active and passive joint movement.

11. Begin skin drag application near the knee or elbow, and work down to the ankle and wrist. Move skin in all directions and end with direction toward the knee or elbow.

12. Apply active and passive joint movement.

13. Redrain upper limb as described in steps 3, 4, and 5.

14. Apply active and passive joint movement.

15. Knead and compress the soft tissue of the wrist and elbow or ankle and knee.

16. Repeat steps 8, 9, 10, 11, and 12.

17. Apply moderately deep, short and long gliding strokes from the wrist to the axilla or from the ankle to the groin.

18. Apply active and passive joint movement.

19. Apply broad-based slow rhythmic, moderately deep compression to the palms of the hands and soles of the feet. Pump the plexus located in these areas for about 60 seconds.

20. Repeat active and passive joint movement.

21. Place client in side-lying position (Figure 13-12).

22. Knead and compress neck tissue to prepare for drain.

23. Begin skin drag methods close to the clavicles and work at the skull. The direction of the force is toward the clavicles.

24. Apply active and passive joint movement to the neck.

25. Use short and long gliding and moderately deep pressure to increase fluid movement in the vessels. Work from the skull toward the clavicles.

26. Repeat steps 24 and 25.

congested, work the legs first, then work the left arm, and then the right arm.

2. Begin with passive and active joint movement in the following sequence: hip, knee, ankle, foot; shoulder, elbow, wrist, hand.

3. Prepare the tissue in the limbs for draining as for the torso. Use gliding, kneading, compression, as well as shaking, to increase pliability of connective tissue and decrease muscle tension. Restriction in these areas interferes with the ability of the fluid to move into the lymphatic capillaries.

4. Repeat passive and active joint movement, as in step 2.

5. Bolster limb above the heart and begin skin drag application close to the torso, in the groin, gluteal, or axilla area. Systematically, gently, slowly, and rhythmically drag the skin in multiple directions, ending in the direction of the

27. Apply broad-based compression to the thorax in a rhythmic pumping manner synchronized with deep breathing (compress on the exhale, release on the inhale) to affect the duct pressure.
28. Repeat steps 23 through 27.
29. Place client in supine position and bolster limbs above the heart.
30. Repeat steps 2 through 18 on each limb.
31. Repeat rhythmic pumping compression of the ribs near the clavicles synchronized with deep breathing. Remember to compress on the exhale and release on the inhale.

Outcome

Full body addressed using massage to mimic natural lymphatic drain process.

STEP-BY-STEP PROTOCOL FOR LYMPHATIC DRAIN MASSAGE FOR SWELLING OF AN INDIVIDUAL JOINT AREA OR CONTUSION (FIGURE 13-13)

Swelling at joints occurs for many reasons. Rheumatoid arthritis is one cause of joint swelling that requires caution when applying massage, and all massage should be closely supervised by the medical team.

Osteoarthritis is another common cause of joint swelling. The fluid build-up is usually protective in nature. Intracapsular fluid inside the joint capsule can serve to keep pain-sensitive bone structures separated and reduce rubbing and friction in the joint. Fluid around the capsule can provide stability for a joint and limit painful motion. In these cases, the goal is not to totally eliminate the fluid, but to keep it moving to reduce the tendency for stagnant edemous tissue to become fibrotic, and to maintain appropriate levels of fluid. As explained, some fluid build-up both in and outside the capsule is beneficial. Too much is detrimental to effective healing. Because it is essential to maintain mobility in arthritic joint maintenance, optimal fluid dynamics in the area is important.

Trauma such as sprains, contusions, breaks, and surgery results in swelling as part of the acute inflammatory response. This tissue fluid must be managed because of its high-protein content as the result of the tissue debris and blood from the injury. This fluid can quickly become fibrotic during the subacute healing phase. The key is to manage the accumulated fluid, and keep it moving without increasing any

inflammatory response or disrupting the healing process. Sometimes the only component of lymphatic drain massage that can be used directly on the site of the trauma is skin drag.

When targeting an isolated area, it may not be necessary to be as meticulous as previously described for full-body lymphatic drain massage. It is helpful to use a shorter and less intense application to the whole body even when targeting a particular joint or area. Passive and active range of motion and some skin dragging are appropriate as part of the general massage application; the increase of fluid movement anywhere in the body influences the movement of all the lymphatics.

Procedure

1. Identify the main area of the trunk that the fluid will move toward. For arm joints and tissue, this would be the axilla and the area around the clavicles. For the joints and tissues in the leg, the destination area would be the groin and lower abdomen.
2. Bolster the entire limb containing the individual target areas to be addressed in a relaxed position above the heart, with the joints in the mid-range, open position.
3. Prepare the tissue in the entire limb with gliding, kneading, compression, and shaking to increase pliability of the connective tissue structures and reduce any muscle tension on the lymphatic vessels.
4. Begin the skin drag close to the torso and meticulously drain to the next distal joint (either the elbow or knee).
5. Apply active and passive joint movement, making sure that the area of either the groin or axilla is effectively compressed in a pumping fashion during the joint movement.
6. Knead and compress the soft tissue of the knee and groin or elbow and axilla with the intent of affecting the deeper interstitial fluid movement.
7. Repeat active and passive joint movement.
8. Repeat steps 4 and 5.
9. Apply gliding strokes of moderate pressure toward the trunk with the intent to increase fluid movement in the lymphatic vessels.
10. Repeat active and passive joint movement.
11. Prepare the tissue in the lower part of the limb (arm or leg) with gliding, kneading, compression, and shaking.
12. Repeat step 4, this time working all the way from the knee or elbow distally to the ankle or the wrist.

FIGURE 13-13

PROCEDURE FOR SWELLING OF AN INDIVIDUAL JOINT AREA OR KNEE CONTUSION

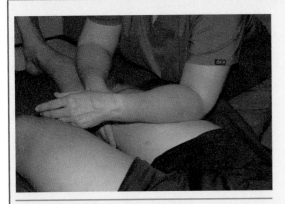

A Bolster and prepare the tissue with gliding.

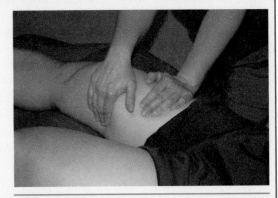

B Prepare the tissue with kneading.

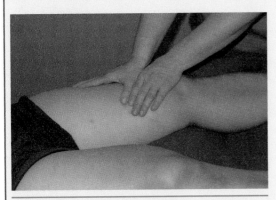

C Apply skin drag method toward the trunk.

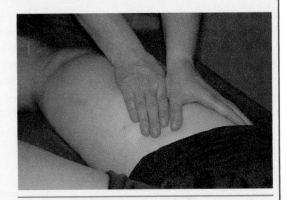

D Continue skin drag method toward the trunk.

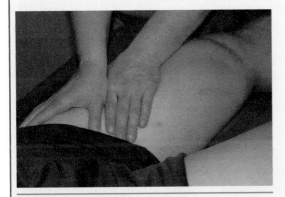

E Complete skin drag method toward the trunk.

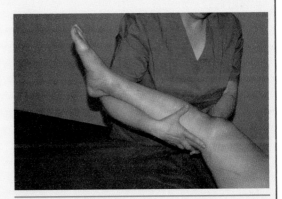

F Take the leg through range of motion.

Continued

FIGURE 13-13 CONT'D

PROCEDURE FOR SWELLING OF AN INDIVIDUAL JOINT AREA OR KNEE CONTUSION

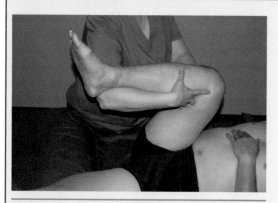

G Take the leg through range of motion.

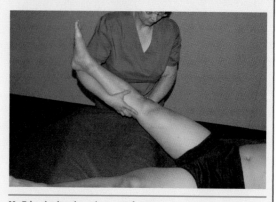

H Take the leg through range of motion.

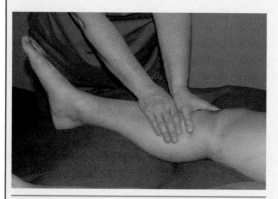

I Prepare the tissue in the lower part of the limb using gliding, kneading, and compression.

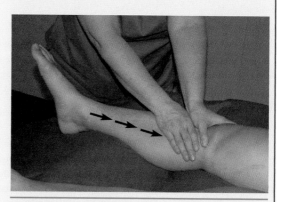

J Using skin drag method.

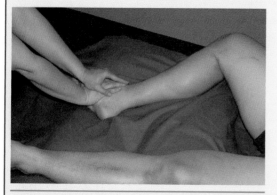

K Foot compression, supine.

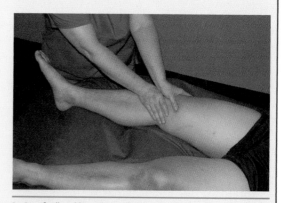

L Specifically address the swollen joint.

13. Repeat steps 5 through 10, including the entire limb from the wrist or ankle to the axilla or groin.
14. Using compression, slowly and rhythmically pump the sole of the foot or the palm of the hand; continue for about 60 seconds.
15. Repeat active and passive joint movement.
16. Specifically address the swollen joint–hip, shoulder, knee, elbow, ankle, wrist, foot/hand, toes/fingers–or contusions by meticulously using skin drag in all directions over the area, unless the skin is damaged. If there is a breach in the skin, then work near the area but not on it.
17. Apply active and passive joint movement.
18. Repeat steps 16 and 17.
19. If the target area is a joint, use compressive action to squeeze and release the tissue surrounding the joint. This should be slow and rhythmic. The smaller joints can be squeezed in the hand; the large joints will require using both hands to surround and squeeze the joint while maintaining the compressive action.
20. Repeat the entire sequence if necessary.

CONNECTIVE TISSUE FOCUS

The quality of the connective tissue can generally be assessed by the pliability of the skin and subcutaneous layers. Thickened, adhered fascia is less mobile, and the skin will glide only a short distance before feeling tight (bind). It is amazing how far healthy tissue can comfortably be stretched in all directions. In the treatment of musculoskeletal problems, the connective tissue of primary concern is the fascia that wraps the muscle fibers into bundles and compartments and then wraps all these together to form the whole muscle. The outer layer of fascia makes up the muscle's sheath, which maintains the overall shape and is smooth on the outside so that the muscle can move freely and independently of other structures. It is not contractile tissue but does have–or should have–the same elasticity as the muscle.

The fascia is subject to trauma through overstretching or impact, and scar tissue and adhesions can form. The main problem, however, comes from chronic changes as a result of long-term strain. The fascia thickens and becomes more fibrous, which makes it less mobile and reduces its pliability. This affects the function of the underlying muscle and may restrict its free movement. Furthermore, if the interstitial fluid cannot pass freely through the fascia, the muscle may not receive an adequate supply of oxygen and nutrients and will be less able to eliminate metabolic waste material.

As well as excessive tension or thickening in the fascia, connective tissue forces affect the autonomic nervous system through a neurofascial reflex. This stimulates local blood flow, and the skin appears red and is warm.

Adhesions and fibrous tissue created by scar tissue cause the most dysfunction. In the early healing stages, scar tissue is quite sticky and fibers can adhere to each other. For a muscle to function properly, the fibers must be able to glide smoothly alongside one another; when stuck together, they cannot do this and the affected area will not function optimally. Over time, a local area of muscle fibers can mat together into a fibrous mass.

The noncontractile soft tissues can also be affected by fibrous adhesion, becoming thick and less pliable. Adhesions can also form between different structures, such as between ligaments and tendons, muscles, and bone. This can lead to a significant restriction in movement and function.

Transverse strokes using shear and bend forces can break down the adhesions by literally tearing the adhesive bonds apart. Once the fibers are separated they are able to functionally slide again. Applied effectively, massage methods targeting connective tissue should create a sensation of burning and localized intense pulling but should not cause any actual damage, because the adhesions themselves contain no blood vessels. If massage is done too heavily or on tissue that is in an early stage of repair, further damage can be caused.

When a large fibrous mat of compacted tissue has formed, there may be little or no circulation running through it, and therefore a natural healing process cannot take place. Massage increases tissue pliability and allows blood to flow more easily through the tissue, stimulating healing.

Massage is able to stretch specific localized areas of tissue in a way that may not be possible with other approaches. Longitudinal (tension force) stroking and kneading (bend and torsion force) can stretch the tissues by drawing them apart and in all possible directions.

In most instances, a lubricant is not used with connective tissue approaches because the drag quality on the tissue is necessary to produce results, and lubricant reduces drag.

FIGURE 13-14

TISSUE MOVEMENT

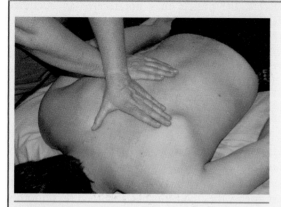

A Begin ease.

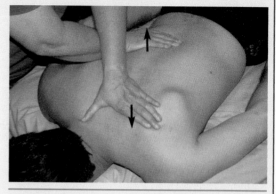

B End bind.

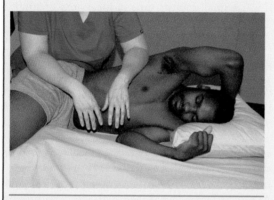

C Begin ease.

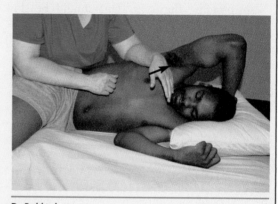

D End bind.

Methods that affect primarily the ground substance require a quality of slow, sustained pressure, tension, and agitation. Most massage methods can soften the ground substance as long as the application is not abrupt. Tapotement and abrupt compression are less effective than slow gliding methods that have a drag quality. Kneading and skin rolling that incorporate a slow pulling action are effective as well. Appropriate application introduces one or a combination of the mechanical forces of tension, compression, bind, shear, and torsion.

Fiber components are affected by stretching methods (either longitudinal or crossfiber) that elongate the fibers past the normal give of the fiber and enter the plastic range past the bind. This either creates a freeing and unraveling of fibers or a small therapeutic (beneficial and controlled) inflammatory response that signals change in the fibers.

TISSUE MOVEMENT METHODS

(Figure 13-14)

The more subtle connective tissue approaches rely on the skilled development of following tissue movements. The process is as follows:

1. Make firm but gentle contact with the skin. This is best accomplished with the tissue in the ease position.
2. Increase the downward, or vertical, pressure slowly until resistance is felt; this barrier is soft and subtle.
3. Maintain the downward pressure at this point; now add horizontal drag until the resistance barrier is felt again.
4. Sustain the horizontal pressure and wait.
5. The tissue will seem to creep, unravel, melt, slide, quiver, twist, or dip, or some other movement sensation will be apparent.

FIGURE 13-14 CONT'D

TISSUE MOVEMENT

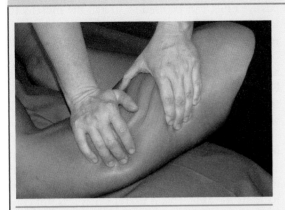

E Twist and release, IT band.

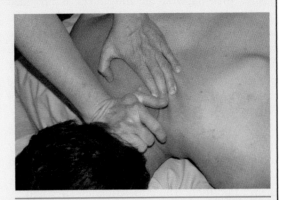

F Twist and release, neck

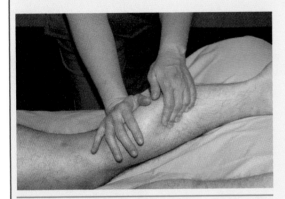

G Twist and release, calf.

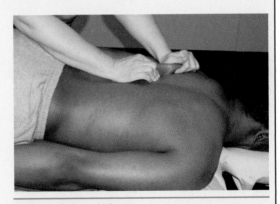

H Twist and release, back.

6. Follow the movement, gently maintaining the tension on the tissues, encouraging the pattern as it undulates though various levels of release.

7. Slowly and gently release first the horizontal force and then the vertical force.

Twist-and-release kneading and compression applied in the direction of the restriction can also release these fascial barriers.

The development of connective tissue patterns is highly individualized, and because of this, systems that follow a precise protocol and sequence are often less effective in dealing with these complex patterns.

The important consideration in all connective tissue massage methods is that the pressure vertically and horizontally (compression and drag) actually moves the tissue to create tension, torsion, shear, or bend, generating forces alteration of the ground substance long enough for energy to build up in it and soften it.

A good grip with the skin is essential, so there must be no lotion or oil present. This grip can be with the hands or forearms. The technique is even sometimes performed with a towel, to provide stronger contact with the skin.

Tissues can be moved toward ease (the way it wants to move) and is held for a few seconds to allow the tissues to soften. The client can add a neurological component by contracting or relaxing the muscle as the massage therapist holds the tissue at ease. The entire procedure can be repeated while holding the tissues at bind (the way it does *not* want to move).

Some varieties of this process have been formalized into modality systems such as active release and deep tissue methods.

ACTIVE RELEASE (Figure 13-15)

In **active release,** the massage therapist applies passive pressure, and the movement is provided by the client. Assessment identifies a local area of fibrotic tissue and/or adhered fibers. Compression is applied to hold the area in a static position. Then the tissues are stretched away from that point. The points where the pressure is applied are often the same as those used for typical trigger points.

The basic method is to start with the muscle relaxed and held in a passive shortened position by moving the associated joint. Focused compression is applied directly into the adhered fibers to fix them in position. The muscle is then stretched by the massage therapist away from this fixed point by moving the joint. Pressure needs to be applied with sufficient force to prevent the target tissues from moving as the stretch takes place.

Active and resisted movements, instead of passive ones, can be used to stretch the muscle. In fact, this may be more effective because the neuromuscular function is involved as well as the focus on connective tissue. The client contracts the antagonist that reciprocally inhibits the muscle being treated and moves the area while the massage therapist maintains focused pressure. An easy way to do this is to have the client move the associated joint areas in a slow circle, or back and forth if the joint is a hinge joint. The tissues can also be stretched away from the pressure point using deep massage strokes made with the other hand or forearm. This is useful when it is not convenient to move the joint—for example when treating the gluteal muscles while the client is in the

---

FIGURE 13-15

EXAMPLES OF ACTIVE RELEASE

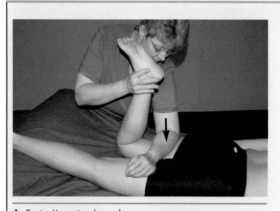

A Begin. Hamstring/move leg.

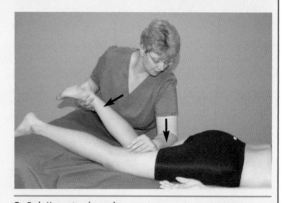

B End. Hamstring/move leg.

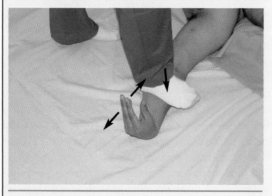

C Supinated forearm/move wrist.

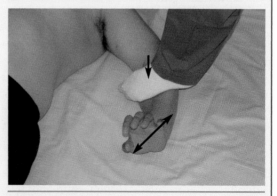

D Pronate forearm/move wrist.

prone position and hip flexion to stretch the muscle would be impossible.

TRIGGER POINTS*

Some confusion exists about the synonymous use of the terms neuromuscular therapy and trigger point therapy. Neuromuscular therapy is an umbrella term that encompasses a variety of treatment approaches, one of which is trigger point therapy. Trigger point therapy is one of many techniques useful in the treatment of neuromuscular and myofascial problems.

A **trigger point** is an area of local nerve facilitation and chemical imbalance of a muscle that is aggravated by stress of any sort affecting the body or mind of the individual. Trigger points are small areas of hyperirritability within muscles (Box 13-1). If these areas are located near motor nerve points, the person may experience referred pain caused by nerve stimulation. The area of the trigger point is often the motor point where nerve stimulation initiates a contraction in a small, sensitive bundle of muscle fibers that in turn activates the entire muscle.

A trigger point area is typically located in a tight band of muscle fibers. Palpation across the band may elicit a twitch response, which is a slight jump in the muscle fibers. This is difficult to detect when the trigger point is in the deeper muscle layers. Any of the more than 400 muscles in the body can develop trigger points. Trigger points are accompanied by the characteristic referred pain pattern and the restriction of motion associated with neuromuscular and myofascial pain.

With classic trigger points, the referred pain pattern can be traced to its site of origin. The distribution of the referred trigger point pain does not usually follow an entire distribution of a peripheral nerve or dermatomal segment.

PERPETUATING FACTORS

Perpetuating factors in the development of trigger points are reflexive, mechanical, and systemic. Reflexive perpetuating factors include:
- Skin sensitivity in the area of the trigger point
- Joint dysfunction
- Visceral dysfunction in the viscerally referred pain pattern
- Vasoconstriction

---

*Recommended text for trigger point therapy: Chaitow L, Delany J: *Clinical applications of neuromuscular techniques,* vols 1 and 2, the upper body, London, 2000, Churchill Livingstone.

| Box 13-1 | THEORY OF TRIGGER POINT FORMATION |

The following progression has been proposed to explain the formation of trigger points:

Dysfunctional motor endplate activity occurs, commonly associated with a strain, overuse, or direct trauma.

Stored calcium is released at the site as a result of overuse or tearing of the sarcoplasmic reticulum.

Acetylcholine (Ach) is released excessively at the synapse because of calcium-charged gates.

High calcium levels present at the site keep the calcium-charged gates open, and Ach continues to be released.

Ischemia develops in the area and creates an oxygen/nutrient deficit.

A local energy crisis develops.

The tissue is unable to remove the calcium ions without available adenosine triphosphate (ATP); therefore Ach continues flowing.

Removal of the superfluous calcium requires more energy than sustaining a contracture; therefore the contracture remains.

The contracture is sustained not by action potentials from the spinal cord but by the chemistry at the innervation site.

The actin/myosin filaments slide to a fully shortened position (a weakened state) in the immediate area around the motor endplate (at the center of the fiber).

As the sarcomeres shorten, a contracture knot forms.

The contracture knot is the "nodule," which is the palpable characteristic of a trigger point.

The remainder of the sarcomeres of that fiber are stretched, thereby creating the usually palpable taut band that also is a common trigger point characteristic.

Attachment trigger points may develop at the attachment sites of these shortened tissues (periosteal, myotendinous) where the muscular tension provokes inflammation.

From Chaitow L, Delany J: *Clinical applications of neuromuscular techniques,* vol 1, *The upper body,* London, 2000, Churchill Livingstone.

Mechanical perpetuating factors include:
- Standing postural distortion
- Seated postural distortion
- Gait distortion
- Immobilization
- Vocational stress (this includes sport activity)
- Restrictive or ill-fitting clothing and shoes

Systemic perpetuating factors include:
- Enzyme dysfunction
- Metabolic and endocrine dysfunction
- Chronic infection
- Dietary insufficiencies
- Psychological stress

ASSESSMENT

It often is difficult to decide whether a tender spot is really a trigger point, a point of fascial adhesion requiring friction, a motor point, or some other irritable reflex point, including an active acupuncture point. Because stretching of trigger point areas is essential for effective treatment, if doubt exists regarding the nature of the point, it should be treated as a trigger point. The stretching can be longitudinal or direct.

The massage therapist usually finds trigger points during palpation or general massage using both light and deep palpation (Box 13-2).

The client is aware of the trigger point but does not initiate protective mechanisms such as guarding (tightening up), breath holding, or flinching during assessment or treatment. The muscle must be relaxed to be assessed effectively. If the pressure is too great, severe local pain may overwhelm the referred pain sensation, making accurate evaluation impossible. Trigger points are so active that referred pain is already being produced; therefore there is no need for exaggerated pressure during assessment.

Box 13-2   PALPATION FOR TRIGGER POINTS

In performing light palpation, the therapist may notice trigger points from the following responses:

Skin changes: The skin may feel tense with resistance to gliding strokes. The skin may be slightly damp as a result of perspiration from sympathetic facilitation, and the therapist's hand will stick or drag on the skin.

Temperature changes: The temperature in a local area increases in acute dysfunction but decreases in ischemia, which indicates fibrotic changes within the tissues.

Edema: Edema is an impression of fullness and congestion within the tissues. In instances of chronic dysfunction, edema is replaced gradually with fibrotic (connective tissue) changes.

Deep palpation: During palpation, the therapist establishes contact with the deeper fibers of the soft tissues and explores them for any of the following:

Immobility
Tenderness
Edema
Deep muscle tension
Fibrotic changes
Interosseous changes

From Fritz S: *Mosby's fundamentals of therapeutic massage,* ed 3. St. Louis, 2004, Mosby.

Palpation for trigger points can aggravate their referred pain activity. Therefore, only muscles that can actually be treated at the same visit should be examined (Figure 13-16).

METHODS OF TREATMENT

Trigger point treatment should not be done for extended periods. It should be incorporated into a more general approach, such as the general protocol in Chapter 14.

All the basic neuromuscular techniques, including muscle energy methods, deal effectively with trigger points if the hyperirritable area within a muscle is hyperstimulated and then lengthened, and the connective tissue in the area is softened and stretched. Direct manipulation of proprioceptors by pushing or pulling on a muscle belly or its attachments is also effective. Positional release with the appropriate stretching is one of the most effective ways to treat trigger points.

After a trigger point has been identified, the massage therapist uses a pressure technique, muscle energy, or a direct manipulation and stretch method to reduce hyperactivity in the point. Intervention progresses from least invasive to most aggressive. Positional release is used first. Positional release consists of identifying the painful point and positioning the body in the easiest position that reduces the pain at the point. Positional release is the first step in the integrated muscle energy method, which introduces muscle contraction before lengthening.

Direct manipulation methods consist of pressing the belly of the muscle together to affect spindle cells and pushing the tendons apart to affect tendon receptors (Figure 13-17). If the belly of the muscle is pressed together and the desired effect is not experienced, the next step should be to separate the tissue from the middle of the muscle belly toward the tendons. Lengthening and direct manipulation are the least invasive and gentlest methods and should be used next. The integrated muscle energy method is more aggressive than positional release or direct manipulation but less aggressive than pressure or pinching methods and should be used next. These methods often are effective and are worth trying before the more intense pressure or pinching techniques.

The local area must be lengthened. This lengthening is performed either directly on the tissues or through movement of a joint.

If the trigger point remains after the less invasive methods have been attempted, pressure techniques can be tried. The pressure may take the form of direct pressure, in which the trigger point is

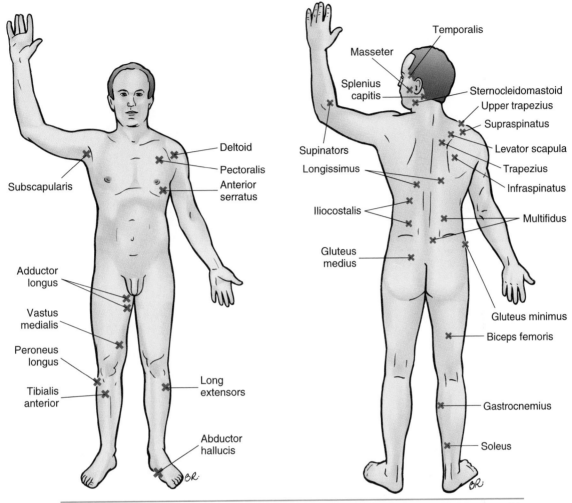

FIGURE 13-16 ■ Common trigger points. (From Fritz S: *Mosby's fundamentals of therapeutic massage,* ed 3. St. Louis, 2004, Mosby.)

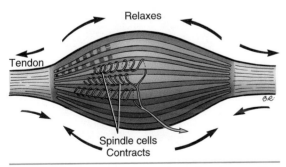

FIGURE 13-17 ■ Direct manipulation of proprioceptors. (From Fritz S: *Mosby's fundamentals of therapeutic massage,* ed 3. St. Louis, 2004, Mosby.)

pressed by the therapist against an underlying hard structure (bone), or pinching pressure, when no bony tissue lies underneath, as in the "squeezing" of the sternocleidomastoid muscle (Figure 13-18).

Pressure techniques can end the hyperirritability by mechanical disruption of the sensory nerve endings mediating the trigger point activity. When using the direct pressure technique, the massage therapist must hold the compression long enough to stimulate the spindle cells.

After the trigger has been located, the time of applied pressure will be different from the time used to locate the trigger. Dr. Chaitow recommends gradually intensifying pressure, building up to 8 seconds, and then repeating the process for up to 30 seconds or as long as 2 minutes. The procedure should end when the client reports that the referred

FIGURE 13-18

EXAMPLES OF TRIGGER POINT PRESSURE AND PINCHING METHODS

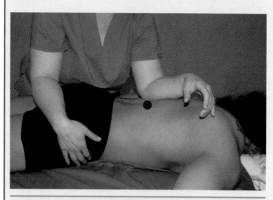

A Direct pressure, posterior serratus inferior.

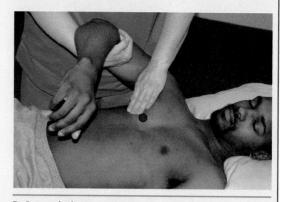

B Positional release, anterior serratus.

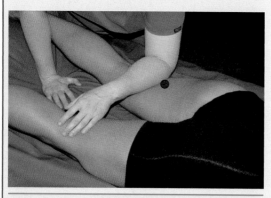

C Direct pressure against bone, hamstring.

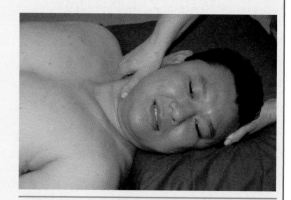

D Pinching pressure for trigger point, sternocleidomastoid.

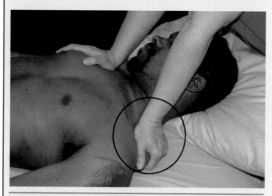

E Local stretching of trigger points.

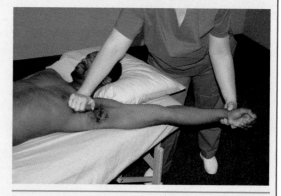

F Joint movement and direct local stretching of trigger point.

pain has stopped or when the massage therapist feels a "release" in the trigger point tissue.

Sufficient duration is determined by the fiber construction of the muscle. Muscles are made up of red (slow-twitch) fibers and white (fast-twitch) fibers. The type of fiber is determined by whether the muscle functions as a postural (stabilizer) muscle or a phasic (mover) muscle and by the demands exerted by the client's lifestyle. It is easier to fatigue phasic muscle fibers than postural muscle fibers. After the muscle is fatigued, a period of recovery ensues in which the fibers will not contract, and the muscle can be lengthened effectively and stretched if necessary.

Dr. Chaitow also recommends variable pressure, rather than constantly held pressure from beginning to end, to avoid further irritation of the trigger area. This is a carefully changing pressure for a specific purpose, which reflects the therapist's sensitivity to what is happening as the tissue responds; the therapist applies more pressure as the tissue shows that it is relaxing and accepting more pressure. When the massage therapist senses that the tissues are becoming tense, pressure is decreased.

As an alternative, deep cross-fiber friction over the trigger point can be effective, followed by lengthening and stretching. This method is beneficial if the massage therapist suspects that the connective tissue around the trigger point has become fibrotic.

Localized treatment of the muscle should always end with lengthening and stretching, either passive or active, of the affected muscle. Gradual, gentle lengthening to reset the normal resting length of the neuromuscular mechanism of a muscle and stretching to elongate shortened connective tissue of the involved muscle must follow any other interventions. Incomplete restoration of the full length of the muscle means incomplete relief of pain. Failure to lengthen and stretch the area results in the eventual return of the original symptoms.

Muscle energy approaches are more effective than passive stretching in achieving the proper response. Trigger points located in deep layers of muscle or in a muscle that is difficult to lengthen by moving the body are addressed with local bending, shearing, and torsion to lengthen and stretch the local area. This is often the most effective method with athletes.

Trigger points in the belly of muscles are usually short, concentrically contracted muscles. Trigger points located near the attachments are usually found in eccentric patterns in long inhibited muscles acting as antagonists to concentrically contracted muscles. Muscle shortening may serve as a response for compensation purposes. Do not treat attachment trigger points; only monitor them. It is best to address trigger point activity in the short tissues first and wait to see if the trigger points in the "long muscles" and at the attachments resolve as the posture of muscle interaction normalizes. Only treat attachment points if tissue remains fibrotic.

Do not overtreat trigger points. Only address the trigger points that recreate or recognize symptoms that the client is experiencing. Remember, anything can feel like a trigger point if pressed hard enough. Only address the trigger point that is most painful, most medial, and most proximal that recreates the client's symptoms. Leave the rest alone. When the posture and function normalize with regular massage, the trigger points will go away on their own.

To balance the long inhibited muscles, the following strengthening procedures can be used.

Isometric Contraction. The muscle is placed in a specific position within its range and the client contracts against resistance, without any actual movement taking place. This is particularly useful in maintaining strength in a muscle that cannot be exercised normally, due to dysfunction in its associated joint. The strengthening effect is greatest in the middle and inner range of movement.

Concentric Movements. This is the most common type of muscle-strengthening activity and involves the contraction and shortening of a muscle by taking it through its active range of movement with a weighted resistance. For example, the biceps muscle concentrically contracts when lifting a weight, by flexing the elbow.

A muscle produces its greatest force in the midrange. If the muscle is only strengthened in the midrange, it will only function in that range and may become chronically short. Therefore it is important to always include exercises with light resistance through the fullest range of both concentric and eccentric function to develop length as well.

The movements should be made slowly to develop control throughout the contraction range. Sudden, quick contractions can lead to injury and are likely to increase muscle tension by overstimulating the nerve receptors.

FIGURE 13-19

MOBILIZATION WITH MOVEMENT ON FINGER

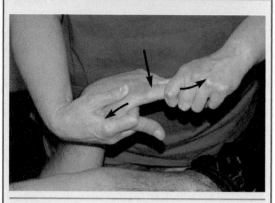

A Traction.

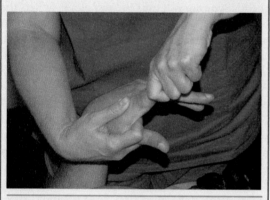

B Ease position.

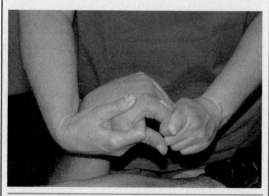

C Assisted movement back and forth.

JOINT PLAY

Synovial joints provide both stability and mobility. Synovial joints are constructed in such a way that there is an inherent movement of the bones inside the joint capsule. This is called **joint play**. It is not uncommon for this natural small movement to become reduced.

In general, all synovial joints have one bone end concave and one convex. The position of the ends of the bones in the joint capsule is a factor in the efficiency of the joint function. Especially with athletes, optimal joint action is necessary, so if the fit of the bone ends is a bit off, this can influence performance. Also, athletes are more likely to get bangs and bumps that jar and jam the joints.

Working with specific joint function is beyond the scope of practice for therapeutic massage and best left in the care of medical team personnel, such as the trainer.

One method that can be used as part of massage to influence proper joint play is an indirect functional technique called **mobilization with movement.** This gentle method uses the ease position of a joint combined with active movement by the client to settle the joint into a more functional position.

To use this method there needs to be a thorough understanding of individual joint structure, the close-packed and loose-packed position of each joint, and the normal range of motion of each joint (Table 13-1).

Before using this method, all soft tissues (muscle, tendons, ligaments), need to be as relaxed and pliable as appropriate to maintain joint stability and produce joint movement.

During assessment, the typical verbage used by the athletic client is "stuck." The client will usually be able identify the stuck area and will describe an event such as jamming fingers while catching a ball, falling, being hit, stepping down hard, stepping in a hole, and so forth, as the cause of the injury.

This method should not cause pain at any time.

Protocol for Mobilization with Movement (Figure 13-19)

1. Normalize all tissue surrounding the joint.
2. Position joint in least-packed position (typically the middle range of motion).
3. Stabilize the most proximal end of the joint and gently pull a straight line traction. Remember, no pain.

4. Maintain the traction while introducing movement in a different direction—up, down–back, forth–rotation, diagonal. Identify the direction of the most ease.
5. Maintain this position, especially the traction, and instruct the client to move the joint through the range of motion. The action of the muscles should pull the joint back into a more functional fit.

If the client is unable to move the joint (including when sleeping), modify the technique by only creating traction and then passively move the joint through pain-free and normal range of motion.

REFLEXOLOGY

Reflexology applies the stimulus/reflex principle to healing the body (Figure 13-20). The foot has been mapped to show the areas to contact to affect different parts of the body. Charts mapping the foot and body relationship areas vary somewhat, but typically, the large toe represents the head, and the junction of the large toe and the foot represents the neck. The other toes represent the eyes, ears, and sinuses. The waist is located about midway on the arch of the foot, with various organs above and below the line. The reflex points for the spine are along the medial longitudinal arch.

It is thought that this stimulus/response reflex is conducted through neural pathways in the body that activate the body's electrical and biochemical activities (Figure 13-21). There is no scientific documentation of this method. It has however consistently showed up in various forms in historical literature. The most thoroughly documented system is in Chinese medicine.

Athletes appreciate having their feet massaged and it does no harm to include these methods.

The foot is a very complex structure. The ankle and foot consist of 34 joints, with many joint and reflex patterns and with extensive nerve distribution. The position of the foot sends considerable postural information from the joint mechanoreceptors through the central nervous system. The sensory and motor centers of the brain devote a large area to the foot and hand.

It is logical to assume that stimulation of the feet activates the responses of the gate control mechanism and hyperstimulation analgesia, with activation of the parasympathetic autonomic nervous system. Many nerve endings on the feet and hands correlate with acupressure points, which, when

TABLE 13-1	LEAST-PACKED POSITIONS OF JOINTS
JOINT(S)	POSITION
Spine	Midway between flexion and extension
Temporomandibular	Mouth slightly open
Glenohumeral	55° abduction, 30° horizontal adduction
Acromioclavicular	Arm resting by side in normal physiologic position
Sternoclavicular	Arm resting by side in normal physiologic position
Elbow	70° flexion, 10° supination
Radiohumeral	Full extension and full supination
Proximal radioulnar	70° flexion, 35° supination
Distal radioulnar	10° supination
Wrist	Neutral with slight ulnar deviation
Carpometacarpal	Midway between abduction/adduction and flexion/extension
Thumb	Slight flexion
Interphalangeal	Slight flexion
Hip	30° flexion, 30° abduction and slight lateral rotation
Knee	25° flexion
Ankle	10° plantar flexion, midway between maximum inversion or eversion
Subtalar	Midway between extremes of range of motion
Midtarsal	Midway between extremes of range of motion
Tarsometatarsal	Midway between extremes of range of motion
Metatarsophalangeal	Neutral
Interphalangeal	Slight flexion

From Magee DJ: *Orthopedic physical assessment*, ed 4. Philadelphia, 2002, Saunders.

stimulated, trigger the release of endorphins and other endogenous chemicals. In addition, major plexuses for the lymph system are located in the hands and feet. Rhythmic compressive forces in these areas stimulate lymphatic movement. Body-wide effects result

METHODS OF MASSAGE FOR THE FOOT

An excellent way to massage the foot is to apply pressure and movement systematically to the entire foot and ankle complex. The pressure stimulates the circulation, nerves, and reflexes. Moving all the

FIGURE 13-20

EXAMPLES OF REFLEXOLOGY

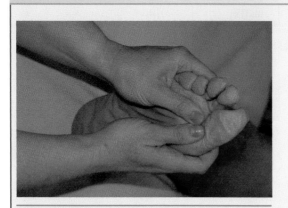

A Neck area.

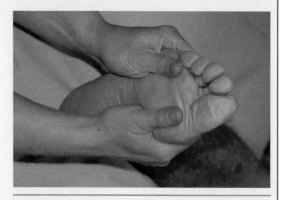

B Lungs and stomach.

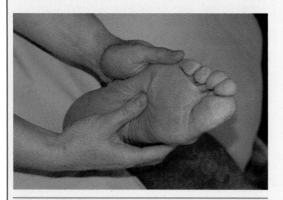

C Liver (right) or heart (left).

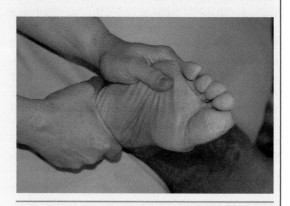

D Shoulder.

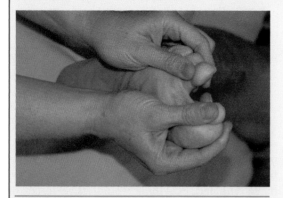

E Sinuses.

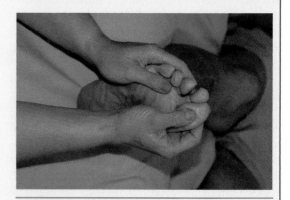

F Hypothalamus, pituitary.

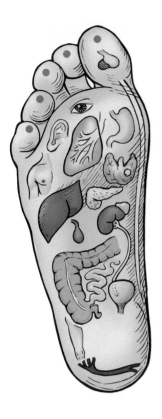
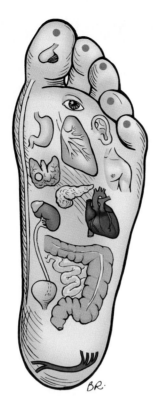

FIGURE 13-21 ■ Generalized reflexology chart. (From Fritz S: *Mosby's fundamentals of therapeutic massage,* ed 3. St. Louis, 2004, Mosby.)

joints stimulates large-diameter nerve fibers and joint mechanoreceptors, initiating hyperstimulation analgesia. The result is a shift in proprioceptive and postural reflexes. The sheer volume of sensory information flooding the central nervous system has significant effects in the body that support parasympathetic dominance. Athletes need effective foot massage. Do not skimp in this area (Figure 13-22).

TRADITIONAL CHINESE MEDICINE

YIN AND YANG

The Chinese perspective considers body functions in terms of balance between complementary forces. These complementary forces, which are often thought of as opposites, are actually a portion of a continuum. **Yin** and **yang** are representations of this concept.

The body physiologically is a closed system. There cannot be areas of "too much" energy in the body without reciprocal areas of "not enough" energy. Just as muscles work in pairs and facilitate and inhibit each other, so do meridians. The tool that helps to make sense of the complex interrelationships in the body is the theory of yin and yang.

The yin/yang theory is a way to recognize and define patterns within highly complex, dynamic systems. It is a tool for perceiving order within supposed chaos and for allowing recognition of patterns of imbalance.

The body can be described in terms of yin and yang: for example, back and front, upper and lower, external and internal. Each part of the body can be further subdivided into yin and yang parts. The internal organs are described as yin/yang characteristics according to their nature and function. Yin and yang manifest in all aspects of the body, interior and exterior interdependently related, allowing internal imbalances to be treated by working externally on the body.

ACUPUNCTURE AND ACUPRESSURE

Acupressure is a modified version of acupuncture that substitutes pressure for needle insertion. The results of acupressure are not as dramatic as those of acupuncture but are still effective, especially if the technique is repeated often with the pressure held long enough. Acupressure has a role in sports massage as an adjunct to the general protocol. It is especially helpful in systemic dysfunction such as a cold or general fatigue.

FIGURE 13-22

METHODS OF MASSAGE FOR FOOT

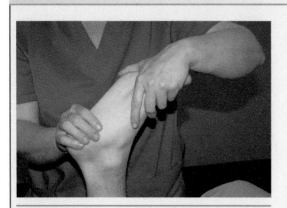

A Move joints.

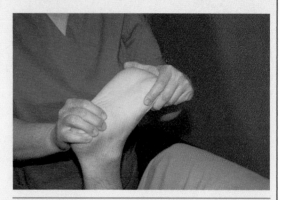

B Stretch.

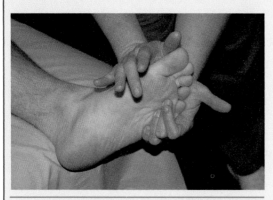

C Eversion/inversion.

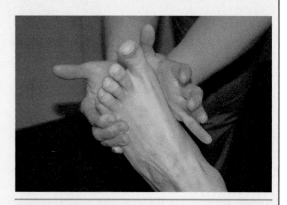

D Eversion/inversion.

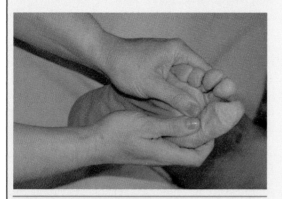

E Point compression to reflex areas.

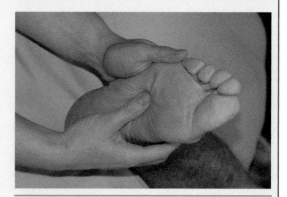

F Direct pressure to muscles.

FIGURE 13-22 CONT'D

METHODS OF MASSAGE FOR FOOT

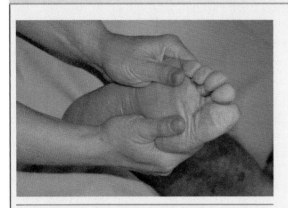

G Stretch and compress.

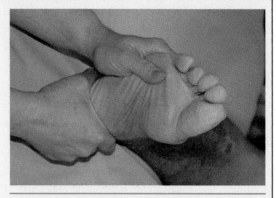

H Stretch, including plantar fascia.

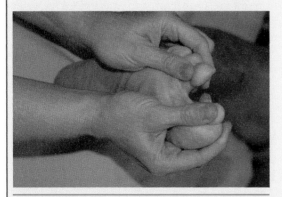

I Toe stretch.

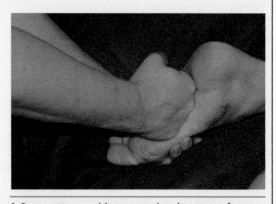

J Prone position—mobilize metatarsals and compress soft tissue.

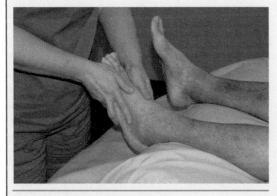

K Supine position—mobilize metatarsals.

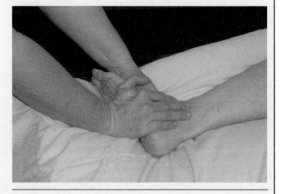

L Compression and mobilization.

Traditional Chinese medicine methods are valued for sound physiologic reasons. It is possible to demonstrate particular effects after acupuncture treatment. Some of these effects involve alteration of the function of organs or systems. There is an analgesic effect and also an anesthetic effect for those that find the physiology of these approaches difficult. It is not necessary to believe that imbalance between yin and yang (the two equal and opposite forces of the universe, which act through qi) causes disease. Instead, the acupuncture benefit can be framed in terms of the body's homeostatic tendency, whereby a stable internal environment is maintained through the interaction of the various body processes and systems.

Stimulating local points is the most basic use of acupressure and probably the most easily accessible for those accustomed to Western methods of treatment. This is, however, only a small part of an ancient system of medical practice that includes needling, herbal therapy, manipulation, exercise, massage, and meditation. Many athletes regularly use these methods.

MERIDIANS

The patterns that **acupuncture points** make on the body's surface have been charted for centuries by practitioners of acupuncture. They have been grouped together in lines called channels, or **meridians**, and have been allocated to the organs or functions upon which they appear to act. In addition to the 12 pairs of bilateral meridians, two meridians lie on the anterior and posterior midline of the trunk and head. Various extra meridians appear to be related to the body's organs and functions. Other points in the ear surfaces, hands, and face have specific reflex effects.

According to tradional Chinese medicine theory, the meridians are internally associated with organs and externally associated with the surface of the head, trunk, and extremities. Meridians seem to be energy flows from nerve tracts in the tissue and are located in the fascial grooves.

There are yin meridians, or channels, and yang meridians, or channels. Yin meridians are associated with parasympathetic autonomic nervous system responses and functions of the solid organs essential to life (e.g., the heart). Yin meridians are located on the inside soft areas of the body and flow from the feet up (Chinese anatomic position with arms lifted into the air).

Yang meridians are associated with sympathetic autonomic nervous system responses and hollow organs whose functions are supportive to life but not essential (e.g., the stomach). Chinese philosophy teaches that a balance must exist between the forces of yin and yang for health to exist. This balance changes according to the weather, seasons, and other rhythms of nature (Figure 13-23).

THE 12 MAIN MERIDIANS

The 12 main meridians are bilateral, symmetrically distributed lines of acupuncture points with affinity for, or effects upon, the functions or organs for which they are named (Box 13-3).

Clinically abundant evidence indicates the existence of reflex links between acupuncture points and specific organs and functions. In fact, no one really knows what an acupuncture point is. There is also a large body of information about acupuncture points, including their nature, structure, function, interrelationships, and interactions, as well as the experience derived from thousands of years of using acupuncture points to treat illness.

The human body has hundreds of acupuncture points. Approximately 360 of the most used points are located on 12 paired and two unpaired centrally located meridians.

METHODS OF TREATMENT USING ACUPUNCTURE POINTS AND MERIDIANS

Acupuncture points and meridians usually lie in a fascial division between muscles and near origins and insertions. A point feels like a small hole, and pressure elicits a "nervy" feeling. Unlike a trigger point, which may be found only on one side of the body, acupuncture meridian points are bilateral (i.e., found on both sides of the body) or may also be located on the central (anterior midline extending up to the mandibular gums) or governing (posterior midline extending over the top of the head to the maxillary gums) meridians. To confirm the location of an acupuncture point, locate the point in the same place on the other side of the body.

The following principles are used (Figure 13-24):
• Light massage of the meridian
• Light or deep massage of a point

To stimulate a hypoactive (not enough energy) acupuncture point, use a short vibrating or tapping action. This method is used if the area is sluggish or if a specific body function needs stimulation.

To sedate a hyperactive (too much energy) acupuncture point for pain reduction, elicit the

| Box 13-3 | THE 12 MAIN MERIDIANS AND NUMBERS OF ACUPUNCTURE POINTS THAT COMPRISE THE MERIDIANS |

Lung (L) meridian (yin) begins on the lateral aspect of the chest, in the first intercostal space. It then passes up the anterolateral aspect of the arm to the root of the thumbnail. 11 points.

Pathologic symptoms: Fullness in the chest, cough, asthma, sore throat, colds, chills, and aching of the shoulders and back.

Large intestine (LI) meridian (yang) starts at the root of the fingernail of the first finger. It passes down the posterolateral aspect of the arm over the shoulder to the face. It ends at the side of the nostril. 20 points.

Pathologic symptoms: Abdominal pain, diarrhea, constipation, nasal discharge, and pain along the course of the meridian.

Stomach (ST) meridian (yang) starts below the orbital cavity and runs over the face and up to the forehead, then passes down the throat, thorax, and the abdomen and continues down the anterior thigh and leg to end at the root of the second toenail (lateral side). 45 points.

Pathologic symptoms: Bloat, edema, vomiting, sore throat, and pain along the course of the meridian.

Spleen (SP) meridian (yin) originates at the medial aspect of the great toe. It travels up the internal aspect of the leg and thigh to the abdomen and thorax, where it finishes on the axillary line in the sixth intercostal space. 21 points.

Pathologic symptoms: Gastric discomfort, bloating, vomiting, weakness, heaviness of the body, and pain along the course of the meridian.

Heart (H) meridian (yin) begins in the axilla and runs up the antermedial aspect of the arm to end at the root of the little fingernail (medial aspect). 9 points.

Pathologic symptoms: Dry throat, thirst, cardiac area pain, pain along the course of the meridian.

Small intestine (SI) meridian (yang) starts at the root of the small fingernail (lateral aspect) and travels down the posteromedial aspect of the arm and over the shoulder to the face, where it terminates in front of the ear. 19 points.

Pathologic symptoms: Pain in the lower abdomen, deafness, swelling in the face, sore throat, and pain along the course of the meridian.

Bladder (B) meridian (yang) starts at the inner canthus, then ascends and passes over the head and down the back and the leg to terminate at the root of the nail of the little toe (lateral aspect). 67 points.

Pathologic symptoms: Urinary problems, mania, headaches, eye problems, pain along the course of the meridian.

Kidney (K) meridian (yin) starts on the sole of the foot. It ascends the medial aspect of the leg and runs up the front of the abdomen to finish on the thorax just below the clavicles. 27 points.

Pathologic symptoms: Dyspnea, dry tongue, sore throat, edema, constipation, diarrhea, motor impairment and atrophy of the lower extremities, pain along the course of the meridian.

Circulation (C) meridian (yin) (also known as heart constrictor or the pericardium) begins on the thorax lateral to the nipple. It runs up the anterior surface of the arm and terminates at the root of the nail of the middle finger. 9 points.

Pathologic symptoms: Angina, chest pressure, heart palpitations, irritability, restlessness, pain along the course of the meridian.

Triple-heater (TH) meridian (yang) begins at the nail root of the ring finger (ulnar side) and runs down the posterior aspect of the arm, over the back of the shoulder, and around the ear to finish at the outer aspect of the eyebrow. 23 points.

Pathologic symptoms: Abdominal distortion, edema, deafness, tinnitus, sweating, sore throat, pain along the course of the meridian.

Gallbladder (GB) meridian (yang) starts at the outer canthus and runs backward and forward over the head, passing over the back of the shoulder and down the lateral aspect of the thorax and abdomen. It passes to the hip area and then down the lateral aspect of the leg to terminate on the fourth toe. 44 points.

Pathologic symptoms: Bitter taste in mouth, dizziness, headache, ear problems, pain along the course of the meridian.

Liver (LIV) meridian (yin) begins on the great toe, runs up the medial aspect of the leg, up the abdomen, and terminates on the costal margin (vertically below the nipple). 14 points.

Pathologic symptoms: Lumbago, digestive problems, retention of urine, pain in lower abdomen, pain along the course of the meridian.

Midline Meridians

There are two midline meridians.

The **conception (or central) vessel (CV) meridian** (yin) starts in the center of the perineum and runs up the midline of the anterior aspect of the body to terminate just below the lower lip (24 points); it is responsible for all yin meridians.

The **governor vessel (GV) meridian** (yang) starts at the coccyx and runs up the center of the spine and over the midline of the head, terminating on the front of the upper gum (28 points); it is responsible for all yang meridians.

From Fritz S: *Mosby's fundamentals of therapeutic massage,* ed 3. St. Louis, 2004, Mosby.

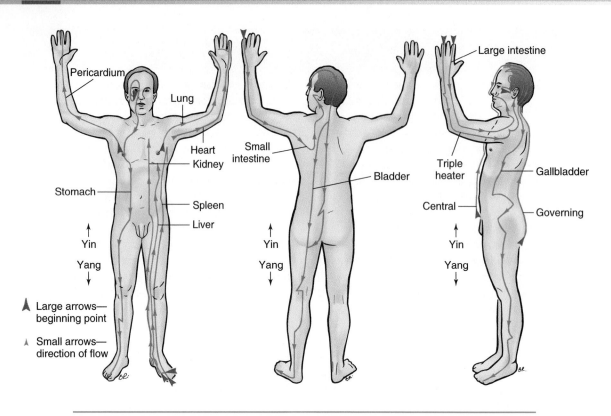

FIGURE 13-23 ■ Typical location of meridians. Meridians tend to follow nerves. Yin and yang meridians are paired as follows:

Yin Meridian	Yang Meridian
Pericardium	Triple heater
Liver	Gallbladder
Kidney	Bladder
Heart	Small intestine
Spleen	Stomach
Lung	Large intestine

(From Fritz S: *Mosby's fundamentals of therapeutic massage,* ed 3. St. Louis, 2004, Mosby.)

pain response within the point itself. Use a sustained holding pressure until the painful excess energy dissipates and the body's own natural painkillers are released into the bloodstream. The pressure techniques are similar to those used for trigger points, but it is not necessary to lengthen and stretch an acupuncture point after treatment.

As with other reflex points, if you are unsure as to the nature of the hypoactive or hyperactive state of the acupuncture point, alternately apply both techniques and allow the body to adjust to the intervention.

It is often difficult to determine whether you are dealing with a trigger point or an acupressure point because the two often overlap. It may be wise to

lengthen and stretch the area gently after using direct pressure methods. The process does not interfere with the effect on the acupressure point, but without it a trigger point cannot be treated effectively.

HEALTH PRESERVATION AND EXERCISE

An important part of traditional Chinese medicine is the discipline of preserving health and extending life (Figure 13-25). Foremost among the various methods that fall in this category are exercise and disciplines aimed at cultivating the inborn treasures of the body, mind, and spirit. Many can benefit from incorporating principles from these methods. These are briefly described.

FIGURE 13-24

EXAMPLES OF USING ACUPUNCTURE POINTS AND MERIDIANS IN GENERAL MASSAGE

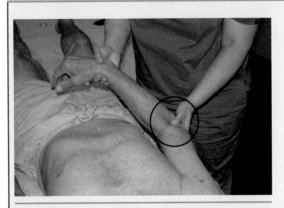

A Sedate acupuncture point with pressure (acupressure).

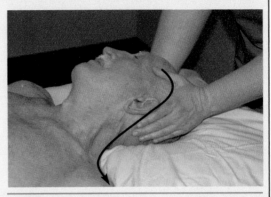

B Meridian massage: general stroking over meridian pathway supporting yin and yang energy flow.

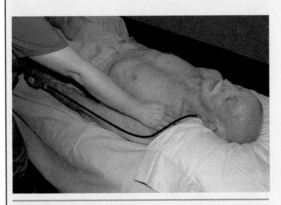

C Meridian massage—Yang flow through shoulder/arm/head.

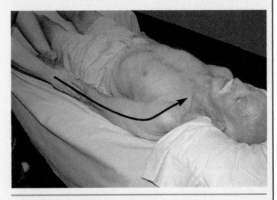

D Yang flow—arms.

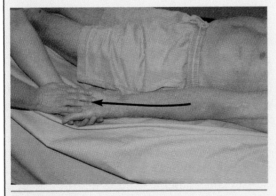

E Yin flow—arms.

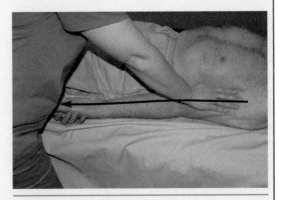

F Yin flow—hand and arms.

Continued

FIGURE 13-24 CONT'D

EXAMPLES OF USING ACUPUNCTURE POINTS AND MERIDIANS IN GENERAL MASSAGE

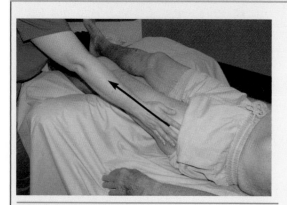

G Yang flow—legs to feet.

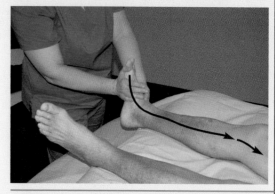

H Yin flow—foot/legs to groin.

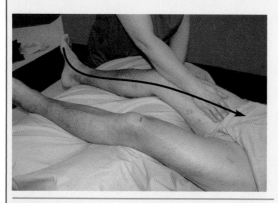

I Yin flow—legs

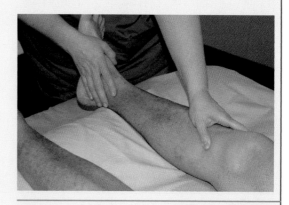

J Sedate acupuncture point with pressure (acupressure).

Qi Gong

Qi gong, or breathing exercise, refers to a variety of traditional practices consisting of physical, mental, and spiritual exercises. The regulation of the breath (qi) is a common feature of such exercise methods. The word *gong* means "achievement; result; skill; work; exercise." It is composed of two radicals. The radical on the left is also pronounced *gong* and means "work." The radical on the right is the word *li* and means "strength" or "force." Qi gong can be understood as exercise designed to strengthen and harmonize the qi, regulate the body and mind, and calm the spirit.

Tai Ji Quan

Tai ji quan (tai chi) is a martial as well as a meditative art. Thus it has complementary aspects that combine in a comprehensive discipline of physical culture and mental and spiritual discipline. The word *quan* means "fist; boxing; punch."

Dao Yin

Dao yin is a discipline involving meditation and breathing exercises that seeks to develop the ability to lead and guide the qi throughout the body for the benefit of the spirit, mind, and body. Dao yin exercises have a long history in China. They consist of bending, stretching, and otherwise mobilizing the extremities and the joints to free the flow of qi throughout the whole body. Like qi gong, dao yin emphasizes control of the breath (qi). Dao yin also includes self-massage techniques that relieve fatigue and prolong life by activating and harmonizing the circulation of blood and qi. These techniques also stress the development of strength in the muscles and bones.

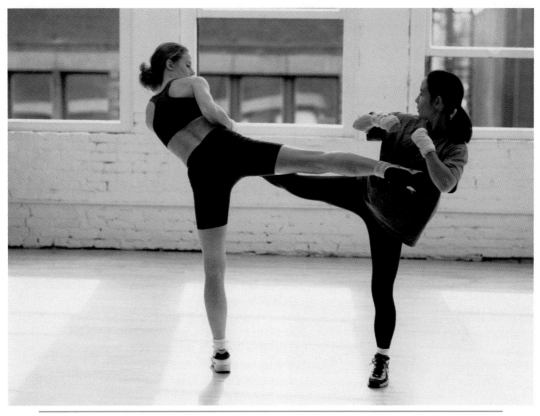

FIGURE 13-25 ■ Exercise is a core part of practicing Chinese medicine.

The vastness of the traditional Chinese medicine model and its elegance are far beyond the scope of this textbook. Therefore no attempt is made to present scaled-down versions of these systems. The reader is directed to the reference list for sources of further study.* Massage therapists who are drawn to these concepts are encouraged to explore them in depth as they continue their path of knowledge.

During the natural course of therapeutic massage, the physical aspects of meridians and points are addressed.

Following are some suggested points to use for problems in the various jointed areas of the body (Table 13-2). It is by no means an exhaustive list.

*Acupressure, Clinical Applications in Musculoskeletal Conditions, Cross R John, Butterworth-Heinemann, © Reed Educational and Professional Publishing Ltd 2000.

13-2 SPECIFIC RELEASES

These individual procedures should be done in the context of a general massage session with an awareness of whole-body compensation patterns. No single muscle functions independently. All muscles are linked into myotactic functional patterns. In order to restore optimal function, all muscles in the pattern must be addressed. Typically when changes in a muscle(s) result in hypertonicity and increased tension, corresponding antagonist patterns will be inhibited and those muscles will weaken. In order to compensate, these same antagonist patterns may also shorten and become fibrotic. The opposite also occurs. Should a muscle(s) become weakened, the antagonist patterns will increase in tension and over time shorten and become less pliable.

It is more effective to think of muscle groups in terms of functioning patterns than to consider individual muscles. Muscles function as flexors,

TABLE 13-2	AREA POINT LOCATION	
AREA	POINT	LOCATION
Hand	P8	Situated in the very middle of the palm.
Foot	Ki 1	Situated on the sole of the foot in the mid-line, two thirds of the way up from the heel.
Elbow	P3	Situated in the middle of the cubital fossa just to the lateral aspect of the biceps tendon.
Knee	Bl 40	Situated in the middle of the popliteal fossa.
Shoulder	LI 15	Situated at the anterior and inferior border of the acromioclavicular joint, inferior to the acromion, when the arm is in adduction.
Hip	GB29 and St 31	There are two points associated with the hip; GB 29 governs the lateral aspect and St 31 governs the anterior aspect. GB 29 is situated midway between the anterior superior iliac spine and the highest point of the greater trochanter of the femur; St 31 is situated directly below the anterior superior iliac spine, in a line level with the lower border of the symphysis iliac spine, in a line level with the lower border of the symphysis pubis bone.
Upper cervical spine	Gov 16	Situated in a depression directly below the occipital protuberance, in the mid-line.
Cervicothoracic spine	Gov 14	Situated between the seventh cervical vertebra and the spinous process of the first thoracic vertebra in the midline.
Thoracolumbar spine	Gov 6	Situated between the spinous processes of the twelfth thoracic and the first lumbar vertebra in the mid-line.
Lumbar spine	Gov 3	Situated between the spinous processes of L4 and L5 in the mid-line.
Sacrum and coccyx	Gov 2	Situated at the junction between the sacrum and the coccyx in the mid-line.

From Cross JR: *Acupressure: clinical applications in musculoskeletal conditions,* Philadelphia, 2000, Butterworth-Heinemann.

extensors, abductors, adductors, internal rotators, and external rotators. These actions are mostly concentrated in the extremities and at the occipital, cervical, thoracic, lumbar, and sacral junctions.

Another important consideration in muscle function is stabilization and maintenance of posture. Stabilizer muscles usually fix the joints above and below the joint being primarily moved. Muscle groups (prime mover and synergist or helpers) can function as stabilizers when the joint they move in is not the primary point of action. All of this must be considered when working with isolated and localized procedures, as described in the following section. The question that needs to be addressed is, "What is the reason for this muscle(s) being dysfunctional?" Until the entire pattern is addressed, the symptoms will continue to return.

The main method for addressing these areas is inhibiting pressure either in the muscle belly or at the attachments to reduce motor tone. These specific procedures address muscles that are often short and in the deeper tissue layers, which makes access difficult.

Remember, perform general massage before and after doing muscle releases.

Most inhibiting pressure is applied to the muscle belly unless it is easier to access the attachments. Use a 45-degree angle to exert pressure on a "hill" instead of a 90 degree contact in a "valley," unless specified as 90 degrees. If you release muscle on the left side, then be sure to release same muscle on the right side, even if it tested tight on only one side. These methods should only be used to achieve outcomes and not routinely incorporated in the massage.

SCALENES (FIGURE 13-26 AND 13-27)

Symptoms

Most symptoms relate to brachial or cervical plexus impingement with symptoms of midthoracic pain near the midscapula, and chest pain. Symptoms include arm pain that is often mistaken for carpal tunnel synrome and occasionally pain that radiates into the head behind the eye.

Assessment

The best positions for assessment are side-lying and supine. Palpate to reproduce symptoms. Systematically apply a flat pressure to the area between the

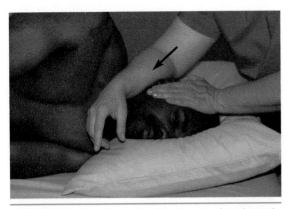

FIGURE 13-26 ■ Specific release performed on the scalenes.

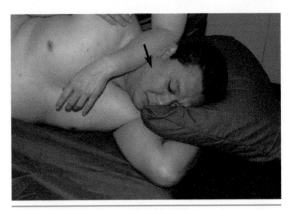

FIGURE 13-28 ■ Specific release performed on the occipital base.

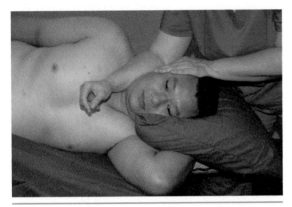

FIGURE 13-27 ■ When assessing the occipitals or sternocleidomastoids, the best position is side-lying or supine.

upper trapezius and the sternocleidomastoid. Starting at the base of the skull, work down toward the clavicles using sufficient pressure to reproduce referred pain patterns. If the pain pattern can be reproduced, the assessment is positive.

The pain is usually caused by a contracted scalene muscle in conjunction with a chain pattern often involving lumbar flexors or lateral flexion. The quadratus or psoas is often involved.

Procedure

1. Use positional release if possible, relying on the position of the lower body to achieve the position of ease.
2. Apply compression at a 45° angle to recreate the symptom. Have the client activate apposing antagonist patterns, either directly (such as the opposite scalene groups) or in the paired pattern (such as the quadratus lumborum) to initiate reciprocal inhibition. As the muscle softens, pinpoint the area of tension. This area will

appear more tense than the surrounding tissue. Then have the client use pulsed muscle energy, using both the muscle and the antagonist against the compression being held, which recreates the symptoms. Let the client rest and lighten pressure every 15 or so seconds. Resume until the tension reduces, but for no longer than 60 seconds. If the area does not release in 60 seconds, it is held by the kinetic chain compensation pattern. Work will need to focus on normalizing this pattern.
3. Once the muscle releases, lengthen it gently if acute and then stretch if the condition has been chronic. The stretching will span several sessions.
4. To stretch, keep the palpating hand in place and slowly move the head and rib cage apart until the palpating hand identifies the longest position of the muscle tissue. The tissue will feel taut in this position. Then stabilize the head and lengthen and stretch from the thorax.

OCCIPITAL BASE (FIGURE 13-28)

Procedure

1. With client in side-lying position, use forearm or foot, for broad-based compression at 45-degree angle.
2. When client rolls eyes, you should feel muscles activate; then hold position for up to total of 30 seconds.

STERNOCLEIDOMASTOID (FIGURE 13-29)

Note: If doing this release before psoas release, find out whether client needs psoas release also by using the test described on page 320.

FIGURE 13-29

SPECIFIC RELEASE PERFORMED ON THE STERNOCLEIDOMASTOID

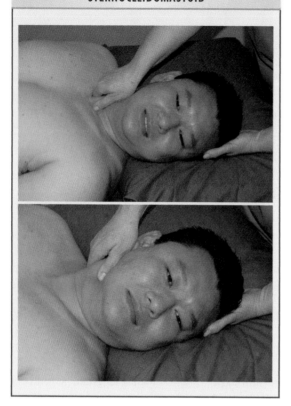

FIGURE 13-30

SPECIFIC RELEASE ON RECTUS ABDOMINIS

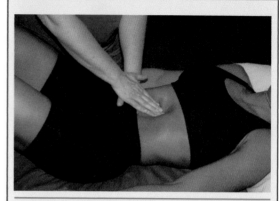

A Specific release performed on the rectus abdominis.

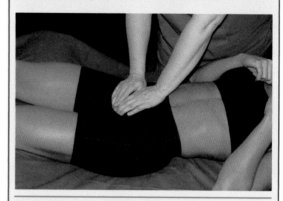

B Inhibiting pressure, symphysis pubis attachment.

Procedure

1. Place client in the supine postion slightly turned; stand above client's head.
2. Hold target muscle between thumb and fingertips and squeeze, starting superior and proceeding to inferior. Client rolls eyes; lifts and depresses chin and legs or bends knees to engage the psoas during release of sternocleidomastoid.

RECTUS ABDOMINIS (FIGURE 13-30)

Explain procedure first and get clear consent from the client because of location of inferior attachments involved. Rule out a hernia before doing this method. If you perform this release, you should also do the hamstrings.

Symptoms

Symptoms mimic those of a groin injury. This abdominal muscle tends to facilitate psoas tightening, because the other three abdominal muscles are inhibited when the rectus abdominis is tight.

Assessment

Palpation of the upper and lower attachments recreates symptoms.

Procedure

1. Start at superior attachments on the lower five ribs. Then shear muscle belly location to loosen middle of rectus abdominis muscle. Caution is required if a female client has had C-section or hysterectomy, because of scar tissue in the muscle.
2. Apply inhibiting pressure on inferior attachments above and below the symphysis pubis for 30 seconds. Work over the client's underwear and hook your fingers around the symphysis pubis for 30 seconds while client raises shoulders as if trying to do a sit-up. If you feel tendons move while client is doing this, you will know your fingers are in the right place.

HAMSTRINGS (FIGURE 13-31)

Symptoms

Pain is felt at proximal and on distal attachments, with a sense of stiffness and aching.

Assessment

Test to see if tight: Can client bend at waist and touch toes while keeping legs straight? Can client flex knees to touch toes and straighten legs?

Procedure

1. Use braced hand to apply inhibiting pressure at proximal and distal attachments. Attachments at the knee are most easily accessed when the knee is flexed.
2. Use broad-based compression on the muscle belly while the client flexes knee. The side-lying position is the most effective.

MULTIFIDI, ROTATORES, INTERTRANSVERSARII, AND INTERSPINALES (FIGURE 13-32)

As a combined group, these muscles produce small, refined movements of the vertebral column. They work in coordination, with each group of muscle fibers contributing to the entire action.

Symptoms

The client often wants to have his or her back "cracked," and yet manipulation does not provide relief. There is stiffness upon initiation of movement, but once the movement begins, the stiffness is reduced. The client is unable to stretch effectively to affect the muscle groups. Aching, as opposed to a sharp pain, is felt.

Assessment

Palpation is the only effective assessment. These are small deep muscles located between and along the edge of the vertebrae. A history of being seated or standing for extended periods of time is common. Palpation, with the client in both the prone and side-lying positions, deep into the spaces between

FIGURE 13-31
SPECIFIC RELEASE PERFORMED ON THE HAMSTRINGS

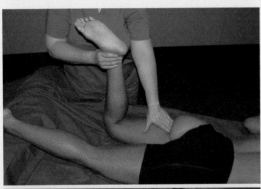

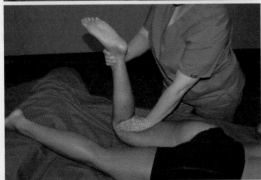

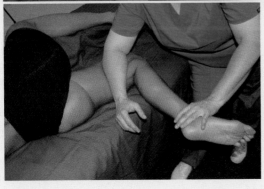

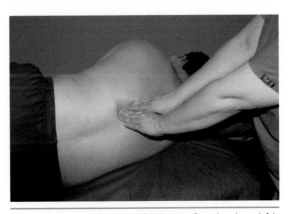

FIGURE 13-32 ■ Specific release performed on the multifidi, rotators, intertransversarii, and interspinalis.

the vertebrae reveals tough tissue bands that will replicate the symptoms. Effective palpation must go deep enough to contact the muscle group and get under the erector spine muscles.

Procedure

Meticulous frictioning of the tight muscle bands combined with tissue stretching using compression is required. Softening and lengthening of the erector spine and associated fascia is necessary before beginning this procedure.

1. Position the client in the side-lying position with the affected side up and with a small amount of passive extension. It may be necessary to get on the table or use a stool to achieve an effective mechanical advantage.
2. Angle in at 45 degrees against the groove next to the spinal column between the transverse and spinous process, using braced double thumbs or a massage tool. Sink in until you can feel the spinous processes.
3. Hold the compression firmly against the affected tissue and have the client slowly move the area back and forth from extension to flexion. Then have the client remain in a slight extension while you move down in a deep scooping action and then out, as if you were digging.
4. After the tissue has softened further, firmly hold the compression and have the client move into spinal flexion very slowly until you feel the tissue become taut, in order to stretch the area. Hold this position until the tissue softens.

SUBSCAPULARIS (FIGURE 13-33)

Symptoms

The client complains of aching or throbbing in the shoulder and upper arm. The wrist may also ache. The client may have been told that he or she has a frozen shoulder. Symptoms include pain or restriction in activities that require any form of external rotation.

Assessment

Visual assessment indicates an internally or medially rotated humerus. When the humerus is placed in external rotation and the client is instructed to move it into internal rotation, pain is usually experienced, but not always. This muscle is usually hypertonic if problems exist. It is part of the whole pattern of the body moving into a forward flexed protective and striking position. A history of over-

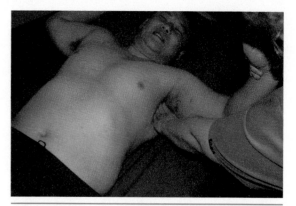

FIGURE 13-33 ■ Specific release performed on the subscapularis.

head throwing, such as in baseball or basketball, or working in horizontal abduction and flexion or over the head with back and forth movements, such as when painting, is common. This pattern of movement is stressed in activities such as driving and raking or shoveling for long periods, especially if the person is not used to the activity.

Palpation of the muscle will reproduce symptoms. With the client in the prone, supine, or side-lying position, the arm is horizontally abducted and externally rotated. Deep palpation in the groove between the latissimus to the back and the pectoralis to the front is required. Taking care to avoid the vessels in this area, weave the supported four fingers in and down at a 45-degree angle until the scapula is felt. Probe in different areas by changing the angle the hand until symptoms are reproduced.

Procedure

1. Once the area of tissue is located that reproduces the symptoms, continue to apply compression while the client moves the arm back and forth from internal to external rotation.
2. Change the position of the humerus from 90 degrees to 130 degrees to access different aspects of the movement pattern as the client moves the humerus into internal and external rotation. This movement can be active, active resisted, or passive, whichever is most effective to access the narrow band of distal attachment of the subscapularis.
3. Keep the pressure on the area and increase the movement at the end of each range to apply the stretch.

Because this is a painful procedure, give the client breaks, but do not loosen the position of the fingers. Avoid the brachial plexus.

RHOMBOID, PECTORALIS MAJOR AND MINOR, ANTERIOR SERRATUS

(FIGURE 13-34)

Symptoms

The client generally complains of pain between the scapulae and that the back feels tight and fatigued. Sometimes there may be a specific tender point or aching in the upper rhomboid area. Often a client will say that he or she is stretching the back, but actually the chest area is being stretched. Breathing is often of the upper chest pattern and/or restricted.

Assessment

The most common problem is increased tension in the pectoralis major and minor and anterior serratus. Palpate these muscle areas for tender points. Usually the client is unaware that these points exist. The scapulae will be difficult to wing, and there will be a forward roll to the shoulders. The client often presents with a history of static position of the arms forward and using small muscle action, such as in computer work. Any activity that requires pushing forward or pulling down will set up or aggravate the symptoms.

Procedure

Reducing tension and restoring length in the pectoralis and anterior serratus will relieve tension on the rhomboids. Pressure held on the tender points in the chest is often effective. If the pattern has become habitual or chronic, the fascia of the chest will need to be stretched.

1. If possible, palpate for the tender points with the client either side-lying or supine. Place one hand in the rhomboid region to feel for the interplay of the pressure applied to the chest involving the pectoralis muscles and anterior serratus. These muscles pull the scapula forward. Compress or squeeze into the area to identify the tender points.
2. Once the tender points are located, apply pressure using various angles against the area to see if a position of release can be found. If not, have the client move around slowly and repeat application of pressure. Once the position of release is located, follow the positional release or integrate the muscle energy procedure.
3. It is important to stretch the area. This is accomplished by manually moving the scapula toward the spine while the client is in the side-lying

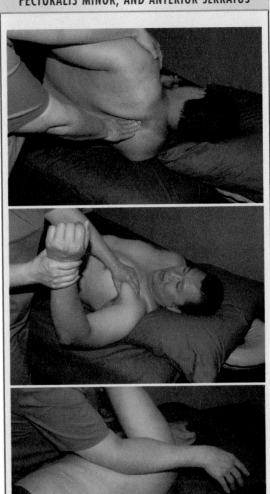

FIGURE 13-34

SPECIFIC RELEASE PERFORMED ON THE RHOMBOID, PECTORALIS MINOR, AND ANTERIOR SERRATUS

position. This is facilitated by either having the client pull the scapula together or using a firm tapotement to the rhomboid, reflexively creating a contraction reflex while pushing the scapula toward the spine.

DIAPHRAGM (FIGURE 13-35)

Symptoms

Client complains of neck and shoulder tension and an aching or pulling at the area of the

FIGURE 13-35

SPECIFIC RELEASE PERFORMED ON THE DIAPHRAGM

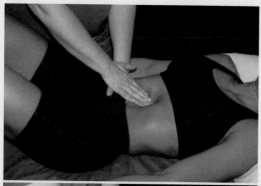

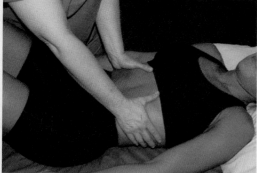

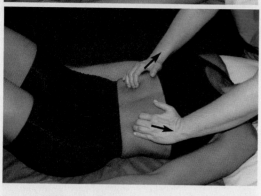

thoracolumbar junction. The symptoms get worse if anything restricts the abdomen, such as tight clothing or pulling in the stomach. Symptoms may also indicate a breathing pattern disorder.

Assessment

Perform assessment for a breathing pattern disorder. In addition, palpate the area of the diaphragm along the edge of the rib cage for tenderness or rigidity.

Procedure

A release of the diaphragm should be done in conjunction with the breathing pattern disorder, psoas, and quadratus lumborum procedures.

1. Client is supine with knees bent. Locate the edge of the rib cage and access with either an overlapping double hand with braced finger contact or with the ulnar side of the hand braced by the opposite hand.
2. While client exhales, slowly let hand sink under the ribs. When resistance is felt, have the client raise arm up and over the head, inhale, and then exhale deeply and slowly.
3. Follow the exhale, taking up any slack. The direction of the compressive force should be at an angle of about 25 degrees along and under the rib cage. Do not press directly down toward the spine. It may be helpful if the client holds the breath to the end of the exhale and, while holding the breath, attempts to push your hand out using the muscles. Be aware of extended breath holding by anyone with high blood pressure.
4. Apply a broad-based alternating rhythmic compression to the lower rib attachments, gently but firmly pushing the rib cage in and out. Do not apply pressure on the xiphoid process. Then hook fingers under ribs and gently stretch up and out.

PSOAS (FIGURE 13-36)

Symptoms

Client complains of generalized lumbar aching, aching into tops of thighs, low-back pain when coughing or sneezing, and pain when lying on stomach or flat on back.

Assessment

Gait stride is shortened, more so on the short side. Externally rotated leg is on short side. Client braces self with hands when sitting down or standing up. Leg is unable to fall into full extension, as in supine "edge of table" test below. Pelvis is anteriorly rotated on short side.

Note: A tight and/or shortened quadratus group and tensor fasciae latae are often found with psoas dysfunction and should be addressed before addressing the psoas muscles. The sternocleidomastoid is also involved.

- *Edge of table test:* Client places the ischial tuberosity on the edge of the table, bringing

FIGURE 13-36

SPECIFIC RELEASE PERFORMED ON THE PSOAS

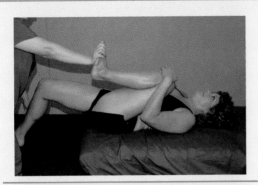

A Stretch position, supine.

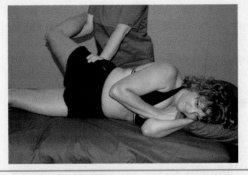

B Stretch position, side-lying.

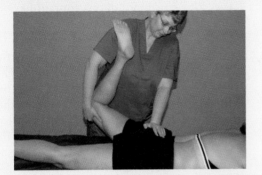

C Stretch position, prone.

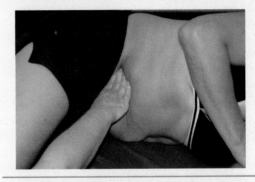

D Direct access, braced hand, side-lying.

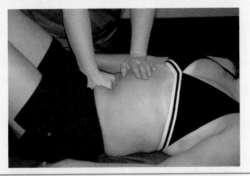

E Direct access, first, prone.

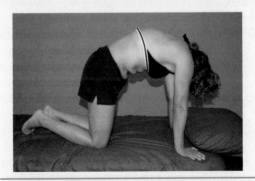

F Sway back, hunchback.

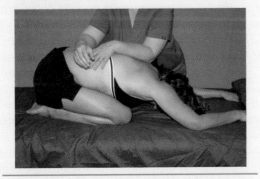

G Stretch knee/chest.

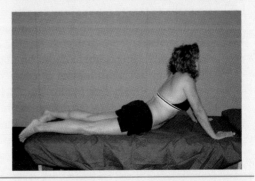

H Stretch/cobra position.

IN MY EXPERIENCE...

Nightmares

I was about three years into working with an NFL Team. Typically about the second week into training camp, and again about November during the season, there seemed to be an epidemic of low-back pain. I think that general fatigue interferes with core stability, resulting in a short psoas. While not a cure, a psoas release can relieve the symptoms at least temporarily. So it was November and it felt like I had done 50 psoas releases that day. The actual count was around 25, but it sure felt like more. Even the best body mechanics won't prevent getting tired after working with that many muscular guys in one day.

That night I had a dream that I was in the massage area at the training facility, and I had a player on the massage table. In my dream I looked down the hall and saw all these guys in different colored helmets. I asked someone who all the guys were. He replied, "It's the entire NFL; they're all here for a psoas release."

Now that was a nightmare!

one leg to the chest and rolling back to lie on the table. When the leg is held tightly to the chest the other leg should lie horizontal with the table. If it is above the table, the psoas is short.

2. Direct access to psoas using hand and/or fist
   a. Client is supine or side-lying, with knees flexed to at least 110 degrees if supine. Both feet are flat on the table. The practitioner stands on the side to be addressed. Either a flat stabilized hand or a loose fist can be used. Decision is based on size and comfort of the client. For the practitioner, the fist position will withstand a longer duration of treatment.
   b. With client side-lying and knees flexed, the practitioner kneels in front of the client and leans in, using stabilized hand or loose fist. The leg top can be used to pull the client toward the pressure.
   c. The muscle location is best accessed midline between the iliac crest and the navel and can usually be found by placing the metacarpophalangeal joint on the iliac crest. The fingers remain straight and the tips of the fingers identify the location of the muscle. This muscle is located deep against the anterior aspect of the lumbar and lower thoracic spine. Slow, deliberate compression into the lower abdomen is required. The abdominal aorta can be palpated as pulsation and also must not be compressed. The small and large intestines will

slide out of the way as downward force is exerted. Identification of the proper location can be confirmed by having the client flex the leg against resistance.

3. A flat sustained compression is applied while client slowly moves the head in large, slow circles. These actions facilitate the psoas and act as a contract/then relax of the muscle.
   a. The psoas can be inhibited by having the client activate the neck extensor by slightly tipping the chin toward the ceiling and pushing the back of the head against the table. Alternating flexion and extension of the neck is valuable while maintaining compression against the psoas. These neck actions can be supplemented with eye movement: eyes look downward during forward flexion, sideways during lateral flexion, and upward during extension.
   b. Additionally, the client can slowly slide the heel of the foot out so that the leg straightens. When the leg is straight, if the client contracts the buttocks the psoas is further inhibited. The client then relaxes the gluteal muscles and slides the heel as close to the buttocks as possible to contract the psoas. This action is repeated while the compression is maintained.

4. Release at the distal attachment: If it is difficult to access the psoas through the abdomen, inhibiting pressure near the distal attachment where the muscle crosses over the pubic bone is possible. Usually the leg is moved into an ease or bind position while the inhibiting pressure is held.

   After the release, the compression of the psoas acts to lengthen and stretch this muscle. Make sure that the client rolls first to the side and then rolls up before getting off the table. Assist client if necessary. Do not let the client sit straight up. It is best to perform the following sequence or after direct pressure on the psoas.

5. Have the client lie prone as a gentle lengthening position for this muscle. Then have the client assume a four-point position by getting on hands and knees.
   a. Have the client assume the cat or sway-back position and the camel or hunchback position.
   b. The client then slides arms in front of them and brings the buttocks back against the hamstrings. Apply broad-based compression.

FIGURE 13-37

SPECIFIC RELEASE AND STRETCH PERFORMED ON THE QUADRATUS LUMBORUM

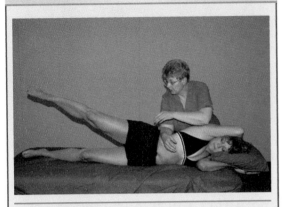

A Release quadratus.

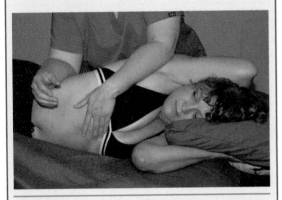

B Stretch again.

c. If the pain in the psoas is not acute, then have the client drop gently in to the cobra position by lifting the head and chest, straightening the arms, and placing the pelvis flat against the table.

e. The client assumes the hands and knees position to get off the table.

QUADRATUS LUMBORUM (FIGURE 13-37)

Symptoms

Symptoms include deep local low-back pain, which may be more intense on one side, and pain radiating into buttocks and down side of leg to knee (nerve entrapment). The client tends to wiggle or attempts to stretch with lateral trunk flexion. The client may have restricted breathing. The leg may be shorter on affected side (may be functional or physical).

Assessment

1. Place client in side-lying position. Palpate with either the forearms or hands in the space between the ribs and the iliac crest. Have the client straighten and then lift the top leg. The area being palpated should not be activated until the leg is raised more than 20 degrees. If it does, the quadratus is tense and short.
2. Have the client lie prone with legs straight and assess leg length. The short leg may indicate a tight quadratus lumborum. If lateral flexion of the torso is restricted or asymmetric, the greatest restriction will be on the short/tense side.

Procedure

1. Position client on side with bottom leg bent slightly and top leg straight and in slight hip extension.
2. While standing behind the client, apply compression into the space between the last rib and the top of the iliac crest. The angle of force is about 90 degrees (heading toward the navel). When resistance is felt in the muscle, have the client lift the top leg up and down. Make sure the hip stays in extension.
3. Alternatively, have the client move neck and head back and forth in lateral flexion and extension. Both of these moves facilitate or inhibit the quadratus lumborum muscles. These neck movements can be supplemented with side-to-side eye movements.
4. After the muscle releases it will need to be lengthened and stretched. Use a manual stretch by exerting force into the low back toward the navel and side-bending the client in extension with both the torso and the leg.
5. Self-help may include the following exercise: fingers are interlaced, palms are turned up, and arms are extended over the head. The pelvis is held stable and rolled forward while the client is standing or on knees. Side-bend and twist into slight flexion.

DEEP LATERAL HIP ROTATORS (FIGURE 13-38)

Symptoms

The foot is externally rotated. The client complains of pain deep in the gluteals, which may be in conjunction with sciatic nerve impingement.

FIGURE 13-38

SPECIFIC RELEASE PERFORMED ON THE DEEP LATERAL HIP ROTATORS

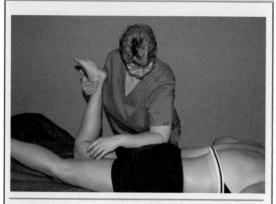

A Compression.

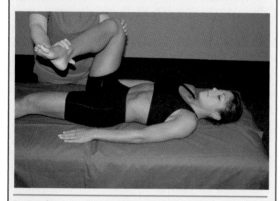

B Stretch.

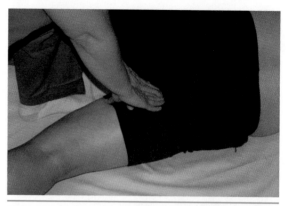

FIGURE 13-39 ■ Specific release performed on the groin area muscle attachments.

GROIN AREA MUSCLES (FIGURE 13-39)

Note: Specific consent is required due to the location of muscle attachments. Perform over clothing or draping.

Symptoms

Sensation of high groin pull, but practitioner is not able to palpate tenderness in the adductor region. Symptoms include restricted breathing, shortened stride, and contralateral shoulder pain.

Assessment

1. Assess by palpation. Have client lie on side with top leg bent and pulled up. Using the supported hand position with flat fingers, contact the ischial tuberosity from an inferior approach on the bottom and slide over it at a downward 45-degree angle, moving superiorly and medially over client's body.
2. Shift direction of force to identify tender areas that recreate symptoms. Tell the client to lift the bottom leg: if you feel the muscle move, you are on right spot.

Procedure

1. Maintain contact with the tender points that create symptoms, increase compressive force, and have client slightly extend and gently adduct bottom leg.
2. Continue pressure until you feel muscle give way and let you in deeper. Be sure to perform this procedure on both right and left sides, or client will feel unbalanced afterward when walking.

Assessment

Perform physical assessment tests for externally rotated foot. Palpate into the belly of the muscle to identify tender points that recreate symptoms.

Procedure

1. Compression with internal and external rotation of deep lateral rotators. Use forearms to apply compression while moving the hip into internal and external rotation. Incorporate muscle energy methods to facilitate release.
2. Stretching while client is in supine position. Due to the placement of the attachments, when the client is in the supine position with the hip flexed to 90 degrees, the leg is externally rotated and pulled toward the chest.

SACROILIAC (SI) JOINT AND PELVIS ALIGNMENT (FIGURE 13-40)

SI Joint

Symptoms

Client reports pain over SI joint, which increases when standing on one leg or while sleeping at night.

Assessment

Apply direct compression over SI joint to determine whether symptoms increase.

Procedure

1. Stabilize the sacrum with the hand, foot, or leg.
2. Have the client, while in the prone position, extend the hips, alternating as if walking backward.
3. In the side-lying position, move the joint by applying compression alternately at the iliac crest and ischial tuberosity to rock the joint back and forth.
4. While client is in the side-lying position, compress sacrum up and down and back and forth.

FIGURE 13-40

SPECIFIC RELEASE PERFORMED ON THE SI JOINT

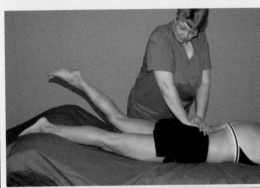
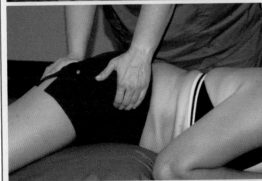
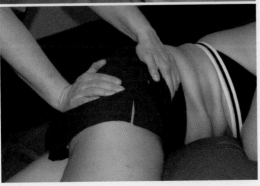

PELVIS POTATION (INDIRECT FUNCTIONAL TECHNIQUE) (FIGURE 13-41)

Symptoms

Client indicates a twisted sensation and may experience pain in the lower back, groin, or hip.

Assessment

First assess for asymmetry by comparing both anterior superior iliac spines (ASIS) while the client is in the supine position. Signs of dysfunction include:

- Bilateral anterior rotation: ASIS palpates as forward and low.
- Bilateral posture rotation: ASIS palpates as backward and high.
- Right or left anterior rotation: ASIS palpates as one low and one high.
- Right or left posterior rotation: ASIS palpates as one low and one high.
- Inflare is left, right, or bilateral: ASIS points toward midline.
- Outflare is left, right, or bilateral. ASIS palpates away from midline.

Procedure

1. **Anterior rotation:** Use leg to rotate pelvis into increased anterior rotation by bringing leg over edge of table. Have client pull leg toward shoulder. Apply moderate resistance and repeat three or four times. On final move, stretch with increasing posterior rotation.
2. **Posterior rotation:** Begin with leg bent toward shoulder, increasing posterior rotation. Have

FIGURE 13-41

EXAMPLES OF INDIRECT FUNCTIONAL TECHNIQUE FOR THE PELVIS—ANTERIOR ROTATION

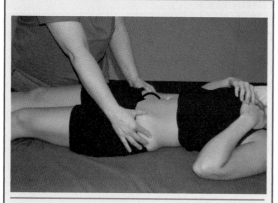

A Assess.

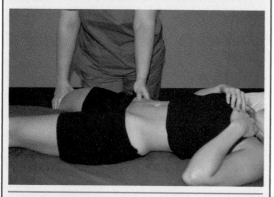

B Increase anterior rotation.

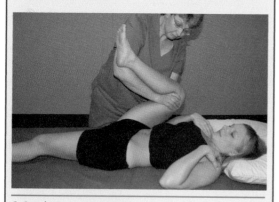

C Stretch into posterior rotation.

client push leg out and down over table. Apply moderate resistance and repeat three or four times. On final move, stretch with increasing anterior rotation.

3. **Inflare:** Position hip in flexion and internal rotation, increasing inflare. Have client push out against moderate resistance. Result is external rotation of hip. Repeat three or four times. On final move, stretch, increasing the outflare.

4. **Outflare:** Position the hip in flexion and external rotation, increasing outflare. Have client move full leg toward midline against resistance. On final move, stretch to increase inflare.

5. Regardless of the corrective procedure, reset the symphysis pubis. Place the client in the supine position, with knees and hips flexed. Have the client firmly push knees together against resistance applied by the massage therapist.

BICEPS TENDON DISPLACEMENT

(FIGURE 13-42)

Symptoms

Symptoms include pain at the biceps attachment and restriction of shoulder and arm extension. The shoulders may be rolled forward.

Assessment

The client recalls that the injury occurred when the biceps were in a slack position and then quickly extended—usually some sort of abrupt trauma.

To identify the displaced tendon, place fingers in the bicipital groove and then have client contract and relax the biceps muscle. You should feel the tendon move in the groove. If not, palpate to the medial side, because this is usually the location of the displacement, and have client contract and relax the muscle.

Procedure

1. Place biceps muscle in as much passive contraction as is necessary to create as much slack as possible. Compress into the area until fingers can wrap under the tendon and gently but firmly lift up.

2. Have the client firmly and forcibly extend the biceps muscle. This action should pull the tendon off your fingers and back into the groove. Repeat if necessary.

3. Lengthen and stretch the muscle afterward to ensure that the tendon does not pull off track again.

FIGURE 13-42

BICEPS TENDON DISPLACEMENT

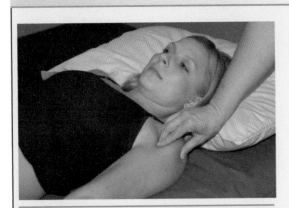

A Palpate biceps tendon.

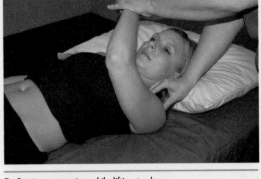

B Passive contraction while lifting tendon.

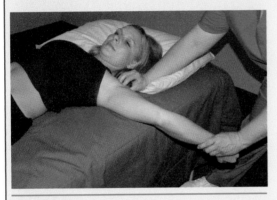

C Extend biceps.

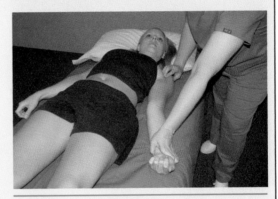

D Stretch.

SARTORIUS DISPLACEMENT (FIGURE 13-43)

Symptoms

Ability to extend the thigh from a flexed position is restricted. The movement is often described as a painful catch. The client reports pain at both attachments.

Assessment

The client may report that the injury occurred when the sartorius was in a slack position and then quickly extended—usually some sort of abrupt trauma.

To identify the displaced tendon, place fingers at the attachment point on the lateral side of the anterior superior iliac spine and then have client contract and relax the sartorius muscle. You should feel the tendon moving. If not, palpate to the medial side, because this is usually the location of the displacement and have client contract and relax muscle.

Procedure

1. Place sartorius muscle in as much passive contraction as is necessary to create as much slack as possible. Compress into the area until fingers can wrap under the tendon, and gently but firmly lift it up.
2. Have the client firmly and forcibly externally rotate hip and extend the sartorius muscle. This action should pull the tendon off your fingers and back into the groove. Repeat if necessary.
3. Lengthen and stretch the muscle afterward to ensure that the tendon does not pull off track again.

FIGURE 13-43

SARTORIUS DISPLACEMENT PROCEDURE

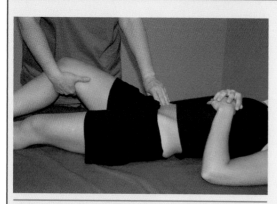

A Assess for position of attachment.

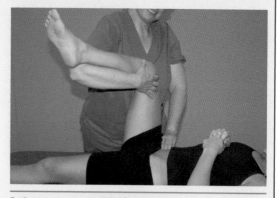

B Passive contraction while lifting tendon.

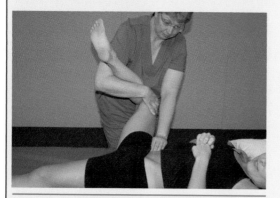

C Extend through resistance.

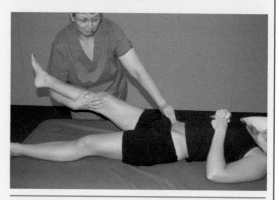

D Stretch.

SUMMARY

The applications discussed in this chapter are usually incorporated into the general massage protocol described in Chapter 14. These methods are intervention approaches used to shift the client's structure or function. As such, they can strain adaptive capacity and therefore should only be used as needed. Do not overuse any of the methods. Think of each of these applications as the seasoning in the main massage soup described in Chapter 14.

In general, the biggest mistake made with massage application is either too much or too little seasoning. A massage that is too straining, or one that is too bland, will not please the client, nor be as therapeutic as it should be. The skilled practitioner strives to get the flavor just right.

For each method described, list at least three situations in which you would use the method.

1 Indirect function technique
    Example: Tissue binds in the lumbar fascia

    _____

2 Arterial circulation focus
    Example: Pre-event massage

    _____

3 Venous return focus
    Example: Long plane ride

    _____

4 General systemic lymphatic drain
    Example: Delayed-onset muscle soreness

    _____

5 Localized lymphatic drain
    Example: Ankle sprain

6 Deep transverse friction

7 Connective tissue mechanics

8 Trigger points

9 Joint play

10 Reflexology

11 Acupressure

12 Scalene/occipital/sternocleidomastoid release

13 Psoas release

14 Quadratus lumborim release

15 Subscapular release

16 Rectus abdominis release

17 Hamstring release

18 Groin attachments of hamstring and adductors

19 Multifidi, rotators, etc

20 Deep lateral rotators

21 SI joint

22 Sartorius displacement

    _____

23 Biceps tendon displacement

    _____

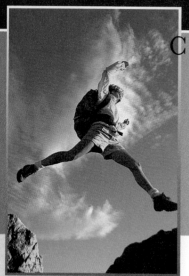

CHAPTER

14

GENERAL PROTOCOL FOR SPORT AND FITNESS MASSAGE

OBJECTIVES

Upon completion of this chapter, the reader will have the information necessary to complete a comprehensive full body assessment and perform a general treatment massage application.

The protocol described in this chapter is used for general maintenance massage for athletes and those involved in fitness programs. Metaphorically it can be considered a weekly or biweekly cleaning. Weekly sessions may provide enough intervention, especially if the client consistently maintains an appropriate stretching program such as yoga. If increased demands are being placed on the client, twice a week is more effective. For the competitive athlete, three times a week would be ideal but is not usually possible. Any of the various positions and method applications found throughout this book can be incorporated into the massage. Do not be limited by the illustrations shown in the examples in this chapter.

PRE-EVENT MASSAGE

Pre-event massage can be considered massage applied 2 days to 2 minutes before an event; the treatment approach will differ greatly according to the time period. A massage given 2 days before an event can be comprehensive and relaxing, so that the athlete gets the maximum restorative benefit. Deep treatment, especially if there are specific problem areas, may take 1 or 2 days to recover from, and should therefore not be given too close to the event. Deep massage can relax the muscles so much that some athletes find that for a time they lose the muscle strength that they may need during competition.

As the time of competition gets closer, massage treatment needs to become more specific to the demands of the sport and the wishes of the athlete. The main muscles used in the event are treated.

Active release
Acupressure
Anterior rotation
Anterior serratus
Biceps tendon displacement
Circulation support massage
Connective tissue application
Deep lateral hip rotators
Diaphragm
Fluid dynamics
Groin area muscles
Hamstrings
Inflare

Indirect functional techniques
Interspinales
Intertransversarii
Joint play
Lymphatic drain massage
Meridian massage
Multifidi
Occipitals
Outflare
Pectoralis minor
Pelvis alignment
Posterior rotation
Psoas

Quadratus lumborum
Rectus abdominis
Reflexology
Rhomboid
Rotatores
Sartorius displacement
Scalenes
Sacroiliac (SI) Joint
Sternocleidomastoid
Subscapularis
Tissue movement methods
Trigger points
Yang Yin

Typically the massage is stimulating, but pre-competition jitters may be reduced if the athlete calms down a little. In these situations, use body rocking and shaking (oscillation) movements rather than work deeply into the tissues. There are sports such as billiards and bowling in which being calm and relaxed is vital for a good performance.

POST-EVENT MASSAGE

The procedures in post-event massage are the same as with any general sports massage, minus the invasive procedures. The post-event time frame is considered 24 hours after activity.

GENERAL PROTOCOL

The general protocol described in this chapter is a comprehensive, repetitive, and sequential approach that is suggested as a basis of massage for the population. It does not need to be performed exactly as presented. However, during comprehensive, full-body massage, all of the anatomic areas described need to be assessed and intervention provided if appropriate.

Due to interconnected fascial networks and neuromuscular reflex patterns, massage in one area influences the entire body, just as dysfunction or compensation in a body area has an influence on the whole body. During the massage session, observation for whole-body influence needs to be maintained.

The application of massage should have pleasurable aspects. It should feel good and effectively produce results. The assessment and massage application should not produce a guarding or flinching response. During active treatment, the sensations can be intense and reproduce symptoms such as trigger point referral pain patterns and a burning sensation resulting from some forms of connective tissue application. Depending on the client goals, there are times when the outcomes require uncomfortable methods to achieve results, and although the actual focused massage application may be intense, the results will indicate improvement. Follow these massage applications with more general pleasurable methods.

The general approach consists of assessing each area and then addressing the outcome goals with appropriate massage methods. As previously mentioned, this protocol should not be used 24 hours or less prior to or following an athletic event. Pre-event and post-event procedures should be used.

The components include:
- Skin, superficial fascia, and edema
- Deeper fascial structures, muscle layers, circulation, and edema
- Tissue density, ground substance, and fluid
- Joint end-feel and intrinsic joint play

- Motor tone
- Reflex mechanisms
- Firing patterns (muscle activation sequences)
- Flexibility

This massage assessment/treatment protocol will require at least 60 minutes, but 90 minutes is more common, and it can take up to 2 hours if the athlete is large or if his or her condition is complex. Remember, athletes can be messy and it takes a while to clean them up.

Rehabilitative methods discussed in Chapter 13 should be incorporated into this general approach to ensure full-body normalization. Although it is appropriate to use some isolated spot work on areas that are injured, the response is improved when incorporated into full-body application. During an active rehabilitation phase, ideally the athlete will have full-body massage every other day, incorporating a specific application for rehabilitation. On alternate days, the focus is on procedures for specific treatment of the injured area.

If the client is massaged frequently, the massage duration can be shorter. If the client receives massage once a week, then the longer 2-hour massage may be required. If the client has two massage sessions a week, 90 minutes may be sufficient, and for three massage sessions a week, 1 hour each is adequate.

The general protocol is presented as follows:
- View of anatomy being targeted.
- Detailed description of the massage application.
- Illustrated examples of the massage application.

 The DVD that accompanies this book further expands the massage approach by application of the general protocol.

FACE AND HEAD (FIGURE 14-1)

Thorough massage of the face and head is very important. It is not uncommon to spend 15 minutes on the head and face.

Many connective tissue structures are anchored and originate in the area. Because there is a fascial connection from the feet to the top of the head, connective tissue bind patterns may either originate in the face and head area or may be the location of the symptom of various tension patterns from other parts of the body.

The muscles of the head and face are highly innervated and some of them, such as the masseter,

are very strong. Many pressure-sensitive structures (nerves, blood, and lymph vessels) are in close proximity to the head and face muscles and connective tissue structures. This sensitivity to pressure, combined with high sensation awareness, often results in pain in the head and face area.

The skull bones need to move in very small increments in response to normal fluctuations in intracranial fluid pressure. If the bones are fixed by tension patterns in the connective tissue or muscles, or both, the result can be a sensation of pressure or aching.

Eye strain and sun glare can cause tensing of the facial and head muscles, and this is common during physical activity. Protective headgear is a compressive element that results in changes in the soft tissue of the head (Figure 14-2). The facial features should look symmetrical with little creasing of the skin from underlying increases in bind, tension, or tone in the myofascial structures.

The scalp should move easily on the skull in all directions. There are connective tissue bands that circle the head. The larger muscles (temporalis, occipital frontalis, and masseter) should be resilient to palpation with no observable or palpable trigger point activity. If there is evidence of sinus congestion, careful work on the small muscles of the face may allow better drainage.

The hair should not pull out during general massage of the scalp. If it does, this could indicate overtraining, fatigue, or nutritional deficiencies and the client should be referred for evaluation by the appropriate specialist.

The skin should be resilient, soft, supple, and mostly free from blemishes. Changes in skin texture are indications of systemic strain. Increased blemishes may indicate increased cortisol and androgen levels, associated with the stress response. If the skin is oily, be cautious about the type of lubricant being used or work without it.

It is appropriate to massage the head and face muscles in all directions. It is interesting that when the muscles of the face that create a smile are activated, the neurochemical response can shift. Therefore, when massaging the face it may be beneficial to stroke in the direction that helps to create the shape of a smile.

PROCEDURES FOR THE FACE

The direction of the lymphatic stroking should be toward the neck and have sufficient drag to gently pull the skin. Address this area with the client in the supine or side-lying position.

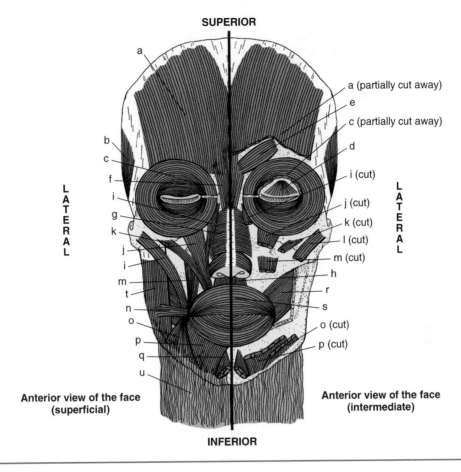

SUPERIOR

a (partially cut away)
e
c (partially cut away)
d
i (cut)
j (cut)
k (cut)
l (cut)
m (cut)
h
r
s
o (cut)
p (cut)

LATERAL

LATERAL

a

b
c
f
i
g
k
j
i
m
t
n
o
p
q
u

Anterior view of the face
(superficial)

Anterior view of the face
(intermediate)

INFERIOR

a. **Occipitofrontalis**
b. **Temporoparietalis**
c. **Orbicularis Oculi**
d. **Levator Palpebrae Superioris**
e. **Corrugator Supercilii**
f. **Procerus**
g. **Nasalis**
h. **Depressor Septi Nasi**
i. **Levator Labii Superioris Alaeque Nasi**

j. **Levator Labii Superioris**
k. **Zygomaticus Minor**
l. **Zygomaticus Major**
m. **Levator Anguli Oris**
n. **Risorius**
o. **Depressor Anguli Oris**
p. **Depressor Labii Inferioris**
q. **Mentalis**
r. **Buccinator**

s. **Orbicularis Oris**
t. **Masseter**
u. Platysma

FIGURE 14-1 ■ Muscles of the face and head—anterior view. (From Muscolino JE: *The muscular system manual,* ed 2. St. Louis, 2005, Mosby.)

- Lightly and systematically, stroke the face to assess for temperature changes, tissue texture, and areas of dampness. If there are identified areas, note them for further investigation.
- Use light compression to assess for bogginess or swelling. If an increase in interstitial fluid is suspected, use lymphatic drain techniques to assist in fluid flow. If in doubt, assume that there is fluid stagnation and perform the method. (Remember, when moving fluid, you cannot push a river. Moving fluid is deliberate work.)
- When the area is drained, re-massage in the direction of the smile.
- Continuing with the face, carefully move the skin to identify any areas of bind in the superficial connective tissue. Be aware of any bind areas that correspond to the areas identified by the light stroking. Pay particular attention

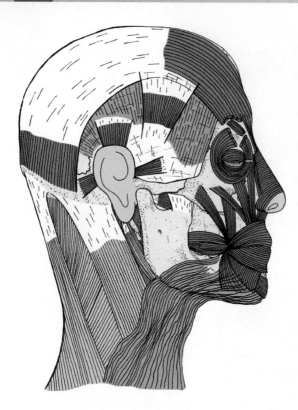

FIGURE 14-2 ■ Connective tissue structures of the head are organized as bands. (Modified from Muscolino JE: *The muscular system manual*, ed 2, St Louis, 2005, Mosby.)

to any areas containing scars, as connective tissue bind is common in areas of scar tissue. Be aware that the soft tissues of the neck weave directly and indirectly into the soft tissues of the head and face. When palpating the soft tissue of the face, observe for tissue movement or bind in the adjacent areas.

- Areas of bind can be addressed by slowly moving the tissue into ease, which is the way it most wants to go. Multiple load directions can be used. For example, if the skin and superficial fascia want to move up and to the right between the eyebrows, then that would be the direction of the forces introduced. Hold the tissue at ease for 30 to 60 seconds and reassess. Usually the area will improve in pliability.
- Treat any remaining areas of superficial fascial bind with myofascial release methods that involve a slow, sustained drag on the binding tissues, with the lines of tension being introduced at each end of the binding tissue.
- Place the finger pad(s) of one hand at one end of the bind and the finger pad(s) of the other hand at the other end of the bind.

- Stretch the tissue gently but firmly and separate the hands, creating a tension force into the binding tissue. Bending force can also be introduced.
- Torsion force is too harsh for this tissue. Maintain the drag on the tissue until the thixotropic nature of the ground substance is affected and becomes more pliable. Subtle changes in the lines of force serve to load and unload the tissue, resulting in hysteresis.
- Next, address the muscle structures. The facial muscles are only one or two layers deep; therefore, light to moderate compressive force is adequate to address the area.
- If muscle tone has increased from sustained isometric contraction, use direct pressure to inhibit the spindle cells and the Golgi tendons. Apply this pressure in a broad-based compression with sufficient intensity to elicit tenderness or reproduce the symptoms, but not so intense that a muscle tenses or breathing changes occur.
- Muscle energy methods can be used in combination with the compression by having the client contract the muscle against the

pressure applied by the hand. It may take a few experimental contractions before the right muscle pattern is discovered. When the correct muscle contracts, the area will tense or seem as if it is pushing against the massage practitioner's pressure. Pulsed muscle energy, where a repeated contract-relax, contract-relax pattern is used, is especially effective for the facial muscles.

- Positional release is possible for these muscles by using eye positions until the pain is reduced in the compressed area.
- Apply pressure to the painful area until the client can feel the tenderness or the reproduced symptoms. Maintain the pressure while the client slowly moves the eyes in different positions until pain, tenderness, or symptom sensation is reduced.
- When the tone begins to reduce, a bending or tension force can then be applied to stretch the muscle fibers. The intent is not to address connective tissue but to mechanically pull the actin and myosin filaments apart to restore normal resting length.
- Address the muscles of the eyes by compressing the eyes gently and having the client move them in slow circles.

- Have the client close the eyes, place their finger pads gently on the eyelids, and slowly press down just a bit. The client should just feel the pressure.
- Use an on/off pumping activation for a moment and then reapply sustained compression while the client move the eyes in circles.

This method both stretches and resets reflexes in the eye muscles. Four small but very sensitive muscles of the eye control eye movement. The proprioceptive feedback from these eye muscles contributes to postural reflexes (Figure 14-3).

Note: Increased fluid pressure in the eyes can be symptomatic of dull aching around the eyes like a tension or pressure headache. If there is any history or trauma to the area around the eyes, coupled with the symptoms described, the client should be immediately referred to a physician for further assessment.

Many athletes chew gum or hold bite plates in their mouth. Pay particular attention to the masseter and other chewing muscles (Figure 14-4). The pterygoids are best reached from inside the mouth. Make sure to use a latex or vinyl glove. Inhibitory pressure on the belly of the muscle is usually sufficient to decrease tone and allows the muscle to be stretched.

a. **Superior Rectus**
b. **Inferior Rectus**
c. **Medial Rectus**
d. **Lateral Rectus**
e. **Superior Oblique**
f. **Inferior Oblique**
g. Levator Palpebrae Superioris

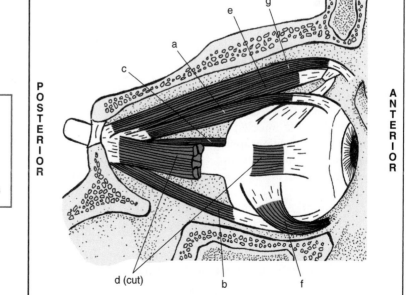

FIGURE 14-3 ■ Muscles of the eye. (From Muscolino JE: *The muscular system manual*, ed 2. St. Louis, 2005, Mosby.)

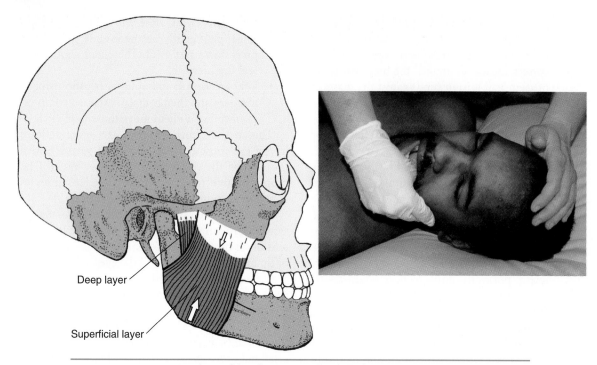

Deep layer

Superficial layer

FIGURE 14-4 ■ Lateral view of the right masseter and methods of treatment. (From Muscolino JE: *The muscular system manual,* ed. 2. St. Louis, 2005, Mosby.)

- Apply a compression force to the chewing muscles by placing the thumb on the inside of the mouth near the temporomandibular joint (TMJ) and the finger pads on the outside on the cheek near the TMJ.
- Pinch the fingers and thumb together to apply inhibitory pressure to the belly of the muscles to affect spindle cell mechanisms or close to the insertions to inhibit the Golgi tendon receptors.
- Muscle energy methods are used by having clients clench their teeth.
- To lengthen the muscles, open the client's mouth wide but do not apply pressure against the lower jaw in an attempt to stretch the muscles. This is too aggressive for the TMJ joint.
- Stretch the area, using the same method that is used when applying inhibitory pressure and introducing a bending force to the tissues.

These are intense methods applied to areas with high levels of neurologic sensitivity. Although the application may be uncomfortable, the client should not tense other body areas or change breathing to endure the approach. Before you begin the application, tell the client to wiggle the whole body to get comfortable, take a deep breath, and exhale slowly.

If the sinuses are problematic, or as a preventive measure, a combination of compression (acupressure) on points with a light rhythmic on/off pressure in about 10 repetitions against the sinus cavities encourages drainage (Figure 14-5).

To finish the face, return to the initial light stroking to reassess for temperature changes. There should be a normalization of areas that were hot, cold, damp, rough, or binding.

Working with the face is relaxing. Therefore, if the face is done first, it can set the stage for a calming whole-body massage; if the face is done at the end of the session, it will gently finish the massage.

Examples of procedures for treatment of the face are shown in Figure 14-6.

FIGURE 14-5

SINUS POINTS AND COMPRESSION AREA

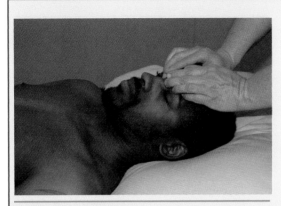

A Eyebrows.

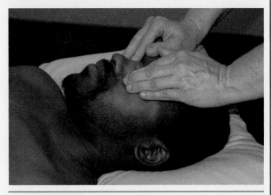

B Bridge of nose.

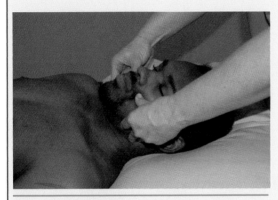

C Edge of nose and maxilla.

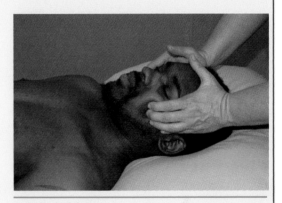

D Under cheek bones.

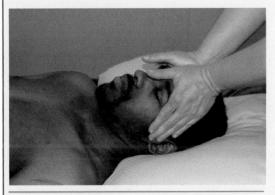

E Forehead and temples.

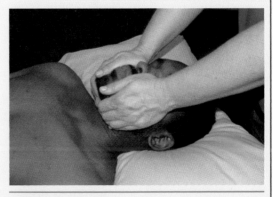

F Cheeks and under jaw.

14-1

FIGURE 14-6

EXAMPLE OF MASSAGE APPLICATION TO THE FACE

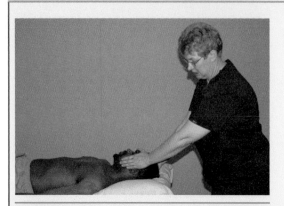

A Stroke the face.

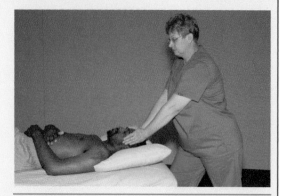

B Drag palpation.

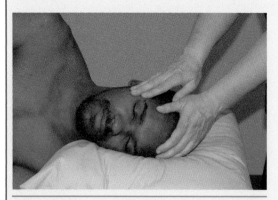

C Compression.

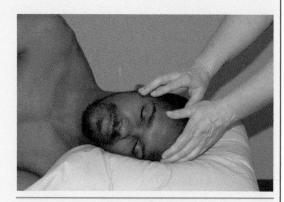

D Assess and treat, using ease and bind.

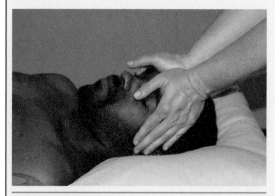

E Tension force.

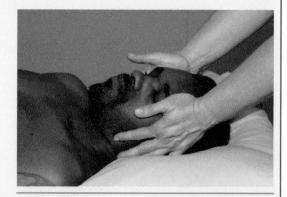

F Tension force.

FIGURE 14-6—CONT'D

EXAMPLE OF MASSAGE APPLICATION TO THE FACE

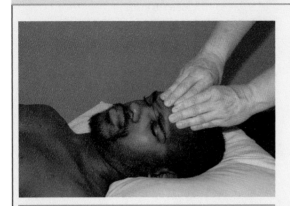

G Bending force.

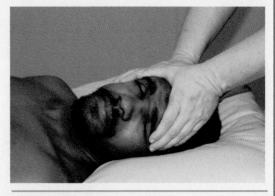

H Broad-based compression to fascial muscles.

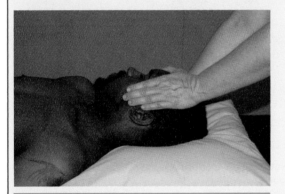

I Chewing muscles.

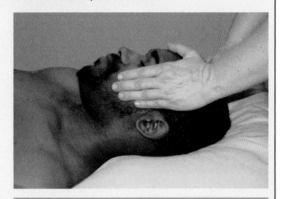

J Finish the face.

PROCEDURES FOR THE HEAD

The musculature of the head is discussed next (Figure 14-7).

Examples of procedures for treatment of the head are shown in Figure 14-8.

The head is next. Caution is necessary with any expensive hair design. This can complicate effective work on the head because the client is not going to want the hair messed up. Various hairstyles that are tight to the head or pull the scalp can be problematic. Heavy hair can also pull on the scalp. Tight bands, such as sweat bands, or restrictive elastic caps used to control or style hair, or sport protective head gear can interfere with circulation of the scalp, restrict cranial bone movement, and put pressure on nerves and vessels in the head. This pulling or compression on the scalp can be the cause of headache, localized fascial restriction, and even body-wide binding and compensation. If this is the case, then a different hairstyle should be used, tight bands and head covering avoided, and protective headgear properly fitted. Shaved heads can be irritated if the massage application rubs against the grain of the hairs as it grows out.

It is important that the scalp moves freely in all directions on the skull to allow cranial bone movement and reduce pressure on muscle, nerves, and vessels. There are distinct fascial bands that circle the head (see Figure 14-2). It is important that these bands are pliable or they will restrict fluid and cranial bone movement.

Address this area with the client in the prone, supine, and side-lying positions.

- Place the hands on either side of the head by the ears. Turning the head to the side facilitates pressure application. Move the scalp in various directions to assess for bind.
- If an area binds, it can be addressed by slowly moving the tissue into ease, dragging it the

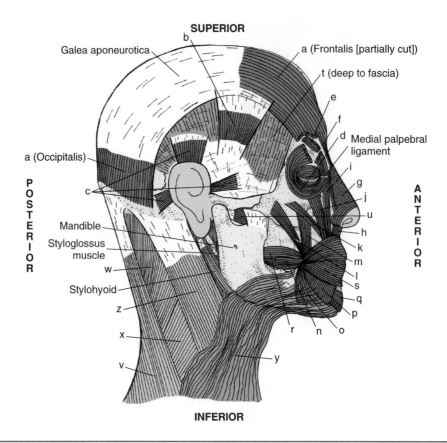

SUPERIOR

Galea aponeurotica

a (Frontalis [partially cut])

t (deep to fascia)

e

f

d Medial palpebral ligament

a (Occipitalis)

i

POSTERIOR

c

g

j

ANTERIOR

u

Mandible

h

Styloglossus muscle

k

m

w

l

s

Stylohyoid

q

z

p

x

r   n   o

v

y

INFERIOR

a. **Occipitofrontalis**	j. **Levator Labii Superioris**	s. **Orbicularis Oris**
b. **Temporoparietalis**	k. **Zygomaticus Minor**	t. **Temporalis**
c. **Auricularis Muscles**	l. **Zygomaticus Major**	u. **Lateral Pterygoid**
d. **Orbicularis Oculi** (partially cut)	m. **Levator Anguli Oris**	v. Trapezius
e. **Corrugator Supercilii**	n. **Risorius**	w. Splenius Capitis
f. **Procerus**	o. **Depressor Anguli Oris**	x. Levator Scapulae
g. **Nasalis**	p. **Depressor Labii Inferioris**	y. Platysma
h. **Depressor Septi Nasi**	q. **Mentalis**	z. Sternocleidomastoid
i. **Levator Labii Superioris Alaeque Nasi**	r. **Buccinator**	

Figure 14-7 ■ Muscles of the head—lateral view. (From Muscolino JE: *The muscular system manual,* ed 2. St. Louis, 2005, Mosby.)

way it most wants to go. Multiple load directions can be used. For example, if the skin and superficial fascia want to move up and to the right, that would be the direction of the forces introduced.

• Once ease is identified, introduce an increased force—tension or shear—and use the force rhythmically to load and unload the tissue to increase pliability of the ground substance. Next, move the tissues into bind and repeat.

• The connective tissue bands (see Figure 14-2) require bend and shear forces to become less

restrictive. Methodically move along the bands, assessing for binding, and address each as it is found. The increase in length and pliability of the connective tissue is small but sufficient to allow normal movement of head structures.

Connective tissue structures in the neck that weave into the scalp can exert pressure into the scalp. In fact, the connective tissue plane that runs from the scalp superficially to the sacrum can create binding in the tissues of the head. Another pattern, from the scalp to the dorsolumbar fascia to the iliotibial (IT) band and then to the foot, can create bind in the scalp. It is necessary to address the entire body to assure appropriate pliability in the fascial structures of the head.

- If there is superficial edema in the head, it should be drained after the connective tissue is addressed. Drain patterns from the head run toward the neck.

The muscle structure of the head is very strong. The temporalis is part of the chewing mechanism and is often increased in tone due to gum chewing, gritting of the teeth, or holding bite plates in the mouth. The suboccipital muscles weave into the posterior neck extensors via connective tissue attachments. The occipital muscles often become locked in isometric contraction patterns and then eventually become fibrotic.

The frontalis and occipitalis are actually one muscle, connected by connective tissues called the *galea aponeurotica*, which attaches at the base of the skull and neck tissues and runs to the forehead. The two portions of this muscle have to be balanced, or an uneven pull force and/or pain can occur. If the occipitalis shortens, then pain can be felt in the forehead, and sometimes there is the sensation that the eyebrows are being pulled back. Squinting and scowling, which can occur when in bright light or when exerting effort during practice or performance, may increase tension in the frontalis and exert a pull on the back of the head.

If muscle tone has increased in any muscles of the head from sustained isometric contraction, use broad-based direct pressure to inhibit the spindle cells and the Golgi tendons.

- Apply pressure using broad-based compression with sufficient intensity to elicit tenderness or reproduce the symptoms, but not so intense that any muscle tensing or breathing changes occur.
- Muscle energy methods can be used in combination with the compression by having the client contract against the pressure applied by the hand or forearm. It may take a few experimental contractions before the right muscle pattern is discovered. When the correct muscle contracts, the area will tense or seem as if it is pushing against the practitioner's pressure.
- Pulsed muscle energy methods, in which a contract/relax, contract/relax pattern is used, are especially effective in the muscles of the head. When the tone begins to reduce, a bending or tension force can be applied to

the muscle fibers. The intent is not to address connective tissue but to mechanically pull the actin and myosin filaments apart to restore normal resting length.

Eye fatigue is common. Systematic pressure on the muscles in the head while the client slowly moves the eyes in circular movements seems to help and certainly will not do harm.

Some clients enjoy having their hair gently pulled. The hair can be used as a handle to pull the scalp away from the skull. Make sure that a large bunch of hair is grasped; a gentle pull is introduced to bind, is held, and is then released. Systematically done, this application addresses the entire scalp.

Compression to the sides and to the front and back of the head, coupled with a scratching motion to the scalp, can be very pleasant. The compression aspect of this sequence can be a typical craniosacral sequence if the massage professional is trained in this bodywork method.

OCCIPITAL BASE (FIGURE 14-9)

This area is the transition point from the head to the neck. Transition areas usually involve fairly mobile jointed areas. The joints in this area are the *atlas* and the *axis*. Local muscles are involved in the stability of this area and consist primarily of the suboccipital group. These muscles also act as proprioceptive feedback stations on the position of the head in relationship to the rest of the body and are involved with the ocular, tonic neck, and pelvic reflexes for maintaining posture and balance. In some instances, the suprahyoid may also work to balance the head, exerting a small counter force to the suboccipitals.

The global muscles that can influence the occipital base are the sternocleidomastoid, platysma, semispinalis, splenius capitis, and trapezius. It is difficult to list individual muscles that can influence any particular area because the body is such an interconnected structure; however, these are the main muscles that affect the local joint stability and proprioceptive information and global movement of this area. The local muscles are deep, and the global muscles, being more superficial, comprise the first and second layers of the tissues.

The cervical plexus and vessels supplying the head are located in this area. Impingement is common. Tissues in this area are often stressed by athletic performance. It is essential that this area function normally to assure proper positional reflexes necessary for agility and precise movement.

14–2

FIGURE 14-8

EXAMPLES OF MASSAGE APPLICATION TO THE HEAD

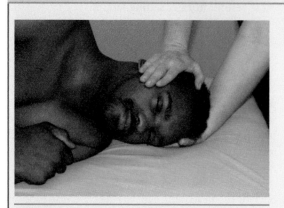

A Assess.

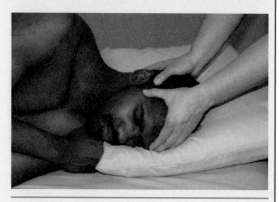

B Connective tissue, ease and bend.

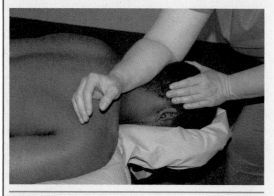

C Occipital.

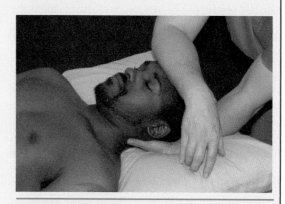

D Frontalis, using forearm.

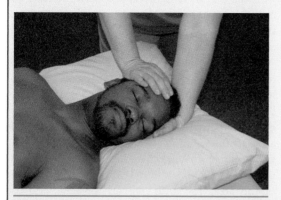

E Temporalis.

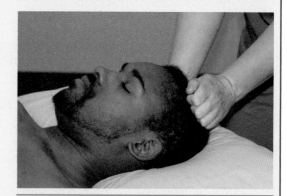

F Mobilize the scalp.

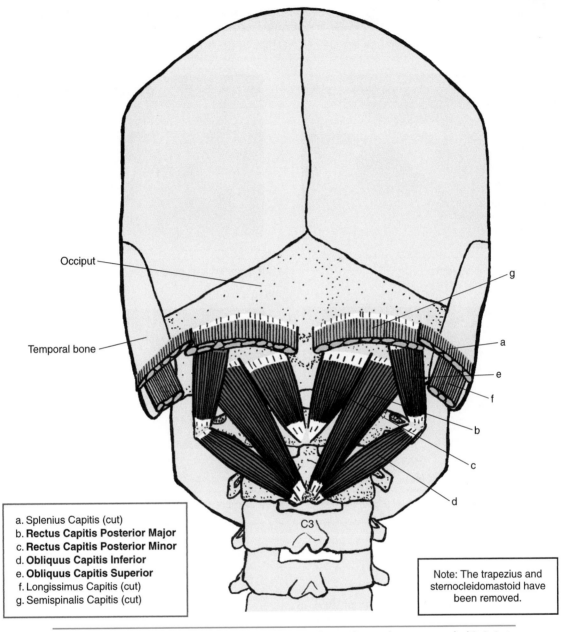

Occiput

Temporal bone

g

a

e

f

b

c

d

C3

a. Splenius Capitis (cut)
b. **Rectus Capitis Posterior Major**
c. **Rectus Capitis Posterior Minor**
d. **Obliquus Capitis Inferior**
e. **Obliquus Capitis Superior**
f. Longissimus Capitis (cut)
g. Semispinalis Capitis (cut)

Note: The trapezius and
sternocleidomastoid have
been removed.

FIGURE 14-9 ■ Muscles of the occipital base. (From Muscolino JE: *The muscular system manual*, ed 2. St. Louis, 2005, Mosby.)

Sympathetic dominance will increase muscle tone in the area. The area most often shows decreased connective tissue pliability.

PROCEDURES FOR THE OCCIPITAL BASE

Examples of procedures for treatment of the neck–occipital base are shown in Figure 14-10. Address this area with the client in the prone and side-lying positions.

- Systematically lightly stroke the area to assess for temperature changes, skin texture, and damp areas. Observe for skin reddening (histamine response) and goose flesh (pilomotor). These signs indicate possible changes in connective tissues, muscle tone, or circulation patterns.
- Increase the pressure slightly and assess for superficial fascial bind, changes in skin pliabil-

14-3

FIGURE 14-10

EXAMPLE OF MASSAGE APPLICATION TO THE OCCIPITAL BASE

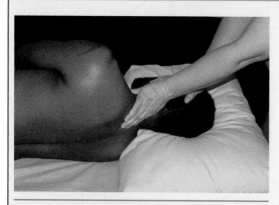

A Client side-lying. Assess/drain.

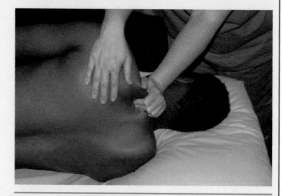

B Assess and bend, global muscles.

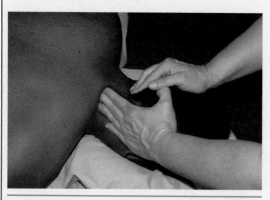

C Assess to make sure tissue layers are not adhered and shear.

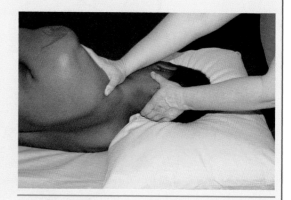

D Myofascial release.

Continued

ity, and accumulation of interstitial fluid, as indicated by boggy or edematous tissue and/or increased skin pressure (like a water balloon).

- If increased fluid pressure is evident, drain the area using a combination of light pressure to drag the skin and deeper rhythmic broad-based compression and kneading to stimulate the deeper vessels.
- Begin with lighter pressure directed toward the collar bone, covering the entire area. Then introduce pumping broad-based compression combined with active and passive movement by having the client slowly rotate the head in circles first one way and then the other.
- Return to dragging the skin and alternate between both methods until the area is

drained, or for about 5 minutes. (Remember, when moving fluid, you cannot push a river.)

- If in doubt about the presence of fluid retention, then assume it is there and drain the area.
- Next, address the superficial fascia by assessing for tissue bind, always observing for involvement in adjacent areas such as the upper back, chest, head, and face.
- Move the skin to identify any areas of bind in the superficial connective tissue. Notice whether any bind areas correspond to the areas of skin reddening or gooseflesh identified by the light stroking. Pay particular attention to any scars, because connective tissue bind is common at these sites.

FIGURE 14-10—CONT'D

EXAMPLE OF MASSAGE APPLICATION TO THE OCCIPITAL BASE

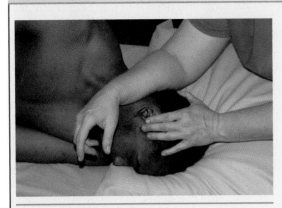

E Compression of deep occipital muscles.

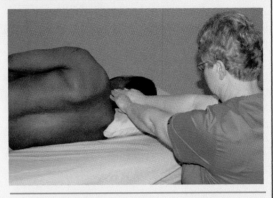

F Friction of deep neck muscles.

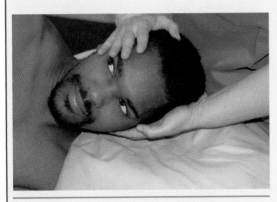

G Muscle energy using eyes to tense muscles (side-lying).

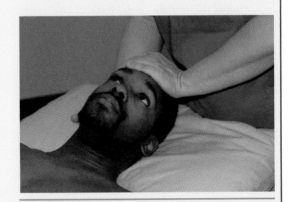

H Muscle energy using eyes to inhibit muscles (supine).

- Address areas of bind by slowly moving the tissue into ease, dragging it the way it most wants to go. Multiple load directions can be used. For example, if the skin and superficial fascia want to move down and to the left at the base of the skull, that would be the direction of the forces introduced. Hold this position for up to 30 seconds and repeat. Reassess.
- Treat any remaining areas of superficial fascial bind with myofascial release methods that involve a slow, sustained drag on the binding tissues, with the lines of tension being introduced at each end of the binding tissue.
- Place your flat hand (finger pads, if hand is too large) at one end of the bind and the other hand at the other end of the bind.
- Contact the tissue gently but firmly, pressing only as deep as the superficial fascial layer,

and separate the hands, creating a tension force into the binding tissue.

Bending force can also be introduced.

- By lifting the tissue much in the way that a mother cat would carry or lift a kitten by the neck, maintain the drag on the tissue until the thixotropic nature of the ground substance is affected and becomes more pliable. Subtle changes in the lines of force serve to load and unload the tissue, resulting in hysteresis.
- Next, grasp as much of the binding tissue as possible and lift it until the bind is identified. Slowly load and unload with torsion and shear force until the tissue becomes warm and more pliable. This method is intense, and the client should feel a pulling or slight burning sensation. The client should not feel the need to tense up or change breathing in order to endure the application.

- Work slowly and deliberately, interspersing lymphatic drain type stroking every minute or so.

The posterior tissue is very thick, and work in this area can be relatively aggressive, whereas the anterior tissue between the chin and hyoid is more delicate, and gentler methods need to be used in this area.

The musculature in the posterior region needs to be addressed in layers, systematically moving from superficial to deep. Depending on the size of the neck, the depth to the suboccipitals can be more than 2 inches.

It is important to make sure that muscle layers are not adhered to each other. One muscle layer should be sheared off the next deeper layer if adhesion exists.

- While client is in the side-lying position, use gliding with a compressive element, beginning at the middle of the back of the head at the trapezius attachments, and slowly drag the tissue to the distal attachment of the trapezius at the acromion process and lateral third of the clavicle.
- With client prone, begin again at the head and glide toward the acromion. Then reverse the direction and work from distal to proximal.
- Next, glide slowly across the fiber direction using enough pressure to ensure that you are affecting muscle fiber. The method addresses both connective tissue and neuromuscular elements of the muscle. Repeat three or four times, increasing the depth and drag each time, and being aware of the muscle moving with the application.
- The upper trapezius area can be grasped, lifted, kneaded, and shaken, all of which will influence the fluid, connective tissue, and neuromuscular elements. Fluid should move more effectively, connective tissue become more pliable, and the muscle tone reduce. Work the upper trapezius tissue all the way to the proximal attachments at the head.
- Address the sternocleidomastoid using sternocleidomastoid release from Chapter 13. Do not use compression, because of underlying pressure-sensitive vessels and nerves. Instead, place the head so that one of the sternocleidomastoids is slackened; then grasp the muscle, lift it slightly, and systematically work with a squeezing motion from the belly to both attachments.
- Repeat slowly while introducing a shear and bend; move just past bind to lengthen the fibers and increase pliability of the connective tissue.
- Gently lift the tissue that includes the platysma and bend it to normalize both neuromuscular and connective tissue elements.

Narrow the focus to address the next layer of muscle; the splenius and semispinalis capitis group. Make sure that more surface muscles slide over these muscles.

- Use a wave-like motion over the area to assess for the sliding. If the tissues are adhered, reintroduce connective tissue methods by grasping the surface layer, lifting it off the underlying tissue, and systematically shearing the tissue until it is freed from the underlying area. If the area is very adhered, it may take many sessions before the layers separate sufficiently to allow proper muscle action. Work for up to 3 minutes on an area or until it gets warm.
- Maintaining a broad-based contact, increase the compressive force and contact the next layer of tissue. Again, glide and drag the tissue from proximal attachment to distal attachment and then reverse. Repeat three or four times.
- Knead and glide and use friction across the muscle fibers, making sure that bending, shear, and torsion forces are sufficient to accurately move the muscles and that they are not adhered to the deeper layer of tissue.

Again, narrow the focus to the suboccipitals. These muscles are too small to use gliding, but they will respond to compression in their belly. This serves to bend the muscle, as well as exerting a tension force at the attachment, to affect the proprioceptors in these locations. When addressing deeper tissue layers, always remember to protect the more superficial muscles by applying pressure gradually and with as broad a base of contact as the area will allow. The side-lying position is best for applying the compression. Supine is too hard on the massage therapist's hands; with the client prone, there is just enough head extension to make the muscles difficult to reach and address. If the head is dropped off the edge of the table into forward flexion, the muscles can be accessed, but the pressure has to be applied through the taut, more superficial tissue. With the client side-lying, the more superficial tissue is passive, and the muscle can be addressed using the forearm; if the area is very small, use the supported fingers. Use suboccipital release from Chapter 13.

Because this area is extremely active in proprioceptive functions, muscle energy methods are effective, especially using motion and position of the eyes. Depending on the situation, use varying degrees of intensity.

The gentlest method is positional release using the eye position to locate the position of release, as follows:

- Locate the tender point and then, while maintaining pressure on the area, have the client slowly move the eyes in circles until the tenderness dissipates.
- Hold for up to 30 seconds.
- Next, if the area is not acutely painful, while maintaining the same pressure contact with the tender area, have the client look hard, moving only the eyes toward the pain. This will initiate a tensing of the muscles.
- Have the client hold this position for a few seconds and then look in the opposite direction; this will activate opposing antagonist patterns and initiate reciprocal inhibition.
- Have the client hold this position for a few seconds and then slowly turn the head in the direction of the eyes, as far away as possible from the pain.
- When the end of range is reached, apply a small overpressure to lengthen the muscles. After a few seconds, apply a bit more tension to the bind and stretch the connective tissue.

The most aggressive muscle energy pattern used in this area involves appropriate facilitation and inhibition of muscle contraction.

- The client's head should be in a natural position. The client can be in the supine, prone, or side-lying position or seated.
- Place hands on either side of the client's head just above the ears and stabilize the head. Instruct the client to push against one of your hands and look hard in that direction. Apply sufficient resistance so that the contraction remains isometric.
- Next, have the client continue to push but to turn only the eyes in the opposite direction, to inhibit the contracting muscles. Apply a slightly increased pressure to determine if the area is inhibited. The client should not be able to hold against the increased pressure unless using other muscles or holding the breath.
- If the area does not inhibit, apply sufficient overpressure to move the head 1 inch. Slowly let go and repeat until the area inhibits easily.

- If a change is not noted in two or three attempts, it is likely that the problem is more global and connected to some other reflex or proprioceptive pattern. Leave it alone.
- Repeat on the other side, then go front to back and on each diagonal. During the treatment, do not let the client recruit other muscles or hold their breath.

This series of moves can substantially reduce the sensation of tightness in the neck, especially the need to "crack" the neck.

Gentle rocking, rhythmic ranges of motion of the area (oscillation) may be used to continue to relax the area. The more global muscles can be re-massaged gently or lymphatic drain massage can complete the procedure.

NECK (FIGURE 14-11)

The neck area includes the cervical vertebrae, particularly C2 to T1. This is an area of many joints that allow flexion, extension, and rotation, and many combinations of these movements, to orient the head and ultimately the eyes, ears, and nose in many different directions. Proper function in the neck region is very important for athletes, in whom a keen sense of the environment is essential. The tissues in this area have to supply stability to maintain the position of the head as well as mobility for both large and small precise movements. The neck has both local and global muscle patterns and the connective tissue of the area is a major factor. The more global muscles have been addressed during massage of the occipital base but will be described again in relation to cervical movement and stability. The local muscles serve to stabilize the cervical vertebrae and guide movement, making it more precise. It is often this deeper layer of muscle that creates a tight neck sensation.

The neck region consists of three or four tissue layers depending how you interpret the anatomy. Besides the muscles that attach to the cervical area, we will also discuss the muscles that do not attach to the head, such as the scalenes, levator scapula, longissimus cervicis, semispinalis cervicis, iliocostalis cervicis, spinalis, longus colli, and infrahyoids, as well as the multifidi, rotatores, interspinales, and intertransversarii at each individual vertebra.

There are many vessels and nerves in this area, including the brachial plexus. Impingement is common, with referral patterns to the neck, down to the chest, and to the arms. This is the area where

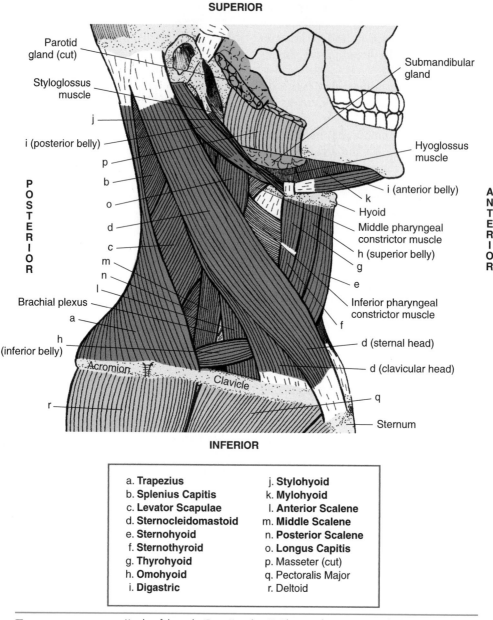

FIGURE 14-11 ■ Muscles of the neck. (From Muscolino JE: *The muscular system manual*, ed 2. St. Louis, 2005, Mosby.)

thoracic outlet syndrome occurs. Preventive care is needed for this condition.

Many athletes get hit (impact trauma) in the head, and the neck absorbs the force and restrains the motion from this trauma. Add the weight of the headgear, and an aching in the neck is understandable.

The neck is involved in many reflex patterns, including the tonic neck reflex. The muscles that insert on the ribs often become short with upper

chest breathing patterns. The outcome of this may be chronic overbreathing and breathing pattern syndrome symptoms.

PROCEDURES FOR THE NECK

Examples of procedures for treatment of the neck are shown in Figure 14-12.

This area is effectively addressed with the client in the supine, prone, side-lying, and seated positions.

14–4

FIGURE 14-12

EXAMPLE OF MASSAGE APPLICATION TO THE NECK

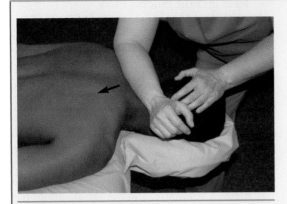

A Glide, proximal to distal.

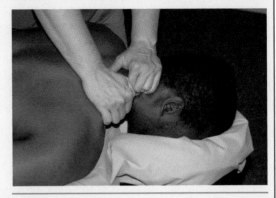

B Knead.

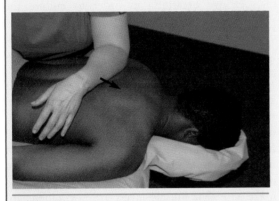

C Glide.

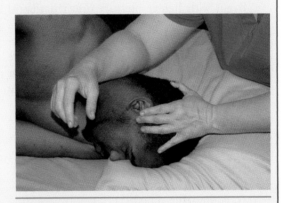

D Compression.

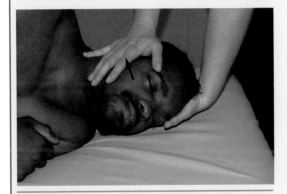

E Post-isometric contraction; eyes look toward top hand.

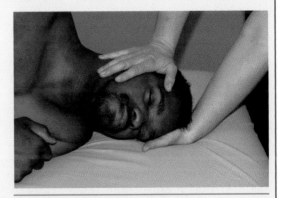

F Lengthen area; eyes look toward bottom hand.

- Systematically lightly stroke the area to assess for temperature changes, skin texture, and damp areas. Observe for skin reddening (histamine response) and goose flesh (pilomotor). These signs indicate possible changes in connective tissue, muscle tone, or circulation patterns.
- Increase the pressure slightly and assess for superficial fascial bind, changes in skin pliability, and accumulation of interstitial fluid, as indicated by boggy or edematous tissue and or increased skin pressure (like a water balloon.)
- If increased fluid pressure is evident, drain the area using a combination of light pressure to drag the skin and deeper rhythmic broad-based compression and kneading to stimulate the deeper vessels.
- Begin with lighter pressure directed toward the collar bone, covering the entire area. Then introduce pumping broad-based compression and kneading combined with active and passive movement by having the client slowly rotate the head in circles, first one way and then the other.
- Return to dragging the skin and alternate between both methods until the area is drained, or for about 5 minutes.
- If in doubt about the presence of fluid retention, then assume it is there and drain the area.

Next, address the superficial fascia by assessing for tissue bind, always observing for involvement in adjacent areas such as the upper back, chest, occipital area, face, and head.

- Move the skin to identify any areas of bind in the superficial connective tissue. Notice whether any bind areas correspond to the areas of skin reddening or gooseflesh identified by the light stroking. Pay particular attention to scars, because connective tissue bind is common in these areas.
- Address areas of bind by slowly moving the tissue into ease, dragging it the way it most wants to go. Multiple load directions can be used. Hold at each position and then reassess.

The remaining areas of superficial fascial bind are treated with myofascial release methods that involve a slow, sustained drag on the binding tissues, with the lines of tension being introduced at each end of the binding tissue.

- Place your flat hand (finger pads, if hand is too large) at one end of the bind and the other hand at the other end of the bind.

- Contact the tissue gently but firmly, pressing only as deep as the superficial fascial layer, and separate the hands, creating a tension force into the binding tissue.

Bending force can also be introduced.

- Maintain the drag on the tissue until the thixotropic nature of the ground substance is affected and becomes more pliable. Subtle changes in the lines of force serve to load and unload the tissue, resulting in hysteresis.
- Next, grasp as much of the binding tissue as possible and lift it until the resistance is identified. Slowly load and unload with torsion, bend, and shear force until the tissue becomes warm and more pliable. This method is intense, and the client should feel a pulling or slight burning sensation. The client should not feel the need to tense up or change breathing in order to endure the application.
- Work slowly and deliberately, interspersing lymphatic drain type stroking every minute or so.

The posterior tissue is very thick. Work in this area can be relatively aggressive, whereas the anterior tissue between the hyoid and the collarbone is more delicate, and gentler methods need to be used here. The musculature in the posterior neck region needs to be addressed in layers systematically, moving from superficial to deep. It is important to make sure that muscle layers are not adhered to each other. If this is occurring, one muscle layer should be sheared off the next deeper layer.

- Use gliding with a compressive element, beginning at the middle of the back of the head at the trapezius attachments, and slowly drag the tissue to the distal attachment of the muscle.
- Begin again at the head and glide toward the acromion. Then reverse the direction and work from distal to proximal.
- Next, glide slowly across the fiber direction, using enough pressure to ensure that you are affecting muscle fiber. This method addresses both the connective tissue and the neuromuscular elements of the muscle. Repeat three or four times, increasing the depth and drag each time, and being aware of the muscle moving with the application.

Narrow the focus to address the next tissue layer, to include the levator scapula and scalenes. Make sure that the surface muscles slide over these muscles.

- Use a wave-like motion over the area to assess for the sliding. If it is not sliding, reintroduce connective tissue methods by grasping the surface layer, lifting it off the underlying tissue, and systematically shearing the tissue until it is freed from the underlying area. If the area is very adhered, it may take many sessions before the layers separate sufficiently to allow proper muscle action.
- Work for up to 2 or more minutes on an area, or until it becomes warm, and then continue with the rest of the area.
- Maintaining a broad-based contact, increase the compressive force. Glide and drag the tissue from proximal attachment to distal attachment and then reverse. Repeat three or four times.
- Knead and glide across the muscle fibers, making sure that bending, shear, and torsion forces are sufficient to accurately move the muscles and to make sure that they are not adhered to the deeper layer of tissue.

Compression is best applied with the client in the side-lying position, using the forearm in the valley of the neck. By changing the angle of the contact, the compression can identify any area where short muscle structures are impinging on the nerves. When such an area is located, the symptoms that are bothering the client will be reproduced.

- First, apply compression; then combine compression with muscle energy methods. Start from the least invasive positional release, using movement of the eyes.
- If there is no release of the target muscle, then progress to positional release, using movement of the head, neck, arms, and pelvis, and finally, to pulsed muscle energy methods.
- If necessary, use the more aggressive reciprocal inhibition and tense-and-relax methods. The goal is to temporarily inhibit the motor tone of the muscle bundle that is problematic so that it can be lengthened to the appropriate resting length that results in reduced pressure on the nerves or vessels.

Again, narrow the focus to the third layer of tissue. These muscles are too small to use gliding but respond to compression in the belly of the muscles. This serves to bend the muscle as well as exert a tension force at the insertion to affect the proprioceptors in these locations. Side-lying is the best position for applying compression. The supine position is too hard on the massage therapist's hands.

The client can be positioned prone with the head dropped slightly into forward flexion. If the superficial tissue is not too taut, the deeper muscle and connective tissue can be addressed. With the client in the side-lying position, the more superficial tissue is relatively passive, and the muscle can be addressed using the forearm, or if the area is very small, using the supported fingers. When addressing deeper tissue layers, always remember to protect the more superficial muscles by applying pressure gradually, with as broad a base of contact as the area will allow.

Neuromuscular reflex patterns can be addressed as follows.

- Have the client's head in neutral position. The client can be in the supine, prone, side-lying, or seated position.
- Place hands on either side of the head just below the ears and stabilize the head. Instruct the client to push against one of your hands and look in that direction. Apply sufficient resistance so that the contraction remains isometric.
- Next, have the client continue to push but turn the eyes and look in the opposite direction; this should inhibit the contacting muscles. Then apply a slightly increased pressure to determine if the area is inhibited. If the area is inhibited, the client will not be able to hold against the increased pressure, unless using other muscles or holding the breath.
- If the area does not inhibit, apply sufficient overpressure to move the head about 2 inches. Let go and repeat until the area inhibits. If a change is not noted in two or three attempts, then it is likely that the problem has a more global connection involving some other reflex or proprioceptive pattern.
- Repeat on the other side, then go from front to back and on each diagonal and in both rotational patterns. Do not let the client recruit other muscles or hold the breath.
- Have the client flex the head and neck by looking toward the navel, and rolling the pelvis toward the navel. Tell the client to hold this position (without using other muscles or holding the breath).
- Apply gentle but firm pressure to the forehead to push the neck into extension. It should hold the contraction easily.
- If it does not hold, have the client maintain the pelvis position while gently performing

pulsing contractions against your hand on the client's forehead; this will stimulate the neck flexors. The flexion should normalize with 10 to 15 pulses.

- Next, have the client look toward his or her navel and roll the pelvis in the opposite direction (which will slightly arch the low back) and hold again, while continuing to breathe normally. Apply a gentle but firm pressure to the client's forehead to push the neck into extension. It should be difficult for the neck flexors to hold the contraction and should let go.
- If the neck flexors do not inhibit, apply a gentle but firm pressure to the forehead to move the neck into extension while the client rocks the pelvis back and forth. Three or four repetitions should reset the reflex.

This series of moves can substantially reduce the sensation of tightness in the neck, especially the need to "crack" the neck.

Use a gentle, rocking rhythmic range of motion to continue to relax the area. The more global muscles can be re-massaged gently, or a lymphatic drain application can be used to complete massage of the area.

ANTERIOR TORSO (FIGURE 14-13)

The anterior torso is best addressed before the posterior torso because it is the location of the structures causing most of the aching and dysfunction in the posterior torso.

This area consists of the rib cage, which protects the vital organs, and the abdominal contents. The muscles in the anterior torso are primarily responsible for breathing. The pectoralis major and pectoralis minor provide the arm and scapula with both movement and stability. The abdominal muscles are layered and quite intricate in design, as well as being extensively encased and supported by fascia structures. This is an important area of core stability, and an understanding of how the abdominal group functions in posture is necessary.

Attachments of the muscles from the neck (platysma, sternocleidomastoid, scalenes) and the connective tissue connections that unify the body are situated in the upper chest. The muscles of the anterior torso are in functional units with the head and neck flexors. The muscles of this area are involved in flexion and adduction movements in the frontal and sagittal plane. The fiber orientation of the muscles and fascia is multidirectional, with a strong diagonal and perpendicular focus.

Three major cross sections of tissue in the transverse plane define this area. First, the muscles of the neck overlap with the muscles of the upper thorax and the back of the neck and torso, to form the thoracic diaphragm. Second, the diaphragm muscle itself separates the upper and lower torso, and third, the pelvic floor is closed by the crisscross design of the pelvic floor muscles. These transverse layers of tissue are involved in stability and respiration.

PROCEDURES FOR THE ANTERIOR TORSO

Examples of procedures for treatment of the anterior torso are shown in Figure 14-14.

Massage begins with superficial work, progresses to deeper tissue layers, and then finishes off with superficial work. Initial applications are palpation assessment to identify temperature and superficial tissue changes. This area can be massaged while the client is side-lying or supine. A combination of both is most desirable.

- Systematically lightly stroke the area to assess for temperature changes, skin texture, and damp areas. Observe for skin reddening (histamine response) and goose flesh (pilomotor). These signs indicate possible changes in connective tissue, muscle tone, or circulation patterns.
- Increase the pressure slightly and assess for superficial fascial bind, changes in skin pliability, and accumulation of interstitial fluid, as indicated by boggy or edematous tissue and or increased skin pressure (like a water balloon.)
- If increased fluid pressure is evident, drain the area using a combination of light pressure to drag the skin and deeper rhythmic broad-based compression and kneading to stimulate the deeper vessels.
- Begin with lighter pressure in the direction of the axilla while working above the waist, or toward the groin while working below the waist, covering the entire area. Then introduce pumping broad-based compression, which can be combined with active and passive movement of the area. (Remember, when moving fluid, you cannot push a river.) To review lymphatic drain, see Chapter 13.

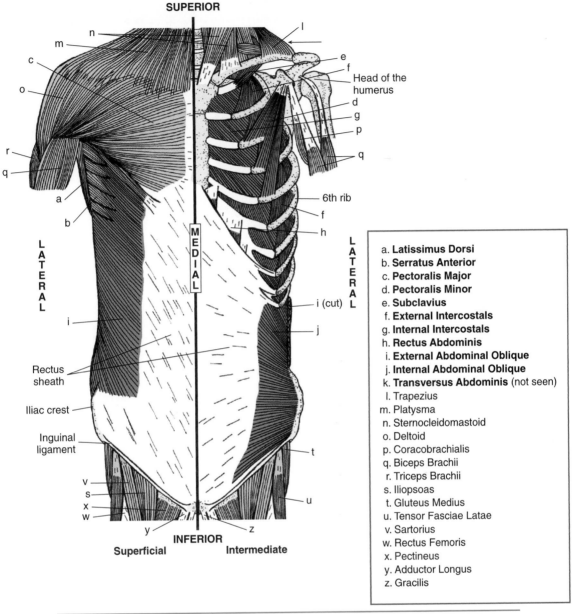

SUPERIOR

n
m
c
o

l
e
f
Head of the
humerus
d
g
p
q

r
q
a
b

LATERAL

MEDIAL

LATERAL

6th rib
f
h

i (cut)

i

j

Rectus
sheath

Iliac crest

Inguinal
ligament

t

v
s
x
w

u

y
INFERIOR
Superficial   Intermediate

z

a. **Latissimus Dorsi**
b. **Serratus Anterior**
c. **Pectoralis Major**
d. **Pectoralis Minor**
e. **Subclavius**
f. **External Intercostals**
g. **Internal Intercostals**
h. **Rectus Abdominis**
i. **External Abdominal Oblique**
j. **Internal Abdominal Oblique**
k. **Transversus Abdominis** (not seen)
l. Trapezius
m. Platysma
n. Sternocleidomastoid
o. Deltoid
p. Coracobrachialis
q. Biceps Brachii
r. Triceps Brachii
s. Iliopsoas
t. Gluteus Medius
u. Tensor Fasciae Latae
v. Sartorius
w. Rectus Femoris
x. Pectineus
y. Adductor Longus
z. Gracilis

FIGURE 14-13 ■ Muscles of the anterior torso. (From Muscolino JE: *The muscular system manual*, ed 2. St. Louis, 2005, Mosby.)

- If in doubt about the presence of fluid retention, then assume it is there and drain the area.

Next, address the superficial fascia by assessing for tissue bind, observing for adjacent areas involved, such as the tissue leading into the shoulder and pelvic girdles.

- Move the skin to identify any areas of bind in the superficial connective tissue. Notice whether any bind areas correspond to the areas of skin reddening or gooseflesh identified by the light stroking. Pay particular attention to any scars, because connective tissue bind is common at these sites.
- Treat areas of superficial fascial bind with myofascial release methods. Address these areas by slowly moving the tissue into ease, dragging it the way it most wants to go.

FIGURE 14-14

EXAMPLE OF MASSAGE APPLICATION TO THE ANTERIOR TORSO

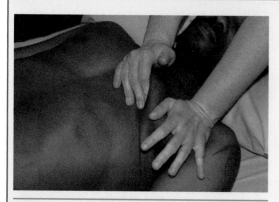

A Massage of anterior torso—assess bend and torsion forces.

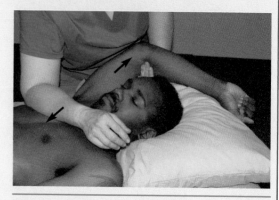

B Fascial stretching (tension force).

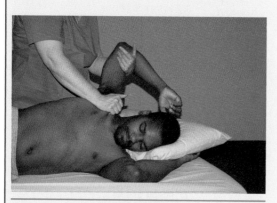

C Address pectoralis major and thorax fascia.

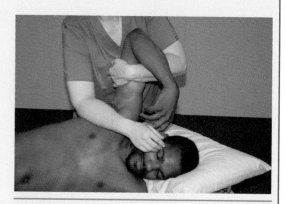

D Gliding.

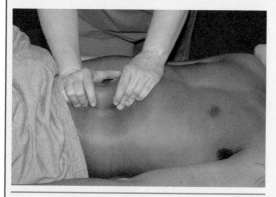

E Rectus abdominis.

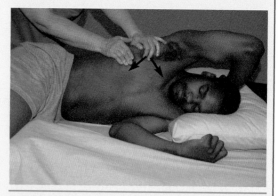

F Multiple direction of ease over trigger point.

FIGURE 14-14—CONT'D

EXAMPLE OF MASSAGE APPLICATION TO THE ANTERIOR TORSO

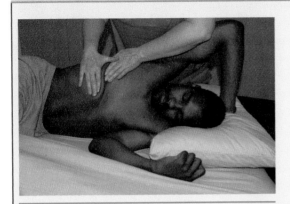

G Direct tissue stretch of trigger point areas.

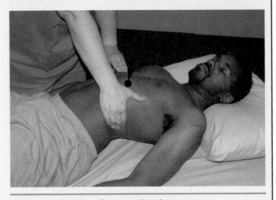

H Position of release of intercostal tender point.

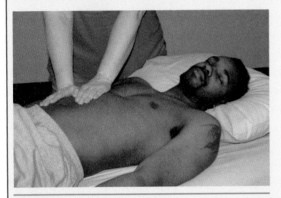

I Lymphatic drain.

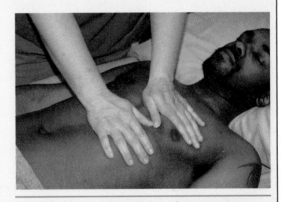

J Reassess tissue using drag palpation and tissue movement.

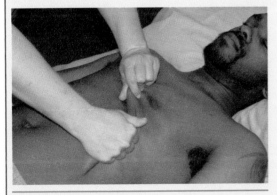

K Shear and bend, adhered tissue.

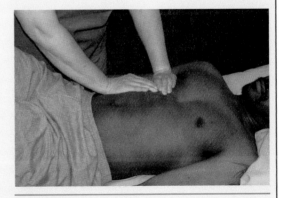

L Compress ribs.

FIGURE 14-14—CONT'D

EXAMPLE OF MASSAGE APPLICATION TO THE ANTERIOR TORSO

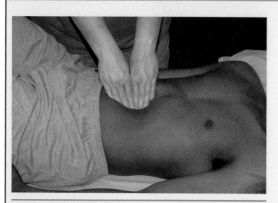

M Compress linea alba.

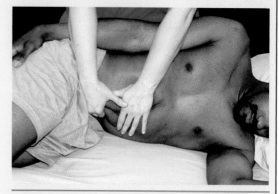

N Abdominal muscles.

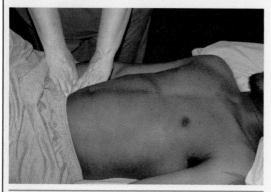

O Psoas.

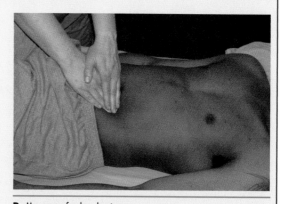

P Massage of colon, begin.

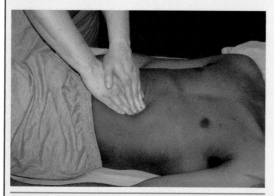

Q Massage of colon, continue.

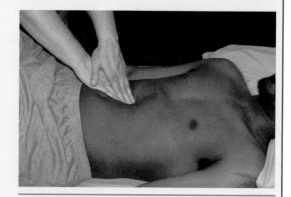

R Massage of colon, end.

- Multiple load directions can be used. For example, if the skin and superficial fascia want to move up and to the right at the sternum, then that would be the direction of the forces introduced. Hold the tissue in ease position until release is felt, or for 30 to 60 seconds.

Next, work into the bind.

- Use a slow, sustained drag on the binding tissues, with the lines of tension being introduced at each end of the binding tissue.
- Place your forearm or flat hand (finger pads if hand is too large) at one end of the bind and the other foreams and hand at the other end of the bind.
- Contact the tissue gently but firmly, pressing only as deep as the superficial fascial layer, and separate the forearms and hands, creating a tension force into the binding tissue.

Bending and torsion forces and joint movement can be introduced as well.

- Maintain the drag on the tissue until the thixotropic nature of the ground substance is affected and it becomes more pliable. Subtle changes in the lines of force serve to load and unload the tissue, resulting in hysteresis.

The musculature in the anterior thorax is addressed in layers, systematically moving superficial to deep. It is important to make sure that muscle layers are not adhered to each other. The most common occurrence is pectoralis major stuck to pectoralis minor. One muscle layer should be sheared off the next deeper layer. It is helpful to place the client so that the surface layer is in a slack position by positioning the attachments of the muscle close together and bolstering the client so that he or she stays relaxed. In some situations, the side-lying position may be more efficient.

Because the fascia in the chest covers the pectoralis major, which extends into the arm, the arm can be used to increase or release the tension force on the tissues. When the arm is passively internally rotated and horizontally adducted, the fascia is slack. When it the torso is stabilized and the arm is externally rotated, abducted, and extended, the fascia is taut. Moving back and forth between these two positions loads and unloads the tissue. Whether using the more direct methods or the movements of the arms, maintain the drag on the tissue until the thixotropic nature of the ground

substance is affected and the area becomes more pliable. Subtle changes in the lines of force serve to load and unload the tissue in various orientations.

- Next, grasp as much of the binding tissue as possible and lift it until the resistance is identified. This application is possible with the pectoralis major and the rectus abdominis.
- Slowly load and unload with torsion and shear force until the tissue becomes warm and more pliable. The arm movements previously described can be combined with the direct lifting of the tissue to introduce multiple forces. This method is intense, and the client should feel a pulling or slight burning sensation. The client should not feel the need to tense up or change breathing in order to endure the application.
- Work slowly and deliberately, interspersing lymphatic drain type stroking every minute or so.
- Use gliding with a compressive element, beginning at the shoulder, and work from the distal attachment of the pectoralis major at the arm toward the sternum, following fiber direction. This can be done in supine or side-lying position with the client rolled. Repeat three or four times, each time increasing the drag and moving slower.
- Move to the abdomen to address the rectus abdominis. If any area binds against the drag, working across the grain of the muscle and in the opposite direction may be beneficial.

Any areas that redden may be housing trigger point activity. Because latent trigger points can cause muscles to fire out of sequence, it is important to restore as much normalcy to the tissue as possible.

- To increase circulation to the area and shift neuroresponses of latent trigger points, move the skin over the point into multiple directions of ease, and hold the ease position for 30 to 60 seconds.
- If this does not relieve the tenderness, positional release is the next option, followed by muscle energy methods, if necessary.

Local lengthening of the tissue containing the trigger points is effective, and authorities have found that it is needed to complete the release of trigger points. Local lengthening is accomplished by using either tension, bending, or torsion force on the tissue with the trigger point and taut band.

Avoid direct pressure or transverse friction, because these methods have the potential for creating tissue damage. If the trigger point does not release with the methods described, then it is part of a compensation pattern that must be dealt with, and the trigger point is likely serving a useful function. Leave it alone.

Once the surface tissue is addressed, then the second layer of muscle is massaged. It is important to make sure that the surface tissue and the fascial separation between muscle layers is not adhered together in any way. Assess by lifting the surface tissue and moving it back and forth in a wavelike movement.

The main muscles being addressed are the pectoralis minor, anterior serratus, and external and internal abdominal obliques.

- Use compresssion with gliding deep enough to address this layer of tissue.
- Broaden the base of contact so that the surface tissue does not tighten to guard against poking.
- Glide in various directions, both with and against the grain of the muscle fibers. Repeat three or four times, with each application slower and at a slightly different angle to access the multiple fiber directions of these muscles.
- Next, knead slowly across the fiber direction, using enough pressure and lift to ensure that you are affecting the muscle fiber in this layer. These methods address both the connective tissue and the neuromuscular elements of the muscle.
- Repeat three or four times, increasing the depth and drag each time and being aware of the muscle moving with the application. Work the entire length of the area, and repeat.

Narrow the focus to address the third tissue layer to include the intercostals. Make sure the surface muscles slide over these muscles.

- Use a wave-like motion over the area to assess for the sliding. If adhesion is identified, reintroduce connective tissue methods by grasping the surface layer, lifting it off the underlying tissue, and systematically shearing or bending the tissue until it is freed from the underlying area. If the area is very adhered, it may take many sessions before the layers separate to allow proper muscle action. Work for

up to 2 or 3 minutes on an area, or until it becomes warm.

- Use the braced finger to contact the tissue between the ribs. Gently and confidently, increase the compressive force and contact this layer of tissue. This is commonly a ticklish area, so do not use a hesitant touch.
- Glide and drag the tissue using the fingers. These are not long moves since the span of these muscles is between ribs.
- Repeat three or four times.
- Tender points are treated with positional release. Many times the position of release can be reached by different compressive force on the ribs to change the shape of the rib cage.

If bones are brittle in this area, be cautious. If direct movement of the rib cage is not possible, moving the hips or shoulders also changes the position of the ribs. It is very important to address these tender points since they can interfere with effective movement of the ribs during breathing. When addressing deeper tissue layers, always remember to protect the more superficial muscles by applying pressure gradually and with as broad a base of contact as the area will allow.

Accessing the Diaphragm Muscle, Psoas, and Colon

The proprioceptors located in the attachments of the diaphragm muscle on the anterior ribs can be stimulated with careful direct pressure by applying compression up and under the rib cage. Care must be taken to protect the liver, stomach, and spleen. See Chapter 13 to review diaphragm release.

Muscle energy methods are introduced by having the client inhale and exhale. There is a possibility that the pelvic floor muscles and diaphragm interact in an antagonist pattern. Recall that these are sheets of muscle that divide the thorax into separate cavities. Even though this muscle interaction has not been verified, it is possible that contracting and relaxing the pelvic floor will affect the tone pattern of the diaphragm. Introduce pelvic floor contraction and relaxation while compression is being applied to the diaphragm's rib attachments.

The diaphragm can also be addressed by applying a compressive or lifting force to the bottom ribs to change the shape of the rib cage. Rib contraindications apply.

Systematic compression into the linea alba has also been used to release the diaphragm.

The inferior attachment of the rectus abdominis to the pubic bone can be addressed at this time if assessment indicates involvement. Shortening of the rectus abdominis can mimic a groin pull. This area should be addressed only if necessary, based on assessment and client goals, with specific informed consent and other prudent cautions, such as having an additional person present.

Likewise, the proximal attachments of the hamstrings and adductors on the ischial tuberosity and pubic bone can be addressed if assessment indicates involvement. This area should be addressed only if necessary, based on assessment and client goals, with specific informed consent and other prudent cautions, such as having an additional person present. This area tends to shorten in the athlete. The quadratus lumborum is addressed when working the anterior torso when the client is in the side-lying position (see specific release in Chapter 13).

The abdominal organs can be rolled to encourage peristalsis. Specific massage to the large intestine can support normal bowl elimination. If assessment identifies psoas symptoms, the psoas muscle can be addressed at this time in Figure 14-15. To complete the area, the following procedures can be used:

- Rhythmic compression of the entire anterior torso area simulates lymphatic flow.
- Assess and correct firing patterns for the abdomen if possible. Usually the area requires therapeutic exercise.

POSTERIOR TORSO (FIGURE 14-16)

The posterior torso consists of the thoracic vertebrae, ribs, lumbar vertebrae, sacrum, and coccyx and the structures that attach to these bones. The most superficial layer of muscle serves to connect, stabilize in force couples, and move the limbs. These soft tissue structures are relatively global. The second, third, and fourth layers of muscle attach intrinsically on the vertebral column and ribs. These muscles and soft tissue structures become progressively more local the deeper they are oriented.

The middle layer of muscles has multiple attachments on the vertebrae and ribs orienting in a direction parallel to the spine. These muscles,

collectively called the sacrospinal or erector spinae, function to extend and stabilize the back. Because the degree of movement for these muscles is limited, the stabilization of posture becomes their primary function. Stabilization involves smaller concentric and eccentric muscle function with sustaining isometric contraction. Therefore these muscles will often feel tense to the client.

Major connective tissue structures begin at the head and cover the entire posterior trunk. These structures spread into the shoulder and pelvis as part of the supporting structures of limbs. Think of a traditional ground-based television or radio broadcast antenna (the spine) supported by its guy wires (connective tissue including fascia).

The deeper layer of muscles—multifidi, rotatores, intertransversarii, and interspinales—are primarily stabilizers with important proprioceptive functions for the position of the spine. The deep muscles, which attach from one vertebra to the next, shorten and become hypersensitive to movement. They are difficult to stretch and tense, and often the client feels as if he or she wants to crack the back.

Many nerves exit the spine, and the potential for entrapment exists. The most common locations where this may occur in the lumbar area are at the lumbar and sacral plexuses.

The quadratus lumborum is a deep muscle that often has trigger point activity, with referred pain to the low back causing difficulty during firing patterns of leg abduction.

The functions of the soft tissue in the posterior torso include extension, rotation, and lateral flexion, but the main function is maintaining an upright posture.

The posterior torso is often the location of many complaints. The reason for the tension, binding, trigger points, and so forth is usually compensatory and adaptive to some sort of postural strain. Direct massage work in the area without also addressing the causal factors is purely palliative and its effects will last only a short period of time. However, there is value in this outcome, especially for pre- and post-event sports massage. Otherwise, a much broader perspective for massage is desirable.

Anterior flexion, internal rotation, and adduction patterns are usually more likely to be involved in the actual cause of backaches because they are pulling forward in the sagittal and transverse planes toward the midline. When these movement

FIGURE 14-15

LOCATION OF THE PSOAS

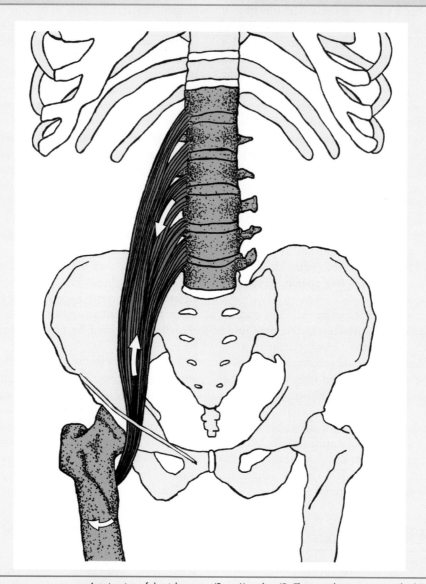

FIGURE 14-15 ■ Anterior view of the right psoas. (From Muscolino JE: *The muscular system manual*, ed 2. St. Louis, 2005, Mosby.)

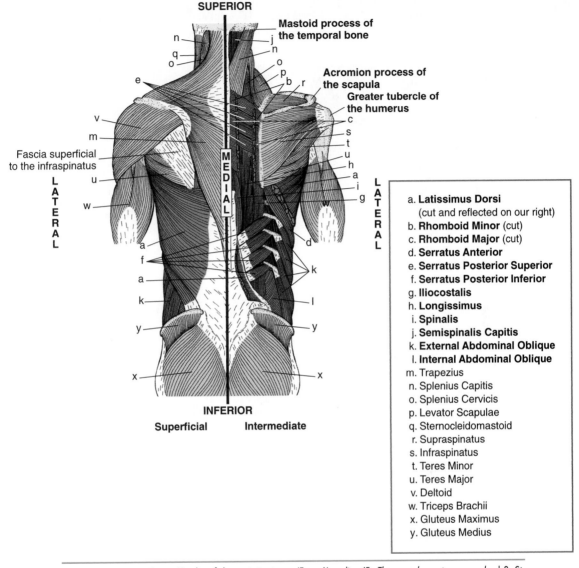

SUPERIOR

Mastoid process of
the temporal bone

Acromion process of
the scapula

Greater tubercle of
the humerus

Fascia superficial
to the infraspinatus

MEDIAL

LATERAL

LATERAL

INFERIOR

Superficial   Intermediate

a. **Latissimus Dorsi**
   (cut and reflected on our right)
b. **Rhomboid Minor** (cut)
c. **Rhomboid Major** (cut)
d. **Serratus Anterior**
e. **Serratus Posterior Superior**
f. **Serratus Posterior Inferior**
g. **Iliocostalis**
h. **Longissimus**
i. **Spinalis**
j. **Semispinalis Capitis**
k. **External Abdominal Oblique**
l. **Internal Abdominal Oblique**
m. Trapezius
n. Splenius Capitis
o. Splenius Cervicis
p. Levator Scapulae
q. Sternocleidomastoid
r. Supraspinatus
s. Infraspinatus
t. Teres Minor
u. Teres Major
v. Deltoid
w. Triceps Brachii
x. Gluteus Maximus
y. Gluteus Medius

FIGURE 14-16 ■ Muscles of the posterior torso. (From Muscolino JE: *The muscular system manual,* ed 2. St. Louis, 2005, Mosby.)

patterns are too strong, posterior thorax structures become inhibited, long, and tight. There are exceptions, usually in the lumbar area, where muscles and connective tissue can shorten.

Be cautious in addressing trigger points and connective tissue bind in inhibited and long muscles of the posterior torso because these conditions may be part of a resourceful compensation pattern. Instead, focus treatment on the anterior thorax and then reassess posterior structures. Use hyperstimulation and counterirritation methods in the inhibited and long areas to reduce symptoms.

PROCEDURES FOR THE POSTERIOR TORSO

Examples of procedures for treatment of the posterior torso are shown in Figure 14-17.

This area is best addressed while the client is in the prone and side-lying positions.

As described previously, massage begins with superficial work, progresses to the deeper tissue layers, and then finishes off with superficial work. Initial applications are palpation assessments to identify temperature and surface tissue changes.

14-6

FIGURE 14-17

EXAMPLE OF MASSAGE APPLICATION TO THE POSTERIOR TORSO

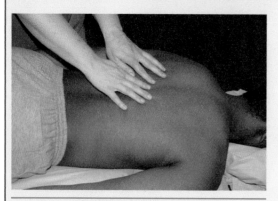

A Assess with surface stroking.

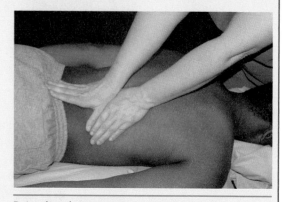

B Lymphatic drain.

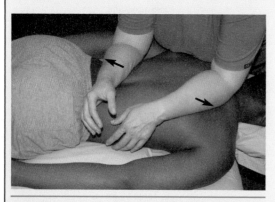

C Myofascial release, to address areas of bind.

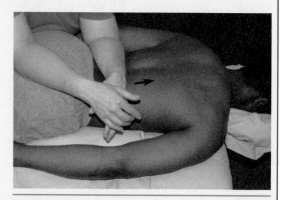

D Glide, prone.

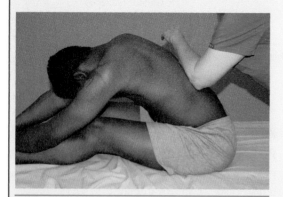

E Glide, seated.

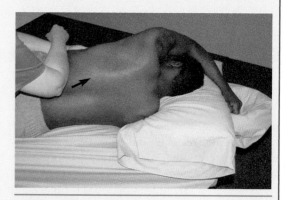

F Glide, side-lying.

FIGURE 14-17—CONT'D

EXAMPLE OF MASSAGE APPLICATION TO THE POSTERIOR TORSO

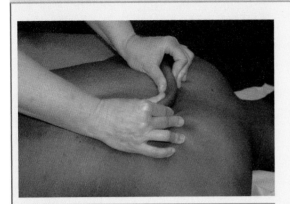

G Skin roll to lift tissues.

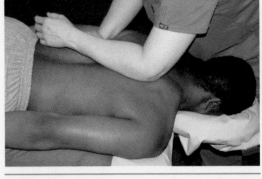

H Glide deep tissue layers.

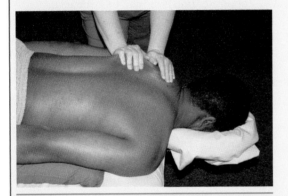

I Kread.

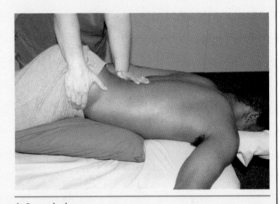

J Postural release.

- Systematically lightly stroke the area to assess for temperature changes, skin texture, and damp areas. Observe for skin reddening (histamine response) and goose flesh (pilomotor). These signs indicate possible changes in connective tissue, muscle tone, or circulation patterns.
- Increase the pressure slightly and assess for superficial fascial bind, changes in skin pliability, and accumulation of interstitial fluid, as indicated by boggy or edematous tissue and increased skin pressure (like a water balloon.)
- If increased fluid pressure is evident, then drain the area using a combination of light pressure to drag the skin and deeper rhythmic broad-based compression and kneading to stimulate the deeper vessels.
- Begin with lighter pressure in the direction of the axilla while working above the waist, and toward the groin while working below the waist, covering the entire area. Then introduce pumping broad-based compression. (Remember, when moving fluid, you cannot push a river.)
- If in doubt about the presence of fluid retention, assume it is there and drain the area.

Next, address the superficial fascia by assessing for tissue bind, always observing for involvement in adjacent areas, such as the tissue leading into the shoulder and pelvic girdles.

- Move the skin to identify any areas of bind in the superficial connective tissue. Notice whether any bind areas correspond to the areas of skin reddening or gooseflesh identified by the light stroking. Pay particular attention to any scars, because connective tissue bind is common at these sites.

- Treat areas of superficial fascial bind with myofascial release methods. Address these areas by slowly moving the tissue into ease, dragging it the way it most wants to go.
- Multiple load directions can be used. For example, if the skin and superficial fascia want to move up and to the right between the scapulae, that would be the direction of the forces introduced. Hold tissue in ease position for up to 30 to 60 seconds.
- Then work into the bind with a slow, sustained drag on the binding tissues and the lines of tension being introduced at each end of the binding tissue.
- Place your flat hand (finger pads if hand is too large) at one end of the bind and the other hand at the other end of the bind.
- Contact the tissue gently but firmly, pressing only as deep as the superficial fascial layer, and separate the hands, creating a tension force into the binding tissue.

Bending force can also be introduced.

- Maintain the drag on the tissue until the thixotropic nature of the ground substance is affected and it becomes more pliable. Subtle changes in the lines of force serve to load and unload the tissue, resulting in hysteresis.
- Next, grasp as much of the binding tissue as possible and lift it until the resistance is identified. Slowly load and unload with torsion and shear force until the tissue becomes warm and more pliable. This method is intense, and the client should feel a pulling or slight burning sensation. The client should not feel the need to tense up or change breathing in order to endure the application.
- Work slowly, interspersing lymphatic drain type stroking every minute or so. The posterior fascia tissue is very thick, especially at the thoracolumbar aponeurosis, and work in this area can be more intense than in other areas of the body.

The musculature in the posterior thorax region needs to be addressed in layers, systematically, moving from superficial to deep. It is important to make sure that muscle layers are not adhered to each other. One layer of muscle should be sheared off the next deeper layer. It is helpful to place the client so that the surface layer is in a slack position, by positioning the attachments of the muscle close together and propping the client so that he or she stays relaxed. In some situations, the side-lying position may be better for this.

- Use gliding with a compressive element, beginning at the iliac crest, and work diagonally along the fibers of the latissimus dorsi, ending at the axilla. Repeat three or four times, each time increasing the drag and moving slower.
- Move up to the thoracolumbar junction and repeat the same sequence on the lower trapezius.
- Then, beginning near the tip of the shoulder, glide toward the middle thoracic area to address the middle trapezius. Repeat three or four times, increasing drag and decreasing speed.
- Begin again near the acromion and address the upper trapezius with one or two gliding stokes to completely cover the surface area.
- If any area binds against the drag, working across the grain of the muscle and in the opposite direction may be beneficial.

Any areas that redden may be housing trigger point activity. Because latent trigger points can cause muscles to fire out of sequence, it is important to restore as much normalcy to the tissue as possible.

- To increase circulation to the area and shift neuroresponses of latent trigger points, move the skin over the latent trigger point into multiple directions of ease, and hold the ease position for 30 to 60 seconds.
- If this does not relieve the tenderness, positional release is the next option, followed by muscle energy methods, if necessary.

Local lengthening of the tissue containing the trigger points is effective, and leading authorities have found it is necessary to complete the release of trigger points. Local lengthening is accomplished by using tension, bending, or torsion force on the tissue with the trigger point and taut band. Avoid direct pressure or transverse friction, because these methods have the potential for creating tissue damage. If the trigger point does not release using these methods, then it is part of a compensation pattern. The trigger point is likely serving a useful function, especially in the posterior muscles that are often in a long and taut state. In this situation, the trigger point areas serve to shorten the tissue and add some counterforce to the areas that are short and pulling.

- Finish off the area with kneading, making sure that the muscle tissue easily lifts off the layer underneath it.
- If adhesions are identified, then introduce a bend, shear, or torsion force until the tissue

becomes more pliable. This method can be intense and create a burning sensation. The client should not guard, display pain behaviors, or hold the breath during application.

• Repeat this sequence bilaterally.

Once the surface tissue is addressed, target the second layer of muscle. It is important to assess to make sure that the surface tissue and the fascial separation between muscle layers is not adhered together in any way.

The main muscles being addressed at this time are the erector spinae, serratus posterior inferior and superior (especially if the client is coughing or sniffing or has signs of any other breathing dysfunction), and rhomboids.

• Begin at the iliac crest and use gliding deep enough to address this layer of tissue, following tissue fiber direction. Maintain a broad base of contact so that the surface tissue does not tighten to guard against poking. Glide toward the scapula, ending just past the rhomboids.

• Repeat three or four times, each stroke slower at a slightly different angle to access the multiple fiber directions of these muscles. Then reverse the direction and work from superior to inferior.

• Next, knead slowly across the fiber direction, using enough pressure and lift to ensure that you are affecting muscle fiber in this layer. These methods address both the connective tissue and the neuromuscular elements of the muscle.

• Repeat three or four times, increasing the depth and drag each time and being aware of the muscle moving with the application. Work the entire length of the area and repeat.

Narrow the focus to address the next layer, which includes the multifidi, rotatores, intertransversarii, and interspinales. Make sure that the more superficial muscles slide over these muscles.

• Use a wave-like motion over the area to assess for the sliding. If the tissues do not slide, reintroduce connective tissue methods by grasping the surface layer, lifting it off the underlying tissue, and systematically shearing or bending the tissue until it is freed from the underlying area. If the area is substantially adhered, it may take many sessions before the layers separate sufficiently to allow proper muscle action.

• Work for up to 2 or 3 minutes on a specific area, or until it becomes warm, and then continue with the rest of the area.

• Maintain a broad-based contact, increase the compressive force, and contact this layer of tissue.

• Glide and drag the tissue, using the forearm and fingers, from the proximal attachment to the distal attachment, and then reverse. These are not long moves, as the span of these muscles is between one and three vertebrae.

• Repeat three or four times. Either the prone or side-lying position can be used successfully.

By changing the angle of the contact, the compression can identify any area in which short muscle structures are impinging on the nerves. When the area is located, the symptoms that are bothering the client will be reproduced. Compression is then combined with muscle energy methods, starting from the least invasive positional release, using the eyes, and then progressing to the more invasive contract, relax, and antagonist contract methods. Rotary movements of the torso while the client is in the side-lying position work well in this area to isolate muscles for muscle energy methods. The goal is to temporally inhibit the motor tone of the problematic muscle bundle so that it can be lengthened to the appropriate resting length and reduce pressure on the nerves or vessels.

After the muscle energy application, lengthen and stretch the area by using rotation.

These small muscles respond to compression in the muscle belly. This serves to bend the belly as well as exert tension force at the insertion, to affect the proprioceptors in these locations. When needed, use specific releases discussed in Chapter 13.

When addressing deeper tissue layers, always remember to protect the more superficial tissue by applying pressure gradually and with as broad a base of contact as the area will allow.

• Address the quadratus lumborum if symptoms indicate (see specific releases in Chapter 13).

• Address muscle firing patterns for hip extension at this time. (See discussion of hip extension firing patterns as in Chapter 12).

• Massage the back in the seated position, using a myofascial release method. Finish the area with superficial work.

SHOULDER (FIGURE 14-18)

The shoulder is a complex musculoskeletal unit. The joint structure is so mobile that it relies more

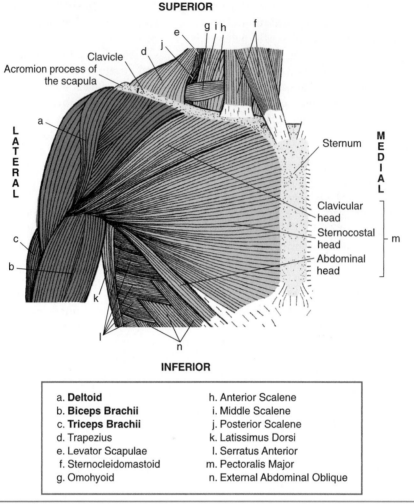

SUPERIOR

Clavicle
Acromion process of
the scapula

LATERAL

MEDIAL

Sternum

Clavicular
head
Sternocostal
head
Abdominal
head

INFERIOR

a. **Deltoid**	h. Anterior Scalene
b. **Biceps Brachii**	i. Middle Scalene
c. **Triceps Brachii**	j. Posterior Scalene
d. Trapezius	k. Latissimus Dorsi
e. Levator Scapulae	l. Serratus Anterior
f. Sternocleidomastoid	m. Pectoralis Major
g. Omohyoid	n. External Abdominal Oblique

FIGURE 14-18 ■ Muscles of the shoulder, anterior view. (From Muscolino JE: *The muscular system manual*, ed 2. St. Louis, 2005, Mosby.)

Continued

than other major joints on muscles and fascia to provide stability. The movement of the scapula, acromioclavicular (AC), sternoclavicular (SC), and glenohumeral joints in a coordinated fashion is necessary for maximal mobility and stability of the area. The inner (local) muscle unit, rotator cuff muscles, and coracobrachialis hold and guide the humerus in the glenoid fossa, using the scapula as a broad-based attachment. The deltoid muscle is expansive and actually functions as three separate units. It also acts as a protective cover for the shoulder. Other muscles of the torso and arm such as the rhomboids, anterior serratus, pectoralis minor, trapezius, and triceps both stabilize and move the scapula, performing a series of muscle actions and working together in force couples.

The pectoralis major and latissimus dorsi form global units that extend the range of motion of the arm.

Muscle/fascial components from the torso and neck affect the stability and mobility of the shoulder. Involvement of gate reflexes necessitates that the shoulders and hip function in coordinated movement patterns.

Nerve impingement of the brachial plexus refers pain to the shoulder and arm.

PROCEDURES FOR THE SHOULDER

Examples of procedures for treatment of the shoulder are shown in Figure 14-19.

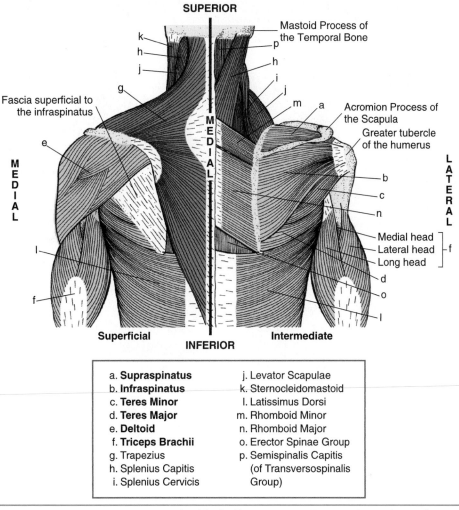

FIGURE 14-18 Cont'd ■ Muscles of the shoulder, posterior view. (From Muscolino JE: *The muscular system manual*, ed 2. St. Louis, 2005, Mosby.)

The shoulder is massaged with the client in the supine, prone side-lying, and seated positions. Massage of the torso and neck naturally progresses to the shoulder.

Assessment of all range of motion patterns and muscle strength will indicate which structures are short and which are long. In addition, gait pattern assessment should provide information about neurologic efficiency and whether muscle activation firing pattern sequences are optimal.

Commencing with the client in the prone position, massage begins with superficial work, progresses to deeper layers, and then finishes off with superficial work. Initial applications are palpation assessment, range of motion, strength, and neurologic assessment, including firing patterns, gait

assessment, and all kinetic chain relationships (see Chapter 12).

- Move the shoulder actively and passively through flexion, extension, internal and external adduction and abduction, and full circumduction. Compare active and passive movements.

- Gently compress the joint to make sure that there is no intercapsular involvement. If pain occurs, refer the client to an appropriate specialist. Massage can still be performed, but be aware that muscle tension patterns may be a guarding response creating appropriate compensation.

It is necessary to make sure that the scapula is mobile on the scapulothoracic junction and that

14-7

FIGURE 14-19

EXAMPLE OF MASSAGE APPLICATION TO THE SHOULDER

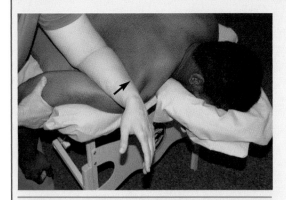

A Assess tissue and range of motion.

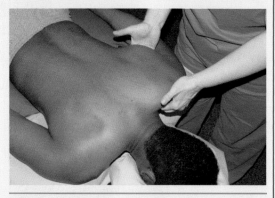

B Assess scapular mobility.

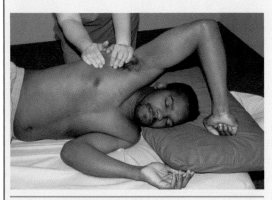

C Knead teres major, latissimus, side-lying.

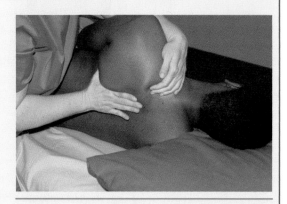

D Mobilize scapula.

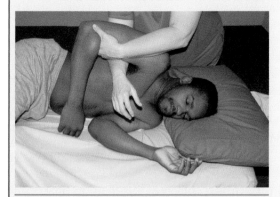

E Active release, shoulder adductors A.

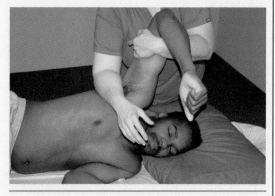

F Active release, shoulder adductors B.

FIGURE 14-19—CONT'D

EXAMPLE OF MASSAGE APPLICATION TO THE SHOULDER

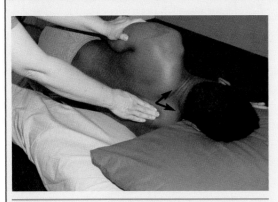

G Rhomboids, anterior serratus attachment A.

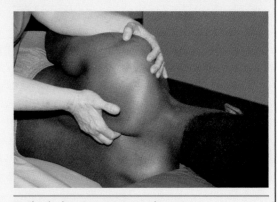

H Rhomboids, anterior serratus attachment B.

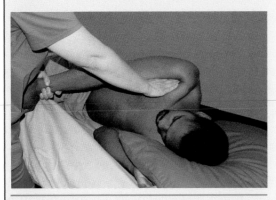

I Pectoralis minor.

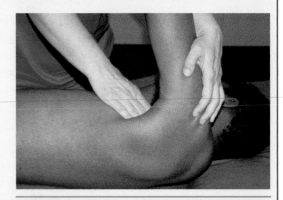

J Subscapularis.

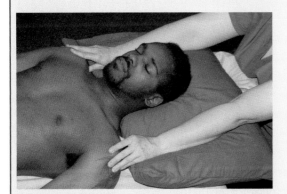

K AC joint, assessment A.

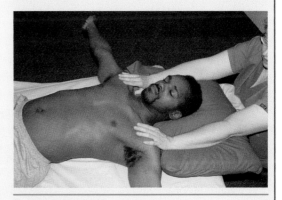

L AC joint assessment B.

FIGURE 14-19—CONT'D

EXAMPLE OF MASSAGE APPLICATION TO THE SHOULDER

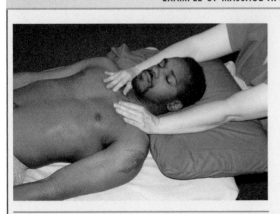

M SC joint, assessment A.

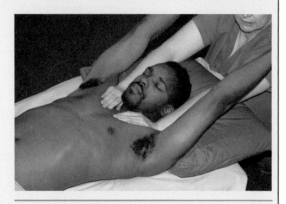

N SC joint, assessment B.

appropriate movement is occurring at the AC and SC joints.

- With the client prone, place one hand under the top of the scapula and the other at the lateral border near the apex.
- With the client relaxed, lift the scapula away from the ribs, and move in various directions. Observation should indicate that the scapula moves easily, but with stability and no winging off the rib cage.

Any areas that are not functioning optimally should be noted and reassessed after they are massaged.

- Systematically lightly stroke the area to assess for temperature changes, skin texture, and damp areas. Observe for skin reddening (histamine response) and goose flesh (pilomotor). These signs indicate possible changes in connective tissue, muscle tone, or circulation patterns.
- Increase the pressure slightly and assess for superficial fascial bind, changes in skin pliability, and accumulation of interstitial fluid, as indicated by boggy or edematous tissue and/or increased skin pressure/turgor (like a water balloon).
- If increased fluid pressure is evident, drain the area, using the lymphatic drain procedure.
- Begin with lighter pressure directed toward the axilla, covering the entire area. Then introduce pumping broad-based compression, which is more efficient when followed by or combined with active and passive movements.

- If in doubt about the presence of fluid retention, assume it is there and drain the area.

Next, address the superficial fascia by assessing for tissue bind. Always observe for superficial fascia involvement in adjacent areas, such as the tissue leading into the torso and neck.

- Move the skin to identify any areas of bind in the superficial connective tissue. Notice whether any bind areas correspond to the areas of skin reddening or goose flesh identified by the light stroking. Pay particular attention to any scars, because connective tissue bind is common at these sites.
- Treat any superficial fascial bind with myofascial release methods. Address these areas by slowly moving the tissue into ease, applying drag to move it the direction it most wants to go.
- Multiple load directions can be used. For example, if the skin and superficial fascia want to move up and to the left on the deltoid, that would be the direction of the forces introduced. Hold ease position up to 30 to 60 seconds. Reassess.

Remaining areas of bind can be treated with the following myofascial release methods.

- Work into the bind using a slow, sustained drag on the binding tissues, with the lines of tension being introduced at each end of the binding tissue.
- Place your flat hand (finger pads if hand is too large) at one end of the bind and the other hand at the other end of the bind.
- Contact the tissue gently but firmly, pressing only as deep as the superficial fascial layer,

and separate the hands, creating a tension force into the binding tissue. Bending forces can also be introduced.

- Maintain the drag and introduce subtle changes in the lines of force, loading and unloading the tissue until it becomes more pliable.
- Next, grasp as much of the binding tissue as possible and lift it until the resistance is identified. Slowly load and unload with torsion and shear force until the tissue becomes warm and more pliable. This method is intense, and the client should feel a pulling or slight burning sensation. The client should not feel the need to tense up or change breathing in order to endure the application.
- Work slowly and deliberately, interspersing lymphatic drain type stroking every minute or so.

The musculature needs to be addressed in layers systematically, moving superficial to deep. It is important to make sure that muscle layers are not adhered to each other. Superficial tissue should be sheared off the next deeper layer. It is helpful to place the client so that the surface layer is in a slack position, by positioning the attachments of the muscle close together and propping the client with bolsters, so that he or she will stay relaxed. In some situations, the side-lying positions may be better for this.

- Begin on the posterior aspect to address the midthorax region that connects with the shoulder. This area is covered by the trapezius (first layer of the muscle). This area was addressed while massaging the torso but now is massaged again in relationship to the shoulder. Carry the strokes into the posterior deltoid.
- Use gliding with a compressive element, from the upper, middle, and lower aspects of trapezius, slowly dragging the tissue toward its distal attachment at the shoulder. Repeat with the latissimus dorsi again in relationship to shoulder function and carry the stroke into the posterior deltoid. If any area binds against the drag, working across the grain of the muscle and in the opposite direction may be beneficial.

Any areas that redden may be housing trigger point activity. Trigger points can cause muscles to fire out of sequence, so it is important to restore as much normalcy as possible.

- To increase circulation to the area and shift neuroresponses of trigger points, move the skin over the point(s) into multiple directions of ease, and hold the ease position for up to 30 to 60 seconds.
- If this does not relieve the tenderness, positional release is the next option, followed by more aggressive muscle energy methods, if necessary.

Local lengthening of the tissue containing trigger points is effective. Local lengthening is accomplished by using tension, bending, or torsion force on the tissues with the trigger point and taut band. Avoid direct pressure or transverse friction, because these methods have the potential for creating tissue damage. If the trigger point does not release using these methods, it is part of a compensation pattern that must be dealt with. The trigger point is likely serving a useful function, especially because the posterior muscles are often in a long and tight/taut state. In this situation, the trigger point areas create stability in the tissues and exert some counterforce to the pulling areas that are short in the anterior.

- Finish the area with kneading, making sure that the muscle tissue easily lifts off the layer underneath it.
- If adhesions are identified, introduce a bend, shear, or torsion force until the tissue becomes more pliable. This can be intense and create a burning sensation. The client should not guard, display pain behaviors, or hold the breath during application.
- Repeat this sequence bilaterally. Once the surface tissue is addressed, the second layer of muscle is massaged. It is important to assess to make sure that the surface tissue and the fascial separation between muscle layers are not adhered together in any way.

The main muscles being addressed in this sequence are the rhomboids, infraspinatus, teres major and minor, subscapularis, and the deeper layers of the deltoid muscle.

- Begin at the vertebral attachments of the rhomboids and use a compressive gliding parallel to the muscle fibers, deep enough to address this layer of tissue. Maintain a broad base of contact so that the surface tissue does not tighten to guard against poking.
- Glide toward the scapula. Repeat three or four times, each time slower and at a slightly different angle.
- Knead slowly across the fiber direction, using enough pressure and lift to assure that you are affecting muscle fiber in this layer. These methods address both the connective tissue

and the neuromuscular elements of the muscle. Repeat three or four times, increasing the depth and drag each time and being aware of the muscle moving with the application.

- Next, address supraspinatus. Glide from the medial border of the scapula toward the acromion. Work above the spine of the scapula to access the supraspinatus. The soft heel of the palm of the hand may fit better in these areas than the forearm. Reverse the direction and then slowly and deeply knead the area. Make sure the upper trapezius is not binding on the supraspinatus.
- Repeat sequence from the medial and lower medial border to address the infraspinatus and the teres major and minor.
- Using gliding and kneading, massage the triceps toward the attachment on the lateral border of the scapula.
- Next, slowly and deeply knead the posterior and medial deltoid.

The side-lying position is effective for addressing the latissimus and teres major and minor attachment on the arm.

- Repeat the sequences described and add placement of the arm over the head.
- Perform active and passive movements while the area is being massaged.
- By positioning the arm as shown in Figure 14-19, *K*, the medial border of the scapula can be lifted and mobilized in rotary movements.
- Massage and compress the attachments of the rhomboids and anterior serratus, both sides.

The pectoralis minor can also be addressed with the client in the side-lying position.

- Use a diagonal compression to move under the pectoralis major from the axilla.
- Place the arm in a passive flexed and adducted position to create slack in the tissues and then slowly follow the contour of the ribs to contact the pectoralis minor. This can be intense, and a confident touch is necessary.

When addressing deeper tissue layers, always remember to protect the more superficial muscles by applying pressure gradually and with as broad a base of contact as the area will allow.

The subscapularis tendon and belly of the muscle can be accessed with the client in either the side-lying or the supine position.

- With the fingers placed, glide posteriorly to access the anterior surface of the scapula. Be cautious of the nerves and vessels in the area.

The belly of the muscle near the shoulder attachment can be reached (see subscapularis release in Chapter 13).

- When symptoms are recreated or bind is felt, use compression against the scapula with internal and external rotation of the arm either passively or actively to release the area.

The attachments of the latissimus dorsi and both teres muscles at the axilla can be reached in the side-lying, prone, and supine positions.

- Combine compression with active or passive or both movements of the arm.
- A slow circumduction of the shoulder tends to access all areas.

The coracobrachialis can be accessed with the client in either the side-lying or supine position. Address this muscle if extension and abduction are limited.

- Place fingers on the muscle belly and have the client flex and adduct the arm. Then reverse the movement.
- If tender points are located, use positional release if possible.

Reassess for firing patterns and gait pattern dysfunction of the shoulder and correct any imbalance that remains.

- Palpate at the AC joint while the client moves the arm through circumduction. (I tell the client to "swim," using an overhand stroke.) The AC joint should easily hinge back and forth. If it does not easily move, increase compression on the joint slightly and have the client repeat the arm movements two or three times.
- Palpation of the SC joint bilaterally should indicate that the clavicles are spinning evenly on the manubrium when the client lifts the arm over the head. If it does not easily move, increase the compression on the joint slightly and have the client repeat the movement two or three times.
- Finish by gliding and kneading the entire area. Add oscillation (shaking and rocking) in various positions.
- As a finishing stroke, drain the area.

ARMS (FIGURE 14-20)

The arm functions as an open chain most of the time. This means that the wrist, elbow, and shoulder joints can function independently of each other. However, even in open chain function, the joints and tissues influence each other. When the

FIGURE 14-20

MUSCLES OF THE ARM

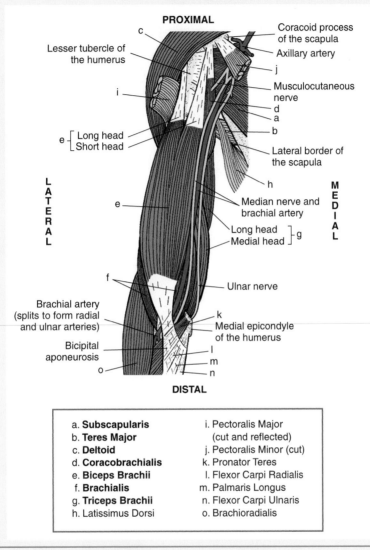

PROXIMAL

Lesser tubercle of
the humerus

c

Coracoid process
of the scapula

Axillary artery

j

Musculocutaneous
nerve

d
a
b

i

e ⎡ Long head
  ⎣ Short head

Lateral border of
the scapula

h

LATERAL

e

MEDIAL

Median nerve and
brachial artery

Long head ⎤ g
Medial head ⎦

f

Ulnar nerve

Brachial artery
(splits to form radial
and ulnar arteries)

k

Medial epicondyle
of the humerus

Bicipital
aponeurosis

l
m
n

o

DISTAL

a. **Subscapularis**
b. **Teres Major**
c. **Deltoid**
d. **Coracobrachialis**
e. **Biceps Brachii**
f. **Brachialis**
g. **Triceps Brachii**
h. Latissimus Dorsi

i. Pectoralis Major
   (cut and reflected)
j. Pectoralis Minor (cut)
k. Pronator Teres
l. Flexor Carpi Radialis
m. Palmaris Longus
n. Flexor Carpi Ulnaris
o. Brachioradialis

A Anterior view of the right arm (superficial).

Continued

FIGURE 14-20 CONT'D

MUSCLES OF THE ARM

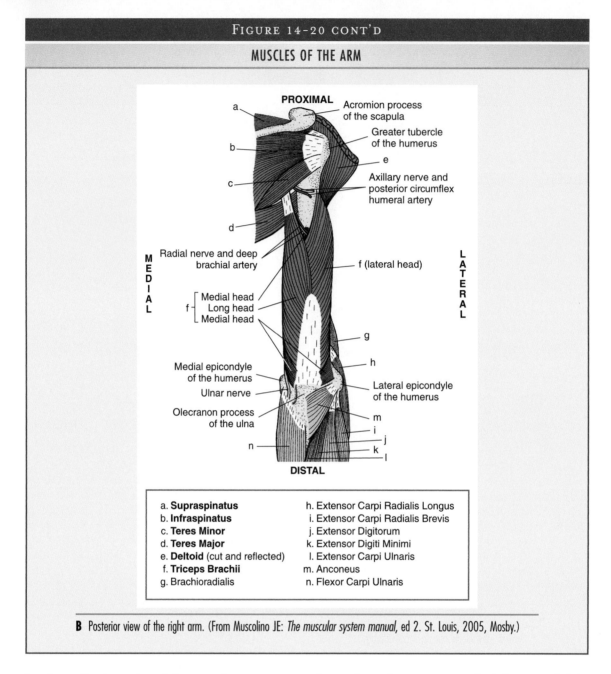

PROXIMAL

a

Acromion process
of the scapula

Greater tubercle
of the humerus

b

e

c

Axillary nerve and
posterior circumflex
humeral artery

d

MEDIAL

Radial nerve and deep
brachial artery

f (lateral head)

LATERAL

f — Medial head / Long head / Medial head

g

Medial epicondyle
of the humerus

h

Ulnar nerve

Lateral epicondyle
of the humerus

Olecranon process
of the ulna

m
i
j
k
l

n

DISTAL

a. **Supraspinatus**	h. Extensor Carpi Radialis Longus
b. **Infraspinatus**	i. Extensor Carpi Radialis Brevis
c. **Teres Minor**	j. Extensor Digitorum
d. **Teres Major**	k. Extensor Digiti Minimi
e. **Deltoid** (cut and reflected)	l. Extensor Carpi Ulnaris
f. **Triceps Brachii**	m. Anconeus
g. Brachioradialis	n. Flexor Carpi Ulnaris

B Posterior view of the right arm. (From Muscolino JE: *The muscular system manual*, ed 2. St. Louis, 2005, Mosby.)

hands are fixed, as when doing a push-up or some sort of handspring, the chain is closed, meaning that the wrist, elbow, and shoulder function in a coordinated movement. When this is the case in athletic performance such as gymnastics, it is essential that all joint function is optimal.

The muscles of the arm primarily work at the elbow. The triceps and biceps cross two joints and function at the shoulder as well. Some of the muscles of the forearm also cross the elbow.

The gait reflexes coordinate interaction between the arms and legs with a flexor, adductor, and internal rotation pattern on the left arm and right leg during forward motion (concentric contraction) working together. Antagonists are functioning eccentrically, decelerating the movement with some inhibition to allow stability and agility during movement. Movement then reverses to the right arm and left leg and the opposite pattern is activated. At the same time, the extensor, abductor, and external rotation pattern is facilitating in concentric contraction in the opposite pattern while the antagonist pattern is functioning eccentrically. This back-and-forth gait movement is necessary for

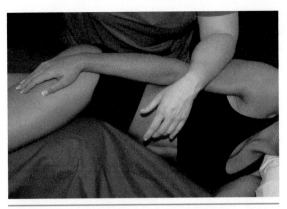

FIGURE 14-21 ■ Side-lying position gives access for best body mechanics when working on the arm and leg pattern.

agility and postural balance. It can become disrupted during injury or repetitive training activities, especially if the movement patterns are altered.

A prime example of this is weight training bilaterally, such as biceps curls, in which both muscles are concentrically contracting during flexion and then eccentrically functioning during extension, without contralateral balancing by leg movement and instead of the normal opposite swing pattern. Although this may increase strength in the arms, it does have a tendency to disrupt gait patterns and can cause an increase in motor tone of the hamstrings.

It is often necessary to work with the arms and legs in some sort of coordinated pattern to increase the effectiveness of massage. For example, the client can actively swing the knee back and forth in an open chain position while massage is being applied to the opposite arm. The flow of the massage application can proceed from the left arm to the right leg, and then from the right arm to the left leg. Another example is to work with the right biceps and the left hamstring, then work with the right triceps and the left quadriceps, and then vice versa. The side-lying position gives the best access for optimal body mechanics, but the supine or prone position can be used as well (Figure 14-21).

The muscles of the arm are in two layers. The two heads of the biceps and the three heads of the triceps are thick muscles, each with attachments on the shaft of the humerus that can bind. The brachialis and anconeus constitute the second layer of muscles.

The arm can be massaged in all basic positions and is often addressed more than once during the massage. The back of the arm is accessible when the client is in the prone position. The lateral and medial aspects can be reached when the client is in the side-lying position. With the client in the supine position, the anterior arm is easily reached, and the lateral, medial, and posterior regions can be massaged as well.

These muscles need to glide over the bone, so it is important to make sure that the tissues roll over the humerus.

For athletes whose arms are highly developed and bulked, in order to obtain adequate pressure without poking it is sometimes necessary to use knees and feet to apply compression while the client is lying on the floor.

PROCEDURES FOR THE ARMS

Examples of procedures for treatment of the arm are shown in Figure 14-22.

Massage of the arm naturally progresses from the shoulder to the forearm and then to the hand. Assessing all range of motion patterns and muscle strength will indicate which structures are short and which are long. In addition, gait pattern and firing pattern assessment should provide information about neurologic efficiency and demonstrate whether patterns are optimal.

The arm can be massaged in the supine, side-lying, or prone position. Massage begins with superficial work and progresses to deeper layers and then finishes off with superficial work. Initial applications are palpation, range of motion, strength, and neurologic assessment. This sequence focuses on massage of the arm in the prone and side-lying positions.

- Move the arm actively and passively through all joint movement patterns. Conpare active and passive movements of the arms for balanced function.
- Gently compress the elbow joint to make sure that there is no intracapsular involvement. If pain exists, refer the client to the appropriate specialist. Massage can be performed, but be aware that muscle tension patterns may be guarding the response, creating appropriate compensation.

Any areas that are not functioning optimally should be noted and reassessed after they are massaged.

- Systematically lightly stroke the area to assess for temperature changes, skin texture, and damp areas. Observe for skin reddening (histamine response) and goose flesh

14-8

FIGURE 14-22

EXAMPLE OF MASSAGE APPLICATION TO THE ARM

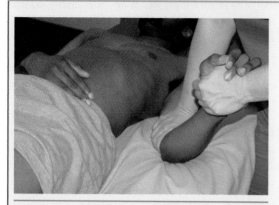

A Compress joint to assess for joint dysfunction.

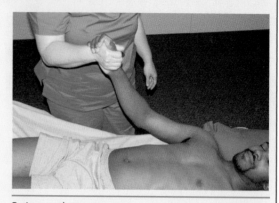

B Assess with joint movement.

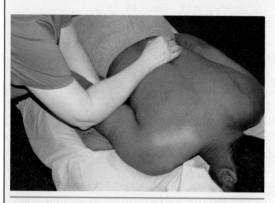

C Glide arm, prone.

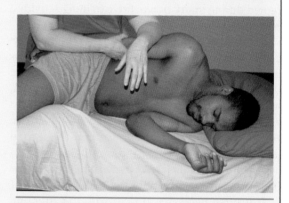

D Compress arm, side-lying.

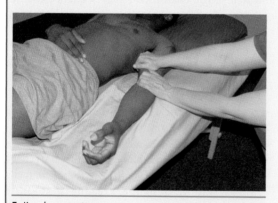

E Knead arm, supine.

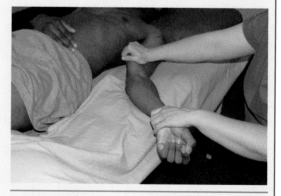

F Combined loading.

(pilomotor). These signs indicate possible changes in connective tissue, muscle tone, or circulation patterns.

- Increase the pressure slightly and assess for superficial fascial bind, changes in skin pliability, and accumulation of interstitial fluid, as indicated by boggy or edematous tissue and or increased skin pressure (like a water balloon.)
- If increased fluid pressure is evident, use lymphatic drain.
- If in doubt about the presence of fluid retention, assume it is there and drain the area.

Next address the superficial fascia by assessing for tissue bind, always observing for involvement in adjacent areas such as the tissue leading into the shoulder.

- Move the skin to identify any areas of bind in the superficial connective tissue. Notice whether any bind areas correspond to the areas of skin reddening or gooseflesh identified by the light stroking. Pay particular attention to any potential connective tissue bind in areas of scar tissue.
- Treat areas of superficial fascial bind with myofascial release methods. Address these areas by slowly moving the tissue into ease, dragging it the way it most wants to go.
- Multiple load directions can be used. For example, if the skin and superficial fascia want to move down and to the right, that would be the direction of the forces introduced. Hold each position for about 30 to 60 seconds.
- Then work into the bind with a slow, sustained drag on the binding tissues, with the lines of tension being introduced at each end of the binding tissue.
- Place your flat hand (finger pads if hand is too large) at one end of the bind and the other hand at the other end of the bind.
- Contact the tissue gently but firmly, pressing only as deep as the superficial fascial layer, and separate the hands, creating a tension force into the binding tissue.

Bending and torsion forces using compression and kneading can also be introduced.

- Maintain the drag on the tissue until the thixotropic nature of the ground substance is affected and it becomes more pliable. Subtle changes in the lines of force serve to load and unload the tissue, resulting in hysteresis.
- Next, grasp as much of the binding tissue as possible and lift it until the resistance is identified.

- Slowly load and unload with bending, torsion, and shear forces until the tissue becomes warm and more pliable.
- Finally, if the arm is small enough, grasp the tissue and twist it around the arm. If the arm is large, or as an alternative, apply a broad-based compression (the foot works well) and have the client roll the arm back and forth.

These methods are intense, and the client should feel a pulling or slight burning sensation but should not feel the need to tense up or change breathing in order to endure the application. Work slowly and deliberately, interspersing lymphatic drain type stroking every minute or so.

The musculature needs to be addressed in layers systematically, moving from superficial to deep. It is important to make sure that muscle layers are not adhered to each other. With the biceps and triceps, it is necessary to make sure that the heads of the muscles are not stuck together, since each part of the muscles has a somewhat different angle of pull. Each muscle layer should be sheared off the next deeper layer. It is helpful to place the client so that the surface layer is in a slack position with the attachments of the muscle close together and bolstering the client, so that he or she stays relaxed. With the client in the prone position, the arm should be in passive extension so that the tissues are on a slack.

- Begin at the elbow, with the client prone. Carry the strokes into the posterior deltoid and into the scapular attachment.
- Reverse the direction, using compression ending at the elbow and then glide again toward the shoulder. Repeat three or four times, each time slower and deeper while maintaining a broad-based contact to protect the more superficial tissue and reduce the potential for guarding.
- If any area binds against the drag, working across the grain of the muscle and in the opposite direction may be beneficial.

Any areas that redden may be housing trigger point activity. Because trigger points can cause muscles to fire out of sequence, it is important to restore as much normalcy to the tissue as possible.

- To increase circulation to the area and shift neuroresponses of trigger points, move the skin over the point into multiple directions of ease, holding the ease position for up to 30 to 60 seconds.
- If this does not relieve the tenderness, positional release is the next option, followed by

more aggressive muscle energy methods, if necessary.

Local lengthening of the tissue containing the trigger points is effective, and authorities have found it is needed to complete the release of trigger points. Local lengthening is accomplished by using either tension, bending, or torsion force on the tissue with the trigger point and taut band. Avoid direct pressure or transverse friction because these methods have the potential for creating tissue damage. If the trigger point does not release with the methods described, it is part of a compensation pattern that must be dealt with and the trigger point is likely serving a useful function. Leave it alone.

- Finish the area with kneading. Make sure that the muscle tissue easily lifts off the layer underneath it and rolls around the bone structure.
- If adhesions are identified, introduce a bend, shear, or torsion force until the tissue becomes more pliable. This can be intense and cause a burning sensation. The client should not guard, display pain behaviors, or hold the breath during application.
- Repeat this sequence bilaterally.

Once the surface tissue is addressed, the deep surface of the triceps muscle is massaged. It is important to make sure that the surface tissue and the fascial separation between muscle segments are not adhered together in any way.

- Use compressive gliding parallel to the fibers and deep enough to address this layer of tissue. Broaden the base of contact so that the surface tissue does not tighten, to guard against poking. Adding passive movement to the compression serves to move the bone a bit against the deep tissue, creating combined loading. Repeat three or four times, each time slower and with a slightly different angle.
- Next, glide and knead slowly across the fiber direction, using enough pressure and lift to ensure that you are affecting muscle fiber and that the tissue can slide around the bone. These methods address both the connective tissue and the neuromuscular elements of the muscle. Repeat three or four times, increasing the depth and drag each time and being aware of the muscle moving with the application.
- With the client in the side-lying position, place the client's arm on the torso. This makes it easier for the therapist to use the forearm to massage the client's arm.

- Systematically lightly stroke the area to assess for temperature changes, skin texture, and damp areas. Observe for skin reddening (histamine response) and goose flesh (pilomotor). These signs indicate possible changes in connective tissue, muscle tone, or circulation patterns.
- Increase the pressure slightly and assess for superficial fascial bind, changes in skin pliability, and accumulation of interstitial fluid, as indicated by boggy or edematous tissue and or increased skin pressure (like a water balloon).
- If increased fluid pressure is evident, drain the area, using a combination of light pressure to drag the skin and deeper rhythmic broad-based compression and kneading.
- Begin with lighter pressure directed toward the shoulder, covering the entire area. Then introduce pumping broad-based compression, combined with active and passive movements, by having the client flex and extend the elbow and shoulder, and then performing passive movement. (Remember, when moving fluid, you cannot push a river.)
- If in doubt about the presence of fluid retention, assume it is there and drain the area. Drainage direction should be toward the axilla.

Next, address the superficial fascia by assessing for tissue bind, always observing for involvement in adjacent areas such as the tissue leading into the shoulder, neck, and forearm.

- Move the skin to identify any areas of bind in the superficial connective tissue. Notice whether any bind areas correspond to the areas identified by the light stroking. Pay particular attention to any scars, because connective tissue bind is common at those sites.
- Treat areas of superficial fascial bind with myofascial release methods. Address these areas by slowly moving the tissue into ease, dragging it the way it most wants to go.
- Multiple load directions can be used. Hold each position up to 30 to 60 seconds.
- Then work into the bind with a slow, sustained drag on the binding tissues, with the lines of tension being introduced at each end of the binding tissue.
- Place your forearm (flat hand if the forearm is too large) at one end of the bind and the other forearm at the other end of the bind.
- Contact the tissue gently but firmly, pressing only as deep as the superficial fascial layer,

and separate the forearms, creating a tension force into the binding tissue. Bending force can also be introduced through kneading. Tension force can be added.

- Have the client actively or passively move the arm into slight flexion and extension and then back into the original position while the massage is applied. Repeat the movement back and forth until a change is noted.
- Maintain the drag on the tissue until the thixotropic nature of the ground substance is affected and it becomes more pliable. Subtle changes in the lines of force serve to load and unload the tissue, resulting in hysteresis.
- Grasp as much of the binding tissue as possible and lift it until the resistance is identified. Slowly load and unload with torsion and shear force, or by having the client move the arm, until the tissue becomes warm and more pliable. This method is intense, and the client should feel a pulling or slight burning sensation. The client should not feel the need to tense up or change breathing in order to endure the application.
- Work slowly and deliberately, interspersing lymphatic drain type stroking every minute or so.

When an area that is bothering the client is located, familiar symptoms will be reproduced. Compression combined with muscle energy methods, from the least invasive of positional release to the more aggressive integrated methods, can be used to create a shift in function. The goal is to temporally inhibit the motor tone of the muscle bundle that is problematic so that it can be lengthened to the appropriate resting length and the client feels reduced pressure on the nerves or vessels.

With the client in the side-lying position, simply by changing the arm position, the lateral, posterior, and anterior areas can be massaged, and range of motion is not limited by the table. When addressing deeper tissue layers, always remember to protect the more superficial muscles, applying pressure gradually and with as broad a base of contact as the area will allow.

The triceps belly and tendon at the scapula are best accessed with the client in the side-lying position.

- Have the client both flex and extend the elbow as well as circumduct the shoulder.
- Combine compression with active, passive, or both movements of the arm. A slow circumduction tends to access all areas.
- Assess firing patterns for the arm.

- Finish by gliding and kneading the entire area in the supine position.
- Add oscillation (rocking and shaking) in various positions.
- As a finishing stroke, drain the area.

FOREARM, WRIST, AND HAND (FIGURE 14-23)

The forearm muscles function to work the wrist and fingers. They also weakly assist elbow movements. This can be an issue when the elbow, wrist, and fingers are functioning as a unit, as while throwing a ball, when the fingers have to grasp (isometric) but the wrist and elbow have to move (concentric and eccentric), thus creating the potential for rubbing at the attachments. The end result from repetitive movements like these can be tendonitis and bursitis. Muscles near the elbow and wrist allow supination and pronation of the hand. Repetitive movement is common for these tissues, as is repetitive strain injury. The goal of the massage is to maintain normal tissue function so that repetitive movement does not become repetitive strain.

The muscles of the forearm are categorized as superficial, intermediate, and deep and are best addressed as three layers that include the supinator, pronator teres, and pronator quadratus. The muscles can also adhere to each other, one on top of the other in the their side-by-side positions. Because the movements of the fingers have a slightly different range than the wrist, it is essential that these muscles glide easily over one another. The superficial muscle layer primarily functions at the wrist, with some activity at the elbow, whereas the deep layers work the fingers, with some activity at the wrist.

The bellies of these muscles are closer to the elbow, and they taper to the tendons in the wrist and fingers. It is important to gauge pressure of the massage, which is more intense along the proximal half of the forearm where the muscle bulk is located. Connective tissue binding often shows up in the distal half of the forearm and into the hand.

Typically, the forearm or flat, soft palm of the hand is used to massage the client's forearm, but the foot also works very well to apply compression. The arch of the foot fits nicely over the muscle bulk, and the client can provide active moment of the wrist and finger while the compression is being applied. This is effective in reducing tone and connective tissue bind in the muscles resulting from repetitive movements.

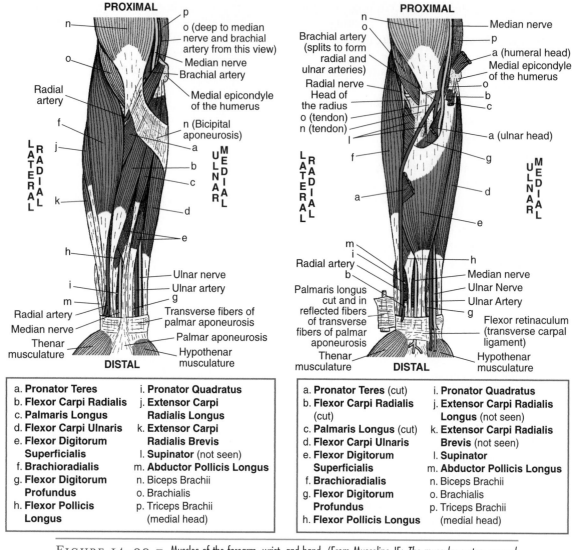

FIGURE 14-23 ■ Muscles of the forearm, wrist, and hand. (From Muscolino JE: *The muscular system manual*, ed 2. St. Louis, 2005, Mosby.)

PROCEDURES FOR FOREARM, WRIST, AND HAND

Examples of procedures for treatment of the forearm, wrist, and hand are shown in Figure 14-24.

The massage pattern is very similar to that presented for all body areas. Massage of the wrist and hand initially involves working with the muscles of the forearm in relationship to the action of the wrist, fingers, and thumb.

- Systematically compress the muscles of the forearm, beginning at the elbow and working toward the wrist while the client moves the wrist and fingers back and forth in circles, or makes and releases the fist.

- To isolate a particular muscle function related to a wrist or finger action, have the client move the wrist or finger in the way that creates the symptom and then palpate the forearm muscles to see which ones are activated. Then use compression or gliding while the client moves the wrist or fingers to affect the identified area. Occasionally, trigger point type application is necessary.

Once this is complete, address the range of motion of the wrist. The wrist is often jammed, with a reduction in joint play. A general method to

14-9   FIGURE 14-24

EXAMPLE OF MASSAGE APPLICATION TO THE FOREARM, WRIST, AND HAND

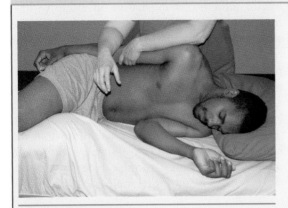

A Forearm gliding, side-lying.

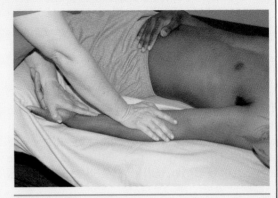

B Forearm gliding, supine.

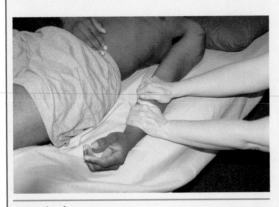

C Kneading forearm.

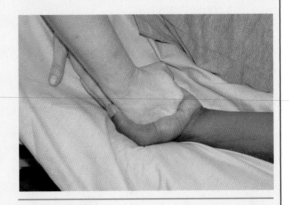

D Compress hand.

restore joint play is to use the "mobilization with movement" sequence described in Chapter 13. This sequence involves the traction of a joint and moving the joint into the ease and pain-free position by the therapist. The client is passive while the position is found. The position is then maintained by the therapist, and the client actively moves the joint through a range of motions. For the wrist, having the client move the wrist in a circle will be effective.

Next, address the intrinsic muscles of the hand.
- Systematically work the area, using compression and gliding of the soft tissues between the fingers and the web of the thumb and on the palm.
- To assist lymphatic movement, use rhythmic compression to stimulate the network of lymphatic vessels in the palm.
- Trigger points are commonly found in the opponens pollicis and other muscles of the palm near the wrist. Positional release works

well: apply compression on the point while the client moves the associated finger or thumb.
- Direct pressure or tapping can stimulate acupuncture points at the side of each nail. An easy way to do this is to squeeze, release, and repeat three or four times, on the lateral and medial side of each finger and thumbnail.
- There is also a major accupuncture point in the web of the thumb used for pain control, nausea, and other dysfunctions. Use rhythmic on/off compression of this point to aid in general homeostasis.
- The many finger and thumb joints often become jammed, and the "mobilization with movement" sequence described in Chapter 13, can be used on the joints of the fingers and thumb. The fingers are hinge joints, as is the distal joint of the thumb. Once traction is applied and the ease position found, the client moves the area back and forth. The

thumb is a saddle joint; therefore circular movement is most effective.

- Finally, address the metacarpal joints. Moving the carpal bones back and forth is effective.
- To finish off, use oscillation (rocking and shaking) and lymphatic drain.

HIP (FIGURE 14-25)

The hip is a complex musculoskeletal unit. The joint structure is mobile, relying on a deep joint capsule, ligaments, muscles, and fascia to provide stability. It is less mobile than the shoulder. The movement of the sacroiliac (SI) and femoral joints in a coordinated fashion is necessary for both maximal mobility and stability of the area.

The inner (local muscle) unit (deep lateral rotator muscles), coupled with an extensive ligament structure, holds and guides the femur in the acetabulum, using the bones of the pelvis as a broad-based attachment point. The gluteus maximus is an expansive outer unit (global muscles) interacting with the contralateral latissimus dorsi and ipsilateral tensor fasciae latae and IT band to provide stability and force closure from the lumbar back and SI joint area down into the knee. Combined with the gluteus medius and minimus, the gluteus maximus can be compared to the deltoid muscle of the shoulder.

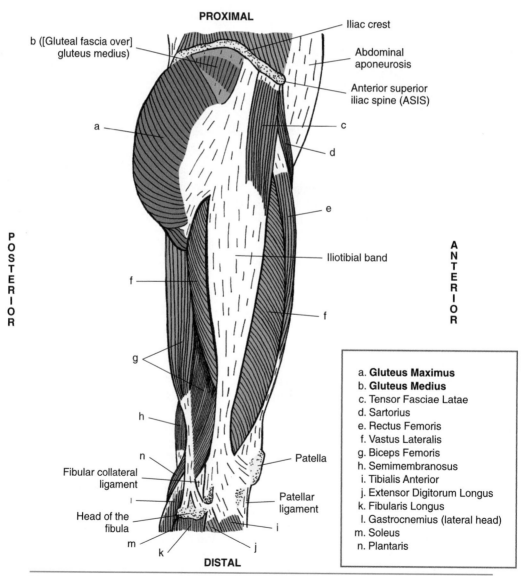

a. **Gluteus Maximus**
b. **Gluteus Medius**
c. Tensor Fasciae Latae
d. Sartorius
e. Rectus Femoris
f. Vastus Lateralis
g. Biceps Femoris
h. Semimembranosus
i. Tibialis Anterior
j. Extensor Digitorum Longus
k. Fibularis Longus
l. Gastrocnemius (lateral head)
m. Soleus
n. Plantaris

FIGURE 14-25 ■ Muscles of the hip. (From Muscolino JE: *The muscular system manual*, ed 2. St. Louis, 2005, Mosby.)

The gluteal muscles interact with the adductors to provide a force couple arrangement during gait.

The psoas and gluteus maximus can become dysfunctional if core stability is inadequate. The gluteus maximus is often inhibited, caused by a short and tight psoas. Muscle activation sequences of the global muscles of the hip are affected if the lower abdominal group does not fire normally. In this type of dysfunction, the psoas and rectus abdominis will fire too soon (synergistic dominance) and inhibit the gluteus maximus. The hip extension firing pattern will in turn become dysfunctional, causing lumbar and hamstring shortening. The knee can be affected. Calf muscles, especially the gastrocnemius, then begin to dominate, leading to both knee and ankle dysfunction.

Muscle fascial components in the torso affect the stability and mobility of the hip. Involvement of gait reflexes necessitates that the shoulders and hips function in coordinated movement.

Nerve impingement by the lumbar and sacral plexus refers pain to the hip and leg.

PROCEDURES FOR THE HIP

Procedures for treatment of the hip are shown in Figure 14-26.

The hip is massaged with the client in the prone and side-lying positions. Massage of the torso naturally progresses to the hip. Assessment of all range of motion patterns and muscle strength will indicate which structures are short and which are long. In addition, gait pattern assessment should pro-vide information about neurologic efficiency and whether firing patterns are optimal. Firing patterns in this area are especially important. Assess patterns for hip extension and abduction (see Chapter 12).

Massage begins with superficial work, progresses to deeper layers, and then finishes off with superficial work. Initial applications are palpation, range of motion, strength, and neurologic assessment. The hip should be first actively and then passively moved though flexion, extension, internal and external rotation, adduction, and abduction as well as full circumduction. This part of assessment can most easily be done, with the least restriction and the greatest range of motion, with the client in the side-lying position. Active and passive movements of the left and right hip should be compared.

- Compress the joint gently to make sure that there is no intracapsular involvement. If there is, refer the client to the appropriate specialist. Massage can be performed, but be aware that muscle tension patterns may be guarding, creating appropriate compensation.

- With the client in the prone, palpate at the SI joint while the prone client circumducts (makes a circle) with the hip; the SI joint should move slightly in a figure-of-eight pattern.

- Continue to palpate the SI joint. Bend the client's knee and internally and externally rotate the leg. Initial movement occurs in the hip joint, and secondary movement occurs at the SI joint. In general, 45 degrees of internal and external rotation in this position indicates normal function. Any alteration in this pattern indicates the potential for both SI joint and hip joint dysfunction.

Any areas that are not functioning optimally should be noted and reassessed after the massage of the area. If the pattern does not normalize, referral to appropriate medical personnel is necessary.

- Systematically lightly stroke the area to assess for temperature changes, skin texture, and damp areas. Observe for skin reddening (histamine response) and goose flesh (pilomotor). These signs indicate possible changes in connective tissue, muscle tone, or circulation patterns.

- Increase the pressure slightly and assess for superficial fascial bind, changes in skin pliability, and accumulation of interstitial fluid, as indicated by boggy or edematous tissue and or increased skin pressure (turgor, like a water balloon). If increased fluid pressure is evident, then drain, using the lymphatic drain method.

- If in doubt about the presence of fluid retention, assume it is there and drain the area.

Next, address the superficial fascia by assessing for tissue bind, always observing for involvement in adjacent areas, such as the tissue leading into the torso and leg.

- Move the skin to identify any areas of bind in the superficial connective tissue. Notice whether any bind areas correspond to the areas of skin reddening or gooseflesh identified by the light stroking. Pay particular attention to any scars because connective tissue bind is common at these sites.

- Treat areas of superficial fascial bind with myofascial release methods. Address these areas by slowly moving the tissue into ease, dragging it the way it most wants to go.

- Multiple load directions can be used. For example, if the skin and superficial fascia want to move up and to the right near the sacrum, that would be the direction of the forces introduced. Hold ease position for up to 30 to 60 seconds.

FIGURE 14-26

EXAMPLE OF MASSAGE APPLICATION TO THE HIP

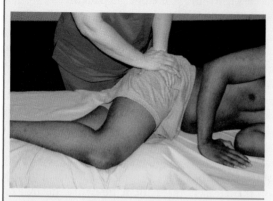

A Compress the hip joint to assess for dysfunction.

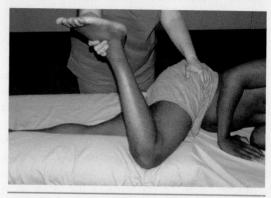

B Range of motion, hip, side-lying.

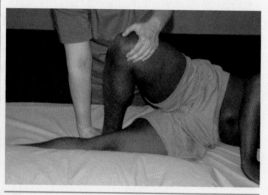

C Range of motion, hip, side-lying.

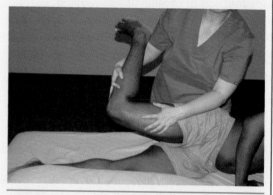

D Range of motion, hip, side-lying.

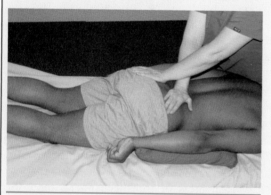

E Multiple loading, ease and bind.

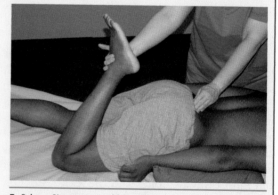

F Palpate SI joint, external hip rotation.

FIGURE 14-26—CONT'D

EXAMPLE OF MASSAGE APPLICATION TO THE HIP

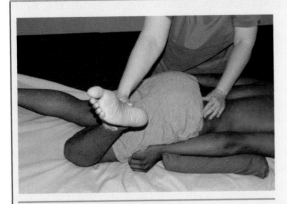

G Palpate SI joint, internal hip rotation.

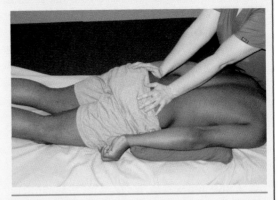

H Tissue stretch.

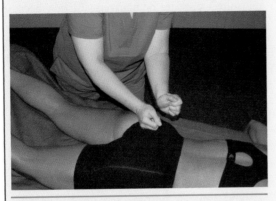

I Percussion on hip.

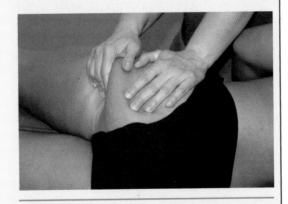

J Knead tissue.

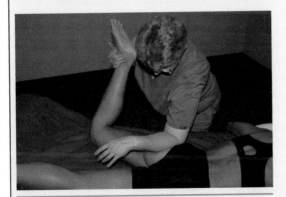

K Compression and movement, hip. Deep lateral hip rotation.

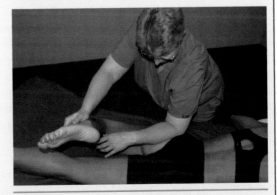

L Compression and movement, hip. Deep lateral hip rotation.

- Then work into the bind with a slow, sustained drag on the binding tissues, with the lines of tension being introduced at each end of the binding tissue. Place your flat forearm or hand at one end of the bind and the other forearm/hand at the other end of the bind.
- Contact the tissue gently but firmly, pressing only as deep as the superficial fascial layer, and separate the forearms or hands, creating a tension force into the binding tissue.
- Maintain the drag on the tissue until the thixotropic nature of the ground substance is affected and becomes more pliable. Subtle changes in the lines of force serve to load and unload the tissue, resulting in hysteresis. Active and passive range of motion can serve to load and unload tissues.
- Next, grasp as much of the binding tissue as possible and lift it until the resistance is identified. Slowly load and unload with torsion and shear force until the tissue becomes warm and more pliable. This method is intense, and the client should feel a pulling or slight burning sensation. The client should not feel the need to tense up or change breathing in order to endure the application. Work slowly and deliberately, interspersing lymphatic drain type stroking every minute or so.

The musculature needs to be addressed in layers, moving from superficial to deep. It is important to make sure that muscle layers are not adhered to each other. If adhesions exist, one muscle layer should be sheared off the next, deeper layer. Layers tend to stick where the gluteus maximus weaves into the IT band at a lengthy musculotendinous junction. Use a wave-like motion to assess the tissue. It is helpful to place the client so that the surface layer is in a slack position with the attachments of the muscle close together, and propping the client so that he or she stays relaxed. In some situations, the side-lying position may be better for this.

Begin on the posterior side to address the lumbar region that connects with the hip. This area was addressed while massaging the torso but now is massaged in relationship to the hip.

- Carry the strokes into the gluteus maximus. Use gliding with a compressive element and drag toward the hip. Repeat with the latissimus dorsi in relationship to hip function.
- Begin at the shoulder and carry the stroke all the way into the opposite gluteus maximus. If any area binds against the drag, working across the grain of the muscle and in the opposite direction may be beneficial.

Any areas that redden may be housing trigger point activity. Because trigger points can cause muscles to fire out of sequence, it is important to restore as much normalcy to the tissue as possible.

- To increase circulation to the area and shift neuroresponses of trigger points, move the skin into multiple directions of ease over the suspected trigger point area and hold the ease position for 30 to 60 seconds.
- If this does not relieve the tenderness, positional release is the next option, followed by muscle energy methods, if necessary.

Local lengthening of the tissue containing the trigger points is effective. Local lengthening is accomplished by using tension, bending, or torsion force on the tissue with the trigger point and taut band. Avoid direct pressure or transverse friction because these methods have the potential for creating tissue damage. If the trigger point does not release with the methods described, it is likely a part of a compensation pattern that must be dealt with, and the trigger point is serving a useful function. Leave it alone.

- Finish the area with kneading, making sure that the muscle tissue lifts easily off the layer underneath it.
- If adhesions are identified, introduce a bend, shear, or torsion force until the tissue becomes more pliable. This can be intense and cause a burning sensation. The client should not guard, display pain behaviors, or hold the breath during application.
- Repeat this sequence bilaterally.

Once the surface tissue is addressed, the second layer of muscle is massaged. It is important to make sure that the surface tissue and the fascial separation between muscle layers are not adhered together in any way. Use either a wave-like motion on the surface muscle to slide it back and forth or lift the muscle tissue up and move it back and forth to assess for adhesion.

The main muscles being addressed are portions of the gluteus medius, gluteus minimus, and deep lateral hip rotators. It is helpful to place the surface layer of tissue in a slack position by passively supporting the hip in extension. This can be done with the client in either the prone or side-lying position.

- Begin at the iliac crest attachments and use a compressive gliding deep enough to address this layer of tissue. Broaden the base of contact so that the surface tissue does not tighten to guard against poking.

- Glide toward the greater trochanter. Repeat three or four times, each time slower and at a slightly different angle.
- Glide and knead slowly across the fiber direction, using enough pressure and lift to ensure that you are affecting muscle fiber in this layer. These methods address both the connective tissue and the neuromuscular elements of the muscles. Repeat three or four times, increasing the depth and drag each time, and being aware of the muscle moving with the application.

Next, address the deep lateral hip rotators.

- With the surface layer still in a slack position, apply a broad-based compression using the forearm into the space between the sacrum and the greater trochanter. This is best accomplished in the prone position.
- Bend the client's knee and move the hip back and forth from medial to lateral rotation. This can be thought of as moving "into the 4 and out of the 4." The action can be active or passive.
- Repeat three or four times, slightly changing the angle. Do not put constant compression on the sciatic nerve. Lighten the compressive force at least every 30 seconds to allow for proper circulation to the area.

The side-lying position is effective for addressing the gluteus medius and tensor fasciae latae on the upper side and the quadratus femoris on the opposite (closer to the table) side. Broad-based compression with the forearm on the gluteus and a stabilized hand position are best when working on the quadratus femoris. Because the quadratus femoris muscle is in the groin area, ask permission before working in this area.

The quadratus femoris is a deep lateral rotator, but unlike the others, which are abductors, it is an adductor and often is short. Active and passive movement can be added while the area is being compressed.

- Assess SI joint by palpating the joint and internally and externally rotating the hip. The hip should be able to move 45 degrees in either direction without feeling binding at the SI joint.
- Perform passive and active mobilization of the SI joint and the symphysis pubis (see specific releases in Chapter 13).
- Assess firing patterns (see Chapter 12).
- Finish by gliding and kneading the entire area. Add oscillation (rocking and shaking) in various positions.
- As a finishing stroke, drain the area.

THIG (FIGURE 14-27)

Lumbar and sacral plexus impingement can cause radiating pain in the legs. The muscles that most often cause impingement are the quadratus lumborum and multifidi. Lumbar plexus impingement causes radiating pain in the thigh, whereas sacral plexus impingement causes radiating pain in the back of the thigh and calf.

The thigh and leg function in a closed chain most of the time, meaning that the hip, knee, and ankle do not function independently of each other. Even in open chain function, these joints and tissues influence each other.

The muscles of the thigh primarily work at the knee. The rectus femoris, hamstring group, and sartorius cross two joints and function both at the hip and knee. Some of the muscles of the leg also cross the knee, such as the gastrocnemius.

The gait reflexes coordinate interaction between the arms and legs with a flexor, adductor, and internal rotation pattern on the left arm and right leg during forward motion (concentric contraction), facilitating with antagonists that are functioning eccentrically for deceleration; then concentric contraction transfers into the right arm and left leg, and the opposite pattern is activated. At the same time, the extensor, abductor, and external rotation pattern is facilitating in concentric contraction in the contralateral side of the body, and the antagonist pattern is functioning eccentrically. This back-and-forth movement of gait is necessary for postural stability, fluid motion, and agility.

Gait function can become disrupted during injury, repetitive training activities, or when competing when fatigued, especially if the movement patterns are altered. A prime example of this is weight training bilaterally, such as hamstring strengthening, in which both left and right are concentrically contracted and then eccentrically contracted at the same time instead of in the opposite swing pattern. Although this may increase strength in the legs, it does have a tendency to disrupt gait patterns, with a corresponding increase in tone in both of the biceps brachii.

It is often necessary to work with the arms and legs in some sort of coordinated pattern to increase effectiveness of the massage. For example, the client can actively bend the elbow back and forth in an open chain position while massage is being applied to the opposite leg, or the flow of the massage application may proceed from the left arm

a. **Tensor Fasciae Latae**
b. **Sartorius**
c. **Rectus Femoris**
d. **Vastus Lateralis**
e. **Vastus Medialis**
f. **Vastus Intermedius** (not seen)
g. **Pectineus**
h. **Adductor Longus**
i. **Adductor Magnus**
j. **Gracilis**
k. Psoas Major
l. Iliacus
m. Gluteus Medius
n. Gastrocnemius
o. Fibularis Longus
p. Tibialis Anterior

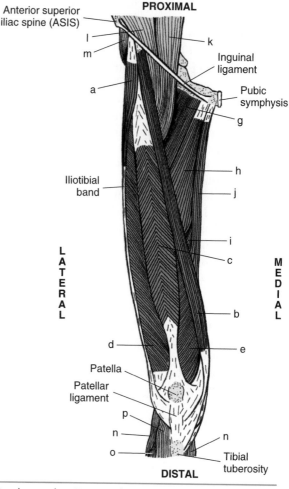

FIGURE 14-27 ■ Muscles of the thigh and anterior leg. (From Muscolino JE: *The muscular system manual*, ed. 2. St. Louis, 2005, Mosby.)

Continued

to the right leg and then from the right arm to the left leg. Another example is to work with the right biceps and the left hamstring, then the right quadriceps and the left triceps, and then vice versa. The side-lying position gives the best access for optimal body mechanics, but the supine or prone position can be used as well.

The thigh muscles are basically two layers. In the superficial layer, the three heads of the hamstrings are thick muscles that superiorly attach in close proximity on the ischial tuberosity and can bind or get stuck together. The four heads of the quadriceps are also thick muscles, three of which have proximal attachments on the shaft of the femur; all four have distal attachments on the tibia, which can become a source of binding if layers are stuck together. The vastus intermedius is the main muscle in the second layer.

The thigh also contains the large group of adductor muscles. This group is very involved in core stability and antigravity function.

The thigh can be massaged in all basic positions and is often addressed more than once during the massage. When the client is in the prone position, the back of the thigh is accessible. With the client in the side-lying position, the adductors and IT band are accessible. With the client supine, the anterior thigh is easily reached, and the lateral, medial, and posterior regions can be assessed from the positions shown in Figure 14-28. The quadriceps muscles are effectively massaged with the client seated.

These muscles need to glide over the bone, so rolling tissues over the femur is important.

When working with athletes in whom the thighs are highly developed and bulked, using your knees

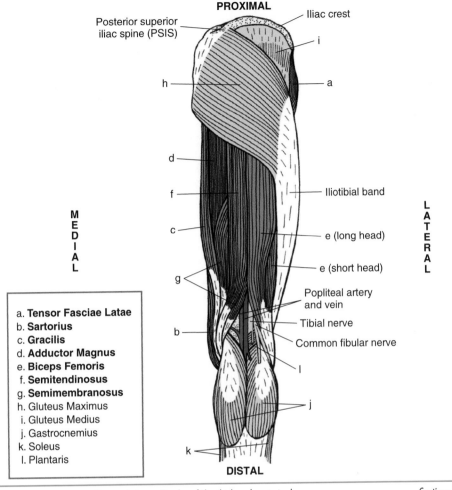

PROXIMAL

Posterior superior
iliac spine (PSIS)

Iliac crest

i

h

a

d

f

Iliotibial band

c

e (long head)

e (short head)

g

**M
E
D
I
A
L**

**L
A
T
E
R
A
L**

Popliteal artery
and vein

Tibial nerve

b

Common fibular nerve

l

j

a. **Tensor Fasciae Latae**
b. **Sartorius**
c. **Gracilis**
d. **Adductor Magnus**
e. **Biceps Femoris**
f. **Semitendinosus**
g. **Semimembranosus**
h. Gluteus Maximus
 i. Gluteus Medius
 j. Gastrocnemius
k. Soleus
 l. Plantaris

k

DISTAL

FIGURE 14-27 Cont'd ■ Muscles of the thigh and posterior leg.   *Continued*

and feet to apply compression while the client is lying on the floor is often advisable.

PROCEDURES FOR THE THIGH

Examples of procedures for treatment of the thigh and leg are shown in Figure 14-29.

Massage of the thigh naturally progresses from hip to calf. Assessment of all range of motion patterns and muscle strength will indicate which structures are short and which are long. In addition, gait pattern and firing pattern assessment should provide information about neurologic efficiency and whether tone patterns are affected.

Like other body regions, massage begins with superficial work, progresses to deeper layers, and then finishes off with superficial work. Initial applications are palpation assessment, range of motion,

strength, and neurologic assessment. Massage should begin with the client in the prone position.

- Move the thigh and knee both actively and passively through flexion, extension, and internal and external rotation. Compare active and passive movements of right and left limbs.
- Gently compress the knee joints to make sure that there is no intracapsular involvement. If there is, refer the client to the appropriate specialist. Massage can still be performed, but be aware that muscle tension patterns may be guarding to create appropriate compensation.

Any areas that are not functioning optimally should be noted and reassessed after the area is massaged.

- Systematically lightly stroke the area to assess for temperature changes, skin texture, and

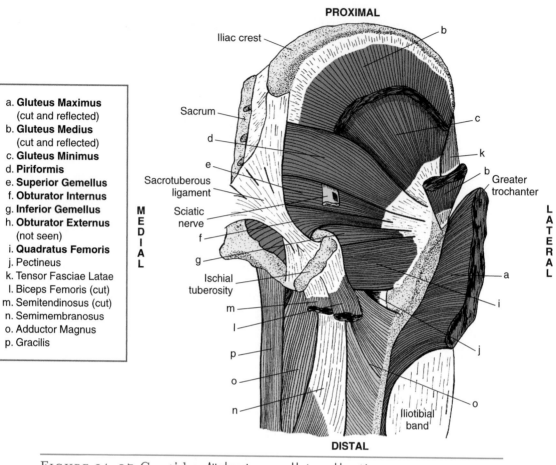

a. **Gluteus Maximus**
   (cut and reflected)
b. **Gluteus Medius**
   (cut and reflected)
c. **Gluteus Minimus**
d. **Piriformis**
e. **Superior Gemellus**
f. **Obturator Internus**
g. **Inferior Gemellus**
h. **Obturator Externus**
   (not seen)
i. **Quadratus Femoris**
j. Pectineus
k. Tensor Fasciae Latae
l. Biceps Femoris (cut)
m. Semitendinosus (cut)
n. Semimembranosus
o. Adductor Magnus
p. Gracilis

FIGURE 14-27 Cont'd ▪ Attachment areas—adductors and hamstrings.

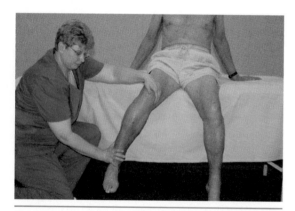

FIGURE 14-28 ▪ Seated position when massaging the thigh.

damp areas. Observe for skin reddening (histamine response) and goose flesh (pilomotor). These signs indicate possible changes in connective tissue, muscle tone, or circulation patterns.

- Increase the pressure slightly and assess for superficial fascial bind, changes in skin pliability, and accumulation of interstitial fluid as indicated by boggy or edematous tissue and/or increased skin pressure (like a water balloon).
- If increased fluid pressure is evident, drain the area using a combination of light pressure to drag the skin and deeper, rhythmic broad-based compression and kneading to stimulate the deeper vessels.
- Begin with lighter pressure directed toward the groin, covering the entire area. Then introduce pumping broad-based compression, combined first with active and then with passive movement by having the client slowly flex and relax the hip.
- Return to dragging the skin, and alternate between both methods until the area is drained (about 5 minutes). (Remember, when moving fluid, you cannot push a river.)

14-11

FIGURE 14-29

EXAMPLE OF MASSAGE APPLICATION TO THE THIGH AND LEG

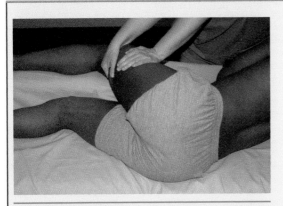

A Knead thigh, side-lying.

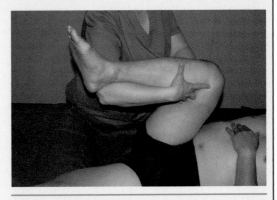

B Joint movement (supine).

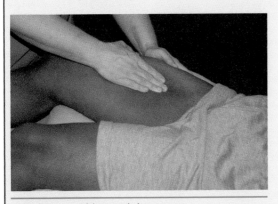

C Thigh supine—sliding muscle layers, supine.

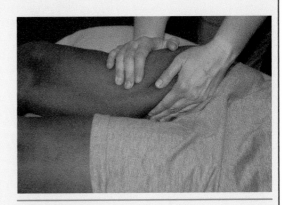

D Knead thigh, supine.

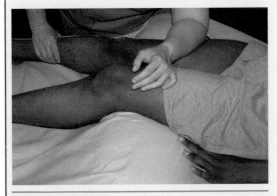

E Glide thigh, supine.

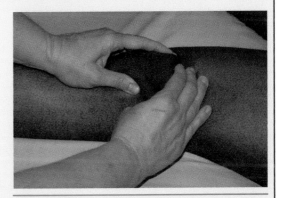

F Move patella.

Continued

FIGURE 14-29—CONT'D

EXAMPLE OF MASSAGE APPLICATION TO THE THIGH AND LEG

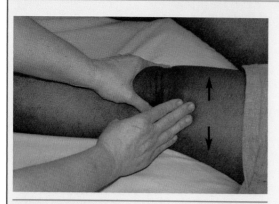

G Friction, vastus lateralis.

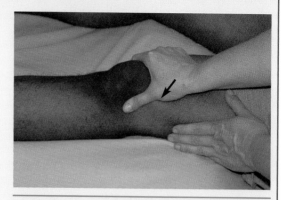

H Compression.

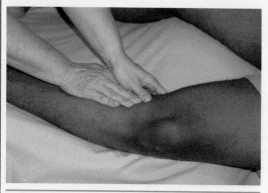

I Pes ansere attachments—friction.

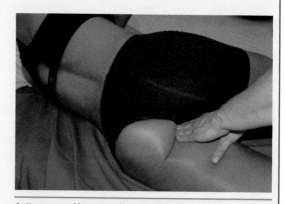

J Hamstring adductor attachments, side-lying.

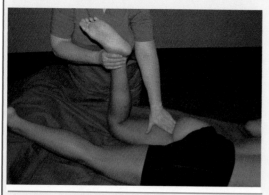

K Hamstring adductor attachments, prone.

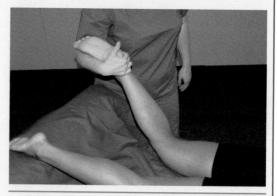

L Oscillation and joint movement, prone.

FIGURE 14-29—CONT'D

EXAMPLE OF MASSAGE APPLICATION TO THE THIGH AND LEG

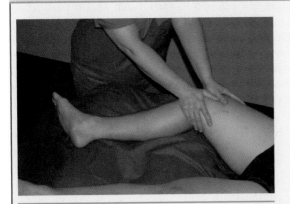

M Thigh adductors, supine.

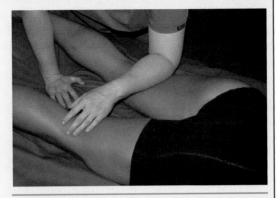

N Thigh gliding, prone.

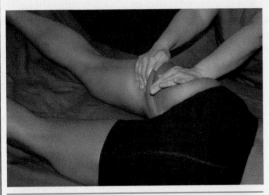

O Thigh kneading, prone. (Body mechanisms, therapist kneeling.)

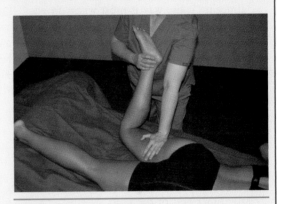

P Thigh compression and movement.

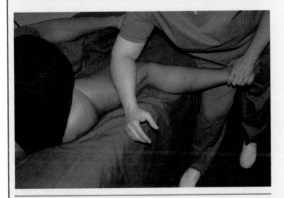

Q Thigh, side-lying. Gliding.

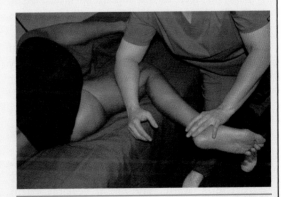

R Thigh compression and movement.

- If in doubt about the presence of fluid retention, assume it is there and drain the area.

Next, address the superficial fascia by assessing for tissue bind, always observing for involvement in adjacent areas such as the tissue leading into the hip and knee. Pay particular attention to the IT band and the junctions of the hamstring and quadriceps in this connective tissue structure.

- Move the skin to identify any areas of bind in the superficial connective tissue. Notice whether any bind areas correspond to the areas of skin reddening or gooseflesh identified by the light stroking. Pay particular attention to any scars, because connective tissue bind is common at these sites.
- Treat areas of superficial fascial bind with myofascial release methods. Address these areas by slowly moving the tissue into ease, dragging it the way it most wants to go.
- Multiple loading directions can be used. For example, if the skin and superficial fascia want to move up and to the right on the IT band, that would be the direction of the forces introduced. Hold the ease position for up to 30 to 60 seconds.
- Then work into the bind with a slow, sustained drag on the binding tissues, with the lines of tension being introduced at each end of the binding tissue. Place your flat hand at one end of the bind and the other hand at the other end of the bind.
- Contact the tissue gently but firmly, pressing only as deep as the superficial fascial layer, and separate the hands, creating a tension force into the binding tissue.

Bending and torsion forces using kneading can be introduced, and these methods are especially effective on the IT band. Subtle changes in the lines of force serve to load and unload the tissue.

- Grasp as much of the binding tissue as possible and lift it until the resistance is identified.
- Slowly load and unload with bending, torsion, and shear force until the tissue becomes warm and more pliable. This method is intense, and the client should feel a pulling or slight burning sensation. The client should not feel the need to tense up or change breathing in order to endure the method. Work slowly and deliberately.
- Do not use tension force application (gliding) with deep pressure over the IT band. Compression of the nerve structures may result. Instead, use kneading.

- Address muscle layers systematically, moving from superficial to deep.

It is important to make sure that muscle layers are not adhered to each other. This is particularly important in the thigh. The most common locations of adherence are at the rectus femoris on the vastus intermedius, at the edges of the two medial hamstrings (semimembranosus and semitendinosus) as they meet in the middle of the posterior thigh, and where the vastus lateralis and lateral hamstring (biceps femoris) weave into the iliotibial band near their distal insertions. In both the quadriceps and hamstrings groups, it is necessary to make sure that the heads of the muscles are not stuck together, as each part of the muscles has a somewhat different angle of pull. One muscle layer should be sheared off the next deeper layer and from the structures next to it. It is helpful to place the client so that the surface layer is in a slack position with the attachments of the muscle close together and bolstering the client so that he or she stays relaxed.

- Begin at the knee. Carry the strokes into the posterior hip. Reverse the direction, using compression toward the knee, and then glide again toward the hip.
- Repeat three or four times, each time slower and deeper, maintaining a broad-based contact to protect the more surface tissue and reduce the potential for guarding.

If any area binds against the drag, working across the grain of the muscle and in the opposite direction may be beneficial.

- Glide slowly across the fiber direction, using enough pressure to be sure that you are affecting muscle fiber. This method addresses both the connective tissue and the neuromuscular elements of the muscle.
- Repeat three or four times, increasing the depth and drag each time, being aware of the muscle moving with the application.

Any areas that redden may be housing trigger point activity. Because trigger points can cause muscles to fire out of sequence, it is important to restore as much normalcy to the tissue as possible.

- To increase circulation to the area and shift neuroresponses of trigger points, move the skin in multiple directions of ease over the area and hold the ease position for 30 to 60 seconds.
- If this does not relieve the tenderness, positional release is the next option, followed by muscle energy methods, if necessary.

Local lengthening of the tissue containing the trigger points is effective. Local lengthening is accomplished by using tension, bending, or torsion force on the tissue with the trigger point and taut band. Avoid direct pressure or transverse friction, because these methods have the potential for creating tissue damage. If the trigger point does not release with the methods described, it is part of a compensation pattern that must be dealt with, and the trigger point is likely serving a useful function. Let it alone.

- Assess for firing patterns for hip extension and knee flexion and correct if necessary.
- Finish the area with kneading, making sure that the muscle tissue easily lifts off the layer underneath it.
- If adhesions are identified, introduce a bend, shear, or torsion force until it becomes more pliable. This can be intense and cause a burning sensation. The client should not guard, display pain behaviors, or hold the breath during application.
- Repeat this sequence bilaterally.

With the client in the side-lying position, the medial, lateral, posterior, and anterior thigh can be massaged, and range of motion is not limited by the table. This is the best position for massage of the medial and lateral thigh. The supine position is most effective for massage of the anterior thigh.

- Systematically lightly stroke the area to assess for temperature changes, skin texture, and damp areas. Observe for skin reddening (histamine response) and goose flesh (pilomotor). These signs indicate possible changes in connective tissue, muscle tone, or circulation patterns.
- Increase the pressure slightly and assess for superficial fascial bind, changes in skin pliability, and accumulation of interstitial fluid, as indicated by boggy or edematous tissue and/or increased skin pressure (like a water balloon).
- If increased fluid pressure is evident, drain the area. (Remember when moving fluid, you cannot push a river.)
- If in doubt about the presence of fluid retention, then assume it is there and drain the area.

Next, address the superficial fascia by assessing for tissue bind, always observing for involvement in adjacent areas such as the tissue leading into the hip and knee.

- Move the skin to identify any areas of bind in the superficial connective tissue. Notice whether any bind areas correspond to the areas of skin reddening or gooseflesh identified by the light stroking. Pay particular attention to any scars, because connective tissue bind is common at these sites.
- Treat areas of superficial fascial bind with myofascial release methods Address these areas by slowly moving the tissue into ease with multiple load directions.
- Work into the bind using a slow, sustained drag on the binding tissues, with the lines of tension being introduced at each end of the binding tissue. Place your forearms (flat hand if forearm is too large) at one end of the bind and the other forearm at the other end of the bind.
- Contact the tissue gently but firmly, pressing only as deep as the superficial fascial layer, and separate the forearms, creating a tension force into the binding tissue.

Bending force can also be introduced through kneading.

- Tension force can be added by having the client actively or passively move the knee into slight flexion and then back into the original position. For passive motion, using the foot and leg to do this is very effective.
- Repeat the movement back and forth until a change is noted. Maintain the drag on the tissue until the ground substance becomes more pliable. Subtle changes in the lines of force serve to load and unload the tissue, resulting in hysteresis.
- Next, grasp as much of the binding tissue as possible and lift until you feel the bind. Slowly load and unload with torsion and shear force, or by having the client move the knee, until the tissue becomes warm and more pliable. This method is intense, and the client should feel a pulling or slight burning sensation. The client should not feel the need to tense up or to change breathing in order to endure the method. Work slowly and deliberately, interspersing lymphatic drain type stroking every minute or so.

When an area is located that creates symptoms that are bothering the client, compression combined with muscle energy methods, from the least invasive positional release to integrated methods, can be used. The goal is to temporarily inhibit the motor tone of the muscle bundle that is problematic so that it can be lengthened to the appropriate resting length and reduce pressure on the nerves or vessels.

When addressing deeper tissue layers, always remember to protect the more superficial muscles by applying pressure gradually and with as broad a base of contact as the area will allow.

The side-lying position allows access to the attachments of the hamstrings and adductors in the groin. Because groin problems often occur, this is an important but difficult area to massage. Compression applied at the attachments, as shown in Figure 14-29, *J*, is effective and can be applied through thin clothing, if necessary.

- With the fingers placed as shown in Figure 14-29, *J*, combine compression with active or passive or both movements of the hip and knee. A slow circumduction tends to access all areas.
- Finish by gliding and kneading the entire area. Add oscillation (rocking and shaking) in various positions.
- As a finishing stroke, drain the area.

LEG, ANKLE, AND FOOT (FIGURE 14-30)

The leg muscles function at the knee, ankle, and foot. Repetitive movement is common for these muscles, as is repetitive strain injury. The goal of the massage is to maintain normal tissue function so that repetitive movement does not become repetitive strain. The muscles of the leg are categorized as superficial, intermediate, and deep. The muscles can adhere to each other in their side-by-side positions and between layers. It is especially important that the popliteus, soleus, and gastrocnemius are not stuck together. The superficial muscle layer primarily functions at the ankle, with some activity at the knee. The intermediate layer functions at the ankle, and the deep layer works the toes, with some activity at the ankle.

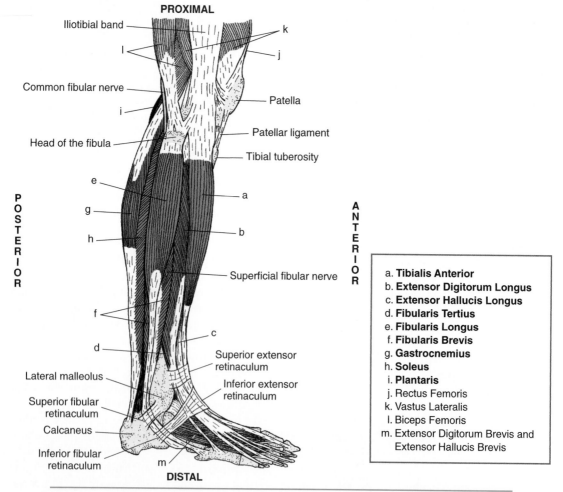

FIGURE 14-30 ■ Muscles of the leg. (From Muscolino JE: *The muscular system manual*, ed. 2. St. Louis, 2005, Mosby.)

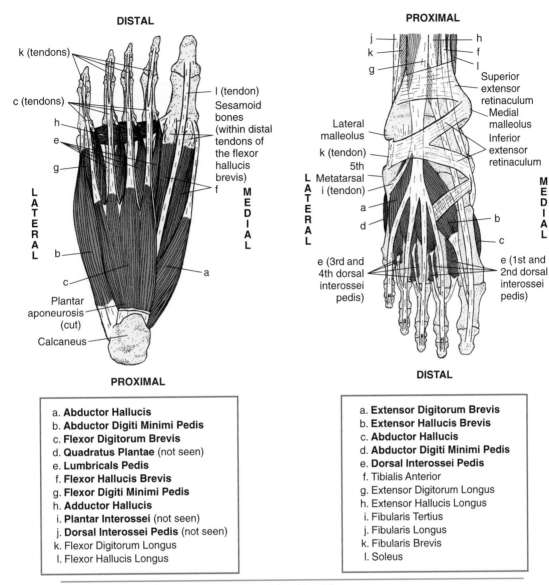

DISTAL

k (tendons)

c (tendons)

h

e

g

l (tendon)
Sesamoid
bones
(within distal
tendons of
the flexor
hallucis
brevis)

f

LATERAL

MEDIAL

b

c

a

Plantar
aponeurosis
(cut)

Calcaneus

PROXIMAL

PROXIMAL

j
k
g

h
f
l

Superior
extensor
retinaculum
Medial
malleolus
Inferior
extensor
retinaculum

Lateral
malleolus

k (tendon)
5th
Metatarsal
i (tendon)

LATERAL

a

d

MEDIAL

b

c

e (3rd and
4th dorsal
interossei
pedis)

e (1st and
2nd dorsal
interossei
pedis)

DISTAL

a. **Abductor Hallucis**
b. **Abductor Digiti Minimi Pedis**
c. **Flexor Digitorum Brevis**
d. **Quadratus Plantae** (not seen)
e. **Lumbricals Pedis**
 f. **Flexor Hallucis Brevis**
g. **Flexor Digiti Minimi Pedis**
h. **Adductor Hallucis**
 i. **Plantar Interossei** (not seen)
 j. **Dorsal Interossei Pedis** (not seen)
k. Flexor Digitorum Longus
 l. Flexor Hallucis Longus

a. **Extensor Digitorum Brevis**
b. **Extensor Hallucis Brevis**
c. **Abductor Hallucis**
d. **Abductor Digiti Minimi Pedis**
e. **Dorsal Interossei Pedis**
 f. Tibialis Anterior
g. Extensor Digitorum Longus
h. Extensor Hallucis Longus
 i. Fibularis Tertius
 j. Fibularis Longus
k. Fibularis Brevis
 l. Soleus

FIGURE 14-30 Cont'd ■ Muscles of the ankle and foot.

IN MY EXPERIENCE...

Feet

Athletes' feet ache. It seems that I am constantly rubbing feet, looking at feet, and assessing feet. As a rule, basketball players have really big feet and gymnasts have little feet. I remember one football player who had big but not huge feet. I massaged his feet every Friday before a game. The problem was that he had ticklish feet. If I touched him with just the littlest bit of hesitancy, he was off the table. I was massaging those feet when he told me that his wife was just diagnosed with breast cancer. You really have to be prepared for the listening art of massage.

The belly of these muscles lies closer to the knee, and they taper to the tendons in the ankle and foot. It is important to gauge pressure. Deeper pressure is used in the proximal half of the lower leg where the muscle bulk is located. Connective tissue binding often occurs in the distal half of the lower leg into the foot. This is common at the Achilles tendon and plantar fascia.

Typically, the forearm or flat hand is used to massage the leg but the foot works very well to apply compression. The arch of the foot fits nicely over the muscle bulk, and the client can provide active movement of the ankle and toes while the compression is being applied. This is effective in reducing tone and connective tissue binding in the tissues.

Anterior view

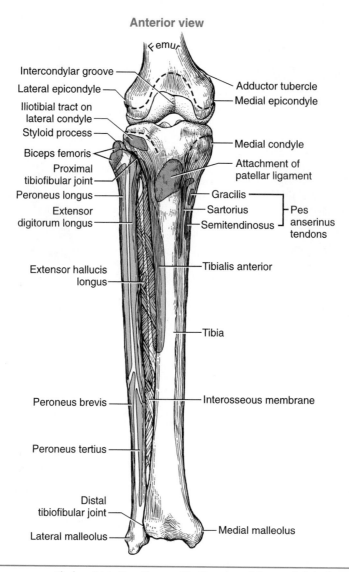

FIGURE 14-31 ■ The knee joint. (From Neumann DA: *Kinesiology of the musculoskeletal system: foundations for physical rehabilitation,* St. Louis, 2002, Mosby.)

PROCEDURES FOR THE LEG, ANKLE, AND FOOT

Examples of procedures for treatment of the ankle and foot are shown in Figure 14-32.

The knee joint is complex (Figure 14-31) and should be addressed by massage of the thigh and lower leg. In addition, make gentle movements of the patella to ensure that it moves freely.

The pes anserinus tendon on the medial aspect of the tibia is where the distal attachments of the sartorius, gracilis, and semitendinosus blend into one structure, just below the knee. Bending can interfere with knee function. Connective tissue application is effective.

The massage pattern is very similar to those presented in other areas. All three basic positions can be used. Massage of the ankle and foot first involves working with the muscles of the lower leg in relationship to the action of the ankle, foot, and toes.

- Apply systematic compression to the muscles of the lower leg, beginning at the knee and working toward the ankle while the client moves the ankle and toes in circles.
- To isolate a particular muscle pain in the ankle or foot action, have the client move

14-12

FIGURE 14-32

EXAMPLE OF MASSAGE APPLICATION TO THE LEG, ANKLE, AND FOOT

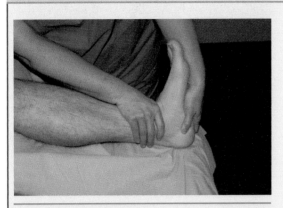

A Assessment, joint movement.

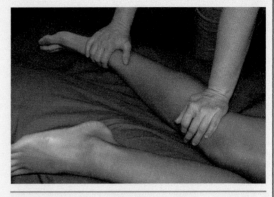

B Leg, side-lying; compression and movement, A.

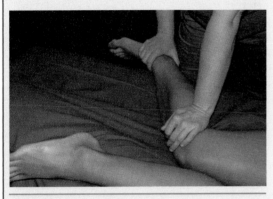

C Leg, side-lying, compression and movement, B.

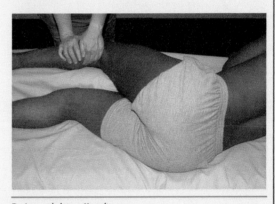

D Leg, side-lying; Kneading.

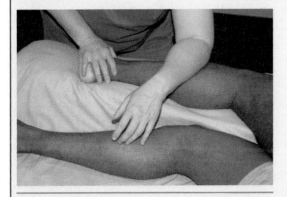

E Leg, side-lying; gliding.

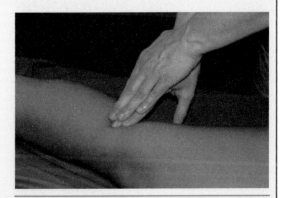

F Friction, pes anserinus tendon.

Continued

FIGURE 14-32—CONT'D

EXAMPLE OF MASSAGE APPLICATION TO THE LEG, ANKLE, AND FOOT

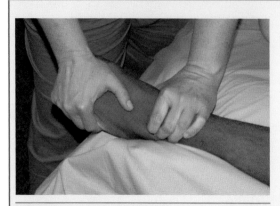

G Ankle range of motion, supine.

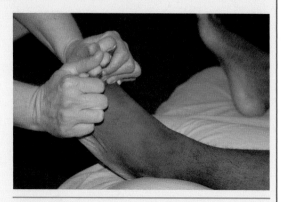

H Toe mobilization, supine.

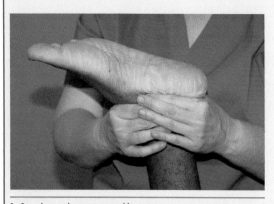

I Stretch muscles, traction ankle, prone.

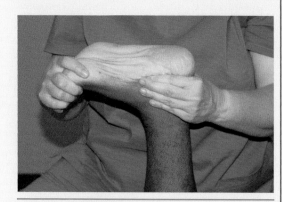

J Stretch plantar fasciae, prone.

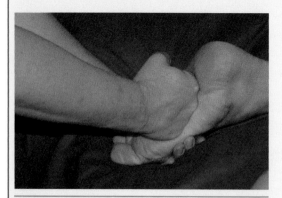

K Foot compression, prone.

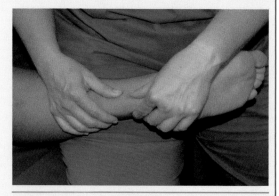

L Shear achilles tendon, side-lying.

FIGURE 14-32—CONT'D

EXAMPLE OF MASSAGE APPLICATION TO THE LEG, ANKLE, AND FOOT

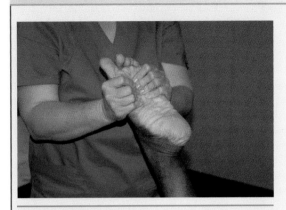

M Mobilize joints, prone.

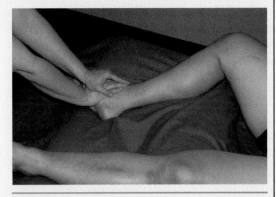

N Compress arch, supine.

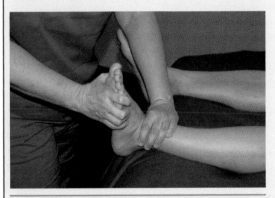

O Foot eversion, supine.

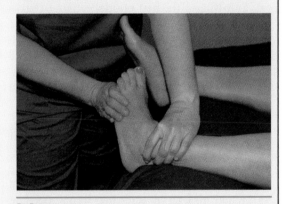

P Foot inversion, supine.

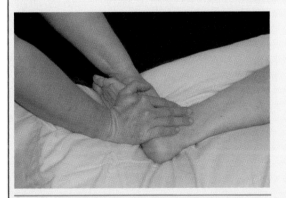

Q Foot eversion, side-lying

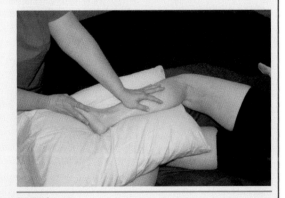

R Finish area.

the ankle or foot in the way that creates the symptom; palpate the muscles to see which ones are activated and then address those muscles.

Once this is complete, attention is given to the range of motion of the ankle. Proper ankle mobility is necessary for knee and hip function. Often, knee pain is related to disruption of ankle function. The ankle may be jammed, with a reduction in joint play. A general method to restore joint play is the "mobilization with movement" sequence described in Chapter 13, which involves traction of a joint and moving the joint into the ease and pain-free position by the therapist. The client is passive while the position is being located. The ease position is maintained by the therapist, while the client actively moves the joint through a full range of motion.

The intrinsic muscles of the foot are addressed next. Side-lying is the best position.

- Systematically work using compression and gliding of the soft tissue of the sole of the foot.
- Rhymic compression of the network of lymphatic vessels in the sole of the foot will assist lymphatic movement.
- Direct pressure or tapping can stimulate acupuncture points at the side of each toenail. An easy way to do this is to squeeze, release, and repeat three or four times, on the lateral and medial side of each nail.
- When the tarsal and toe joints become jammed, joint play methods can increase mobility in this area. The toes are hinge joints and once traction is applied and the ease position found, the the client moves the area back and forth.
- To finish off, use oscillation and lymphatic drain.

Thorough and specific massage of the foot is essential for athletes. Awareness of reflexology (see

IN MY EXPERIENCE...

I have performed some variation of this protocol at least 20,000 times over the last 25 years of practice. It really is the same thing over and over, moving from one region of the body to another and only changing the names of the bones, joints, and muscles. However, there are specific cautions and suggestions for particular regions, and textbooks have a vital role as reference sources as well. I believe many readers will use specific sections of this protocol during massage, either while learning or later on, to recall details. So this is a deliberate strategy: you can find what you need about any particular region of the body with this protocol. This protocol in all its variations is what I consider my "weekly house-cleaning massage."

Chapter 13) is helpful and integrating it into the massage is appropriate.

SUMMARY

This chapter presented a detailed, comprehensive and repetitive approach to massage. Hopefully, upon completing this chapter the reader realizes that regardless of the body area, the general sequence of the massage is the same. It is not necessary to use the protocol exactly as presented. Applications can be incorporated or deleted. More often an approach will be modified based on the client's goals, initial client positioning, and other contributing factors. As described, specific areas should be addressed as needed. The protocol is a basic, general maintenance massage approach used for performance and recovery massage. It is too intense for pre-event application and should be simplified if the client is ill or especially tired.

1 Review the general protocol and identify the repeating sequences. Then list the components of the sequence.

_____

_____

_____

_____

_____

2 Rewrite the general protocol in a way that best makes sense to you. In the space provided, describe the thought process used to write this protocol.

_____

_____

_____

_____

_____

3 List the illustrations in the entire text that demonstrate ways to massage the following:

a. The Face

_____

_____

_____

b. The Head

_____

_____

_____

c. The Occipital Base Area

_____

_____

_____

d. The Neck

_____

_____

e. The Anterior Torso

_____

_____

_____

f. The Posterior Torso

_____

_____

_____

g. The Shoulder

_____

_____

_____

h. The Arm, Wrist, and Hand

_____

_____

_____

i. The Hip

_____

_____

_____

j. The Thigh

_____

_____

_____

k. The Leg, Ankle, and Foot

_____

_____

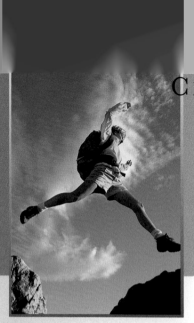

15
UNIQUE CIRCUMSTANCES AND ADJUNCT THERAPIES

OBJECTIVES

Upon completion of this chapter, the reader will have the information necessary to do the following:

1 Alter massage application to work effectively with a sleeping client.

2 Alter massage application to adjust to unique draping concerns, hairstyles, and clothing.

3 Provide massage in various environments and in context of typical sports schedules.

4 Adjust massage to respect habitual behavior.

5 Use simple and safe application of adjunct therapies to support the massage outcome.

This final chapter of Unit Two discusses some of the specific circumstances often encountered while working with the sport population. The information is based on years of professional experience. I hope the suggestions will help you understand athletes a little better and provide ideas to address these issues.

This population can present unique situations that require ingenuity, flexibility, creativity, and a sense of humor. As mentioned in the beginning of this textbook, many different situations arise that can stretch one's ability to carry out an effective massage. The main challenges are the sleeping client, draping considerations, clothing and hair, distractions, restroom needs, body size, the massage location, scheduling, and habitual behavior.

The sport and fitness community is open to using essential oils, homeopathy, and **magnets.** The massage therapist needs to be ethical and informed about these approaches. Many of these products are expensive and may have little value beyond placebo affect. The methods are possibilities for self-help treatment or to support or extend the effects of massage.

Arnica montana
Aromatherapy
Balsam fir
Chamomile, German
Epsom salt soaks
Eucalyptus
Gauss
Geranium

Helichrysum
Hydrotherapy
Juniper berry
Lavender
Lemongrass
Magnets
North pole
Peppermint

Pine
Rescue remedy
Rosemary
Ruta graveolens
South pole
Tea tree
Thyme

This chapter provides information on adjunct therapy such as **aromatherapy,** hydrotherapy, and magnet therapy. Hydrotherapy is well researched and is used extensively by those involved in sport fitness and rehabilitation. Aromatherapy (essential oils) is also a useful method, and more valid research is providing insight into its mechanism and effects. This chapter describes the oils that I have found most useful and that are generally safe.

Magnet therapy and other energetic methods such as homeopathy are less solid in their research base, but many athletes use magnets, so it is important to understand the current theories. My own personal experience indicates that several homeopathic remedies are helpful, especially arnica. **Rescue remedy** is a Bach flower remedy that also seems to help with the ongoing trauma and shock these clients experience.

THE SLEEPING CLIENT

Athletes commonly fall asleep during the massage. Because restorative sleep is so important, the ability to adapt massage application to accommodate sleep and continue to achieve outcomes is important. The most obvious challenges are active assessment and use of methods that require active participation. Altering the flow of massage application so that these methods are used at the beginning of the massage and after massage usually will solve the problem.

Extra blankets and pillows and bolsters usually are required. Clients' circulation alters during sleep and massage, and they become cool. Changing the position of the client needs to be gentle and smooth so that they are disturbed as little as possible.

Use rhythmic rocking to settle the athlete if they are aroused a bit from sleep. This usually will allow them to go back to sleep. This can occur during position change, using passive range of motion, and stretching methods, or if the method applied is unexpectedly painful.

Attempt to do most of the massage with the client in the side-lying and supine position. The prone position can cause the sinuses to clog up and strains the lower back. Use it when the client is most wakeful, and bolster the lower legs and under the abdomen to reduce lumbar strain.

The massage needs to be given in a confident rhythmic manner. All movement should be secure and stabilized appropriately. The massage professional needs to be focused, observant of client responses, and quiet. Passive methods, such as lymphatic drain and other fluid dynamic methods, are easy to apply during sleep.

Some of the more active applications and assessment procedures can be altered and applied passively by the skilled massage therapist.

In general, assessment is primarily observation and palpation. For more active assessment methods such as assessing firing patterns, alter the assessment process. When you sense heat and muscle tension, this can indicate a synergistic dominance pattern. If in doubt, assume the firing pattern is synergistic dominant. Methods applied can be focused to reduce tone in the misfiring muscles while more stimulating methods are applied to the inhibited muscles.

To address gait patterns with the passive or sleeping client, work opposite arm and legs in a sequence as follows:

1. Left biceps with left quadriceps and right hamstrings
2. Left triceps with left hamstring and right quadriceps
3. Right biceps with right quadriceps and left hamstrings
4. Right triceps with right hamstring and left quadriceps
5. Left wrist and finger flexors with left foot dorsiflexors and evertors and right plantar flexors and invertors
6. Left wrist and finger extensors with left foot plantar flexors and invertors and right foot dorsiflexors and evertors
7. Right wrist and finger flexors with right foot dorsiflexors and evertors and left plantar flexors and invertors
8. Right wrist and finger extensors with right foot plantar flexors and invertors and left foot dorsiflexors and evertors
9. Left hand with right foot
10. Right hand with left foot

Restoring joint play is done by applying traction to the joint and moving it passively within the normal range of motion.

The passive application is usually less effective than active participation of the client but benefits still are achieved when sleep is also an important goal. Indirect functional techniques become a primary treatment method. Passive application of the ease/bind tissue movement method replaces the more invasive connective tissue methods and trigger point application. Pay attention to the sleep cycle, which naturally fluctuates about every 45 minutes, and time the massage to end about when the client would begin to wake up.

DRAPING, CLOTHING, HAIR, AND ENVIRONMENT CONSIDERATIONS

Ideal draping procedures are presented thoroughly in *Mosby's Fundamentals of Therapeutic Massage*, and certainly the skilled massage practitioner has been able to incorporate effective modifications based on need. The athlete does present some draping challenges that can go a bit contrary to the typical draping recommendations.

The reasons for draping are to respect the boundaries and modesty of the client and to provide warmth. Many athletes are hypersensitive to skin stimulation and find the drape irritating.

They can wear loose shorts and or a tee shirt instead. Other athletes cannot stand to feel wrapped up, so a very loose draping style is necessary. Athlete clients seem to be hot or cold and usually end up cold before the massage is over. It is common for athletes not to want a drape to start and to prefer to wear some sort of loose shorts and by the end of the massage to be buried in sheets and blankets. Make sure you have extra draping materials and blankets available. Continually monitor skin temperature and add draping as needed to keep the client warm. This is especially important if the client is fatigued and tends to fall asleep during the massage.

Typically, each area to be massaged is undraped, worked with, and then redraped. However with a cold client, it may become necessary to work under the drapes. Pay attention to where your hands and forearms are and if by mistake you touch the genital or breast area acknowledge it and apologize.

Athletes commonly are very modest and not only want precise draping but also wear restrictive undergarments. Most common are sports bras, compression shorts, and athletic supporters. Many athletes leave their socks on because they have athletes' foot, their feet get cold, or they think they have weird feet. Some athletes wear elastic-type hats that protect or control their hair, and others just want to leave their hats on. Massage needs to be altered to work through these garments, and the massage therapist needs to understand that there is some sort of benefit to the client from wearing these clothing items.

Just as common are the athletes who are not modest because of ongoing focus on their body or even the type of sport (bodybuilding, for example) where they regularly display their body. This usually manifests as disrobing while the massage practitioner is in the area or showing the massage therapist the location of some area they want addressed during the massage. The massage therapist should not interpret this as sexual and should maintain a matter-of-fact, anatomy-is-just-anatomy approach. Because groin injury is common, the massage professional needs to become comfortable with working in this area.

When working with male clients, the genitals can get in the way of accessing the area needing treatment. Use the drape to move tissue around, or ask the client to reposition the genitals. Male clients often get erections while receiving massage because of the increase in circulation and parasympathetic response. Young athletes are more susceptible and more embarrassed by this physiologic response. The drape moving in the area can stimulate the erection response as can working in the groin, buttock, and low back area. Athletes often sleep during massage, and it is common for an erection to occur. Do not use a draping method that would increase awareness of this response and increase the embarrassment of the athlete. This is one of the reasons why male athletes wear athletic supporters and compression shorts during massage.

Keep the drapes loose in the genital area and use an extra towel over the groin if necessary. Be prepared to discuss this issue in a matter-of-fact and physiologic way. If the massage therapist is embarrassed too, then the situation is even more difficult for the client. One of the reasons that young male athletes prefer middle-aged (40 and older) female massage therapists is because they are most comfortable with these types of physiologic responses with the "mother-aged" person. The author's experience is that young male athletes tend to avoid younger female and male massage practitioners because of concerns and misinterpretation of this natural body function.

The buttock area needs effective massage for all clients, but any one who runs or jumps will especially require effective work in this area. Being comfortable working in this area is absolutely necessary for the massage therapist.

When working with female athletes, the breasts are literally in the way of accessing the anterior thorax. Because this is such an important area, especially for supporting effective breathing, the massage therapist needs to be comfortable working in this area, both with positioning the client and moving the breast tissue so that is out of the way. Do not use the hands to move breast tissue. Use the sheet or forearm. No therapeutic reason exists to massage the actual breast tissue if it is normal.

Because athletes drink a lot of fluid they have to urinate frequently. They may be embarrassed to ask to use the restroom. The massage therapist should ask whether the client needs to use the restroom at least half way through the massage. A good time is when changing positions. It is impossible to relax with a full bladder.

Athletes also consume food and supplements that produce intestinal gas. The sports massage professional cannot react adversely if the client passes gas during the massage. The high-protein and soy-based sport drinks can make the gas particularly

IN MY EXPERIENCE...

I cannot resist telling the following story. One of the athletic clients with whom I work has a precocious young daughter. At the time this event occurred, she was about 6 years old. She was in the massage area with me, helping me set up. She asked me if her daddy passed gas when he got a massage (her term was "make fluffies"). I asked her why she thought this might be so, and she said, "My daddy passes gas when he is asleep. He sleeps when he gets a massage, so he must pass gas when he gets a massage." How can you argue with this logic? Every time I think of this conversation, I smile. I could not resist disclosing this conversation to my client. We both got a good laugh. A while later, he asked me if he did indeed pass gas when he got a massage. My answer was, "Who doesn't. I am gas tolerant."

odoriferous (smell strong), so if a person finds intestinal gas especially disgusting, they may have difficulty with this population.

Athletes sweat, and while the author's personal experience is that most athletes are meticulous about hygiene, the massage therapist at times may have to work with perspiring clients. Keep a towel available to dry the skin.

Perspiration may create a body odor. This is just part of the process, and the massage therapist cannot be disturbed by these types of normal body odors.

Athletes shower and bathe a lot. In addition, they often soak in hot and or cold tubs and use saunas. Constant exposure to the soap, water, and chlorine dries the skin, and they may need more lubricant during the massage than the general population. Use only hypoallergenic lubricants. An athlete who has to compete with a skin rash from a reaction to lubricant will not be pleased.

Many athletes shave their heads, keep their hair short, or braid it. The various braid designs can be intricate and expensive, so it is not appropriate to mess them up during massage. Use compression instead of kneading and remove lubricant from your hands before working in the hair. Shaved heads present unique challenges. Massage only with the grain of the hair. Do not go in a direction where you feel stubble because this will irritate the area. This recommendation also applies to shaved bodies.

Most athletes are of normal size, but some are large and do not fit on standard massage tables comfortably. They usually are most comfortable on a mat. I have used duct tape to connect two massage tables together to make it wide enough. If tall (basketball players for example), the athletes hang off the ends of the massage table. They often need some sort of support for their arms, and although some massage tables are equipped with armrests, unless the armrests are adjustable, they are not in the right position. The large, round exercise balls work well when placed at the end of the table. A short stool, chair, or ottoman can work. Usually large and tall athletes will not fit comfortably in the massage chairs.

Large athletes need large bolsters. The bolsters that come with most massage tables are too small. Some creative solutions are rolled exercise mats, two king-size pillows taped together, rolled blankets, and sofa cushions.

Various environmental distractions can occur: massage in a public environment, the client talking on the phone, text messaging, listening to music with or without headphones, fellow athletes, or family members in the area. The massage therapist needs to remain focused and flexible.

Many athletes watch television or movies while getting a massage. The massage therapist must allow them to be able to see the screen. Position the massage table or mat on a diagonal where the television screen is visible. When prone, the client should be able to turn his or her head to see the television. Then turn the lies on the side so the client is facing the screen. When it is time to massage the other side completely, have the client switch ends of the table so his or her head is where the feet were. When the client lies on the other side to be massaged, the client still will be facing the television. When in the supine position, the client again can turn the head slightly to see the screen.

When one is working with athletes, massage commonly is provided in locations other than the typical private massage office. Instead, massage may be given in the locker room, playing field, or whatever corner is available.

If athletes can afford it, they often want massage in their home, which presents all the challenges of an on-site massage, that is, privacy; distractions; attention to confidentiality; discretion; arriving, setting up, and leaving efficiently; and many other situations. If the athlete is traveling, hotel rooms are cramped, and it is difficult to find enough room for the massage table. In these situations you just have to do the best you can and have a sense of humor.

SCHEDULING

The athlete's schedule also can present unique challenges. Often massage appointments are early in the morning or late at night. Depending on the type of sport, scheduling of massage sessions at the same time consistently may not be possible. On occasion, the massage therapist may have to travel with the athlete. If this population is the massage therapist's main focus, then specific scheduling times will be difficult. For example, most of the football players with whom I have worked want a massage on Tuesday night at 8 PM or 9 PM in their home. Tuesday is the typical day off, and they want to get the children in bed before the massage. The other popular times are Friday night after 9 PM to be ready before the final game practice or on Saturday or Monday morning early before practice. The football players will settle for late evening appointments on the other nights, but it is not their preference. Taking this into account, it is impossible for one massage therapist to see more than six to eight football players as clients during the season.

Basketball, baseball, soccer, and hockey are even worse for scheduling because the game schedule changes days, times, and frequency. For example, basketball players and baseball players can play two games in a row, have 3 days off, play an afternoon game, and 2 days later play a night game. They will schedule a massage when they can, which is often at the last minute.

Individual athletes such as tennis players, golfers, and bowlers may have a bit more control of their schedules, but availability is dictated by when events occur. Even if the massage professional is employed by an athletic organization, meetings and practice schedules make scheduling difficult.

Because of these scheduling issues, working with a large population of athletic clients on a schedule of 9 to 5, 5 days a week is difficult. The most difficult scheduling demands are with the professional athlete and the least with the client pursuing fitness or involved in physical rehabilitation. The massage therapist needs to consider these issues carefully when targeting this population. A life with a standard routine is usually not possible. Difficult scheduling issues may prohibit a massage therapist form working with professional athletes. They cannot easily alter their schedule and often request on-site massage at odd hours. Working for a fitness or rehabilitation center provides the most stable scheduling options. If your career goals target professional athletes, be prepared for an erratic schedule.

HABITUAL BEHAVIOR

Many athletes are highly disciplined and have habitual behaviors. For the internal and external daily sequence of events to be predictable is important, even with the erratic schedules previously described. The athlete responds best to familiarity. This manifests as the same general massage sequence, the same location if possible, the same draping materials and blankets, the same uniform worn by the massage therapist, and the same lubricant. The massage therapist must honor this.

Because of this habitual/ritual behavior, referring the athletic client to a different massage therapist is difficult. If athletes are happy with a massage therapist's work, they commonly will be unwilling for anyone else to work with them. This can place demands on the massage therapist.

IN MY EXPERIENCE...

While working with a professional athlete during the playoffs toward a world championship, my life revolved around schedules until the team finally won. He was just not in a position at this critical juncture to adapt to another massage therapist's style. Remember, even though this particular athlete is considered a world-class champion, the person recovering from a hip replacement is no less stressed and vulnerable and needs to be supported by familiarity.

HYDROTHERAPY

Hydrotherapy is a separate and distinct form of therapy that combines well with massage. Water is a near-perfect natural body balancer and is necessary for life. It accounts for the largest percentage of our body weight.

The effects of water are primarily reflexive and are focused on the autonomic nervous system. The addition of heat energy or dissipation of heat energy from tissues can be classified as a mechanical effect. In general, cold stimulates sympathetic responses, and warmth activates parasympathetic responses. Short- and long-term applications of hot or cold differ in effect. For the most part, short cold applications stimulate and vasoconstrict, with a secondary effect of increased circulation as blood is channeled to the area to warm it. Long cold applications depress and decrease circulation.

Short applications of heat vasodilate vessels and depress and deplete tone, whereas long heat applications result in a combined depressant and stimulant reaction.

Different water pressures can exert a powerful mechanical effect on the nerve and blood supply of the skin. Techniques that are used include a friction rub with a sponge or wet mitten and pressurized streams of hot and cold water directed at various parts of the body (Box 15-1).

Diffusion is a principle of hydrotherapy by which water moves across a permeable or semipermeable membrane from a low mineral salt concentration to a high concentration to equalize the solution.

If the water used for hydrotherapy application is lower in salt content than body fluids, water moves from the outside of the body to the inside through the semipermeable superficial tissue of the skin and superficial fascia. If the salt content of the water external to the skin is higher, such as when mineral salt baths are used, water from the body moves into the external soak water. When this happens, surface edema is reduced.

In organized sports and physical therapy, the athletic trainer or physical therapist applies hydrotherapy (usually ice). To support hydrotherapy treatment, do not massage an area that has been iced. Let the body restore circulation to the area to warm it.

Hot and cold contrast hydrotherapy is effective in supporting fluid movement. **Epsom salt soaks** and salves can assist in managing surface edema. Cold is most effective for just about everything, and ice application is part of acute care in the PRICE system (protection, relative rest, ice, compression, elevation). When in doubt, put ice on it. Real ice is safer than chemical ice packs. Immersion of an area in ice water is especially effective for injuries such as sprains and strains. Heat is more for palliative effect and a surface muscle relaxer. If injury is not present, a general rule can be ice joints and heat muscles. Heat may be best before competition and ice afterward. Warm applications, such as the rice or seed bags, which go in the microwave, are pleasant during the massage, especially on the feet.

ESSENTIAL OILS

Essential oils are the highly concentrated oils of aromatic plants.

BOX 15-1   EFFECTS OF HYDROTHERAPY USING HEAT, COLD, AND ICE APPLICATIONS

Effects of heat
- Increased circulation
- Increased metabolism
- Increased inflammation
- Increased respiration
- Increased perspiration
- Decreased pain
- Decreased muscle spasm
- Decreased tissue stiffness
- Decreased white blood cell production

Application of hydrotherapy
As a *sedative*, water is an efficient, nontoxic, calming substance. It soothes the body and promotes sleep.

Techniques: Use hot and warm baths to quiet and relax the entire body. Salt baths, neutral showers, or damp sheet packs can be used to relax certain areas.

For *elimination,* the skin is the largest organ, and simple immersion in a long, hot bath or a session in a sauna or steam room can stimulate the excretion of toxins from the body through the skin. Inducing perspiration is useful in treating acute diseases and many chronic health problems.

Techniques: Use hot baths, Epsom salt or common salt baths, hot packs, dry blanket packs, and hot herbal drinks.

As an *antispasmodic,* water effectively reduces cramps and muscle spasms.

Techniques: Use hot compresses (depending on the problem), herbal teas, and abdominal compresses.

Effects of cold and ice
Cold
- Increased stimulation
- Increased muscle tone
- Increased tissue stiffness
- Increased white blood cell production
- Increased red blood cell production
- Decreased circulation (primary effect); increased circulation (secondary effect)
- Decreased inflammation
- Decreased pain
- Decreased respiration
- Decreased digestive processes

Ice
- Increased tissue stiffness
- Decreased circulation
- Decreased metabolism
- Decreased inflammation
- Decreased pain
- Decreased muscle spasm

Application type
- Ice packs
- Ice immersion (ice water)
- Ice massage
- Cold whirlpool
- Chemical cold packs
- Cold gel packs *(use with caution)*

Contraindications for ice
- Vasospastic disease (spasm of blood vessels)
- Cold hypersensitivity; signs include the following:
  Skin: Itching, sweating
  Respiratory: Hoarseness, sneezing, chest pain
  Gastrointestinal: Abdominal pain, diarrhea, vomiting
  Eyes: Puffy eyelids
  General: Headache, discomfort, uneasiness
- Cardiac disorder
- Compromised local circulation

Precautions for ice
- Do not use frozen gel packs directly on the skin.
- Do not use ice applications (cryotherapy) for longer than 30 minutes continuously.
- Do not do exercises that cause pain after cold applications.
- Do not use cryotherapy on individuals with certain rheumatoid conditions or on those who are paralyzed or have coronary artery disease.

Applications of hydrotherapy
Ice is a primary therapy for strains, sprains, contusions, hematomas, and fractures. It has a numbing, anesthetic effect and helps control internal hemorrhage by reducing circulation to and metabolic processes within the area.

For *restoration* and *increasing muscle strength* and *increasing the resistance of the body to disease,* cold water boosts vigor, adds energy and tone, and aids in digestion.

Techniques: Use cold water treading (standing or walking in cold water), whirlpool baths, cold sprays, alternate hot and cold contrast baths, showers and compresses, salt rubs, apple cider vinegar baths, and partial packs.

For *injuries,* the application of an ice pack controls the flow of blood and reduces tissue swelling.

Technique: Use an ice bag in addition to compression and elevation.

As an *anesthetic,* water can dull the sense of pain or sensation.

Technique: Use ice to chill the tissue.

For *minor burns,* water, particularly cold and ice water, has been rediscovered as a primary healing agent.

Technique: Use ice water immersion or saline water immersion.

To *reduce fever,* water is nature's best cooling agent. Unlike medications, which usually only diminish internal heat, water lowers temperature and removes heat by conduction.

Technique: Use ice bags at the base of the neck and on the forehead and feet, cold water sponge baths, and drinking of cold water.

From Fritz S: *Mosby's fundamentals of therapeutic massage,* ed 3. St. Louis, 2004, Mosby.

evolve Aromatherapy is the art of using these oils to promote healing of the body and the mind and combines well with massage. Log on to the Evolve web site that accompanies this book to learn more about the essential oils used in massage.

IN MY EXPERIENCE...

Essential Oils

Persons in general seem to enjoy pure essential oils as part of the massage. I typically carry around a mood mix "happy oil," a sleepy mix (sedative), an antiinflammatory analgesic mix (ouchy oil) an upper respiratory mix (snotty nose oil), and energizing stimulatory (energizer oil). These various mixes basically are made from the suggestions provided in the chapter. The funny names are easy to remember. These oil mixes are like the "big squash" massage for general all-over recovery and the "squeeze the sponge" massage for fluid retention. Anyway, because I work with a lot of football players, I am careful to make sure the essential oil mix does not smell like grandma's perfume. I usually do this by adding some sort of fir (pine, cypress, or juniper) to the mix. One of my favorite happy oil mixes is lavender, orange, and rose. This mix is calming and mood regulating.

It was a Monday after a particularly bad performance in the football game on Sunday. Needless to say, the coaches were not pleased. The players were scheduled for massage Monday morning, and then after lunch there was going to be an important team meeting. When the players asked for essential oil, I pulled out the lavender, orange, and rose mix, and just about every player wanted some on them. After awhile, I realized that I had not softened the flowering scent. I had left out the fir. Off went a majority of the football team to this big meeting smelling like grandma's perfume. From what I heard later, the meeting did not go as anticipated. The coaches for some reason could not seem to maintain a stern demeanor. I later confessed to the essential oil intervention, and the coach looked at me and said, "So that is what I was smelling." We had a good laugh about it. As I remember this event, I now wonder if I forgot the fir on purpose. Oh well, it all worked out fine.

The oils are found in different parts of the plant such as the flowers, twigs, leaves and bark, or in the rind of fruit. Because of the large quantity of plant material required, pure essential oils are expensive, but they are also highly effective—only a few drops at a time are required to achieve the desired effect. Essential oils are chemicals that interact with the body physiology. Although in general their influences are subtle, the massage therapist needs to take care when using them. Specific therapeutic treat-

ment should be provided only by a qualified aromatherapist.

Most essential oils are volatile (they quickly evaporate), and the molecules are passed readily into the bloodstream.

Essential oils have an immediate impact on the sense of smell. When essential oils are inhaled, olfactory receptor cells are stimulated, then the hypothalamus is stimulated, and the impulse is transmitted to the emotional center of the brain, or limbic system. Recent research has determined that the hypothalamus has neurotransmitter and neuroendocrine activity. The hormones found there are being traced to find out where they go in the body and what effects they have.

The limbic system is connected to areas of the brain linked to memory, breathing, and blood circulation, as well as the endocrine glands, which regulate hormone levels in the body. The properties of each oil, the fragrance and its effects, determine stimulation of these systems. The active chemicals in the oil also are absorbed directly by the mucous membranes in the nose.

When used in massage, essential oils are not only inhaled but also absorbed through the skin. They penetrate the skin and find their way into the bloodstream where they are transported to the organs and systems of the body.

Essential oils have differing rates of absorption, generally between 20 minutes and 2 hours, so it is probably best not to bathe or shower directly following essential oil use to ensure maximum effectiveness.

Simply think of these properties of the oils: antibacterial, antiviral or antifungal, antiinflammatory, effect on body fluids, analgesic (reduce pain), and stimulant or sedative.

For example:

- If a client has just increased training intensity and has delayed-onset muscle soreness, which is a combination of inflammation and fluid retention, then use German chamomile and juniper berry.
- If a client has a bruise, then use helichrysum.
- If a client is fatigued but having trouble sleeping, use balsam fir and lavender.
- If a client is getting a cold, use eucalyptus, tea tree, and thyme.
- If a client feels achy and stiff, use black pepper and lemongrass.
- If a client has a mild ankle sprain, use helichrysum, German chamomile, and rosemary. If a client has joint aching such as arthritis, use eucalyptus, lemongrass, and peppermint.

• If the client has a headache, use peppermint and lavender. The list goes on and on. If you do not know what to use, have the client smell the oils, pick two or three that they really like, and mix them together. The massage therapist will find it interesting to do this and then compare the properties of the oils to the client's symptoms and outcome goals.

The following list of essential oils has focused benefits for the athlete. They are reasonably safe when used in small quantities and mixed in a carrier oil. Good carrier oils for athletes are high-quality olive oil and almond oil.

The essential oil also can be mixed into melted food-grade coconut oil. When the coconut oil resolidifies, the result is like an ointment. Typically 10 drops of essential oil in an ounce of carrier oil is all that is necessary. It is best to blend no more than three essential oils together. Do not have a total of more than 15 drops of essential oil per ounce of carrier oil. Target the essential oil to the goals of the massage. The client can use the mixed oil as a self-help measure. When in doubt about skin sensitivity, use the oil mixture on the bottoms of the feet.

An ounce of mixed oil will last a while because only a small amount is used at a time. When purchasing essential oils, buy only pure, high-quality essential oils from well-known suppliers.

The essential oils recommended are:

Balsam fir: It has a fresh balsamic odor.
Uses: To relieve muscle aches and pains; relieve anxiety and stress-related conditions; fight colds, flu, and infections; and relieve bronchitis and coughs.

Black pepper: It has a warm, peppery aroma.
Uses: To energize; increase circulation; warm and relieve muscle aches and stiffness; and fight colds, flu, and infections. Use with care. Only a small amount, 3 to 5 drops, in an ounce of carrier oil is required.

Chamomile, German: It has a strong, sweet and warm herbaceous aroma and is blue. German chamomile has many of the same properties as Roman chamomile, with a much higher azulene content, so its antiinflammatory actions are greater.
Uses: To relieve muscular pain; heal skin inflammations, acne, and wounds; as a sedative, to ease anxiety and nervous tension and help with sleeplessness. German chamomile should be avoided during early pregnancy and may cause skin reactions in some persons. Before using, do a small

test on a small area of skin, such as the medial ankle.

Eucalyptus: It has a strong camphorous odor.
Uses: For colds; as a decongestant, to relieve asthma and fevers; for its bactericidal and antiviral actions; and to ease aching joints. Avoid if you or your client have high blood pressure or epilepsy.

Geranium: It has a leafy rose scent.
Uses: To reduce stress and tension; ease pain; balance emotions and hormones; relieve premenstrual syndrome; relieve fatigue and nervous exhaustion; lift depression; and lessen fluid retention.

Helichrysum: It has an intense, honey, tealike aroma.
Uses: To heal bruises (internal and external), wounds, and scars; to detoxify the body, cleanse the blood, and increase lymphatic drainage; heal colds, flu, sinusitis, and bronchitis; and relieve melancholy, migraines, stress, and tension.

Juniper berry: It has a fresh, pine needle aroma.
Uses: To energize and relieve exhaustion; ease inflammation and spasms; improve mental clarity and memory; purify the body; lessen fluid retention; and disinfect. Juniper berry should be avoided during pregnancy or if the client has kidney disease.

Lavender: It has a sweet, fresh scent.
Uses: To balance emotions; relieve stress, tension, and headache; promote restful sleep; heal the skin; lower high blood pressure; help breathing; and disinfect.

Lemongrass: It has a powerful, lemon-grass aroma.
Uses: To relieve athlete's foot; tone tissue; relieve muscular pain (sports-muscle pain); increase circulation; relieve headaches, nervous exhaustion, and other stress-related problems. Use with care, only using a small amount if necessary, 3 to 5 drops per ounce of carrier oil. Avoid in pregnancy.

Peppermint: It has a sweet, mint aroma.
Uses: To boost energy; brighten mood; reduce pain; help breathing; and improve mental clarity and memory. Peppermint may irritate sensitive skin, so do a skin test. Avoid during pregnancy.

Pine: It has a strong, coniferous, woody aroma.
Uses: To ease breathing, as an immune system stimulant, to increase energy, and for relieving muscle and joint ache.

Rosemary: It has a camphorlike aroma.
Uses: To energize; relieve muscle pains, cramps, or sprains; brighten mood and improve mental clarity and memory; ease pain; relieve

headaches; and disinfect. Avoid during pregnancy, if the athlete is epileptic, or if the client or massage therapist has high blood pressure.

Tea tree: It has a spicy, medicinal aroma. Tea tree oil is one of the most scientifically researched oils.

Uses: An immunostimulant, particularly against bacteria, viruses, and fungi; relieve inflammation; and disinfect.

Thyme: It has a sweet, intense herb-medicinal odor.

Uses: To inhibit infectious diseases; treat colds and bronchitis; relieve muscle aches and pains; aid concentration and memory; and relieve fatigue.

Caution: Not all essential oils are safe:

- Oils that *are not suitable for use* include, but are not restricted to, cinnamon, clove, hyssop, and sage.
- Oils that *should not be used during pregnancy* include, but are not restricted to, basil, clove, cinnamon, fennel, hyssop, juniper, lemongrass, marjoram, myrrh, peppermint, rosemary, sage, and white thyme.
- Oils that *should not be used with steam* include, but are not restricted to, bay, clary sage, ginger, juniper, pine, and tea tree.
- Oils that are *photosynthesizing* include, but are not restricted to, lemon, bergamot, lime, and orange. Do not go out into the sun for at least 2 hours after applying these oils to your skin.

The cautions listed pertain to client and therapist because oils are absorbed not only through the skin but also through the olfactory bulb and hypothalamus. If you are using multiple oils during massage work, it is advisable to ground and center yourself before using the oils and afterward. Otherwise, aromatic effects can distort your thinking, judgment, and sensations as a therapist.

VIBRATION METHODS

Vibration methods are based on the frequency of the vibration on the body. Many therapeutic methods are included in this aspect of treatment, including sound, color, and light. Two safe and appropriate methods are a Bach flower remedy and homeopathy.

RESCUE REMEDY

Rescue remedy is a Bach flower that is specific for trauma. Why this remedy is appropriate for athletes is obvious. Rescue remedy consists of a premixed flower essence combination that can be applied as a first aid measure in emergencies of all kinds. The solution consists of the following flower essences:

- Star of Bethlehem for shock
- Rock rose for acute fear and panic
- Impatiens for inner tension and stress
- Cherry plum for fear of breaking down and despair
- Clematis for the feeling of being "not completely here"

Rescue remedy is appropriate when a situation appears threatening to the individual or indeed might be life threatening. The theory is that a state of shock paralyzes the energetic system; the conscious mind has the tendency to withdraw itself from the body or in extreme cases even to leave it. In such cases, the body is left completely on its own and is therefore unable to activate self-healing energy. Rescue remedy is said to remove the energetic block quickly and enable the regulatory system of the body to initiate the necessary measures for emergencies.

Because rescue remedy is an energetic interaction that is being held in the water molecules, it is safe. One to 4 drops in a glass of water or water bottle cannot hurt and may help. If the person does not want to take the remedy internally, then the remedy can be rubbed on the skin.

HOMEOPATHIC REMEDIES

Homeopathic remedies are usually in the form of small pellets (which are sweet-tasting and dissolve easily), liquids, or tablets. They are prepared from pure, natural substances (animal, vegetable, or mineral) that are listed in the *Homœopathic Pharmacopœia of the United States.*

Homeopathic remedies are prepared by obtaining the source in its most concentrated form and then, through a long process of dilution, preparing a remedy with a potency sufficient to effect a physiologic change by vibrational or energetic means. The potency describes the measure of the dilution of the remedy and is denoted by the number that follows the name of the medicine itself. The higher the number, the greater the dilution (up to 1 part remedy to 1 trillion parts diluent), and the stronger the effect.

Because of the minute doses used in homeopathic remedies, they are safe and nonaddictive and have no unwanted side effects.

These remedies cannot harm the client and may have a potential for benefit. The remedy may do nothing, but it also may help. These remedies are especially useful in the acute stages of injury and before and after surgery. Combined homeopathic remedies also are available for specific for sport-related conditions and can be helpful. They can be found at health food stores for about $5 to $10 a bottle. Homeopathy for specific conditions is a complex discipline, and referral to a qualified professional is necessary.

Arnica Montana

Arnica montana is a natural homeopathic remedy that athletes frequently take in oral pellet form to help reduce bruising and swelling. Grown in mountain regions, this homeopathic herb is said to help reduce bruising and swelling, promote healing, and lessen postoperative pain and discomfort.

Arnica montana also may aid in the prevention of bruising and muscular fatigue.

Ruta graveolens is a homeopathic remedy for trauma to the ligaments and for stiffness and bruising to the limbs and joints.

MAGNETS

In general, magnets seem to help manage pain, especially acute pain. Magnets also may support tissue healing. The effects may just be a placebo. If appropriate cautions are followed, magnets are safe and noninvasive. The following information is presented to help the massage therapist educate the client.

No research indicates that the expensive specialty magnets work any better than inexpensive ones. Just do not drop magnets, which can demagnetize them. The application is similar to ice or heat: about 20 minutes 2 or 3 times a day, or the magnets can be strapped, taped, or wrapped on the body for extended use.

Magnet power is measured in terms of **gauss,** the line of force per unit area of the pole. The gauss rating of a magnet determines the speed with which it works, and the thickness determines the depth of penetration. The surface of the earth is approximately 0.5 gauss. Many manufacturers rate their products using internal gauss and external gauss to indicate strength. The following list shows typical magnetic strength classifications:

Low gauss = 300 to 700 gauss
Medium gauss = 1000 to 2500 gauss
High gauss = 3000 to 6000 gauss
Super gauss = 7000 to 12,000 gauss

Surface gauss rating also refers to the external strength of the magnet.

Gauss depends on the size, shape, polarity, and grade of the magnetic material. Some experts in magnet therapy begin treatment at low gauss and gradually increase strength as necessary. Some companies list their products by internal gauss, and others use the external gauss rating. A quick rule of thumb in determining proper gauss strength is to take the external gauss rating, with 800 gauss being appropriate. To get the internal gauss, multiply this number by 3.9 (approximate). Magnets at 800 gauss external strength also can be considered 3120 gauss internal rating (approximate). Do not be misled into believing you are getting a higher-strength product; both are correct ratings for the same magnet.

About as many types of magnets are available as there are body parts. Magnetic mattresses and pads are designed to be slept on; magnetic insoles fit inside shoes; block magnets can be placed under mattresses, pillows, or seat cushions; and back supports are even available with slots for magnet insertion.

Other magnets are made as body wraps with velcro closures, jewelry, and magnetic foil.

Most magnets are made of ferrites, which are iron oxides combined with cobalt, nickel, barium, and other metals to make a ceramic-like material. The flexible types of magnets are combined with plastic, rubber, or other pliable materials. The strongest magnets are those made from neodymium (a rare earth element).

Claims of therapeutic effects of magnets still should be regarded with considerable skepticism. Most of the testimonials to the effectiveness of magnetic therapy devices can be attributed to placebo effects and to other effects accompanying their use. For example, the magnetic back braces used may help ease back pains through providing mechanical support, through warming, and a constant reminder to not overexert the muscles. All these effects are helpful with or without magnets.

Most valid research does not support benefits from magnet use. One highly publicized exception is a double blind study done at Baylor College of Medicine, which compared the effects of magnets and sham magnets on the knee pain of 50 postpolio patients. The experimental group reported a significantly greater reduction in pain than the control group. No replication of the study has been done. The results of the Baylor study, however, raise the possibility that at least in some cases, topical application of magnets indeed may be useful in pain relief.

Although not scientifically proven and controversial, theories suggest that magnets do not heal but rather stimulate the body to heal naturally.

An important aspect of magnet use is magnet polarity. This relates to the direction in which the magnet is placed. The **north pole** corresponds to yin, or negative polarity. The **south pole** corresponds to yang, or positive polarity. The chart shows the magnetic influences of the south and north poles by example:

North Pole	South Pole
Characteristics: sedation, cooling	Characteristics: stimulation, heating
Negative: yin	Positive: yang
Acute headaches	Fibrosis
Arthritis	Numbness
Bursitis	Paralysis
Fractures	Scars
Inflammation	Tingling
Low back pain	Weak muscles
Sharp pain	
Tendonitis	

If the body appears to lack positive and negative energies to heal, then two magnets can be used to apply the north and south poles (known as bipolar) simultaneously. Bipolar magnet therapy may be used to heal fractures or treat chronic pain. Unipolar magnets also are on the market, and which pole is used is not a factor. These magnets tend to be more expensive. When in doubt, use the **north pole of the magnet.**

As with any treatment, there are cautionary measures to follow. Magnets should not be used during pregnancy, on patients with a history of epilepsy, while taking blood-thinning medications, on bleeding wounds, or if internal bleeding exists. Magnets should never be used on a client with a pacemaker or who has metal implants that could be dislodged by magnet use. Many athletes have had broken bones that are pinned or screwed together. Do not use the magnet on these areas.

From an ethical standpoint, it is probably not the best professional practice to sell these products to clients. Too much potential exists for conflict and dual roles. The products are obtained easily, and the client can find and purchase them easily on his or her own.

Essential oils can be mixed and given to the client as self-help. I strongly suggest that the oils not be "sold" to the client but instead be part of therapeutic massage application.

SUMMARY

A conditioned response occurs with repetitive behavior and familiarity. The response is comfortable, safe, and reassuring. All the unique circumstance that arise when the massage therapist is working with the sport population cannot be described. I personally could tell stories for a long time and still laugh, cry, and marvel over the process. If you are reading this text, at some level you are considering working with this population. As previously discussed, your massage therapy skills, professional behavior, and internal and external coping skills need to be excellent.

I hope this chapter, combined with Chapter 1, reinforces realistic expectations for a career path in this area.

1 Develop a strategy for addressing each of the following:

   a. A large client who wants to watch television during the massage. The client typically falls asleep.
   b. A client who wants the massage therapist to work with her while training at the gym.
   c. The client is a race horse.
   d. The client has a headache, an expensive hair design with braids, and is cold; no massage table is available.
   e. The only time the client has available is 10 PM at her home, with no babysitter, and she is breast-feeding.

   a._____
   _____

   b._____
   _____

   c._____
   _____

   d._____
   _____

   e._____
   _____

2 Develop an appropriate essential oil treatment for each of the following.

   a. Fatigue
   b. Anxiety over competition
   c. The inability to concentrate on paperwork
   d. Headache and upset stomach
   e. Grade one ankle sprain

   a._____
   _____
   _____

   b._____
   _____
   _____

   c._____
   _____

   d._____
   _____

   e._____
   _____

3 Describe a situation in which you might use or recommend each of the following.

a. Cold hydrotherapy _____

b. Warm hydrotherapy _____
_____

c. Hot and cold contrast hydrotherapy
_____

d. Epsom salt soak _____

e. Aromatherapy _____

f. Rescue remedy _____

g. *Arnica* _____

h. *Rula graveolens* _____

i. North pole magnet _____

j. South pole magnet _____

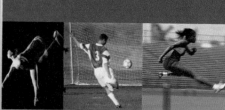

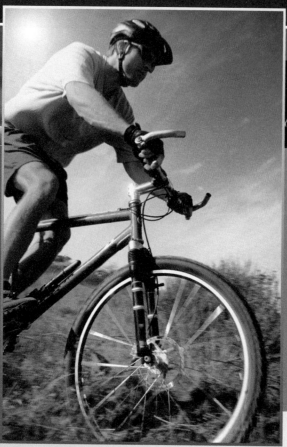

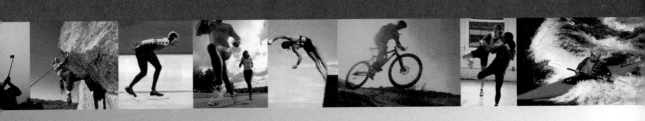

STORIES
from the field
SCOTT

All persons—athletes included—have a story. Each individual's story shapes his or her life. Because when working with so-called celebrities, one commonly focuses on what they do instead of who they are, I have included a few stories of individuals, who are also athletes, to put into perspective the importance of the professional relationship the massage therapist achieves and maintains with this type of client. We do not provide massage to a football player or basketball player or golfer. We support individuals in their own personal quest for achievement. The stories I have chosen to tell are about those with whom I have spent the most time and therefore know the best. The stories are from my point of view and with their permission.

Scott grew up in football. His dad had a long football career with the Detroit Lions. His mom continues to work in the Detroit Lion's office.

Scott played professional football with the Lions for most of his career, which spanned years. When I met Scott, he was entering his peak years. Scott is a wild man. His major claim to fame was as a special teams player, which is one of the craziest jobs in football. Scott cannot sit still, talks a mile a minute, and had trouble even lying on the massage table to get a massage in the early years. He would bounce around and then just get up in the middle of the massage and walk off. I can remember working on his neck while he was walking down the hall.

Scott is married to a great person—Michelle. He has two daughters. The one I know the best is Emma. One of my greatest stories of all is when Scott was asleep on the sofa, Emma painted his toenails pink. Scott never noticed and went into practice with bright pink toenails. He came in for one of his "just get my neck" massages, and there he stood with pink toenails. This was just a priceless moment.

Emma is her own personality and has her dad wrapped right around her finger. She likes to help do the massage and would rub her dad's feet with lots of massage cream. One of her favorite movies

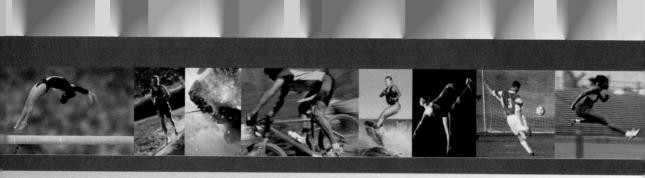

is *Shrek,* and I think Scott, Emma, and I watched it 50 times. Actually, Emma watched the movie, Scott talked constantly during the massage about everything, and I attempted to put him back together week after week from the wear and tear of playing football. If his neck felt good, then his back was killing him. When the back felt better, then his neck was driving him crazy, and back and forth it went.

The story I really want to tell about Scott is how he put his life together after football. He is still working on it. It was hard for him. His entire life had involved sports. Remember, his dad played professional ball. Who was he going to be when he was no longer a football player? He struggled. It did not help that it was not his choice to retire. He was cut from the team during a yearly reorganization period and did not get picked up by another team.

He looked into coaching. See, for Scott, being the wild man that he is, the thrill of game day—the intensity of professional sports—is like a tonic for him. He did not know how he was going to replace that aspect of his life. Now, as is Scott's style, he talks and talks, and I massage and listen. He got professional help too. I was really proud of him for that. He has tried different things, and he has made it through to the other side (mostly). He is still young—mid-30s—but it is coming together for him. He will continue to be on the edge of professional sports, likely for the rest of his life. He does a radio show, plays in lots of charity/celebrity golf tournaments, and is involved with the Lions in helping players make the transition to the rest of their life. His neck still drives him crazy and will likely need further medical intervention. He will always be a wild man, and that is just fine.

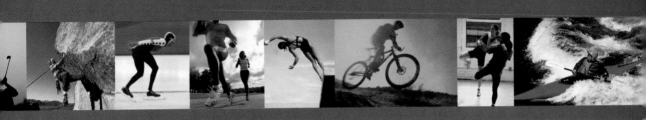

The content of Unit Three describes the transition from performance and recovery to rehabilitation massage. Rehabilitation is a medical specialty, and massage therapists working with sport injury will need to be able to function as a contributing part of a multidisciplinary medical team.

Therapeutic massage, provided as an integrated aspect of health care, has its own unique knowledge base and performance standards. The massage therapist needs to undrstand the implications of massage when combined with medication, surgical procedures, and rehabilitation protocols. This unit cannot possibly describe all of this content. It is important for the massage therapist to respond to the directives of doctors, nurses, physical therapists, and athletic trainers; maintain appropriate medical records; and only work within the parameters of treatment orders. ■

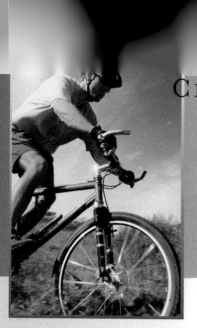

16

INJURY IN GENERAL

OUTLINE

OBJECTIVES

Upon completion of this chapter, the reader will have the information necessary to do the following:

1 List the common causes of physical activity injuries.

2 List injury prevention strategies.

3 Define trauma.

4 List the three healing phases.

5 Describe acute and chronic inflammation and relate the inflammation process to the three stages of healing.

6 Define illness.

7 Estimate general healing time for various injuries and illnesses.

8 Perform PRICE application.

9 Create effective strategies for massage application for acute, subacute, and remodeling phases of healing to support the recovery process.

The focus of the first unit of this book was on sport function and fitness, including an anatomy and physiology review and research relevant to sports and fitness massage. Unit Two covered the benefits of massage for recovery, performance enhancement, and injury prevention and provided a detailed series of massage applications. This third unit describes the application of massage therapy for sport injury recovery, including rehabilitation protocols featuring massage. All the methods to address the injuries in this unit were presented in Unit Two, and the specific sequences for applying these methods are found in this unit.

Unfortunately, athlete injury is common. Various injuries are the major reason that persons participate in physical rehabilitation programs. Those who are deconditioned; overtrain, especially when fatigued; or practice and play fatigued are more prone to injury and **illness.**

Acute reinjury of a chronic condition
Age
Backward-tilting (posterior) pelvis
Breathing
Cardiorespiratory fitness
Cervical lordosis
Chronic inflammation
Chronic or overuse trauma
Comparative weakness
Complete rupture
Direct trauma
Elevation
Fatigue
Forward-tilting (anterior) pelvis
Ice
Illness

Inappropriate training
Indirect trauma
Joint pain
Kyphosis
Lifestyle
Linear region
Lumbar lordosis
Major failure region
Muscle weakness
Neuromuscular
   control/proprioception/kinesthesis
Numbness and tingling
Pathomechanics
Posture deviations
PRICE therapy
Progressive failure region

Progressive relaxation
Protection
Reduced range of motion
Regeneration and repair
Remodeling
Rest
Rotated (left or right)
Sport-specific demands
Strength
Swayback (hyperextended) knees
Swelling
Tenderness at a specific point
Toe region
Trauma
Vascular
Visualization

The usual experience in conventional treatment is to restore normal function when someone is injured. But in sport, there is no acceptance of "normal" function in terms of **strength,** speed, or movement. Most athletes continually try to push themselves to new limits, and no matter how carefully they train, they inevitably will get an injury from time to time.

The actual treatment of an injury may be the same for the athlete and nonathlete if the pathologic condition is the same, but the thinking behind the treatment of a sports injury is different. If someone sustains an injury falling downstairs, the event probably will not happen again. Once healing occurs, the injury event can be forgotten. However, if an overuse injury caused by some component in a sports activity or if a traumatic injury such as an ankle sprain occurs, effective treatment alone will not necessarily prevent it from recurring. Identification and changing of any component in training that may be causing the overuse or injury potential is vital to prevent a recurrence of the injury. In many ways, this is the most challenging part of the massage therapist's assessment process, because it requires careful questioning and a detailed understanding of the training methods used.

Most athletes hope to reach a level of performance slightly beyond that which they will ever actually achieve. They want to be "better," not "normal," and the massage therapist must be aware of this goal of the athlete. The overall aim of treatment therefore must always be to strive to enhance performance, regardless of the current status of the athlete. A major risk in the quest for enhanced performance is injury.

The primary therapeutic massage outcome is to prevent injury, as described in Unit Two. Sports massage has great potential in this area and this is why many top competitors use it as an integral part of their training regimen. With regular massage treatment, the athlete is more able to sustain high levels of performance without getting injured. The massage therapist should measure success, not by how well he or she treats an injury, but by how few actual injuries the therapist treats. The great preventative benefits of massage are not yet widely exploited by the recreational athlete, and this is something that needs to be developed through education and greater public exposure.

COMMON CAUSES OF PHYSICAL ACTIVITY–RELATED INJURIES

If a massage therapist is going to be working with injured athletes or those in physical rehabilitation, first the therapist needs to understand the different factors that contribute to creating injury potential.

FATIGUE

Doing too much of a particular exercise fatigues the tissues and can cause damage. This should never occur in training (even though it often does), but it can happen easily during competition, when the athlete pushes to the limit and overexerts. Similarly, problems can arise if training sessions are too frequent and time is insufficient for the tissues to recover fully between practice sessions.

INAPPROPRIATE TRAINING

Inappropriate training occurs when a particular aspect of training leads to injury. The best training for a particular sport is actually to do that sport, because the musculoskeletal system naturally develops in a balanced way in relation to the demands placed on it. Weight training or other gym work that adds to the particular strengths and skills needed in that sport is also recommended. Problems occur if the main power muscles have been strengthened, but the smaller muscles, which have a synergistic or stabilizing function in the activity, have not also been strengthened. Injury occurs because the increased demands cause **fatigue** and natural movement patterns become affected, leading to other problems. Many of these problems are due to compensatory patterns that arise.

Injury potential increases when athletes mix their training styles.

Endurance athletes, for example, often do some anaerobic training to improve their speed; or sprint athletes do some endurance training to improve their stamina. However, if this is overdone, using different energy systems and working the muscles in a way that might not be best suited to them can cause damage.

Different types of exercise are certainly not a bad thing and are a vital part of many athletes' training schedules, but they need to be incorporated appropriately. The situation also can occur if a person participates in two or more different sport activities—for example, basketball and golf, or soccer and bowling.

WARM-UP AND COOLDOWN

Warming up and cooling down is another area that commonly is neglected, which can result in injury. The particular tissues involved in the activity, as well as the general systems of the body, must be prepared for the stresses of athletic activity.

A proper cooldown, which again is sport specific, is also important. It helps the recovery process to begin properly following hard exercise. After anaerobic activities, for example, maintaining activity at about 50% intensity for a short period is believed to be the best way of facilitating the breakdown of accumulated lactic acid. Stretching is also an important part of a cooldown because it helps realign muscle fibers and prevent the natural tightness and stiffness that often follow hard exercise.

AGE

The aging process alters metabolic processes involved in recovery after activity. Tendons become less well lubricated and so are more prone to damage. Repetitive training over a time span can cause wear and tear on the joints. The older athlete basically needs to put more effort into helping the natural recovery processes work better. This usually means longer recovery periods between training sessions, more stretching, and proper warming up and cooling down. Massage is especially beneficial for the older athlete.

POSTURAL DEVIATIONS

Postural deviations are often a major underlying cause of sports injuries. Postural misalignment may be the result of unilateral (one side of the body) muscle and soft tissue asymmetries or bony asymmetries. As a result, the athlete engages in poor mechanics of movement (**pathomechanics**).

Common postural imbalances include the following:
- **Cervical lordosis:** Short upper erector spinae. This is usually a postural compensation for a thoracic curvature. The sternocleidomastoid muscles may not be weak, although they may shorten and become tense.
- Thoracic **kyphosis:** Weak erector spinae; short abdominal and sternocleidomastoid
- **Lumbar lordosis:** Short lower erector spinae; weak abdominal muscles
- **Forward-tilting (anterior) pelvis:** Short gluteus maximus and rectus femoris; weak abdominal muscles, hamstrings, and iliopsoas
- **Backward-tilting (posterior) pelvis:** Short hip extensors, abdominal muscles, iliopsoas, and hamstrings; weak rectus femoris
- **Rotated (left or right):** Short and tight structures in the concave areas; long taut and inhibited muscles and structures in the convex areas
- **Swayback (hyperextended) knees:** Short calf muscles and rectus femoris; weak hamstrings

Distortions can occur in many lateral and rotational directions as well. These distortions involve imbalance between the postural muscles on either side of the body and also reciprocal imbalances in muscles of the torso. None of these postural imbalances occurs in isolation. An imbalance in one area generally leads to imbalances developing in adjacent areas as they compensate. The combined positional distortion patterns are the upper crossed, lower crossed, and pronation distortion syndrome. The patterns can occur singularly or in combination with each other (see Chapter 12).

Muscle imbalance can lead to problems in the bone structure. Structural bone problems lead to muscle imbalance. Both problems need to be addressed, and although the massage therapist cannot treat the bone structures directly, working with the soft tissue can be beneficial.

No single answer exists to these postural problems. Significant improvements usually require a variety of specialized skills to rectify muscle balance, structural alignment, and joint function.

MUSCLE WEAKNESS

Muscles may become weak because of a combination of injury, lack of use, and nerve inhibition. Once the root cause of the problem has been resolved, then normal use, or exercise, should be able to restore muscle strength. However, the body learns to adapt and compensate for small areas of weakness. Because of the complexity of the muscular system, altered movement patterns avoid using weak muscles but still allow performance of daily activities. The weak muscle does not get the exercise it needs and does not improve.

Whether nerve stimulation is the cause or the consequence, the nerve stimulation to a weak muscle is reduced, and eventually nerve function becomes poor. Nerve conductivity improves quickly when the muscle is stimulated. This is why initially great improvement occurs in apparent strength when one starts a new sport or activity. The increased nerve stimulation, rather than true strength, is responsible. By isolating the specific muscle that is weak and making it work, the nerves are stimulated and this rapidly improves its function. In fact, a real improvement usually can be felt after only four or five contractions, and the functional effect sometimes can be remarkable. The client immediately feels better movement and therefore uses the muscle(s) more normally. Correcting gait reflexes and firing patterns as

described in Unit Two is an example of neural stimulation.

In the chronic situation, nerve conductivity may have become so poor that the client has real difficulty in creating any movement and feels that he or she does not even know how to move the area. It becomes necessary to address the situation with passive movements, with the client feeling and experiencing the movement. The massage therapist then moves the area with the client assisting and watching the movement before progressing to the full active method.

IN MY EXPERIENCE...

I have seen this commonly occurring with turf toe to the point that athletes break a sweat trying to move the big toe, and the experience really can be disturbing.

THE LIFE STYLE

The general environment in which the athlete lives, practices, and plays can involve unduly high levels of stress, which can have a direct effect on the structure of the body and contribute to injury. Increased mental demand and worry can drain energy and lead to muscular fatigue and tension. A poor practice or a competitive environment that is cold, damp, or noisy can add to the physical stress. Inadequate or ill-fitting equipment also can be a factor. Prior injury history creates a potential for a future reinjury. Lack of sleep, being distracted and having unrealistitc performance expectations, and poor nutrition and taking dangerous substances such as ephedra increase injury potential. Any and all aspects of life may play a part in contributing to an injury situation.

Psychological/Emotional Factors

Psychology and emotion play a part in all aspects of life, and injury is no exception. In some clinical situations, despite good and apparently effective treatment, the client continues to suffer painful symptoms. Some persons seem to suffer continually from one injury or another. A person may hold on to an injury because it satisfies other needs (secondary gain). The injury may provide the client with support and sympathy from the persons around him or her. The injury also provides an excuse to avoid activities or to avoid failure. It makes a good excuse for poor performance. Continuing in the sport or activity, despite the pain, makes the athlete appear to be a martyr. Therefore these clients will have had the problem for a long time and will have been to other therapists. Massage treatment alone may give slight improvement in the symptoms for a few sessions, but then the client usually moves on to another therapist and starts again.

Although there may be physical or medical reasons for the client's symptoms, underlying psychological factors also may be influencing the situation. Although this is not an area in which the massage therapist should attempt to work, it is important to be aware of the possibility of these emotional influences. The massage therapist must accept that the pain the client feels is usually real, and to say that there is not a problem would be wrong. The massage therapist should not attempt to deal with the psychological aspect of the injury and should refer the client to the appropriate specialist. However, being an empathetic listener sometimes can help the client see the problem for himself or herself.

INJURY PREVENTION

Injury prevention is possible if the athlete is prepared for activity physically and mentally. The athlete should not overtrain and do more than the trainer allows. A balance of training with **rest** is important to avoid overuse injuries. The following tips can help the athlete avoid sports injuries:
- Wear and use proper gear for the sport, including helmets, pads, shoes, sunglasses, gloves, and layered clothing where appropriate.
- Warm up slowly before activity. This is especially important in sports that require quick, dynamic movements, such as basketball and soccer.
- Always use proper body mechanics and skill training in sports involving repetitive stress to the upper extremities (tennis, baseball, golf).
- The athlete should use specific skills to train to prepare for the sport.
- Moderate cross-training for overall conditioning allows specific muscles to rest. Cross-training also will alleviate training boredom.
- The athlete should listen to the body. Pain is a warning sign of injury. The athlete should not work through pain but stop or slow activity until the pain subsides.

- Anyone who is not fit is more likely to sustain an injury. Being fit really means choosing a healthful **lifestyle** in which one is able to express emotions effectively; have good relations with others; and be concerned about decision-making abilities, ethics, values, and spirituality. Paying attention to aspects of a healthful lifestyle such as physical fitness, adequate nutrition, stress management, control of alcohol consumption and avoidance of drug abuse, smoking cessation, and weight control management can contribute to preventing injury.

Coaches and athletic trainers recognize that improper conditioning is one of the major causes of sports injuries. Coaches and athletic trainers work cooperatively to supervise training and conditioning programs that minimize the possibility of injury and maximize performance. It takes time and careful preparation to bring an athlete into competition at a level of fitness that will reduce injury potential. Therapeutic massage should be part of this program.

TRAUMA

Many factors produce mechanical injuries or **trauma** in sports and exercise. *Trauma* is defined as a physical injury or wound sustained in sport and produced by an external or internal force. Trauma triggers the healing mechanism. Healing mechanisms work through the inflammatory response and resolution of the inflammatory response. Different tissues heal at different rates. Skin heals fast, whereas ligaments heal slowly. Stress can influence healing by slowing the repair process. Sleep and proper nutrition are necessary for proper healing. Medication use, particularly analgesics for pain and antiinflammatory drugs, is common and their effects need to be considered. Pain medication reduces pain perception so the athlete can continue to perform before healing is completed. This interferes with successful healing. Antiinflammatory drugs may slow the healing process, particularly connective tissue healing.

Understanding sports injuries and appropriate massage application requires knowledge of tissue susceptibility to trauma and the mechanical forces involved.

Tissues have relative abilities to resist a particular load. A load can be singular or a group of outside or internal forces acting on the body. A *force* can be defined as a push or pull. The resistance to a load is called a mechanical stress, and the internal response is a deformation, or change in dimensions. *Deformation* also is defined as a mechanical strain. The stronger the tissue, the greater magnitude of load it can withstand. All human tissues have viscous and elastic properties, allowing for deformation.

Tissue such as bone is brittle and has fewer viscoelastic properties compared with soft tissue such as muscle. The loads (forces) applied to bone and soft tissues that can cause injury are tension, compression, bending, shearing, and torsion. Interestingly, these same forces are created by massage application. When tissue is deformed to the extent that its elasticity is almost fully exceeded, a yield point has been reached. When the yield point has been exceeded, mechanical failure occurs, resulting in tissue damage.

Because these same forces are applied therapeutically during massage to encourage tissue repair, the massage therapist needs to take care not to superimpose extensive force during massage that may increase the injury. The choice of which type of force offers the most therapeutic value also is important. In general, during acute and subacute phases, do not use the same force as the one that loaded the tissue and produced the injury. For example, if a sprain occurs from a torsion load, then kneading that applies a torsion force may not be the best choice until healing is progressing and stability is restored in the area. In chronic injury, it may be necessary during the massage to introduce the same force that caused the injury to achieve results. Therefore if an ankle sprain caused by a torsion force healed badly, massage reintroduces torsion force (kneading) to restore normal tissue function.

Injuries to soft tissue can be described by a stress/strain arc. *Stress* is defined as the force per area applied to the tissue, and *strain* as the percent change in length. The degree of damage to the soft tissues is affected not only by the force. The higher the acceleration, the greater the damage. This explains the whiplash phenomenon, in which low speed but high acceleration can cause damage to the soft tissues.

FIVE DEGREES OF SOFT TISSUE FAILURE

The five degrees of soft tissue failure are as follows (Figure 16-1):
• **Toe region:** If the stress is small, the tissue returns to its normal length. This is represented

by the toe region of the curve. Tissue may be loaded with a 1.5% to 2.5% strain and return to normal. This ability decreases with age because the amount of connective tissue crimp decreases with age. Athletes often will describe this as "tweaked."
• **Linear region:** If the strain is between 2.5% and 4%, all of the fibers have straightened out, and the collagen tears at its outermost fibers first. This is called **microfailure**. This degree of injury is represented by the linear area of the curve. The tearing of collagen is like a rope that frays from its outer fibers to the center. The client complains of stiffness when using the injured area. Microfailure can occur within the normal physiologic range if there is repetitive stress on an already damaged structure. This is a grade one injury.
• **Progressive failure region:** A strain between 4% and 6% is called the yield point, at which major tearing occurs. This is a grade two injury.
• **Major failure region:** A strain of more than 6% involves many points of rupture. This is a grade three injury.
• **Complete rupture:** An 8% strain causes the collagen fibers to tear completely apart. This can be classified as a grade three, four, or five injury.

Even with microfailure, the cells, fibers, and ground substance matrix are now damaged, and an inflammatory response is initiated. The injury also affects the sensory nerves in the connective tissue, causing pain. Repair and regeneration of the tissue is carried out through the process of inflammation and repair.

INJURY CLASSIFICATION

Injury can be classified simply as traumatic or repetitive strain. A sprained ankle is an example of traumatic injury. Typically, a causative event is identifiable. Repetitive injury results from an accumulation of minor trauma and overuse. Symptoms occur when adaptive processes are no longer effective. Bursitis and plantar fasciitis are examples. Traumatic injury is easier to treat than repetitive injury. Traumatic injury generally is classified as mild, grade one; moderate, grade two; or severe, grade three. The most common injuries are contusions, sprains, muscle pulls and tears, strains, dislocations, fractures, and nerve impingements.

The four types of trauma are the following:

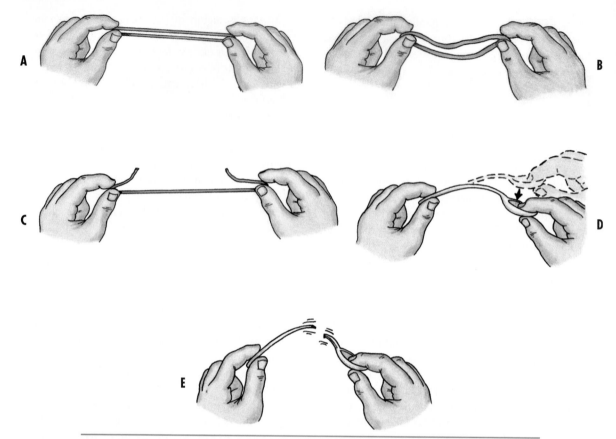

FIGURE 16–1 ■ Properties of connective tissue. **A–C,** Elastic deformation. Stress applied to a rubber band. When stress is removed, the rubber band returns to its original length. If the stress exceeds the strain capabilities of the band, it can break. **D, E,** Plastic deformtion. A low degree of stress is applied to a plastic spoon. The spoon will deform slowly and accommodate to a new shape. If stress is applied suddenly and with great force, the spoon will break. (From Shankman GA: *Fundamental orthopedic management for the physical therapist assistant,* ed 2, St Louis, 2004, Mosby.)

- **Direct trauma:** blunt trauma such as from contact sports and car accidents
- **Indirect trauma:** trauma that occurs with sudden force overloading
- **Chronic or overuse trauma:** trauma that results from repeated overload, frictional resistance, or both
- **Acute reinjury of a chronic condition:** trauma that results from a sudden tear of a persistent lesion.

STAGES OF INFLAMMATION AND REPAIR

Inflammation protects the body from infection and repairs damaged tissue by stimulating new cell growth, which then synthesizes new fibers for repair.

The inflammatory process can be described in the following three phases.

Vascular—Acute

Acute vascular inflammation typically lasts 24 to 48 hours. In some cases, however, it may last up to a week. Dilation of the arteries, veins, and capillaries occurs, producing redness, heat, and escape of blood plasma, causing edema. The number of fibroblasts and macrophages increases. The fibroblasts increase in size and synthesize ground substance and collagen. This process begins within 4 hours of injury and can last 4 to 6 days. Collagen initially forms a weak, random mesh of fibers. Pain is produced by the pressure from the **swelling** and by the chemical irritation that stimulates the pain receptors.

Regeneration and Repair—Subacute

The process of regeneration and repair usually begins 2 to 6 days after injury and lasts 3 or 4 weeks.

New capillaries are formed and are laid down in a random orientation unless the area is mobilized. Fibroblastic activity and collagen formation increase. Scar tissue at this stage is highly cellular and fragile.

In the acute and subacute stages, collagen is laid down in a random, disorganized pattern, usually in a plane perpendicular to the long axis, and therefore has little strength. The collagen develops abnormal cross-links, leaving the tissue with less flexibility. Immature connective tissue is less dense and therefore is injured more easily. The massage therapist must take care with the amount of pressure applied in a massage.

Remodeling

In the early stages of **remodeling,** the collagen matures into a lattice that is completely disorganized in a gel structure. The collagen can be palpated as thickened or fibrous tissue. Relative decrease in cellularity and vascularity occurs as collagen density increases.

After about 2 months, fibroblastic activity decreases and there is less collagen synthesis. Random orientation of collagen provides little support for tensile loads unless appropriate rehabilitation is provided.

Two months to 2 years later, collagen may develop a functional linear alignment in response to stimuli provided by movement and use patterns.

Ineffective rehabilitation and immobilization during all inflammatory healing phases will lead to significant adhesion formations; osteoporosis or loss of bone density; and atrophy of muscle, joint capsules, and ligaments.

CHRONIC INFLAMMATION

Chronic inflammation can result from repeated episodes of microtrama or chronic irritation to the tissue. The process is an inflammation that is no longer productive.

Chronic inflammation leads to stimulation of pain receptors that cause compensatory adaptations that facilitate muscles, causing hypertonicity, or inhibit muscles, causing weakness. Typically, with joint inflammation, the flexors of the joint become hypertonic, and the extensors become inhibited. The innate subconscious logic of the body is apparent: the flexed position affords more joint capsule space for the increased fluid present and avoids the greater pressure and pain that would occur if the joint were in an extended position. Extended positions are often, but not always, associated with increased force because of weight bearing, so flexion occurs subconsciously as a form of guarding.

Chronic inflammation can cause sensitization of the mechanoreceptors, and normal mechanical stimuli cause the mechanoreceptor to be a pain producer.

Repetitive strain injuries frequently result in limitation or curtailment of sports performance. Most of these injuries in athletes are related directly to the dynamics of running, throwing, or jumping. The injuries may result from constant and repetitive stresses placed on bones, joints, or soft tissues; from forcing a joint into an extreme range of motion; or from prolonged strenuous activity. Overuse and repetitive stress injuries may be relatively minor; still, they can be disabling. General massage is used to manage pain and edema and to restore mobility. Rest is important in treatment of microtrauma and overuse conditions with chronic inflammation. Massage used to create parasympathetic dominance helps to support restorative sleep.

Careful and targeted use of methods that superimpose acute inflammation can help resolve chronic inflammation. The key is to create just enough acute reinjury to jump-start the resolution of the inflammatory process. This can be considered therapeutic inflammation. Friction is the most common massage method used to create these controlled acute inflammation areas.

Chronic inflammation and repetitive injury is difficult to treat. Onset is gradual, and the acute, subacute, and remodeling healing stages are not defined clearly. Both types of injury, traumatic and repetitive, can become chronic if the healing process is not completed successfully. A concept of chronic injury symptoms is an injury healing process that for whatever reason has not been able to resolve and is stuck in the later stages of the subacute healing stage. The common causes for this include impaired injury repair process, return to activity too soon after rehabilitation, and inappropriate rehabilitation.

Of the traumatic injuries, those to the ligaments and cartilage are most difficult to heal. If treated properly, bone fractures heal the best. Mild and moderate injury is most suitable to massage being part of the active treatment process. Severe injury requires medical intervention and possibly surgery. Massage becomes more supportive, instead of direct care, until rehabilitation begins (Box 16–1).

ILLNESS

Illness involves some sort of pathogenic invasion that causes infection (bacteria, funguses, or viruses), immune system dysfunction (hyperactivity or hypoactivity), or organ and system failure. Examples of illnesses are colds, sinus infection, digestive upset, cardiovascular disease, Epstein-Barr virus, diabetes, multiple sclerosis, and fibromyalgia. Illnesses can be acute, subacute, or chronic.

Box 16-1   MASSAGE APPROACH
                   DURING HEALING

Massage during Acute Phase
Manage pain.
Support sleep.

Massage during Subacute Phase—Early
Manage pain.
Support sleep.
Manage edema.
Manage compensation patterns.

Massage during Subacute Phase—Later
Manage pain.
Support sleep.
Manage edema.
Manage compensation patterns.
Support rehabilitative activity.
Support mobile scar development.
Support tissue regeneration process.

Massage during Remodeling Phase
Support rehabilitation activity.
Encourage appropriate scar tissue development.
Manage adhesion.
Restore firing patterns, gait reflexes, and neuromuscular responses.
Eliminate reversible compensation pattern.
Manage irreversible compensation patterns.
Restore tissue pliability.

Box 16-2   ANTIINFLAMMATORY DIET

EAT fruit, vegetables, whole grains, omega 3 eggs, fish, chicken, yogurt (unsweetened) with live cultures, extra virgin olive oil, and flaxseed oil.

AVOID dairy (except yogurt), pork, beef, processed meat, refined grains and sugar, artificial food, and most fats and oils, especially hydrogenated oils.

FOODS AND HERBS are especially valuable in controlling inflammation include: ginger, turmeric, cumin, pineapple, and papaya.

Massage is appropriate during illness if applied correctly. The typical treatment plan is a general nonspecific full-body massage that supports sleep and restorative mechanisms, particularly parasympathetic dominance. Energy-based modalities can be used during infection in an adult who is generally healthy. A temperature up to 102° F might not be treated with medicine but instead supported with increased fluid intake and rest. Artificially reducing productive fever (fever that results from an unimpeded healing process, also referred to as low-grade inflammatory response) can prolong infection. A temperature higher than 103° F needs to be evaluated by a doctor.

Autoimmune disease often involves an increased, sustained, and/or inappropriate inflammatory response. Antiinflammatory support includes an antiinflammatory diet (Box 16-2), possible use of antiinflammatory medications, and other antiinflammatory treatment strategies, such as cold hydrotherapy.

Massage is appropriate for autoimmune disease as long as the application does not generate inflammation and does not strain adaptive capacity. The general massage protocol described in Unit Two of this text is appropriate with caution for overuse of mechanical force targeting connective tissue. Be especially cautious with shearing forces (friction) and compressive force application that could cause tissue damage such as bruising.

REALISTIC EXPECTATIONS FOR RECOVERY

The idea of "good as new" after injury recovery is misleading. Even the best healing outcome results in some sort of compensation adaptation. Injured areas are prone to tissue changes, such as decreased connective tissue pliability in the area; altered firing patterns with tendency to synergistic dominance; reflexive activity to other aspects of the kinetic chain function; susceptibility to subclinical (chronic) inflammation and swelling; tendency to develop traumatic arthritis/arthrosis; and changes in muscle size and strength patterns.

Massage is effective as part of a treatment plan for all of these issues. If an athlete has experienced only a few minor injuries, then performance is likely not to be affected. However, recovery from repeated injury eventually takes its toll. Adaptive mechanisms become strained, and performance is affected. Massage therapy that supports appropriate training, rehabilitation, and ongoing maintenance can reduce the adaptive strain of cumulative compensation on the body. For example, if a client has had three or four ankle sprains in the mild to moderate range, the ongoing treatment plan for the athlete would always include attention to the ankle.

Massage is effective at this level of maintenance care.

HEALING TIME

Healing of illnesses and sports injuries can take some time. After swelling is reduced, healing depends on blood supply. A good blood supply will help move nutrients, oxygen, and infection-fighting cells to the damaged area to work on repair. Athletes tend to have a better blood supply and heal faster than those with chronic illness, smokers, or those with sedentary lifestyles. Ultimately, healing time varies from person to person, and the athlete cannot force healing.

For someone who is reasonably fit, the following are the average lengths of healing time for various injuries and illnesses:

Fractured finger or toe: 3 to 5 weeks
Fractured clavicle: 6 to 10 weeks
Sprained ankle—minor: 5 days; severe: 3 to 6 weeks
Mild contusion: 5 days
Strains/muscle pulls: a few days to several weeks, depending on the severity and location of the injury
Mild shoulder separation: 7 to 14 days
Major shoulder separation: 6 to 12 months
Common viral infection—cold and flu: 7 to 14 days
Common bacterial infection: 14 days

Healing time for any injury or illness can take longer if the athlete returns to activity too soon. The athlete should never exercise the injured area if there is pain during rest. When the injured area no longer hurts at rest, the athlete may start exercising it slowly with simple range of motion exercises. If the athlete feels pain, he or she should stop and rest. Over time the athlete can return to activity at a low intensity and build up to the previous level. The athlete can increase intensity of exercise only when he or she can do the activity without pain.

The athlete may find that the injured area is more susceptible to reinjury, and closer attention to warning signs of overdoing it should be observed. Soreness, aching, and tension must be acknowledged, or the athlete may end up with an even more serious injury in the future. An athlete is more prone to injury or reinjury when ill.

Knowing when to return to activity after illness is more difficult. Typically, illness symptoms above the clavicle (i.e., head cold or sinus problems) are less serious. Activity is okay but should not cause fatigue. More serious illnesses should be supervised by the physician.

The massage therapist has different roles in the injury and illness rehabilitative process than in the maintenance and recovery process described in Unit Two. These roles include support of general healing and restorative processes, management of soreness related to rehabilitation, conditioning programs, and managing compensation patterns from the injury or from protective gear.

Various treatments are used during injury rehabilitation. Therapeutic modalities consist of mechanical, electric, and thermal interventions used by athletic trainers and physical therapists. These modalities control or reduce swelling, reduce pain, and help maintain strength. Standard therapies such as ultrasound, electric stimulation (E-Stim or transdermal electric nerve stimulation), paraffin baths, and hot/cold whirlpool and massage have a proven track record for lessening the time lost to injury. Acupuncture has been shown to produce some positive effects as well.

Swelling is particularly problematic because it contributes to a spinal cord reflex that inhibits muscle function and interferes with rehabilitative exercise (i.e., joint motion, shock absorption, and balance). Massage supports lymphatic drainage and is especially beneficial in the management of swelling located outside the joint capsule. The lymphatic drain application is time consuming, and the massage therapist typically has more time than the trainer to apply the method. Some facilities have pneumatic compression devices that rhythmically compress and release against the tissue. These devices are helpful in encouraging fluid movement.

Some modalities are beneficial by influencing blood flow to the injured area and modifying the pain response. Massage is especially effective in this regard. At times, too much emphasis is placed on therapy when the greatest healing methods are time, rest, and proper nutrition. The massage therapist, along with others treating the injury, needs to respect the body and not "overdo" treatment.

PRICE THERAPY

The acronym PRICE describes the standard procedure for addressing an injury in the acute phase. The massage therapist should be supportive of this treatment procedure.

The first treatment indicated for any acute injury is reducing any swelling. Swelling causes pain and loss of motion, which in turn limit use of the muscles, which then can weaken, shorten, and resist repair.

Never apply heat to an acute injury. Heat increases circulation and increases swelling.

PRICE therapy consists of the following:

Protection. Immobilize the affected area to encourage healing and to protect it from further injury. The athlete may need to use elastic wraps, slings, splints, crutches, or canes.

Rest. Avoid activities that increase the pain or swelling. Rest is essential to tissue healing. But it does not mean complete bed rest. The client can do other activities and exercises that do not stress the injured area. Swimming and water exercise may be well tolerated.

Ice. To decrease pain, muscle spasm, and swelling, apply ice to the injured area. Ice packs, ice massage, or slush baths can help. Twenty-minute applications, 4 to 6 times a day, are recommended.

Compression. Because swelling can result in loss of motion in an injured joint, compress the area until the swelling has ceased. Wraps or compressive (Ace) elastic bandages are best.

Elevation. To reduce swelling, raise the affected area above the level of the heart, and above jointed areas that lie between the injury and the heart. For example, a sprained ankle would be elevated above the knee, which in turn would be placed higher than the hip. Use of this position is especially important at night.

Avoid the use of nonsteroidal antiinflammatory drugs if possible. They interfere with the normal healing response and can cause nausea, stomach pain, stomach bleeding, or ulcers. In rare cases, prolonged use can disrupt normal kidney function. The risk of these conditions increases with age. Individuals with liver problems should consult their physician before using products containing acetaminophen.

When injury occurs and the athlete is forced to miss training time, levels of **cardiorespiratory fitness** may decrease rapidly. The client needs to rest the injured body part and work the rest of the body during the recovery stage, especially during the playing season. Alternative activities that allow the athlete to maintain existing levels of cardiorespiratory fitness need to begin as early as possible in the rehabilitation period. Depending on the nature of the injury, a number of activities can help the athlete maintain fitness levels. When a lower extremity injury occurs, non–weight-bearing activities should be incorporated, such as pool activities. Cycling also can maintain cardiorespiratory fitness. Because these activities may require using muscles different from those the athlete typically uses, postexercise soreness can occur. Massage is appropriate to help manage soreness and therefore support the cardiorespiratory fitness regimen.

Continued rehabilitation of the injured area is important, even though the symptoms may seem to have resolved. Symptoms may reduce significantly during the second stage of healing; however, the area is not healed fully until the third stage, called remodeling, has been completed. A saying that rings true is that healing takes time (often as much as a year to be complete).

When the athlete begins to practice and compete, ongoing rehabilitation using hydrotherapy, massage, and electric modalities can prevent or manage recurrence of swelling and soreness.

RECOVERY PROCESS

Whether the person is a competitive athlete or a recreational exerciser or is recovering from a traumatic injury, viral infection, or heart attack, healing presents a challenge. How the person understands and responds to pain and limitation is an individual experience based on many factors. However, certain responses and psychological skills can help most persons take an active role in their own recovery. See Unit One for more information.

Individuals often initially feel overwhelmed by an injury. The ability to cope improves greatly if the athlete or rehabilitation client works closely with the doctor, trainer, and other health care providers to develop a clear plan for recovery.

Successful rehabilitation begins with the client becoming informed about the injury. The client must know the extent of the injury, anticipated recovery time, and the plan to recover safely and effectively. The client must see himself or herself as an active participant in rehabilitation planning and the treatment process. The client may not understand every scientific aspect of recovery, so careful and accurate explanation of massage method application, how it affects underlying physiology, and its relationship to the total rehabilitation program is necessary. The information must not conflict with explanations of other health care professions. Be ready to answer the athlete's questions respectfully, but keep answers within the scope of massage practice. If the question is outside that scope, suggest that the athlete consult someone with more training.

How the athlete responds to the injury is also important. Although certain sports or activities have greater risk for injury than others, an injury generally is not expected and is never planned or welcomed. Injuries have different meaning for different persons. For some, an injury might be life-threatening or career ending. For others, an injury might take them away from a team or social structure that gives them a sense of identity and community. An injury also can interfere with a job or responsibilities at home. Therefore the athlete or rehabilitation client must understand the coping skills required to help them through the loss using professional help if necessary. This was described in Unit One. Directing or redirecting the athlete's or rehabilitation client's response to the injury may aid recovery. At the very least, it can help the client maintain a positive outlook during healing. A few suggestions include the following:

- Consider the pain and injury as something that will go away and will heal.
- Mentally and physically befriend the pain as a guide to recovery. Pushing too hard may cause reinjury, but fearing pain may lead to too passive of an approach.
- Be positive every day about the ability to cope with and recover from injury.
- Use the desire to recover to help integrate the sense of self and mental and physical healing power.
- Connect with emotions and let them guide through the healing process: If the client becomes emotionally overwhelmed, encourage activity that is enjoyable and distracting. When the client feels emotionally strong, that energy should be used to progress in recovery.

The athlete or rehabilitation client should express the needs and concerns about the rehabilitation progress directly to the health care team. However, these discussions often likely will occur first with the massage therapist, because massage therapists tend to spend longer uninterrupted time with athletes, and they experience blood chemistry changes (lower cortisol, increased serotonin, dopamine, endorphins, and oxytocin) that promote personal bonding during massage. Although our hands are busy, we are able to listen when they are relaxing and ready to talk. Identify any negative mental responses to injury, and then reframe them to promote a positive approach to

IN MY EXPERIENCE...

I have worked with many persons recovering from injury. Rehabilitation is a physical and emotional roller coaster. I recall a young soccer player who was in a severe auto accident. He sustained a horrible injury in which the soft tissue was scraped from the lateral side of one of his lower legs. Skin grafts were necessary, and the scarring was awful. He was experiencing foot drop from the nerve injury and entrapment and would likely never play soccer again. I taught one of my advanced students how to do scar tissue release. My student and this teenage athlete worked together, and little by little the texture of the scar became more pliable. Eventually the nerve function returned. I am happy to report that this young man is playing soccer again. In fact, he recently invited the student who worked with him to attend his first game after the rehabilitation. The emotions just on my part as the teacher were anger, frustration, fear, determination, hope, and when I was told he would play soccer again, tears of joy. Although we cannot let our work affect our professional judgment and performance, who says we do not ever become emotionally involved?

healing. If you do not know how to do this, then do not say anything and refer the client to someone who is proficient in these types of communication skills. If you have advance permission from the client, describe the particular significant circumstances, if any, during the massage when the client's questions surfaced in order to assist this communication process with the professional to whom you have referred the client. Then let go, and just be supportive of the medical team, knowing that you chose to refer when appropriate.

Help the client be creative, humorous, and positive in the approach to the daily inconveniences caused by injury. The person in rehabilitation needs to ask for and receive help and be surrounded by emotionally and physically supportive persons.

Several specific mental techniques also can aid in the recovery. The methods usually are presented by the psychologist but are supported by the massage therapist. See Unit One for more detailed information for these methods. The methods are as follows:

- **Progressive relaxation.** Direct the client to start with the head and work down, alternate flexing the muscles in each body part (producing tension), then relaxing them. Have the client mentally and physically memorize the feeling of relaxation.

- **Breathing.** Breath control can help modify stress and response to pain. Massage can support a functional breathing pattern.
- **Visualization.** Use of imagery can enhance healing by creating a positive internal atmosphere by focusing on a scene that creates a positive, nurturing, and healing state of mind during the massage. During practice of this technique, use music that the athlete finds peaceful to reinforce the imagery. The massage therapist usually does not guide the visualization but can support the effectiveness of the method. The relaxed client can concentrate on total body healing and can visualize a color or sound that represents healing as it moves slowly through the entire body, cell by cell. Others prefer to focus on the injured area, create a healing image such as blood vessels sending out healing roots, hold the image, and "see" the area healing. Some persons combine these techniques and images.

Some persons prefer to visualize only, whereas others like to combine visualization with mental statements such as, "I am healing," "I am calm," or "I will get better." The massage therapist also can visualize and use an energetic intention for healing during the massage process.

Visualization is also helpful as a form of distraction from pain. Use imagery to pull away from the body to a scene or favorite experience. Additionally, this technique may be helpful to facilitate sleep.

Remember that the prospect of prolonged recovery from an injury can be daunting for anyone. The successful completion of a rehabilitation program challenges physical and psychological capacities to the fullest. Patience, commitment, and persistence are necessary for any professional working in a rehabilitation setting. The massage therapist requires solid emotional stability and a bit of detachment to allow the possible emotional storms of the client to not affect him or her personally.

IN MY EXPERIENCE...

I recall a conversation with an athlete's wife. The player had surgery to remove a loose body from his knee. The procedure was successful, but the mood swings of the player were difficult, to say the least. The wife asked me how I could stand even being around her husband. I gave her a knowing smile and replied, "He pays me."

Remember the rehabilitation process is about the *client*—not about you.

After an athlete sustains an injury, he or she must move forward through the psychological and physical stages of healing. Psychological stages include shock, realization, mourning, acknowledgment, and coping. Physically, an athlete must progress through the stages of initial pain, swelling, and loss of the previous level of control of the injured limb or body part. The athlete also faces the challenge of reestablishing strength, balance, coordination, and confidence to a safe level before returning to competition. Once the symptoms resolve or the medical staff feels it is safe to return to activity, the athlete first must achieve fitness gradually, then sport performance, and finally be able to demonstrate, to the satisfaction of the medical staff, that he or she is able to participate without the potential of further damage to the injured area. The medical staff may require the athlete to wear protective padding, bracing, or other modifications to protect the injured area.

The team physician should be ultimately responsible for deciding that the athlete is ready to return to practice or competition. That decision should be based on collaborative input with the physical therapist/athletic trainer and from the massage therapist, the coach, and the athlete.

WHEN TO RETURN TO TRAINING AND COMPETITION

Appropriate functional assessment indicates that the extent of recovery is sufficient to allow successful performance. Typically, the following types of assessments are used:

Strength: Power, strength, or muscular endurance is great enough to protect the injured structure from reinjury.

Neuromuscular control/proprioception/kinesthesis: The athlete has "relearned" how to use the injured body part.

Cardiorespiratory fitness: The athlete has been able to maintain aerobic fitness at or near the level necessary for competition.

Sport-specific demands: The demands of the sport or a specific position will not predispose the athlete to reinjury.

Once the athlete has demonstrated sufficient physical recovery, prophylactic strapping, bracing, and padding that provide additional support may be necessary for an injured athlete who is not quite healed to return to activity.

The responsibility of the athlete involves the ability to listen to his or her body, to recognize a potential reinjury situation, and to be able to understand the importance of continuing to engage in conditioning exercises that will reduce the chances of reinjury.

Psychological factors also influence the athlete's return to activity and competition at high levels without fear of reinjury. The role of the massage therapist is to continue to support the healing process for up to 1 year and to manage any lingering pain or compensation.

ASSESSMENT OF INJURY

Some sports injuries are immediately evident; others can creep up slowly and progressively get worse. The massage therapist needs to recognize possible injury and refer the athlete for diagnosis and treatment.

Signs of injury include the following:

Joint pain. Joint pain, particularly in the joints of the knee, ankle, elbow, and wrist, should never be ignored. Because these joints are not covered by muscle, acute joint pain is rarely primarily of muscular origin. Joint pain requires a trainer or physician evaluation.

Tenderness at a specific point. If the pain can be recreated at a specific point in a bone, muscle, or joint, there may be a major injury. Compare the painful area with the same spot on the other side of the body. If pain sensations are different, refer the athlete for diagnosis.

Swelling. Swelling is a sign of injury. Swelling will cause pain and stiffness or may produce a clicking sound as the tendons snap over one another because they have been pushed into a new position because of the swelling. Refer the athlete to a physician to determine the cause.

Reduced range of motion. If pain occurs with passive or active motion, refer the athlete to a physician. Again, compare one side of the body with the other to identify major differences. If there are any, make a referral.

Comparative weakness. Comparing one side with the other for **muscle weakness** can identify significant injury. If this situation exists, make a referral.

Numbness and tingling. Often related to nerve compression, numbness or tingling may indicate serious injury and should always be evaluated by the trainer or physician.

The massage therapist should always refer to a physician if the athlete has the following:
- An injury that does not heal in 3 weeks.
- An infection with pus, red streaks, a fever, or swollen lymph nodes
- Severe pain, or if pain persists for more than 2 weeks in a joint or bone
- Pain that radiates to another area of the body

SUMMARY

This chapter has discussed injury in general, the types of injury, progress of healing, predisposition to injury, injury prevention, and the massage therapist's role when working injury rehabilitation. Also discussed were illness and appropriate massage treatment for someone who is ill. Because most injury and illness involve pain, the next chapter specifically addresses this issue.

1 Using the information about the common causes of injury, develop an injury prevention strategy for each of the following situations. Include massage if appropriate, explain how massage would be applied, and the expected outcomes.

   Example: Fatigue–Restorative sleep supported by general massage targeting parasympathetic response, reduce training/competition schedule, and improve self regulation.

   a. Inappropriate training

   _____

   _____

   b. Warm-up/cooldown

   _____

   _____

   c. Age

   _____

   _____

   d. Posture deviations

   _____

   _____

   e. Muscle weakness

   _____

   _____

   f. Lifestyle

   _____

   _____

   g. Psychological/emotional factors

   _____

   _____

   _____

   _____

   _____

2 Write three case studies, fictional or real, that describe a client in the acute, subacute, and remodeling stage of healing.

   Example: Acute–68-year-old female fell 1 day ago while race walking. She has various bruises and abrasions on her right arm and leg. There appears to be a mild lateral right ankle sprain. Otherwise, she is fine.

   Case 1

   _____

   _____

   _____

   _____

   _____

   Case 2

   _____

   _____

   _____

   _____

   _____

   _____

   Case 3

   _____

   _____

   _____

   _____

   _____

   _____

3 Based on your cases, develop an appropriate massage treatment plan to address the client.

Example: General nonspecific massage lasting 45 minutes, avoiding areas of abrasion. Lymphatic drain applied over the bruises with skin drag only. Light touch energy-based application on right ankle. Suggest arnica and rescue remedy. Offer lavender essential oil as part of the massage with helichrysum over the bruises.

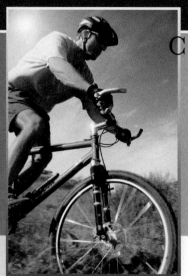

17

PAIN MANAGEMENT

OBJECTIVES

Upon completion of this chapter, the reader will have the information necessary to do the following:

1 Describe pain in relationship to injury and rehabilitation.
2 Apply massage targeting pain management mechanisms.

PAIN

Pain is a major issue for the athlete and those in rehabilitation. Pain management is most effective as a multidisciplinary intervention. Clients involved in physical rehabilitation likely have pain from the injury and the rehabilitation. Athletes often play and practice with pain. Massage coupled with other pain management strategies is essential for exercise compliance, persistence in training protocols, and enhancing performance.

Pain is a universal experience. The degree to which a person reacts to pain comes from biologic, psychological, and cultural makeup. Past encounters with painful injury or illness also can influence pain sensitivity. Athletes who are prone to recurring injury in the same area can experience increasing pain sensation for the same or even less degree of injury.

When pain persists beyond the time expected for an injury to heal or an illness to end, it can become a chronic condition. No longer is the pain just the symptom of another disease, but it is a separate condition unto itself. Unfortunately, pain coexists with athletic training, performance, and competition. The massage therapist must understand pain and use massage methods effectively to manage pain. This information expands on content in Units One and Two and provides specific massage strategies for pain management.

WHAT IS PAIN?

Pain basically results from a series of exchanges involving three major components: **peripheral nerves,** spinal cord, and brain.

Acute pain
Adrenaline
Chronic pain
Cortisol
Counterirritation

Dopamine
Endorphin
GABA
Hyperstimulation analgesia
Nociceptors

Noradrenaline
Peripheral nerves
Serotonin
Substance P

PERIPHERAL NERVES

Peripheral nerves encompass a network of nerve fibers that branch throughout the body. Attached to some of these fibers are special nerve endings (nociceptors) that can sense an unpleasant stimulus, such as a cut, burn, or painful pressure.

Millions of nociceptors reside in the skin, bones, joints, and muscles and in the protective membranes around the internal organs. Nociceptors are concentrated in areas more prone to injury, such as the fingers and toes. As many as 1300 nociceptors may be present in just 1 square inch of skin. Skin stimulation during massage that is intense enough to stimulate the "good hurt" response causes the nociceptors to fire. This is one of the mechanisms of **counterirritation.** This is also a major component of massage benefits for pain management.

Muscles, protected beneath the skin, have fewer nerve endings. Internal organs—protected by skin, muscle, and bone—have even fewer. Some nociceptors sense sharp blows; others sense heat. One type senses pressure, temperature, and chemical changes. Nociceptors also can detect inflammation caused by injury, disease, or infection.

Massage that addresses these receptors must have enough depth of pressure to elicit a neuroresponse.

When nociceptors detect a harmful stimulus, they relay their pain messages in the form of electric impulses along a peripheral nerve to the spinal cord and brain. The speed with which the messages travel can vary as described in Unit Two. Sensations of severe pain are transmitted almost instantaneously. Dull, aching pain—such as an upset stomach, earache, or aching joint—is relayed on fibers that transmit at a slower speed.

When pain messages reach the spinal cord, they meet up with specialized nerve cells that act as gatekeepers, which filter the pain messages on their way to the interpretive areas of the brain where the pain is felt and understood and coping strategies are developed.

For severe pain that is linked to bodily harm, the "gate" is wide open and the messages take an express route to the brain. Nerve cells in the spinal cord also respond to these urgent warnings by triggering other parts of the nervous system into action, especially the motor nerves to signal muscles to move away from harm, a process described as a reflex arc. Weak pain messages, however, such as from a scratch, may be filtered or blocked out by the gate. Often athletes do not realize they have these minor injuries, and the massage therapist is the first to notice them. Athletes can be unaware of even major injury in the excitement of the competition.

SPINAL CORD

Within the spinal cord, the messages also can change. Other sensations may overpower and diminish the pain signals. This is called counterirritation or **hyperstimulation analgesia.** Again, massage is an effective intervention to create counterirritation or hyperstimulation analgesia to suppress pain sensation (Figure 17–1).

Nerve cells in the spinal cord also release chemicals such as endorphins or **substance P** that amplify or diminish the strength of a pain sig-nal that reaches the brain for interpretation. Massage can influence these chemical responses, although research has not yet identified the exact mechanism.

BRAIN

When pain messages reach the brain, they are processed first by the thalamus, which is a sorting and switching station. The thalamus quickly interprets the messages as pain and forwards them simultaneously to three specialized regions of the brain: the physical sensation region (somatosensory cortex), the emotional feeling region (limbic system), and the thinking (cognitive) region (frontal cortex). Awareness of pain is therefore a complex

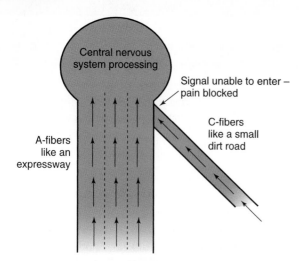

Touch, pressure, movement or moderate acute pain purposefully applied = counterirritation which may provide hyperstimulation analgesia.

FIGURE 17—1 ■ Gate-control theory of pain (based on Melzack and Wall's gate-control theory of pain). (From Fritz S: *Mosby's essential sciences for therapeutic massage: anatomy, physiology, biomechanics, and pathology,* ed 2, St Louis, 2004, Mosby.)

experience of sensing, feeling, and thinking. Pain tolerance comes from the interplay of these functions. Athletes *must* have a high pain tolerance to sustain performance and the length of the career. Massage can influence all these areas: that is, somatic sensation through nerve stimulation, limbic system by calming sympathetic dominance and nurturing, and the cognitive areas through education, thus reframing and providing symptom relief.

The brain responds to pain by sending messages that trigger the healing process. Signals are sent to the autonomic nervous system, which then sends additional blood and nutrients to the injury site. Pain-suppressing chemicals sends stop-pain messages to the injury site. The use of pain-suppressing medication that mimics the chemicals of the body is controversial and may even slow healing. However, the stress of severe **acute pain** can slow the healing process, and intractable **chronic pain** suppresses the immune system. In these cases, pain medication is appropriate.

PAIN SENSATION

Pain comes in many forms of physical sensations: stiff, achy, tight, stuck, heavy, sharp stabbing, tearing, tingling, numbing, picky, throbbing, hot, gripping, cramping.

These pain sensations were described in the assessment section of Unit Two. Pain also varies

from mild to severe. Severe pain grabs your attention more quickly and generally produces a greater physical and emotional response than mild pain. Severe pain can be incapacitating, making it difficult or impossible to function.

The location of pain can affect the response to it. A headache that interferes with the ability to focus or work may be more bothersome than, for example, arthritic pain in the ankle. Therefore the headache would receive a stronger pain response.

The emotional and psychological state, memories of past pain experiences, upbringing, and attitude also affect how persons interpret pain messages and tolerate pain.

The emotional state also can work by improving the tolerance to severe pain. Athletes condition themselves to endure pain that would incapacitate others. However, simple insignificant pain areas, especially if involved in performance, also can bother athletes more than seems reasonable. Athletes may not realize the difference between the good and bad hurt during massage, making them vulnerable to tissue damage and injury from too intense a massage application. Also, the athlete's misconception of "no pain, no gain" interferes with appropriate pain response.

IN MY EXPERIENCE...

It is amazing to me how contact sport athletes can run and bang into each other and hardly notice it. Then during their massage appointment, their first response is, "Don't hurt me." I also wonder about the athlete who has a big gash in the calf, a huge bruise on the thigh, and a grade one shoulder separation but complains about that "stuck fat sensation" in the elbow. The more elite athletes seem to be more sensitive to smaller irritations and somehow ignore the pain from major trauma. I believe therapeutic massage that targets the seemingly "small stuff" that other health care professionals might disregard is one of the greatest benefits massage therapists offer to clients.

DIFFERENCES IN ACUTE AND CHRONIC PAIN

Acute pain is triggered by tissue damage. Acute pain is the type of pain that generally accompanies illness, injury, or surgery and is location specific. Acute pain may be mild and last just a moment, such as from an insect sting, or it can be severe and last for weeks or months, such as from a burn, pulled muscle, or broken bone.

In a fairly predictable period and with treatment of the underlying cause, acute pain generally fades away. Massage targets acute pain with symptom management and healing support. Such pain is fairly easy to treat.

Chronic pain is different. It lingers after the injury is healed. The pain may remain constant, or it can come and go. The original injury shows every indication of being healed, yet the pain remains—and may be even more intense.

Chronic pain also can occur without any indication of injury. The cause of chronic pain is not well understood, and there may be no evidence of disease or damage to the body tissues that doctors can link directly to the pain. This is extremely frustrating for the medical team and client. Massage is one of the more effective interventions for managing chronic pain.

MASSAGE AND PAIN MANAGEMENT

Various mechanisms influencing pain are affected during massage. The neurotransmitters that perpetuate and inhibit the pain response are affected by massage application. The neurochemical most recognized by athletes is **endorphin.** Endorphins are part of a group of peptides that act as the internal pain modulator of the body, like morphine. Endorphins have become recognized as part of the "runner's high" phenomenon. Actually, a combination of neurotransmitters and hormones works together to alter pain perception, inhibiting it and/or enhancing it. Massage seems to alter the chemical interaction. The pain-inhibiting chemicals influenced by massage are from the entire endorphin class, as well as **serotonin,** gamma-aminobutyric acid **(GABA),** and **dopamine.** The pain-facilitating chemicals influenced by massage are **adrenaline, noradrenaline, cortisol,** and substance P. The research is still scant on just how this all works, but what we understand is sufficient for strategic development and justification of massage for pain modulation.

Massage also influences the nervous system, central and peripheral (somatic and autonomic). Application of massage that results in counterirritation and hyperstimulation analgesia functions by activating the gate control for transmission of pain signals (Figure 17–1).

Reducing mechanical pressure on peripheral somatic nerves by increasing pliability in the tissues modulates pain sensation. Massage can reduce stimulation of nociceptors in tissues. Massage can inhibit the proprioceptors. When this occurs, joint function and the muscle length/tension relationship normalizes, decreasing pain. Supporting parasympathetic dominance increases pain tolerance.

Reducing hydrostatic pressure of edema using lymphatic drain application reduces excessive accumulation of interstitial fluid and decreases pressure on pain receptors. Similar results occur when tissue density is reduced, using connective tissue methods to increase ground substance pliability or to reduce adhesion from random connective tissue fiber distribution.

Pain also can occur if circulation is not appropriate. Ischemic tissues are sensitized to pain. Massage exerts a powerful influence on blood movement. Arterial and venous circulation is involved, and massage can target normalization.

Massage also has a compassionate and comforting quality that can increase pain tolerance.

PAIN MANAGEMENT MASSAGE STRATEGIES

Massage application targeted to pain management incorporates the following principles:

1. General full-body application is given with a rhythmic and slow approach as often as feasible with 45- to 60-minute durations. Goal: Parasympathetic dominance with reduced cortisol.

2. Pressure depth is moderate to deep with compressive, broad-based application. No poking, frictioning, or pain-causing methods are used. Goal: Support serotonin and GABA, and reduce substance P and adrenaline.

3. Drag is slight unless connective tissue is being targeted. Drag is targeted to lymphatic drain and skin stimulation. Goal: Reduce swelling and create counterirritation through skin stimulation.

4. Nodal points on the body that have a high neurovascular component are massaged with a sufficient depth of pressure to create a "good hurt" sensation but not defensive guarding or withdrawal. These nodal points are the location of cutaneous nerves, trigger points, acupuncture points, and reflexology points. The feet, hands, and head, as well as along the spine, are excellent target locations. Goal: Gate control response, endorphin and other pain-inhibiting chemical release.

5. Direction of massage varies but deliberately targets fluid movement. Goal: Circulation

6. Mechanical forces of shear, bend, torsion, and others are introduced with an agitation quality to "stir" the ground substance and not create inflammation. Goal: Increased tissue pliability and reduced tissue density.

7. Mechanical force application of shear, bend, and torsion is used to address adhesion or fibrosis but needs to be targeted specifically and to be limited in duration. Goal: Reduce localized nerve irritation or circulation reduction.

8. Muscle energy methods and lengthening are applied rhythmically and gently and are targeted to shortened muscles. Goal: Reduce nerve and proprioceptive irritation and circulation inhibition.

9. Stretching to introduce tension force is applied slowly, without pain, and targeted to shortened connective tissue. Goal: Reduce nerve and proprioceptive irritation.

10. Massage therapists are focused, attentive, and compassionate but maintain appropriate boundaries. Goal: Support entrainment, bioenergy normalization, and palliative care.

Additional methods that modulate pain sensation and perception that can be incorporated into the massage are simple applications of hot and cold hydrotherapy, analgesic essential oils, calming and distracting music, and (maybe) north side magnet application. These methods were discussed in Unit Two.

SUMMARY

Massage is effective at managing acute and chronic pain and supports other pain treatments such as medication, ultrasound, and hydrotherapy. The massage therapist needs to really understand the concept of management. A common error is to think of massage targeting pain reduction as therapeutic change. Massage to manage pain is palliative. Massage that is too aggressive, causes inflammation, and creates excessive pain during application that persists beyond the actual massage is incorrect.

Massage therapists need to learn to back off. Massage targeting pain management as presented in this chapter is an appropriate strategy.

1 List the physiologic mechanisms that currently are considered influenced by massage application.

_____
_____
_____
_____
_____

2 Describe the difference between massage treatment for the following:

Acute pain _____.

Chronic pain _____.

3 Justify the benefits of using massage as an active part of a comprehensive pain management program.

_____
_____
_____
_____
_____
_____
_____
_____
_____

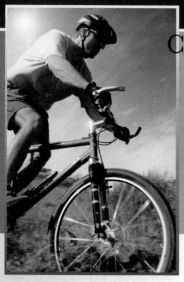

OBJECTIVES

Upon completion of this chapter, the reader will have the information necessary to do the following:

1 Describe and apply appropriate massage for the following common syndromes and injury categories:

  a. Overtraining syndrome

  b. Muscle soreness and stiffness

  c. Muscle cramp, spasm, and guarding

  d. Contusions

  e. Wounds

  f. Strains

  g. Sprains

  h. Chronic muscle injury

  i. Degenerative joint disease

  j. Dislocation

  k. Bone injury

  l. Nerve injury

This chapter categorizes similar injuries into general treatment protocols. What changes are the targeted locations. For example, a sprained knee or wrist is similar, and only the anatomy is different. A wound on the leg or the foot is still a wound. Specific treatment strategies are provided for these general categories, which then are applied to specific injuries by region in Chapter 21. The student will need an orthopedic injury text for further research.

Acute bone fractures
Arthrosis
Articular crepitus
Atrophy
Bone injuries
Bursitis
Capsulitis
Chronic joint injuries
Compression
Contracture

Degenerative joint disease
Diastasis
Disk herniation
Dislocation
Entrapment
Epiphyseal conditions
Luxation
Nerve impingement
Nerve injuries
Nerve root compression

Osteochondrosis
Periostitis
Stress fractures
Subluxation
Synovitis
Tendonitis
Tendonosis
Traumatic osteoarthritis

OVERTRAINING SYNDROME

A problem in physical conditioning and training is overexertion. A gradual pattern of overloading the body is necessary for training effects; however, many athletes and training personnel still believe that if there is no pain, there is no gain. Overtraining occurs when athletes work too hard to improve performance and train beyond the ability of the body to recover.

Overtraining is reflected in muscle soreness, decreased joint flexibility, and general fatigue 24 hours after activity. Four specific indicators of possible overexertion are acute muscle soreness, delayed-onset muscle soreness, muscle stiffness, and muscle cramping and spasms.

The common warning signs of overtraining include the following:

- Mild leg soreness, general aching
- Pain in muscles and joints
- Washed-out feeling, tired, drained, lack of energy
- Sudden drop in ability to run "normal" distance or times
- Insomnia
- Headaches
- Inability to relax, fidgety
- Insatiable thirst, dehydration
- Lowered resistance to common illnesses such as colds and sore throat

The massage professional needs to be aware of these warning signs. Proper diagnosis by the physician rules out potentially serious problems. Interventions include rest, drinking plenty of fluids, alteration of diet if needed, and general nonspecific massage that is even less targeted and intense than the pain management protocol in the previous chapter. Massage supports parasympathetic dominance, pain management, fluid movement, and sleep. Do not overmassage someone with overtraining syndrome. Adaptive capacity already is strained, and massaging too much (for example, too aggressively or by pursuing too many outcomes in a single session) can add strain to the client's adaptive ability.

MUSCLE SORENESS AND STIFFNESS

Overexertion during strenuous muscular exercise often results in muscular soreness. Most persons, at one time or another, have experienced muscle soreness, usually resulting from some physical activity to which they are unaccustomed. The older a person gets, the more easily muscle soreness seems to develop.

ACUTE-ONSET MUSCLE SORENESS

Acute-onset muscle soreness accompanies fatigue. This muscle pain is transient and occurs during and immediately after exercise. The pain is caused by lack of oxygen to the muscles and buildup of metabolic waste from anaerobic functions. The pain dissipates as oxygen is restored and metabolic wastes produced are removed from muscle tissue and are eliminated or converted. Massage is not especially effective in treating acute-onset muscle soreness. If massage is used immediately after exercise, the focus is arterial and venous circulation. Do not attempt to stretch or aggressively treat. Cramping usually will occur.

DELAYED-ONSET MUSCLE SORENESS

Delayed-onset muscle soreness becomes most intense after 24 to 48 hours and then gradually subsides so that the muscle becomes symptom free after 3 or 4 days. Delayed-onset muscle soreness leads to increased muscle tension, swelling, stiffness, and resistance to stretching. Delayed-onset muscle soreness is thought to result from several possible causes. It may occur from small tears (microtrauma) in the muscle tissue, which results in an inflammatory process and seems to be more likely with eccentric or isometric actions. Soreness also may occur because of disruptions of the connective tissue that holds muscle tendon fibers together. Another contribution to delayed-onset muscle soreness is increased interstitial fluid resulting in hydrostatic pressure on pain-sensitive structures.

Muscle soreness can be produced by many types of muscular activities. A major impairment of physical activity is postexercise soreness from movements that produce tension as the involved muscles are forced to lengthen. The muscle actions needed for these movements are known as "eccentric" or "negative" actions. These types of movement activities include movements that resist gravity or forward momentum, such as downhill running, lowering heavy barbells, and the downward phase of push-ups or sit-ups; movements that resist forces exerted by stronger opponents, such as a pin or a hold in wrestling and a block in football, are also eccentric actions.

Popular explanations for muscle soreness include lactic acid accumulation, muscle spasms, or muscle damage. Lactic acid and muscle spasms have been largely discredited as reasons, but the muscle damage explanation has a sound scientific basis.

Movements that cause muscle soreness have been shown to produce localized damage to the muscle fiber membranes and contractile elements. Chemical irritants such as histamine are released from damaged muscles and can irritate pain receptors in the muscle.

Muscle damage often causes swelling of the muscle tissue, which creates enough fluid pressure to stimulate pain receptors. Swelling has been shown to persist long after the muscle soreness has disappeared. The pain receptors gradually adapt to the swelling or to some other factors present that reduce pain perception. Because no effective treatment for muscle soreness has been identified, training programs should be designed to minimize or prevent soreness.

Typical recommendations for treatment of delayed-onset muscle soreness include gentle stretching, topical application of analgesic creams and/or ice, submersion in hot baths, hot and cold contrast exposure, Epsom salt soaks, and sauna. Each of these treatments may provide temporary relief, but none is effective for long. The use of aspirin or other antiinflammatory drugs may provide some relief, but scientific studies show that this treatment is controversial. Several studies have found that taking aspirin after exercise reduces muscle soreness and improves the athlete's range of motion a day or 2 days later, whereas others believe the side effects outweigh the benefit. Delayed-onset muscle soreness is common and annoying but not serious. The athlete can do many things to prevent, avoid, and shorten delayed-onset muscle soreness:

- Warm up thoroughly before activity and cool down completely afterward.
- Use easy stretching after exercise.
- Start an exercise program with easy to moderate activity and build up intensity over time.
- Avoid making sudden major changes in the type of exercise.
- Avoid making sudden major changes in the amount of time exercising.

Soreness will go away in 3 to 7 days with no special treatment, and the athlete should avoid any vigorous activity that increases pain. The individual should allow the soreness to subside thoroughly before performing any vigorous exercise. Easy, low-impact aerobic exercise will increase blood flow to the affected muscles, which may help diminish soreness.

Treatment of delayed-onset muscle soreness usually involves general massage with a lymphatic drainage focus. Muscle soreness can be treated with ice applied within the first 48 to 72 hours.

Gentle stretching of the affected area with gentle massage helps. Do not overmassage, work aggressively, or use any methods that would increase swelling or cause tissue damage.

Almost all professional teams use various ointments and liniments on sore athletes, but sports doctors do not fully understand how liniments work. The massaging action of rubbing in the liniment and working it into muscles may be what actually relaxes the muscle and may be part of the mechanism of action.

There are two basic types of ointments/liniments. The first typically contains menthol and an aspirin-like chemical, methyl salicylate. When the liniment is massaged on the skin, the skin becomes slightly irritated, which causes an increase in blood flow to the area. This also produces heat, which relaxes stiff muscles. Some salicylate may enter the bloodstream. Because salicylate is the active ingredient in aspirin, it also may have some pain-relieving effect. A counterirritant action occurs as well.

The second type of ointment depends on a substance called capsicum, which is the active ingredient in jalapeño and other hot peppers. An extract of this chemical now is being used as a prescription ointment for arthritis pain, which is an indication that these ointments really do work. These hotter ointments have a much stronger irritating effect on the skin to stimulate blood flow and give off so much heat that they can cause a burn, so caution is required. Do not allow these preparations to come into contact with any mucous membranes or the eyes.

Make sure the client has no skin sensitivity to an ointment that will cause an allergic reaction.

MUSCLE STIFFNESS

Muscle stiffness does not produce pain. Stiffness occurs when a group of muscles have been worked hard for a long period of time. The fluids that collect in the muscles during and after exercise are absorbed into the bloodstream at a slow rate. As a result, the muscle becomes swollen, shorter, and thicker and therefore resists stretching. Light exercise, lymphatic drainage type of massage, and passive mobilization assist in reducing stiffness. Stiffness also results with decreased pliability of connective tissue. This occurs as the ground substance thickens as part of an enzyme process during sympathetic dominance.

Massage is effective for muscle stiffness, particularly in the management of the fluid retention. See the discussion on lymphatic drainage in Unit Two. All pain management approaches are appropriate. Massage to restore connective tissue pliability and hydration helps reduce the stiffness. These conditions are not an increase in muscle tone but rather an issue of fluid dynamics. Do not use aggressive massage.

MUSCLE CRAMPS AND SPASM

Muscle cramps and spasms can lead to muscle and tendon injuries. A cramp is a painful involuntary contraction of a skeletal muscle or muscle group.

Cramps often occur because of a lack of water or other electrolytes, from muscle fatigue, and from an interruption of appropriate neurologic interaction between opposing muscles. A spasm is a reflex reaction caused by trauma of the musculoskeletal system.

The two types of cramps or spasms are the clonic type, with alternating involuntary muscular contraction and relaxation in quick succession, and the tonic type, with rigid muscle contraction that lasts a period of time. The massage therapist applies compression firmly in the belly of the cramping muscle and gently massages, moves, and stretches the surrounding joint areas. If cramps recur, send the client for hydration and electrolytes. Cramps and spasm respond to proper hydration and rest.

MUSCLE GUARDING

Following injury, the muscles that surround the injured area contract in effect to splint that area, thus minimizing pain by limiting movement. Often this splinting is referred to incorrectly as a muscle spasm. *Muscle guarding* is a more appropriate term for the involuntary muscle contractions that occur in response to pain following musculoskeletal injury. Muscle guarding is appropriate during the acute and subacute healing process. Massage application *should not* attempt to reduce muscle guarding until the later stages of the subacute phase. Use gentle massage to reduce pain sensation.

CONTUSIONS

A bruise, or contusion, occurs because of a sudden traumatic blow to the body. The severity of a contusion can range from superficial and minor to extremely serious with deep tissue compression and hemorrhage.

The extent to which an athlete may be hampered by this condition depends on the location of the bruise and the force of the blow. This type of injury is common in contact sports. An impact to the muscles can cause more damage than might be expected and should be treated appropriately. The muscle is crushed against the bone, and if the injury is not treated correctly or if it is treated too aggressively, then myositis ossificans may result. The speed of healing of a contusion, as with all soft tissue injuries, depends on the extent of tissue damage and internal bleeding.

The three types of contusions are intramuscular, intermuscular, and bone bruise.

Intramuscular contusions are a tearing of the muscle within the sheath that surrounds it. This means that the initial bleeding may stop early (within hours) because of increased pressure within the muscle; however, the fluid is unable to escape because the muscle sheath prevents it. The result is a considerable loss of function and pain, which can take days or weeks to recover. The typical bruise discoloration may not appear with this contusion type—especially in the early stages. Because a bruise is not seen, the severity of the injury may not be recognized. The typical bruise may appear finally in the subacute phase and indicates progressive healing.

Intermuscular contusions are tearing of the muscle and part of the sheath surrounding it. The initial bleeding will take longer to stop. Recovery is often faster than intramuscular contusions because the blood and fluids can flow away from the site of injury through tears of the muscle sheath. Bruising discoloration occurs with this type of contusion.

A bone contusion can penetrate to the skeletal structures, causing a bone bruise. Bone bruises are painful and require a fairly extensive healing time.

Symptoms of contusions are the following:
- Pain
- Swelling
- Discoloration
- Restricted movement

If after 2 to 3 days the swelling has not gone, then it is likely to be an intramuscular injury. If the bleeding has spread and has caused bruising away from the site of the injury, then the injury is likely to be intermuscular.

Contusions are grade 1, 2 or 3 depending on the severity (Box 18-1).

Caution is necessary when providing massage over contusions. Compressive force and depth of pressure need to be modified to prevent further injury. Lymphatic drainage types of applications are usually appropriate. Once the bruising dissipates, in all three grades of contusion, kneading is used to prevent fibrosis. Over the next 3 to 6 months, continue to apply the bending and torsion forces of kneading to support the remodeling stage of healing.

WOUNDS

The first concern with any wound is to control bleeding. Concerning first aid, this usually means use of a pressure bandage. The next concern is to prevent wound contamination by cleaning the wound and applying a sterile bandage and possibly

Box 18-1   CONTUSION GRADES

Grade 1
Tightness
Minor swelling
Nearly a full range of motion
  Treatment includes PRICE and lymphatic drainage massage with skin drag methods only.

Grade 2
Painful movement
Swelling
Compression causes pain
Limited range of movement
  Treatment consists of ultrasound and electric stimulation, lymphatic drainage massage application using skin drag methods only, and a rehabilitation program consisting of stretching, strengthening, and a gradual return to full function.

Grade 3
Severe pain
Immediate swelling
Isometric contraction will be painful and might produce a bulge in the muscle.

Treatment
  PRICE: Seek medical attention immediately.
  Use ultrasound and electric stimulation.
  Peform lymphatic drainage massage using skin drag methods only. Wait at least 48 hours before applying massage.
  Operate if needed to relieve pressure.

an antibiotic ointment. Lastly, immobilization of the injured part, along with medical intervention, is needed. Many wounds will need to be sutured or stitched.

The purpose of suturing is to pull the tissue together just enough so that there will be no dead spaces below the skin where blood and fluid can accumulate. If there is space, it eventually will be a breeding ground for an infection. Wounds heal better when the edges are close together.

Generally speaking, the deeper the wound, the more serious the consequences. With minor wounds, the outer layer of skin, the epidermis, is scraped away or opened up to permit bacteria and materials to enter. In a more severe wound, the next layer downward, the dermis, is injured. This contains connective tissue, sweat glands, hair follicles, nerves, and lymph and blood vessels, and the potential for infection to spread increases.

Box 18-2   TYPES OF WOUNDS

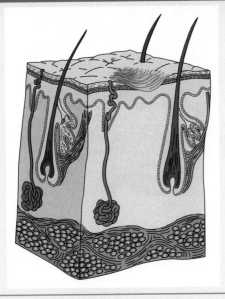

Abrasion. (From Young AP, Kennedy DB: *Kinn's the medical assistant: an applied learning approach*, St Louis, 2003, Saunders.)

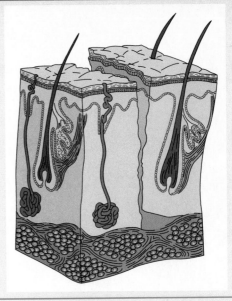

Laceration. (From Young AP, Kennedy DB: *Kinn's the medical assistant: an applied learning approach*, St Louis, 2003, Saunders.)

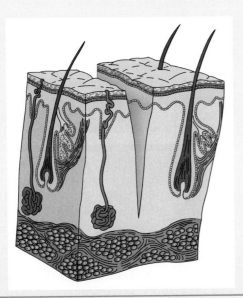

Incision. (From Young AP, Kennedy DB: *Kinn's the medical assistant: an applied learning approach*, St Louis, 2003, Saunders.)

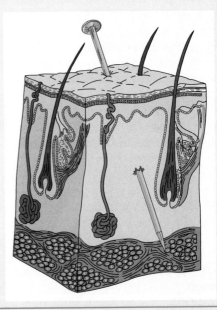

Puncture. (From Young AP, Kennedy DB: *Kinn's the medical assistant: an applied learning approach*, St Louis, 2003, Saunders.)

Continued

Box 18-2   TYPES OF WOUNDS—Cont'd

Avulsion. (From Young AP, Kennedy DB: *Kinn's the medical assistant: an applied learning approach,* St Louis, 2003, Saunders.)

Wounds can be classified as follows (Box 18-2):
- *Abrasion.* In this wound the outer surface of skin has been scraped away. Usually some minor oozing of blood and serum occurs.

Depending on how the injury was obtained, dirt or foreign matter usually is ground into it. To treat an abrasion such as a scraped knee, the wound first must be cleaned to remove dirt that will cause an infection and therefore impair healing.

Once cleaned, the wound should be blotted dry with a sterile gauze, and pressure should be applied over the injured site for a few minutes for the purpose of controlling bleeding. The application of a first aid or antibiotic cream to the abrasion could help to prevent infection and keep the bandage from sticking to the raw wound. For the best protection, the bandage should cover an inch beyond the wound. An ice pack over the final bandage can serve to reduce swelling and ease some of the discomfort.
- *Incision.* This wound type is made from a sharp, knifelike object that leaves a cut with smooth edges. Incisions are often part of surgical care procedures.
- *Laceration.* This wound type is similar to an incision but with jagged edges caused by a tear. Because incisions and lacerations go beyond the outer layer of skin and into the deeper layers that contain blood vessels, there is a lot of bleeding. If the wound is deep enough to cut an artery,

blood will squirt out with each heartbeat because of the high pressure in these vessels. Care involves applying pressure dressing and getting the victim to medical care where sutures usually are needed to close the wound fully or partially.
- *Puncture.* As its name implies, a puncture occurs when a foreign object is pushed into the skin. The wound can be superficial or deep. Minimal bleeding is evident externally, but there could be internal bleeding. A deep puncture wound requires medical care, and a tetanus injection may be required. Some arthroscopic surgical procedures produce wounds that are more like punctures than incisions.
- *Avulsion.* In this injury the skin is pulled or torn off. The severed tissue should be saved and taken to the hospital. A pressure dressing is applied over the wound until medical care is received. Once a dressing is applied, leave it alone and do not take it off to check the wound.

18-1 THERAPEUTIC MASSAGE APPLICATION FOR WOUNDS

Follow these guidelines for therapeutic massage for wounds (Figure 18-1):

Massage Applied Days 1 to 3
Sanitation and infection prevention are essential.

Avoid the area during massage to protect the wound from contamination.

FIGURE 18-1

THERAPEUTIC MASSAGE APPLICATION FOR WOUNDS

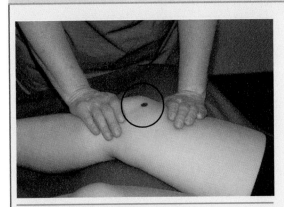

A Wound, acute (1 to 3 days).

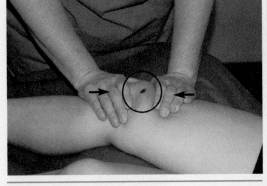

B Wound, subacute early (3 to 5 days).

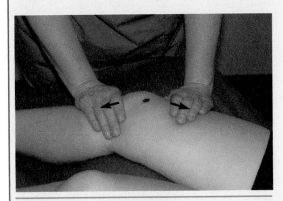

C Wound, subacute early (5 to 7 days).

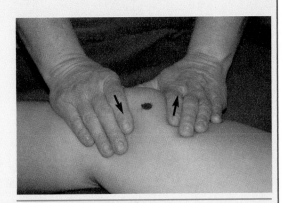

D Wound, subacute middle (7 to 10 days).

Continued

Lymphatic drainage can be used above and below the wound. Do not perform drainage if any signs of infection are present: heat, swelling, red color (especially any type of red streaking), pus, or sour smell.

Day 3

Use bend, shear, and tension forces around the wound far enough away to prevent any chance of contamination. The goal is to drag the skin gently in multiple directions to prevent adhesions from forming. The connective tissue formation is random at this time. Do not disturb the wound edges.

Increase the intensity and depth of the forces in the area that has been treated and move closer to the wound. Decrease intensity and gently apply bend, shear, and stretch (tension) force to the tissue. Do not disturb the wound edges.

Day 7

Again increase the intensity in the previously treated areas and then move closer to the wound. At this point the wound should be moving a bit from the forces loading the adjacent tissue, but the wound edges must not be disturbed. Progressively increase intensity daily by moving closer and closer to the wound.

As soon as the wound is healed completely (14 days is typical, but it can take longer), begin to bend and shear the scar tissue and stretch it with tension.

The wound must be healed completely before working directly on it. Before working on the scar,

FIGURE 18-1 CONT'D

THERAPEUTIC MASSAGE APPLICATION FOR WOUNDS

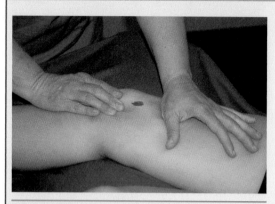

E Wound, subacute end (10 to 14 days).

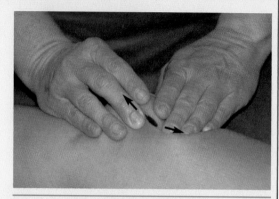

F Wound, remodeling (14 days up to 6 months).

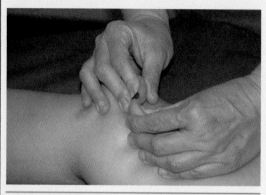

G Wound, remodeling (14 days up to 6 months).

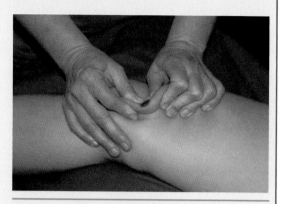

H Wound remodeling (14 days up to 6 months)

address the tissue surrounding the wound. Address this tissue after the acute phase has passed. Usually this happens after 2 to 3 days. Maintain ongoing attention to the scar for at least 6 months. These methods can be taught to the client or family member.

OLD SCARS

Old scars that are adhered to underlying tissue can be softened and stretched. All mechanical forces are used in multiple directions on the scar each session until the scar tissue and tissue at least 1 inch away from the scar become warm and slightly red. The intensity should be enough so that the client experiences a burning stretching sensation (Figure 18-2). A small degree of inflammation is desired and the area may be a bit tender to the touch after the massage but not painful to movement. Ideally, treatment would

occur every other day, allowing the tissue to recover in the alternate days. These methods can be taught to the client or family member.

STRAINS

Note: Specific massage treatment protocol for strain and sprains is on p. 458.

A strain is a stretch, tear, or rip in the muscle or adjacent tissue such as the fascia or muscle tendons (Figure 18-3). Strains also are called pulls and tears. The cause of muscle strain is often not clear. Often a strain is produced by an abnormal muscular contraction during reciprocal coordination of the agonist and antagonist muscles. This type of injury often occurs when muscles suddenly and powerfully contract. Possible explanations for the muscle

FIGURE 18-2

OLD SCARS

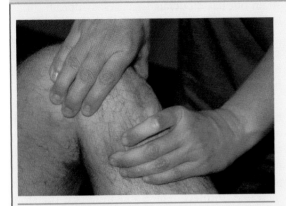

A Old scar—tension force.

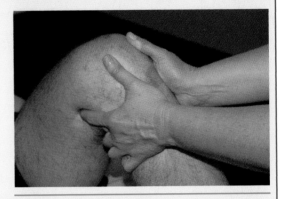

B Old scar—tension force.

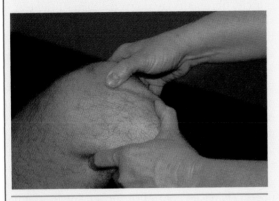

C Old scar—shear force.

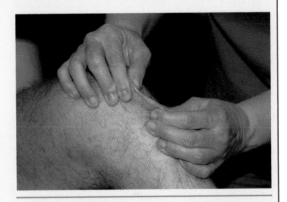

D Old scar—shear force.

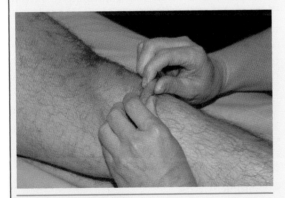

E Old scar—bending force.

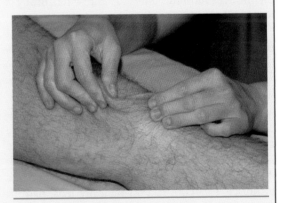

F Old scar—torsion force.

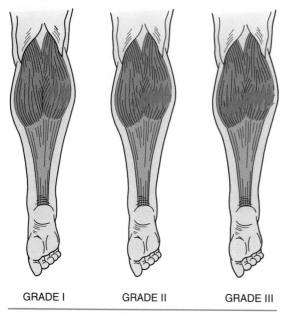

GRADE I   GRADE II   GRADE III

FIGURE 18-3 ■ Calf pull with degrees of severity. (From Salvo SG, Anderson SK: *Mosby's pathology for massage therapists*, St Louis, 2004, Mosby.)

imbalance may be related to a mineral imbalance caused by profuse sweating, fatigue, metabolites collected in the muscle itself, or a strength imbalance between agonist and antagonist muscles. A muscle may become strained or pulled—or may even tear—when it stretches unusually far or abruptly. A muscle strain may occur while slipping on the ice, running, jumping, throwing, lifting a heavy object, or lifting in an awkward position.

A strain may range from a tiny separation of connective tissue and muscle fibers to a complete tendinous avulsion (breaking away from the bone) or muscle rupture. The resulting pathologic condition is similar to that of the contusion or sprain, with capillary or blood vessel hemorrhage. Typically, persons with a strain experience pain, muscle guarding, and muscle weakness. They also can have localized swelling, cramping, or inflammation and, with a minor or moderate strain, usually some loss of muscle function. Clients typically have pain in the injured area and general weakness of the muscle when they attempt to move it. Severe strains that partially or completely tear the muscle or tendon are usually very painful and disabling.

GRADES OF MUSCLE STRAIN

A grade 1 (mild) strain is accompanied by local pain, which is increased by tension of the muscle, and minor loss of strength. Mild swelling and local tenderness occur.

A grade 2 (moderate) strain is similar to the mild strain but has moderate signs and symptoms, mild bruising, and impaired muscle function.

A grade 3 (severe) strain has signs and symptoms that are severe, with a loss of muscle function and bruising, and commonly a palpable defect (small hole) in the muscle.

Injuries usually occur at the junction where the muscle and tendon meet, called the musculotendinous junction, or where the tendon attaches to the periosteum of the bone, called the tenoperiosteal junction. Junction sites of ligament, tendon, and joint capsules are relatively vascular and have an increased stiffness. These junctions are therefore more prone to injury.

After a tear of the connective tissue of the muscle, fibroblasts lay down collagen. If the tear is significant, adhesions often form in the connective tissue layers. Because of the development of abnormal cross-links in the collagen and adhesions within the fascia of the muscle during healing, a muscle that has had a strain injury typically shortens and loses some of its extensibility. After a tear of the muscle fiber, satellite cells help myoblasts develop into muscle fibers. The regeneration is usually complete in 3 weeks. Immobilization causes decreased cellular activity, decreased collagen formation in the fascia, and loss of muscle fibers. Therefore controlled movement is essential for optimal healing.

Muscle dysfunctions that contribute to susceptibility to muscle strain include sustained hypertonicity, sustained inhibition, abnormal position, or abnormal torsion in the soft tissue. These contractions are caused by the following:

- Poor posture
- Static stress (nonproductive isometric contraction)
- Muscle injury
- Joint dysfunction
- Emotional or psychological stress: anxiety and anger
- Chronic overuse
- Disuse-deconditioned syndrome

Massage addresses muscle dysfunction by reversing the inappropriate soft tissue adaptation in response to these conditions.

The muscles that have the highest incidence of strains in sports are the hamstring group, sacrospinalis group of the back, deltoid, and rotator cuff group of the shoulder. Contact sports such as soccer, football, hockey, boxing, and wrestling put athletes at risk for strains. Gymnastics, tennis, rowing, golf, and other sports that require extensive gripping can increase the risk of hand and forearm muscle strains. Elbow muscle strains sometimes occur in persons who participate in racquet sports, throwing, and contact sports.

Muscle strain usually causes a protective muscle guarding response. The guarding should not be reduced by massage because it protects the area from further injury.

Massage needs to target the following during muscle strain injury repair:
- Minimize adhesion formation.
- Promote circulation.
- Increase lubrication of the tissues.
- Promote proper alignment of collagen fibers.
- Support movement to stimulate replacement of connective tissue and regeneration of the muscle fibers.

TREATMENT FOR STRAINS

18-1 Treatment for strains has two stages (see also p. 458). The goal during the first stage is to reduce swelling and pain. Use PRICE–protection, rest, ice, compression, and elevation–for the first 24 to 48 hours after the injury. Severe strains may require surgery to repair the torn muscle or tendons. Surgery usually is performed by an orthopedic surgeon. The doctor also may recommend an over-the-counter or prescription nonsteroidal anti-inflammatory drug, such as aspirin or ibuprofen, to help decrease pain and inflammation, but this can slow healing, so use should be questioned. Gentle massage around the area encourages circulation, and lymphatic drainage manages swelling and supports healing. During the acute and subacute phases, the soft tissue should be massaged in the direction of the fibers and crowded toward the site of the injury to promote reconnection of the ends of the separated fibers (Figure 18-4). Depth of pressure, duration, and intensity need to be adjusted during the various healing phases. Once the acute phase of healing is complete, the methods that support mobile scar formation can be introduced, including moving the tissue away from the injury site and massaging across the fibers.

The second stage of treating a strain is rehabilitation, with the overall goal to improve the condition of the injured part and restore its function with an exercise program designed to prevent stiffness, improve range of motion, and restore the normal flexibility and strength.

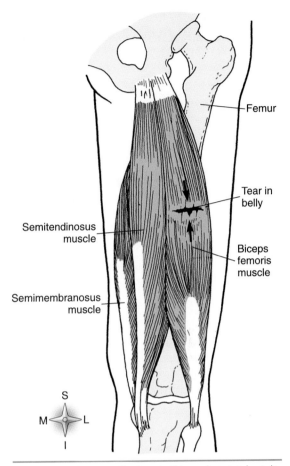

FIGURE 18-4 ■ Muscle strain. This muscle strain is located in the biceps femoris muscle of the hamstring group (in this case, a tear in the midportion of the belly of the muscle). Arrows show direction of massage stroke. (From Thibodeau GA, Patton KT: *The human body in health and disease*, ed 2, St Louis, 1997, Mosby.)

SPRAIN

Note: Specific massage treatment protocol for strain and sprain is found on p. 458 (Box 18-3).

A sprain is an injury to a ligament and/or a joint capsule, resulting in overstretching or tearing. A sprain can result from a fall, a sudden twist, or a blow to the body that forces a joint out of its normal position. Typically, sprains occur when persons fall and land on an outstretched arm, slide, land on the side of their foot, or twist a knee with the foot planted firmly on the ground. One or more ligaments can be injured during a sprain. The severity of the injury depends on the extent of injury to a single ligament (whether the tear is partial or complete) and the number of ligaments involved, and if any fractures are involved. Effusion of blood and synovial fluid into the joint

Box 18-3 EXAMPLES OF SPRAINS

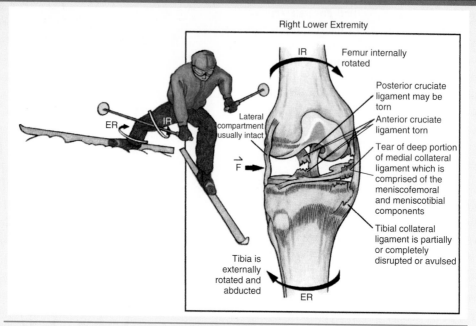

Right Lower Extremity

Femur internally rotated

Posterior cruciate ligament may be torn

Anterior cruciate ligament torn

Tear of deep portion of medial collateral ligament which is comprised of the meniscofemoral and meniscotibial components

Tibial collateral ligament is partially or completely disrupted or avulsed

Lateral compartment usually intact

Tibia is externally rotated and abducted

Anterior cruciate and medial collateral tear with tibial collateral sprain. (From Saidoff DC, McDonough AL: *Critical pathways in therapeutic intervention: extremities and spine,* St Louis, 2002, Mosby.)

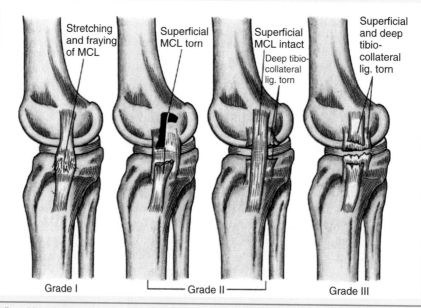

Stretching and fraying of MCL

Superficial MCL torn

Superficial MCL intact

Deep tibio-collateral lig. torn

Superficial and deep tibio-collateral lig. torn

Grade I — Grade II — Grade III

Medial collateral ligament sprains. (From Saidoff DC, McDonough AL: *Critical pathways in therapeutic intervention: extremities and spine,* St Louis, 2002, Mosby.)

Box 18-3 SPRAINS—Cont'd

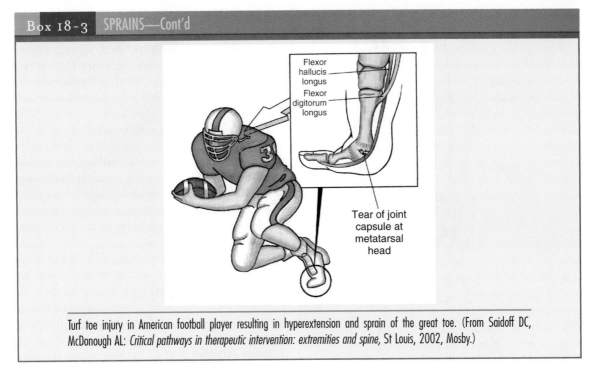

Flexor hallucis longus

Flexor digitorum longus

Tear of joint capsule at metatarsal head

Turf toe injury in American football player resulting in hyperextension and sprain of the great toe. (From Saidoff DC, McDonough AL: *Critical pathways in therapeutic intervention: extremities and spine*, St Louis, 2002, Mosby.)

cavity during a sprain produces joint swelling, local temperature increase, pain or point tenderness, and skin discoloration. Ligaments and joint capsules heal slowly because of a relatively poor blood supply. Nerves in the area often produce a great deal of pain.

Although sprains can occur in the upper and lower parts of the body, the most common site is the ankle. Ankle sprains are the most common injury in the United States and often occur during sports or recreational activities. About 1 million ankle injuries occur each year, and 85% of them are sprains.

The talus bone and the ends of two of the lower leg bones (tibia and fibula) form the ankle joint. This joint is supported by several lateral and medial ligaments. Most ankle sprains happen when the foot turns inward as a person runs, turns, falls, or lands on the ankle after a jump. This type of sprain is called an inversion injury. One or more of the lateral ligaments are injured, usually the anterior talofibular ligament. The calcaneofibular ligament is the second most frequently torn ligament. A more serious ankle sprain often is called a high ankle sprain. This happens when the ankle rolls over the foot and the membrane between the tibia and fibula is damaged (Figure 18-5).

The knee is another common site for a sprain. A blow to the knee or a fall is often the cause. Twisting also can result in a sprain.

Sprains frequently occur at the wrist, typically when persons fall and land on an outstretched hand.

The usual signs and symptoms of a sprain include pain, swelling, bruising, and loss of the ability to move and use the joint (functional ability). These signs and symptoms vary in intensity, depending on the severity of the sprain. Sometimes a person feels a pop or tear when the injury happens.

In general, a grade 1 or mild sprain causes overstretching or slight tearing of the ligaments with no joint instability. A person with a mild sprain usually experiences minimal pain, swelling, and little or no loss of functional ability. Bruising is absent or slight, and the person usually is able to put weight on the affected joint. Persons with mild sprains usually do not need an x-ray exam, but one sometimes is performed if the diagnosis is unclear.

A grade 2 or moderate sprain causes partial tearing of the ligament and is characterized by bruising, moderate pain, and swelling. A person with a moderate sprain usually has some difficulty putting weight on the affected joint and experiences some loss of function. An x-ray exam may be needed to determine whether a fracture is causing the pain and swelling. Magnetic resonance imaging is used occasionally to help differentiate between a significant partial injury and a complete tear in a ligament.

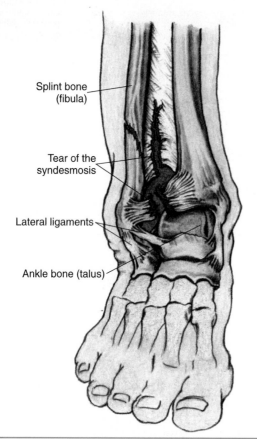

Splint bone (fibula)

Tear of the syndesmosis

Lateral ligaments

Ankle bone (talus)

FIGURE 18-5 ■ High ankle sprain. Sprain of the distal tibiofibular syndesmosis, injury to the deltoid or lateral ligaments of the ankle joint. (From Peterson L, Renstrom P: *Sports injuries: their prevention and treatment,* Chicago, 1983, Year Book Medical.)

A grade 3 or severe sprain completely ruptures ligaments. Pain, swelling, and bruising are usually severe, and the patient is unable to put weight on the joint. An x-ray film usually is taken to rule out a broken bone. The injury may be difficult to distinguish from a fracture or dislocation.

When diagnosing any sprain, the doctor will ask the person to explain how the injury happened and will examine the affected joint and check its stability and ability to move and bear weight. For persons with a severe sprain, particularly of the ankle, a hard cast may be applied.

Rehabilitation includes different types of exercises, depending on the injury. For example, persons with an ankle sprain may be told to rest their heel on the floor and write the alphabet in the air with their big toe. A person with an injured knee or foot will work on weight-bearing and balancing exercises. Rehabilitation commonly lasts for several weeks.

Another goal of rehabilitation is to increase strength and regain flexibility. Depending on the individual rate of recovery, this process begins about the second week after the injury. During this phase of rehabilitation, the client progresses to more demanding exercises as pain decreases and function improves.

The final goal is the return to full daily activities, including sports when appropriate. Sometimes persons are tempted to resume full activity or play sports despite pain or muscle soreness. Returning to full activity before regaining normal range of motion, flexibility, balance, and strength increases the chance of reinjury and may lead to a chronic problem.

The amount of rehabilitation and the time needed for full recovery after a sprain depend on the severity of the injury and individual rates of healing. For example, a moderate ankle sprain may require 3 to 6 weeks of rehabilitation before a person can return to full activity. With a severe sprain, it can take 8 to 12 months before the ligament is healed fully.

MASSAGE APPLICATION: STRAINS AND SPRAINS

The following strategies describe how to manage muscle tears and tendon strains and ligament sprains as well as incisions and skin wounds, and why they are addressed in a similar fashion.

Regardless of the soft tissue type and area of the injury, these injuries result in tissue and fiber separation. For treatment purposes, the injured area can be explained simply as a hole in the tissue created during the injury. Healing involves closing the hole and restoring function.

Appropriate massage application occurs after the medical team makes a diagnosis. These types of injuries typically are graded as first, second, and third degrees or as mild, moderate, and severe. Grade 1 (mild) is a little hole, grade 2 (moderate) is a medium-sized hole, and grade 3 (severe) is a big hole.

Other tissue injuries such as punctures, abrasions, cuts, ulcers, and surgical incisions are "holes" as well. Bone breaks can be conceptualized in the same simple manner.

The healing of these injuries follows a typical pattern in terms of acute, subacute, and remodeling phases (Table 18-1).

TABLE 18-1	STAGES OF TISSUE HEALING AND MASSAGE INTERVENTIONS		
	STAGE 1: ACUTE INFLAMMATORY REACTION	STAGE 2: SUBACUTE REPAIR AND HEALING	STAGE 3: CHRONIC MATURATION AND REMODELING
Characteristics	Vascular changes Inflammatory exudate Clot formation Phagocytosis, neutralization of irritants Early fibroblastic activity	Growth of capillary beds into area Collagen formation Granulation tissue; caution necessary Fragile, easily injured tissue	Maturation and remodeling of scar Contracture of scar tissue Collagen aligns along lines of stress forces (tensegrity)
Clinical Signs	INFLAMMATION Pain before tissue resistance	DECREASING INFLAMMATION Pain during tissue resistance	ABSENCE OF INFLAMMATION Pain after tissue resistance
Massage Intervention	PROTECTION Control and support effects of inflammation: PRICE. Promote healing and prevent compensation patterns: • Passive movement midrange • General massage and lymphatic drainage with caution Support rest with full-body massage. 3 to 7 days	CONTROLLED MOTION Promote development of mobile scar: • Cautious and controlled soft tissue mobilization of scar tissue along fiber direction toward injury • Active and passive, open- and closed-chain range or motion, midrange Support healing with full-body massage. 14 to 21 days	RETURN TO FUNCTION Increase strength and alignment of scar tissue: • Cross-fiber friction of scar tissue coupled with directional stroking along the lines of tension away from injury • Progressive stretching, and active and resisted range of motion; full range Support rehabilitation activities with full-body massage. 3 to 12 months

From Fritz S: *Mosby's fundamentals of therapeutic massage,* ed 3, St Louis, 2004, Mosby.

Massage can offer support during all stages of the healing process. Tissue healing involves two main processes: regeneration and replacement. Regeneration occurs when functional tissue cells regrow. Bone is active regenerative tissue. "Holes" in bone heal well if the ends of the broken bones are lined up and held in that position. Skin heals well, especially if deep, large wounds are sutured.

Muscle tissue does not regenerate well. However, the closer the ends of the breach in the tissue (the hole), the better potential for muscle cell regeneration to occur.

Most "holes" heal through the replacement process. The connective tissue that fills up an injury is called a scar.

The healing goal is to create an environment where the least amount of scar tissue is needed to repair the injury. Therefore strategies to make the "hole" as small as possible are appropriate. Interventions such as sutures, casts, and immobilization accomplish the goal by sewing the ends of the tissue together or positioning the injured tissues so that they approximate (touch). Little surgical "holes" are one of the major benefits of arthroscopic and laparoscopic surgical procedures and have been a major advancement in medical treatment.

Understanding the tissue regeneration or replacement process is important in the acute and subacute stages of healing. Any application or activity that brings the ends of the healing tissue apart will prolong the healing and increase scar formation. Because scar tissue is nonfunctional tissue and has a tendency to shorten and become nonpliable, the smaller the scar, the better the tissue should function after healing is complete. One of the major errors made during massage is to create forces that disrupt healing by pulling apart the ends of the healing tissue. During any tissue breach, the surrounding muscle tissue contracts to pull the ends of the injured tissue together and prevent the ends from separating. This is called muscle guarding. Massage must *not* interfere with this appropriate protective response. This appropriate guard response often is mistaken for muscle tension or trigger point activity that should be eliminated. To the contrary, reducing the muscle activity and lengthening and stretching the tissue

FIGURE 18-6

EXAMPLES OF MASSAGE OF LATERAL ANKLE SPRAIN

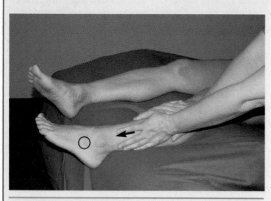

A Acute, 24 to 48 hours. Crowd tissue toward injury. Example: grade 1+ lateral ankle sprain.

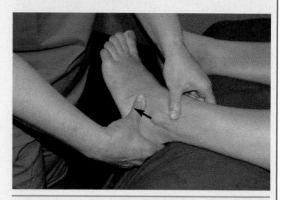

B Acute. Glide tissue into injury—approximate ends of injured tissue.

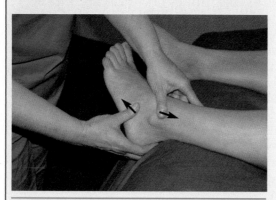

C Subacute. Tension force.

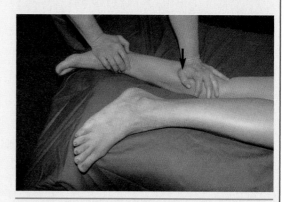

D Subacute. Reduce guarding.

is ineffective and has the potential to prolong, disrupt, and negatively affect the healing process and increase the likelihood of excessive scar tissue forming.

The guarding process typically involves cocontractions of agonist and antagonist muscle groups around the injured area. This appropriate process further stabilizes the area, protecting the healing area, and keeps the torn tissue ends close together. The result is a temporary reduction in the range of motion of the area and a sensation of stiffness or a knot. Again, this process must not be disturbed during the acute and early subacute healing stages. Stretching and aggressive joint movement techniques are inappropriate at this time.

Frictioning and compressing in the early stage of tissue healing are inappropriate as well. This approach to massage is contraindicated during the acute and early subacute stages. Error in massage

applications is to mistake grade 1 and 2 injury, particularly in the deeper layers of muscle, as trigger point activity or to apply these methods too soon during the healing process. Friction will disturb the healing tissue formation, and compression into the injured area *also spreads* the fibers and disturbs the tissue formation.

TREATMENT STRATEGIES

Methods that are appropriate during the acute and early subacute phases of healing include general full-body massage as described in this text to support the restorative capacity. Perform massage as often feasible, with every other day being ideal. Include in the general massage at the area of the injury the following (Figure 18-6):

- Acute phase: During the first 24 hours, PRICE should be used. Because it is assumed that the medical team has evaluated the injury, the

FIGURE 18-6 CONT'D

EXAMPLES OF MASSAGE OF LATERAL ANKLE SPRAIN

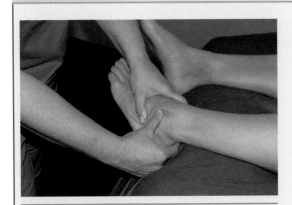

E Remodel using shear force.

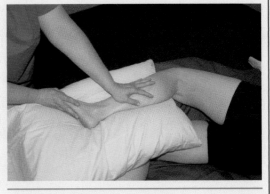

F Remodeling, reduce guarding, ease position.

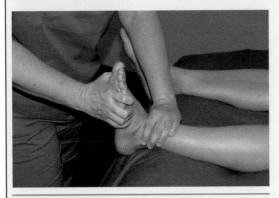

G Remodeling. Move tissue into ease and bind.

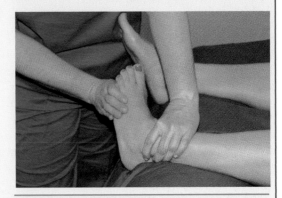

H Move tissue into ease and bind.

massage therapist should follow all recommendations. If pain medication is prescribed, the therapist needs to evaluate and factor into the treatment approach the possible interaction with massage. Pain medication and antiinflammatory drugs alter pain mechanisms. Therefore the therapist must monitor pressure levels carefully. Massage application must not produce pain in the injured area during this stage.

With medical team approval, massage can be applied to the injured tissue in a specific and precise manner to approximate (push together) the ends of the torn tissue. This method should be applied only to tissue that can be accessed easily from the body surface around joints, such as ankle and knee, or to pulls and tears in surface muscles (Figure 18-7). The method is ineffective for muscle tears in the deeper layers and for tendons and ligaments that are deep to surface tissue. The approach works because injured tissue is sticky

during the first 48 hours after injury. Massage is applied to push the tissue together mechanically with the intention of decreasing the size of the "hole" by approximation of the injured tissues of the hole to encourage the torn ends to stick together. This should be a beneficial strategy because the smaller the hole, the faster the healing.

Identification of the exact location of the injury site is necesssary. This usually is indicated by a painful point, and the athlete can best locate this spot if the trainer or other medical personnel have not located it for you. Understanding the anatomic structure of the area is essential because a deliberate stroke is applied in the direction of the tendon, ligament, or muscle fibers so that the sticky ends of the new injury touch. The application must not be painful, create additional inflammation, or specifically touch the injury. The method is repeated for up to 5 minutes and is applied slowly and rhythmically. The hand is lifted and reposi-

FIGURE 18-7

TREATMENT STRATEGIES FOR QUADRICEPS STRAIN—APPROXIMATE TISSUE

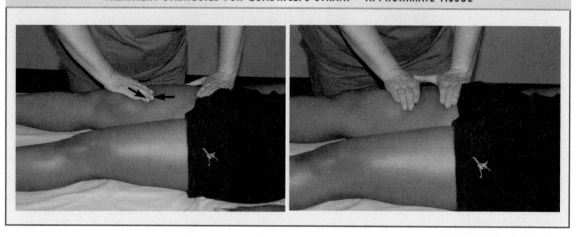

tioned for each stroke, allowing crowding of the tissue ends together. The method can be repeated 3 to 4 times per day within the first 3 days of the injury. If during the acute injury phase the area surrounding the injury becomes excessively stiff and painful, then the area can be shaken rhythmically and gently for up to 10 minutes. This repetitive movement will decrease swelling and guarding just a bit, making the client more comfortable.

- Subacute phase: Massage in the subacute phase is best given every other day and involves full-body massage to address any compensation from the body protecting the injury. This can occur as guarding, changes in gate from limping, or altered sleep patterns. Applying massage to corresponding reflex areas as indicated can help manage pain, normalize some tension, and reduce mild compensation (Figure 18-8).

Massage also can begin to reduce tension by 50% in the muscles that are guarding at the injury site. Work on the larger surface muscles in the area. Do not massage the deeper stabilizing groups, because these muscles are still providing a protective function.

Continue with strokes at the injury site in the opposite direction, gradually increasing pressure and drag over the typical 10-day subacute period. Light cross-fiber (bend and shear) force can be applied 5 to 7 days after injury. This application should not cause pain.

- Remodeling phase: Massage 2 to 3 times per week.

The injured area should be filled completely with connective tissue and some tissue regenera-

tion. Muscle guarding is still present, particularly in the deep stabilizing muscles, but movement in the midrange with a moderate resistance load applied should not be painful. The intent of massage at this point is to encourage strength and function of the new tissue. Gradually, over the next 4 weeks, the tension in the deep stabilizing muscles should be reduced as muscle strength increases in the injured area. Massage is applied across the grain of the fibers to encourage scar mobility and reduce adhesion. This massage application can be mildly painful but not so intense to cause flinching or inflammation.

The massage is applied across fiber direction to the entire length of the injured structure, be it a ligament or tendon and attached muscle. The pressure, drag, and force introduced to the healing area gradually increase over the 4-week interval. The area should not be painful during movement the next day. However, it may be a bit sore to touch. This massage application is included in the context of full-body general massage with continued awareness of compensation patterns.

At the end of this treatment phase, 6 to 8 weeks have passed. It takes up to 6 months for a grade 1 to 2 injury to heal fully and 6 to 12 months for a grade 2 to 3 injury to heal fully. During this time, the massage therapist should address the area periodically with the cross-fiber massage process previously described.

This procedure sequence can be used for any wound, sprain, or strain. The method is most effective for grade 1 and 2 injuries. Grade 3 injuries take longer to heal and may have had some sort of

FIGURE 18-8

EXAMPLES OF MASSAGE OF REFLEX AREAS

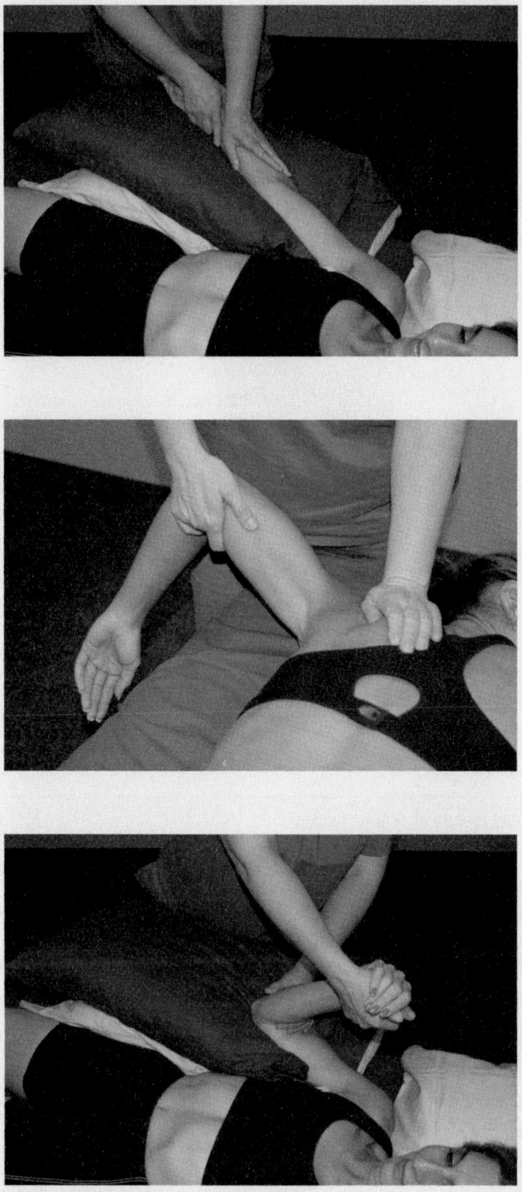

fore the actual tissue damage is minimized. Arthroscopic surgery is a wonderful advancement in joint surgery; however, during the procedure, fluid is introduced into the joint capsule, which helps separate the joint, allowing for the procedure to wash away any debris and keep the field of vision clear for the surgeon. The body has to remove any water left in the joint cavity after the procedure is complete. Restoring range of motion as quickly as possible helps the body absorb and eliminate the intracapsular fluid, which helps the joint heal after the procedure. Swelling in all injuries beyond the acute phase must be managed, and lymphatic drainage massage is one of the most effective methods. Lymphatic drainage is described in Unit Two.

With the more severe injuries, massage treatment needs to be more focused to manage compensation patterns and edema from body adjustment to the injury and rehabilitation activities such as weight training and range-of-motion activities. Scar mobility and return to function are the goals.

CHRONIC SOFT TISSUE INJURIES

Chronic soft tissue injuries consist of a low-grade inflammatory process with a proliferation of fibroblasts and scarring. An acute injury that is managed improperly or an athlete who returns to activity before healing is complete can cause chronic injury.

MYOSITIS AND FASCIITIS

In general, the term *myositis* means inflammation of muscle tissue. More specifically, it can be considered a fibrositis, or connective tissue inflammation. Fascia that supports and separates muscle also can become chronically inflamed after a traumatic or repetitive injury. A typical example of this condition is plantar fasciitis.

TENDON INJURIES

The tendon contains wavy parallel collagenous fibers that are organized in bundles surrounded by a gelatinous material that decreases friction. A tendon attaches a muscle to a bone and concentrates a pulling force in a limited area. Tendons can produce and maintain a pull from 8700 to 18,000 pounds per square inch. When a tendon is loaded by tension, the wavy collagenous fibers straighten in the direction of the load; when the tension is

medical intervention such as surgery, casting, or other stabilization. Each of the three healing stages is longer with severe injuries, and the acute phase may last up to a week. The swelling that occurs with these types of injuries is managed with lymphatic drainage. Surgery creates swelling just as traumatic injury does, but it is much more controlled, there-

FIGURE 18-9

TENDON INJURIES

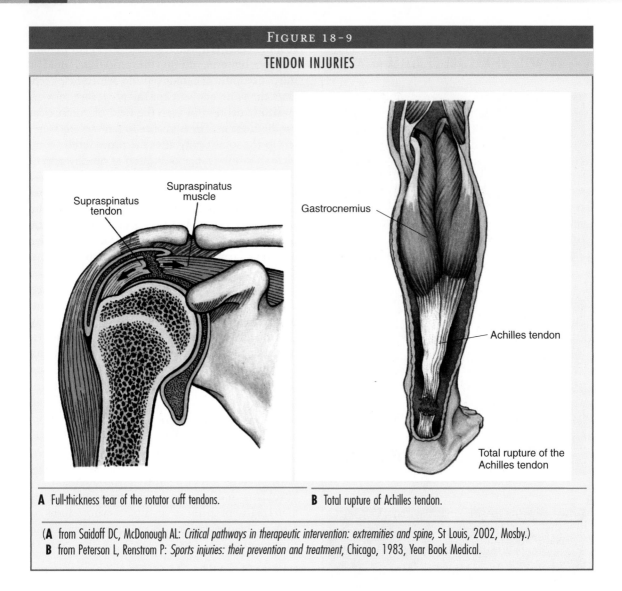

Supraspinatus muscle

Supraspinatus tendon

Gastrocnemius

Achilles tendon

Total rupture of the Achilles tendon

A Full-thickness tear of the rotator cuff tendons.

B Total rupture of Achilles tendon.

(**A** from Saidoff DC, McDonough AL: *Critical pathways in therapeutic intervention: extremities and spine,* St Louis, 2002, Mosby.)
B from Peterson L, Renstrom P: *Sports injuries: their prevention and treatment,* Chicago, 1983, Year Book Medical.

released, the collagen returns to its original wavy shape. In tendons, collagen fibers will break if their physiologic limits have been exceeded. A breaking point occurs after a 6% to 8% increase in length. Because a tendon is usually double the strength of the muscle it serves, tears most commonly occur in the muscle belly, musculotendinous junction, or bony attachment (Figure 18-9).

Tendon injuries usually progress slowly over a long period of time. Repeated acute injuries can lead to a chronic condition. Constant irritation caused by poor performance techniques or an ongoing stress beyond physiologic limits eventually can result in a chronic condition.

Repeated microtraumas from overuse can evolve into chronic muscle strain resulting in reabsorption of collagen fibers and eventual weakening of the tendon or other connective tissue structures. Col-

lagen reabsorption also occurs in the early period of sports conditioning. During reabsorption, collagenous tissues are weakened and susceptible to injury; therefore a gradually paced conditioning program process is necessary.

Tendonitis is inflammation or irritation of a tendon. Tendonitis has a gradual onset, diffuse tenderness because of repeated microtraumas, and degenerative changes. Obvious signs of tendonitis are swelling and pain.

The condition, which causes pain and tenderness just outside a joint, is most common around the shoulders, elbows (tennis elbow) and knees, but it also can occur in the hips and wrists.

Tendons usually are surrounded by a sheath of tissue similar to the lining of the joints (synovium). They are subject to wear and tear, direct injury, and inflammatory diseases. The most common cause of tendonitis is injury or overuse. Occasionally, an infection within the tendon sheath is responsible for the inflammation. The condition also may be associated with diseases such as rheumatoid arthritis. Tenosynovitis is inflammation of the synovial sheath surrounding a tendon. In its acute stage there is rapid pain onset, **articular crepitus** (crackling noise or vibration produced during joint movement), and diffuse swelling. In chronic tenosynovitis, the tendons become locally thickened, with pain and articular crepitus present during movement.

Tendonitis produces pain, tenderness, and stiffness near a joint and is aggravated by movement. The type of tendonitis typically is named for the associated joint. For instance, tennis elbow causes pain on the outer side of the forearm near the elbow when the forearm is rotated or when the hand is gripping, which involves the wrist. Achilles tendonitis causes pain just above the heel. Adductor tendonitis leads to pain in the groin, patellar tendonitis causes pain just below the kneecap, and biceps tendonitis leads to shoulder pain. If the tendon sheath becomes scarred and narrowed, it may cause locking of the tendon, such as in trigger finger.

Risk factors for developing tendonitis include excessive repetitive motions of the arms or legs. For instance, baseball players, swimmers, tennis players, and golfers are susceptible to tendonitis in their shoulders, arms, and elbows. Soccer and basketball players, as well as runners and dancers, are more prone to tendon inflammation in their legs and feet.

Improper technique in any sport is one of the primary causes of overload on tissues, including tendons, that can contribute to tendonitis. The incidence of tendonitis increases with age as muscles and tendons lose their elasticity.

Tendonitis may become chronic and can lead to the rupture of a tendon. Tendonitis also can cause permanent damage to the tissue that makes up the tendons.

Sometimes the discomfort of tendonitis disappears within a matter of weeks, especially if the joint area is rested and iced. In elderly persons and those who continue to use the affected area, tendonitis often heals more slowly and is more likely to progress to a chronic condition termed **tendonosis.** This condition often involves a change in the structure of the tendon to a weaker, more fibrous tissue.

If tendonitis is severe and leads to the rupture of a tendon, surgical repair may be required. This is almost certainly the case if the rupture is in the Achilles tendon. Usually rest and medications to reduce pain and inflammation are the only treatments required. The pain of tendonitis is usually worse with activities that use the muscle that is attached to the involved tendon. Appropriate massage that can support healing is described on p. 466

ATROPHY AND CONTRACTURE

Two complications of muscle and tendon conditions are **atrophy** and contracture. Muscle atrophy is the wasting away of muscle tissue. The main cause of atrophy in athletes is immobilization of a body part, inactivity, or loss of nerve stimulation. A second complication is muscle contracture, an abnormal shortening of muscle tissue in which there is a great deal of resistance to passive stretch. A contracture is associated with a joint that, because of muscle injury, has developed unyielding scar tissue. Whether there is inflammation or fibrosis determines the type of massage used. Inflammation can be caused by rubbing short structures, and massage should focus on restoring normal length to the muscles and connective tissue in the area. Therapeutic exercise to strengthen muscles that have been inhibited is necessary. If tissue has become fibrotic, then connective tissue methods are used to restore pliability.

TREATMENT

The goals of tendonitis treatment are to relieve pain and reduce inflammation. Tendonitis is treated with PRICE.

Steroid injection into tissue or around a tendon may be used to relieve tendonitis. Injections of cortisone reduce inflammation and can help ease pain. These injections must be used with care because repeated injections may weaken the tendon or cause undesirable side effects. *Do not massage over an injection site.* The steroid works by pooling around the inflamed area. Massage disperses the medication.

Research has shown that persons with tendonitis and tendonosis also may be helped by a program of specific exercise designed to strengthen the force-absorbing capability of the muscle-tendon unit. When a tendon is torn, a reconstructive operation may be necessary to clean inflammatory tissue out of the tendon sheath or to relieve pressure on the tendon by removing bone. Surgeons can repair tendon tears to reduce pain, restore function, and in some cases, prevent tendon rupture.

To avoid a recurrence of tendonitis, warming up before exercising and cooling down afterward are important. Strengthening exercises also may help prevent further episodes of tendonitis.

BURSITIS, CAPSULITIS, AND SYNOVITIS

The soft tissues that are an integral part of the synovial joint can develop chronic problems.

Bursitis. The bursas are fluid-filled sacs found in places at which friction might occur within body tissues (Figure 18-10). Bursas provide protection between tendons and bones, between tendons and ligaments, and between other structures where there is friction. Sudden irritation can cause acute **bursitis.** Overuse of muscles or tendons and constant external compression or trauma can result in chronic bursitis.

The signs and symptoms of bursitis include swelling, pain, and some loss of function. Repeated trauma may lead to calcific deposits and degeneration of the internal lining of the bursa. Bursitis in the knee, elbow, and shoulder is common among athletes. Massage can be used to lengthen the shortened structures, reducing friction. Muscle energy methods, lengthening, and inhibiting pressure at the belly or muscle attachments affect muscle tension. Connective tissue application to increase pliability is beneficial. Ice applications and rehabilitative exercise are indicated. Short-term use of antiinflammatory medication may be helpful. Steroid injections at the site are a common treatment. Massage is contraindicated in the area of steroid injection until the medication is absorbed completely by the body. Five to 7 days is a safe waiting period for massage. Massage application should not increase inflammation in the area.

Capsulitis. **Capsulitis** is an inflammation process affecting the joint capsule. Usually associated with capsulitis is **synovitis,** which is inflammation of the synovial membrane. Synovitis occurs acutely, but usually chronic conditions arise with repeated joint injury or with joint injury that is managed improperly. Chronic synovitis involves active joint congestion with edema. As with the synovial lining of the bursa, the synovium of a joint can undergo degenerative tissue changes. Several movements may be restricted, and there may be joint noises such as grinding or creaking. Again, massage is focused on pain management and supporting mobility without creating irritation. Mechanical force application to increase pliability of the joint capsule is a possible massage application in these conditions as long as the inflammatory response is not increased.

Acute Synovitis. The synovial membrane of a joint can be injured acutely by a contusion or sprain. Irritation of the membrane causes an increase in fluid production, and swelling occurs in the capsule. The result is joint pain during motion, along with skin sensitivity from pressure at certain points. In a few days, with proper care the excessive fluid is absorbed, and the swelling and pain diminish. This condition is managed best by the athletic trainer.

MASSAGE STRATEGIES FOR TENDONITIS AND BURSITIS

Observe the following massage strategies for clients with tendonitis and bursitis:

1. Initially the inflamed tendon or bursa area is not directly massaged. Instead the area is iced. Massage is targeted to reducing the reason for the inflammation by lengthening the shortened tissue.

   A progressively deep gliding is applied from the least affected muscle attachment over the muscle belly and stops just before the area of inflammation is reached. For example, Achilles tendonitis would be treated with gliding beginning at the knee and ending at the Achilles attachment. The depth of pressure and drag gradually increases, with the method applied up to 10 times during each massage session. The corresponding reflex areas also are addressed (i.e., ankle, wrist, and forearm).

2. The next step is to apply sustained compression in the muscle belly of the inflamed tendon while the client moves the affected jointed area in a slow range of motion, usually a circle, but sometimes back and forth. This method is followed by the gliding as described in step 1. These strategies are typically are used for 3 to 10 sessions.

3. Once no significant improvement is noted, add connective tissue methods as described in Unit Two. Active release and kneading are effective. Do not massage the directly on the specific location of the inflammation. Treatment should be combined with steps 1 and 2 and spans several sessions.

4. If after a reasonable treatment period (6 to 10 weeks) the tendon or bursa remains painful, then controlled use of deep transverse friction can be attempted. Friction would be applied along with the first three steps of this protocol and would be repeated every other day for 1 to

FIGURE 18-10

MAJOR LOCATION OF BURSAS

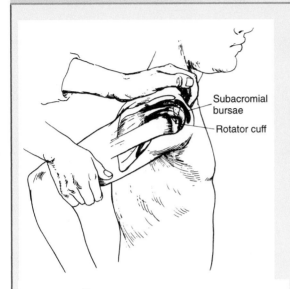

Subacromial
bursae

Rotator cuff

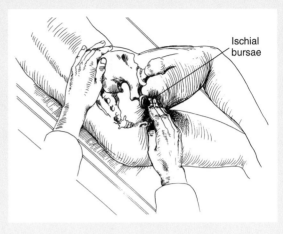

Ischial
bursae

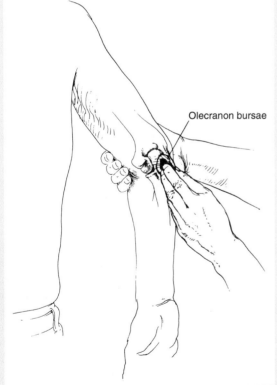

Olecranon bursae

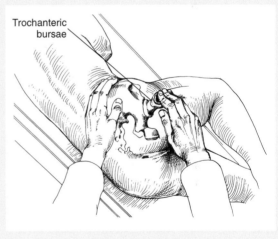

Trochanteric
bursae

From Hoppenfeld: *Physical examination of the spine and extremities*, Upper Saddle River, N.J., 1976, Pearson Education.

Continued

FIGURE 18-10 CONT'D

MAJOR LOCATION OF BURSAS

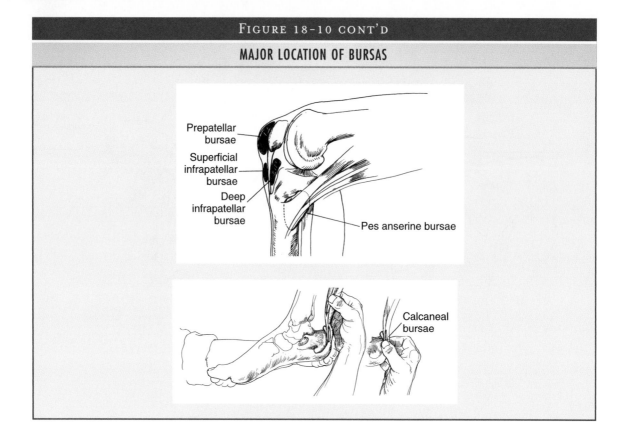

CHRONIC JOINT INJURIES

DEGENERATIVE JOINT DISEASE

Like other chronic physical injuries or problems, chronic synovial joint injuries stem from microtraumas and overuse. The two major categories are **osteochondrosis** and **traumatic osteoarthritis.** A major cause of **chronic joint injuries** is failure of the muscles to control or limit deceleration during eccentric function. Athletes can avoid such injuries by avoiding chronic fatigue and training when tired and by wearing protective gear to enhance absorption of impact forces (Figure 18-11).

Traumatic arthritis is usually the result of accumulated microtraumas. With repeated trauma to the articular joint surfaces, the bone and synovium thicken, and pain, muscle spasm, and articular crepitus (grating on movement) occur. Joint wear leading to arthritis can come from repeated sprains that leave a joint with weakened ligaments. Joint wear can arise from misalignment of the musculoskeletal structure, which stresses joints, or it can arise from an irregular joint surface from repeated articular chondral injuries. Loose bodies that have been dislodged from the articular surface also can irritate and produce arthritis. Athletes with joint injuries that are immobilized improperly or who are allowed to return to activity before proper healing has occurred eventually may be afflicted with arthritis. Massage applications for chronic joint injury are managed with palliative care to control pain and the following protocol added during the general massage protocol.

MASSAGE FOR ARTHROSIS AND ARTHRITIS

Repetitive impact and joint trauma predispose the joints to arthritic development. Therapeutic massage has benefits as part of a comprehensive treatment program for chronic joint pain and

2 weeks and then reduced to every third day. Improvement should be noted in the first 2 weeks to justify continued use of deep transverse friction.

The client needs to ice the area consistently, be involved in appropriate rehabilitation, and be consistent with massage sessions for the massage strategies to be successful.

FIGURE 18-11

DEGENERATIVE JOINT DISEASE EXAMPLES

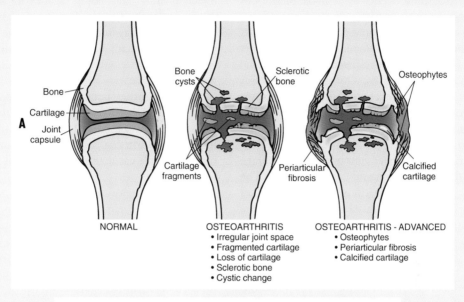

A

Bone

Cartilage

Joint capsule

Bone cysts

Sclerotic bone

Cartilage fragments

Osteophytes

Periarticular fibrosis

Calcified cartilage

NORMAL

OSTEOARTHRITIS
• Irregular joint space
• Fragmented cartilage
• Loss of cartilage
• Sclerotic bone
• Cystic change

OSTEOARTHRITIS - ADVANCED
• Osteophytes
• Periarticular fibrosis
• Calcified cartilage

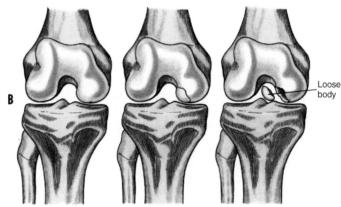

B

Loose body

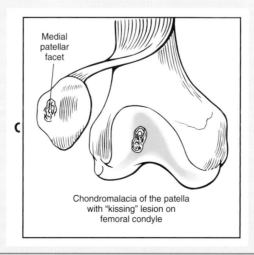

C

Medial patellar facet

Chondromalacia of the patella with "kissing" lesion on femoral condyle

A from Damjanov I: *Pathology for health-related professions*, ed 2, Philadelphia, 2000, Saunders. B and C from Saidoff DC, McDonough AL: *Critical pathways in therapeutic intervention: extremities and spine*, St Louis, 2002, Mosby.

mobility. The neuromuscular involvement is of two types: guarding response and inhibition.

Guarding is the response of the body to protect the joint. Guarding occurs with an isometric co-contraction of the muscles that surround an affected joint. The strategy is a good one if it occurs during the acute phase of an injury for a short period of time but is problematic with chronic problems such as arthritis. Guarding compresses the joint space, reduces mobility, and causes an uneven force distribution through the joint, which over the long term aggravates the arthritic condition.

An arthritic joint needs mobility to encourage synovial fluid production and cartilage health. The cocontraction of the guarding response reduces mobility by increasing muscle shortening in the agonist/antagonist muscles that surround the joint, compressing the bone ends in the joint capsule.

Also, because flexors, internal rotators, and adductor muscle groups exert more pull than extensors, external rotators, and abductors during cocontraction, the joint fit is altered because the flexors, internal rotators, and adductors are compressing the bone ends more than the extensors, external rotators, and abductors. Anytime the joint does move, the bone end can rub, increasing the inflammation and damaging the cartilage further.

Massage can manage the guarding response and encourage more normal neuromuscular function. Normalizing gate and muscle activator firing pattern sequences is important. The short, tense muscles can be inhibited with muscle energy methods and lengthening. Compression applied at the muscle belly or at the attachments affects spindle cells or Golgi tendon receptors, allowing the motor tone to reduce and muscles to lengthen to a more normal resting length. Trigger point activity specifically located in the muscle belly of short muscles can be addressed with trigger point methods. Do not treat trigger points in a long inhibited muscle. Address reflex areas in paired joints such as knee/elbow, ankle/wrist, toes/fingers, hip/glenohumeral joint, sacroiliac joint/sternoclavicular joint.

Arthritic joints tend to display increased edema. Extracapsular fluid around the joint limits movement and can inhibit normal muscle function, especially firing patterns. Lymphatic drainage methods are effective. An increase in intracapsular fluid (effusion) is an attempt to keep bone ends separated, and under most conditions it should be left untreated during massage. If the fluid inside of the capsule becomes excessive, treatment is best left to the doctor. Needle aspiration can relieve the pressure. Synvisc, or artificial synovial fluid, can be injected into the joint space if insufficient intracapsular fluid exists. Treatment of arthritis is a condition management situation because the guarding and edema usually recur. Ideally, massage would be given every other day, but 2 times per week is effective.

Pain is another issue with arthritic joints. All pain management massage methods are appropriate, with massage creating counterirritation and hyperstimulation analgesia. Use of a counterirritant ointment with capsicum is also helpful if the skin will tolerate it.

Antiinflammatory medications are commonly prescribed. Side effects and symptoms affect the heart, kidney, liver, and gastrointestinal system. These medications can thin blood, and bruising is more likely. Massage pressure and intensity need to be altered. Make sure compression during massage is broad based and avoid friction. Massage methods should not increase inflammation. Antiinflammatory essential oils mixed in with the massage lubricant are appropriate.

Hydrotherapy is effective for arthritic joints. See Unit Two. In general, ice goes on the joint, and heat on the surrounding soft tissue.

All methods to treat degenerative joint disease seek to reduce pain and increase mobility, but not reduce stability. In the rare situation that steroid injection is used, massage is contraindicated in the area.

Note: Rheumatoid arthritis is a systemic disease and is not discussed in this text.

DISLOCATION AND DIASTASIS

Dislocations are second to fractures in terms of disabling the athlete (Figure 18-12). A dislocation is an injury in which the ends of the bones that form a joint are forced from their normal positions. The cause is usually trauma, such as a hard blow to a joint or a fall. In some cases, an underlying disease such as rheumatoid arthritis may cause dislocation of a joint.

The highest incidence of dislocations involves the fingers and the shoulder joint. Dislocations, which result primarily from forces causing the joint to go beyond its normal anatomic limits, are divided into two classes: **subluxation** and **luxation.** Subluxations are partial dislocations in which an incomplete separation between two articulating bones occurs. Luxations are complete dislocations, presenting a total disunion of bone apposition between the articulating surfaces.

A **diastasis** is of two types: a disjointing of two bones parallel to one another, such as the radius and ulna and tibia and fibula (usually called a high ankle sprain), and the rupture of a "solid" joint, such as the symphysis pubis. A diastasis commonly occurs with a fracture.

Dislocations are common injuries in contact sports, such as football and hockey and in sports that may involve falls, such as downhill skiing, gymnastics, and volleyball.

Dislocations may occur in the major joints—shoulder, hip, knee, elbow, or ankle—or in smaller joints such as a finger, thumb, or toe. The injury temporarily deforms and immobilizes the joint and may result in sudden and severe pain.

Signs and symptoms of a dislocation may include the following:
- A deformed and immovable joint
- Swelling
- Intense pain
- Tingling or numbness near the injury

At times, x-ray examination of the dislocation, as with a fracture, is the only absolute diagnostic measure. First-time dislocations or joint separations may result in a rupture of the stabilizing ligamentous and tendinous tissues surrounding the joint and in avulsion, or pulling away from the bone. Trauma is often so violent that small chips of bone are torn away with the supporting structures (avulsive fracture), or the force may separate growth epiphyses or cause a complete fracture of the neck in long bones. These possibilities indicate the importance of administering complete and thorough medical attention to first-time dislocations.

Treatment

A dislocation requires prompt medical attention, returning bones to their proper positions without damaging the joint structure. Depending on the amount of pain and swelling, a local anesthetic may be administrated before manipulation.

Surgery is required if the blood vessels or nerves are damaged, or if the doctor cannot move the dislocated bones back into the correct positions. Surgery also may be necessary because lax joint capsules or ligaments stretched during the injury cause predisposition to recurring dislocations.

The doctor may immobilize the joint with a splint or sling and prescribe a pain reliever and a muscle relaxant. After the splint or sling is removed, a slow and gradual rehabilitation program that is designed to restore the stability, range of motion, and strength of the joint is completed. The client should avoid strenuous activity involving the injured joint until full movement is regained and normal strength and stability of the joint are achieved.

It often has been said, "Once a dislocation, always a dislocation." In some cases this statement is true because once a joint has been partially or completely dislocated, the connective tissues that stabilize and hold it in its correct alignment are stretched to such an extent that the joint will be vulnerable to subsequent dislocations. Chronic, recurring dislocations may take place without severe pain because of the slack condition of the stabilizing tissues. The massage practitioner needs to be aware of any history of dislocation. Increased muscle tension and connective tissue formations may occur around the dislocated joint as an appropriate stabilization process. The massage therapist need to take care to maintain joint stability while supporting mobility. Do not lengthen the shortened structures to the point that the joint is vulnerable to another dislocation.

With a fairly simple dislocation without major nerve or tissue damage, the joint likely will return to

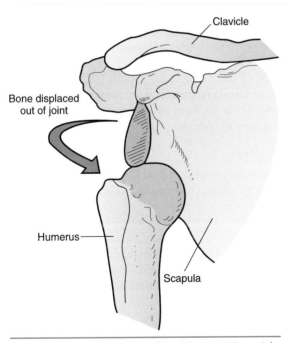

FIGURE 18-12 ■ Shoulder dislocation. (From Salvo SG, Anderson SK: *Mosby's pathology for massage therapists*, St Louis, 2004, Mosby.)

a near or fully normal condition. As with most injuries, returning to activity too soon may cause reinjury to the joint or dislocate it again. Massage therapists must acknowledge the instability of dislocated joints. Muscle guarding around the joint provides stability. Massage manages muscle tension that is excessive without interfering with joint stability. Typically, the massage application is inhibiting compression in the belly of the excessively short muscle without stretching. The lengthening response is enough to reduce pain and increase mobility. If lengthening or stretching is necessary, the massage is applied only directly to the tissue. Movement of the joint to stretch the area is not recommended. Also, massage the corresponding reflex areas such as the shoulder/hip and elbow/knee.

BONE INJURIES

Because of its viscoelastic properties, bone will bend slightly. However, bone is generally brittle and is a poor shock absorber because of its mineral content. This brittleness increases under tension forces more than under compression forces. **Bone injuries** generally can be classified as **periostitis, acute bone fractures,** and **stress fractures.**

PERIOSTITIS

An inflammation of the periosteum can result from various sports traumas, mainly contusions or attachment of short soft tissue structures. Periostitis often appears as skin rigidity of the overlying muscles. It can occur as an acute episode or can become chronic. Lymphatic drainage type of massage is indicated.

ACUTE BONE FRACTURES

A bone fracture can be a partial or complete break of a bone. Fracture can occur without external exposure or can extend through the skin, creating an external wound (open fracture). Because of normal tissue remodeling, a bone may become vulnerable to fracture during the first few weeks of intense physical activity or training. Weight-bearing bones undergo bone reabsorption and become weaker before they become stronger.

Fractures can result from direct trauma, and the bone breaks directly at the site where a force is applied. A fracture that occurs some distance from where force is applied is called an indirect fracture. A sudden, violent muscle contraction or repetitive abnormal stress to a bone also can also cause a fracture (Figure 18-13).

STRESS FRACTURE

Another type of bone break is a stress fracture. The exact cause of stress fracture is not known, but there are a number of likely possibilities, such as an overload caused by muscle contraction, an altered stress distribution in the bone accompanying muscle fatigue, a change in the ground traction force such as movement from a wood surface to a grass surface, or the performance of a rhythmically repetitive stress such as distance running.

Early detection of the stress fracture may be difficult. Because of their frequency in a wide range of sports, stress fractures always must be suspected in susceptible body areas that fail to respond to usual treatment. The most common sites of stress fracture are the tibia, fibula, metatarsal shaft, calcaneus, femur, lumbar vertebrae, ribs, and humerus (Figure 18-14).

The major signs of a stress fracture are swelling, focal tenderness, and pain. In the early stages of the fracture, the athlete complains of pain when active but not at rest. Later, the pain is constant and becomes more intense at night. Percussion by light tapping on the bone at a site other than the suspected fracture will produce pain at the fracture site.

The management of stress fractures varies with the individual athlete, injury site, and extent of injury. Stress fractures that occur on the concave side of bone heal more rapidly and are managed more easily compared with those on the convex side. Stress fractures on the convex side can rapidly become a complete fracture.

Treatment

Bone is an active tissue that regenerates well. It heals completely as long as initial treatment is appropriate. Treatment of fractures typically involves realignment of the broken segments of bone (reduction). Some fractures, such as stress fractures, do not require reduction. Simple fractures can be treated with closed reduction and immobilization (cast). More complicated fractures may require more complicated surgical repair that may include using various pins, screws, and plates. Infection is a great concern if the bone penetrates the skin. The massage practitioner needs to be aware of the potential of stress fractures and refer the client if necessary.

FIGURE 18-13

FRACTURE TYPES

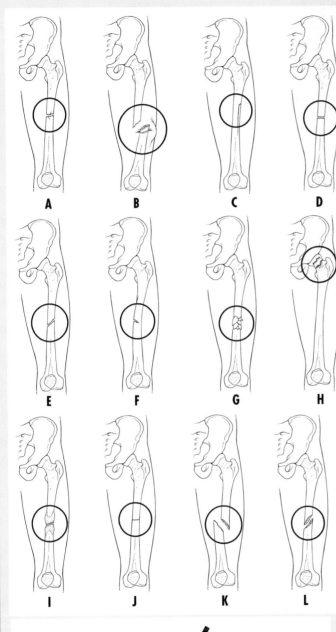

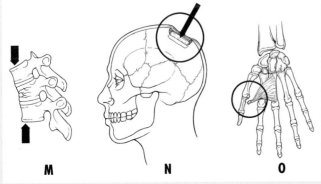

A, Closed, or simple. **B,** Open, or compound. **C,** Longitudinal. **D,** Transverse. **E,** Oblique. **F,** Greenstick. **G,** Comminuted. **H,** Impacted. **I,** Pathological. **J,** Nondisplaced. **K,** Displaced. **L,** Spiral. **M,** Indirect compression. **N,** Direct compression. **O,** Avulsion. (From Salvo SG, Anderson SK: *Mosby's pathology for massage therapists,* St Louis, 2004, Mosby.)

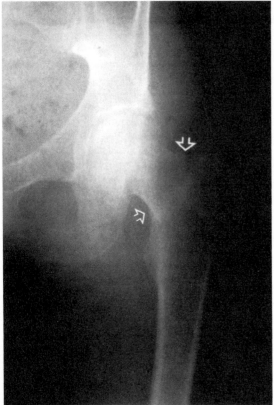

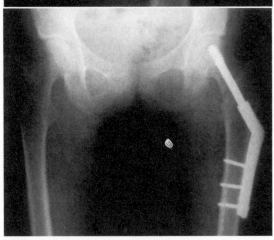

FIGURE 18-14 ■ Femoral neck stress fracture in a female distance runner. (From Anderson K, Strickland SM, Warren R: Hip and groin injuries in athletes, *Am J Sports Med* 29:521–533, 2001.)

Complete fracture healing takes a minimum of 6 weeks and much longer if the injury is complex. Bone heals well if conditions are present that support healing such as proper nutrition, appropriate rehabilitation from qualified medical professionals, stress management, and restorative sleep.

MASSAGE APPLICATION TO SUPPORT FRACTURE HEALING

Massage application does not address bone fractures directly. Instead massage supports general healing and any compensation from changes because of use of various types of immobilization, crutches, changes in gait, or postural stabilization.

When applying massage during the first week or 2 weeks, generally avoid the area of the fracture and as always be attentive to sanitation during the massage. The massage should be relaxing, non-painful, and focused to support parasympathetic dominance. Sufficient pressure needs to be used during the general massage to generate a serotonin and endorphin response to aid in pain management.

As the client becomes more mobile, compensation develops in response to the fracture, treatment, and rehabilitation. General massage can be expanded to address the areas that are sore and aching. These adaptations often occur in the neck, shoulder, and low back areas in the postural muscles. Muscle guarding commonly occurs around the fracture area. This tension pattern will not shift while the area is in acute and subacute healing phase. General pain control measurements are used to help the client be more comfortable. Avoid any deep or aggressive methods. Repetitive light stroking or gentle holding of the tissues that are aching in response to the guarding can generate hyperstimulation analgesia. Massage in the corresponding reflex areas can increase comfort. For example, if the break is in the right lower leg (fibula), then massage the left forearm.

In theory, placing the hands above and below the break generates an electric current that would affect the piezoelectric quality of bone and support tissue regeneration. This type of energy-based modality is noninvasive, can be applied over the cast, will do no harm, and has the potential for benefit.

Once the immobilization (cast or other) is removed and with approval from the medical team, soft tissue mobilization around the break can begin. The forces used are applied so as not to disturb the healing bone. Instead, the tissues generally are moved around the bone. Tension and torsion forces are used to increase soft tissue pliability in the area of immobilization where tissue often becomes atrophied and dense. The process is gentle at first, moving the tissues in and out of bind. The drag is increased over the following weeks of rehabilitation. Therapeutic exercises will reverse the atrophy of the surrounding muscles. If surgical areas exist, the same approach is used in the specific incision areas and scar tissue management.

NERVE INJURIES

The two main forces that cause major nerve injury are compression and tension. As with injuries to other tissues in the body, nerve injury may be acute or chronic. Injured peripheral nerve tissue can heal over time (Figure 18-15).

Any number of traumas directly affecting nerves can produce a variety of sensory responses, including pain. For example, a sudden nerve stretch or pinch (burners, stingers) can produce muscle weakness and a sharp burning pain that radiates down a limb. Neuritis, a chronic nerve problem, can be caused by a variety of forces that usually have been repeated or continued for a long period of time. Symptoms of neuritis can range from minor nerve problems to paralysis.

Pain felt at a point of the body other than its actual origin is known as referred pain. Another potential cause of referred pain is a trigger point, which occurs in the muscular system. Massage applications for **nerve injuries** are palliative to reduce pain. If the nerve is being impinged by short muscles and fascia, massage can be used to restore normal length of these tissues and reduce pressure on the nerve.

NERVE IMPINGEMENT

Nerve impingement commonly is called a pinched nerve. Two types of impingement exist: **entrapment** and compression.

Entrapment results when soft tissue (e.g., muscles and ligaments) exerts inappropriate pressure on nerves; compression occurs when hard tissue (e.g., bone) exerts inappropriate pressure on nerves. Regardless of what is impinging (pressing) on the nerve, the symptoms are similar; however, the therapeutic intervention is different. Therapeutic massage is beneficial in entrapment but less so with compression.

Tissues that can bind and impinge on nerves are the skin, fascias, muscles, ligaments, and bones. Shortened muscles and connective tissue (fascia) often impinge on major and minor nerves, causing discomfort. Because of the structural arrangement of the body, these impingements often occur at major nerve plexuses. The specific nerve root, trunk, or division affected determines the condition, producing disorders such as thoracic outlet syndrome, sciatica, and carpal tunnel syndrome (Figure 18-16).

If the cervical plexus is impinged, the person most likely will have headaches, neck pain, and breathing difficulties. The muscles most responsible for pressure on the cervical plexus are the suboccipital and sternocleidomastoid muscles. Shortened connective tissue at the cranial base also presses on these nerves. Many cutaneous (skin) branches of the cervical plexus transmit sensory impulses from the skin of the neck, ear area, and shoulder. The motor branches innervate muscles of the anterior neck. Impingement causes pain in these areas.

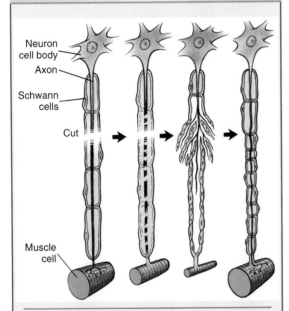

FIGURE 18-15

REPAIR OF A PERIPHERAL NERVE FIBER

Neuron cell body
Axon
Schwann cells
Cut
Muscle cell

A, An injury results in a cut nerve. **B,** Immediately after the injury occurs, the distal portion of the axon degenerates, as does its myelin sheath. **C,** The remaining neurilemma tunnels from the point of injury to the effector. New Schwann cells grow within this tunnel, maintaining a path for regrowth of the axon. Meanwhile, several growing axon sprouts appear. When one of these growing fibers reaches the tunnel, it increases its growth rate, growing as much as 3 to 5 mm per day. (The other sprouts eventually disappear.) **D,** The connection of the neuron with the effector is reestablished. (From Thibodeau GA, Patton KT: *Anatomy and physiology,* ed 5, St Louis, 2003, Mosby.)

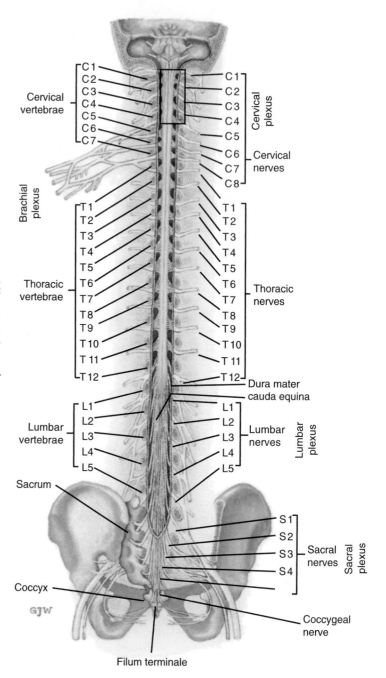

FIGURE 18-16 ■ Spinal nerves. (Each of 31 pairs of spinal nerves exits the spinal cavity from the intervertebral foramens. Notice that after leaving the spinal cavity, many of the spinal nerves interconnect to form networks, called plexuses.) (From Chipps EM, Clanin JJ, Campbell VG: *Neurologic disorders*, St Louis, 1992, Mosby.)

The brachial plexus is situated partly in the neck and partly in the axilla and consists of virtually all the nerves that innervate the upper limb. Any imbalance that increases pressure on this complex of nerves can result in pain in the shoulder, chest, arm, wrist, and hand. The muscles most often responsible for impingement on the brachial plexus are the scalenes, pectoralis minor, and subclavius muscles. The muscles of the arm also occasionally impinge on branches of the brachial plexus.

Brachial plexus impingement is responsible for thoracic outlet symptoms, which often are misdiagnosed as carpal tunnel syndrome. Whiplash injury, stingers, and burners often cause impingement on the brachial plexus.

Carpal tunnel syndrome is caused by compression of the median nerve as it passes under the transverse carpal ligament at the palmar aspect of the wrist. The syndrome can occur when fluid retention causes swelling of the hand and wrist. The syndrome is common in persons who use their hands in repetitive movements, usually because of inflammation that results in compression on the nerve. The symptoms are palmar by pain and numbness in the first three digits. Sometimes surgically opening the transverse carpal ligament can help relieve the pain.

Impingement on the lumbar plexus gives rise to low back discomfort, which is marked by a beltlike distribution of pain and by pain in the lower abdomen, genitals, thigh, and medial lower leg. The main muscles that impinge on the lumbar plexus are the quadratus lumborum, multifidi, and the psoas. Shortening of the lumbodorsal fascia exaggerates a lordosis and can cause vertebral impingement on the lumbar plexus.

The sacral plexus has about a dozen branches that innervate the buttock, lower limb, and pelvic structures. The main branch is the sciatic nerve. Impingement on this nerve by the piriformis muscle is a cause of sciatica. Shortened ligaments that stabilize the sacroiliac joint can affect the sacral plexus. Pressure on the sacral plexus can cause pain in the gluteal muscles, leg, genitals, and foot.

Various forms of massage reduce muscle spasm, lengthen shortened muscles, and soften and stretch connective tissue, restoring a more normal space around the nerve and alleviating impingement. When massage is combined with other appropriate methods, surgery is seldom necessary. If surgery is performed, the massage practitioner's role is to manage adhesions to prevent reentrapment of the nerve in the future and to maintain soft tissue suppleness around the healing surgical area. As healing progresses, extend the therapeutic massage focus to deal with the forming scar more directly. Before doing any work near the site of a recent incision, the practitioner must obtain the physician's approval. In general, work close to the surgical area can begin after the stitches have been removed and all inflammation dissipates. Follow the massage strategies for wounds.

NERVE ROOT COMPRESSION

Many different conditions can result in compression of the nerve root, including tumors, subluxation of vertebrae, and muscle spasms (entrapment) and shortening. Disk degeneration is a common cause. As the degeneration progresses and the fluid content of the disk decreases, the disk becomes narrower. As a result, the amount of space between vertebrae is reduced. Because spinal nerves exit and enter in the spaces between the vertebrae, this situa-

tion increases the likelihood of **nerve root compression.** The condition most commonly occurs in the areas where the spine moves the most: C6 to C7, T12 to L1, L3 to L4, and L5 to S1 (*C*, cervical; *T*, thoracic; *L*, lumbar; *S*, sacral). The result is radiating nerve pain often associated with protective and stabilizing muscle guarding, weakness, or both.

DISK HERNIATION

Disk herniation occurs when the fibrocartilage surrounding the intervertebral disk ruptures, releasing the nucleus pulposus. The resultant pressure on spinal nerve roots may cause pain and may damage the surrounding nerves. This condition most often occurs in the lumbar region and involves the L4 or L5 disk and L5 or S1 nerve roots. This particular back pain radiates from the gluteal area down the lateral side or back of the thigh to the leg or foot. Back strain or injury often causes disk herniation, but occasionally coughing and sneezing may precipitate the condition. Improper form during weight lifting is a common source of injury in the athlete.

The symptoms of herniation are similar to those produced by a compressed disk but often are more severe. In extreme cases, surgical intervention may be necessary; otherwise, conservative care is used. Conservative treatment consists of rest, exercise, and other methods, including massage to reduce spasm. Traction can be beneficial.

MASSAGE TREATMENT

Various forms of massage are important for managing the muscle spasm and pain associated with the nerve irritation from the herniated disk. The muscle spasms/guarding response serves a stabilizing and protective function. Without some protective muscle guarding, the nerve could be damaged further, but too much muscle contraction increases the discomfort. Therapeutic intervention seeks to reduce pain and excessive tension and to restore moderate mobility while supporting resourceful compensation produced by the muscle tension pattern.

Athletes often experience nerve impingement, and physical rehabilitation exercises are used to treat nerve impingement in the general population. Repetitive strain, posture changes, and compensation from traumatic injury are common causes. The elderly are prone to cervical and lumbar nerve impingement because of age-related tissue and bone changes. Nerve pain usually radiates in a line following the tract of the nerve. Massage applied to reduce soft tissue binding on the nerve needs to address the soft tissue effectively but *not* irritate the underlying nerve. If the impingement is entrapment and compression, the muscle tension actually may be protective, attempting to stabilize the bony structures and prevent further compression on the nerve. Massage application addressing the soft tissue, combined with repositioning the underlying structure with manipulation and therapeutic exercise, is required for effective treatment.

Massage methods used to treat entrapment vary depending on what is impinging the nerve:

Muscle shortening: Use muscle energy methods including positional release and lengthening. Direct inhibiting pressure at the spindle cell and/or Golgi tendon organs combined with application of tension and bend force will lengthen the muscle.

Connective tissue: Mechanical force, bend, torsion, and compression force increase ground substance pliability. Adhesion/fibrosis can be addressed with bend, shear, torsion, and tension force to encourage more appropriate fiber alignment.

Fluid: Lymphatic drainage combined with passive and active joint movement.

Bone: Compression usually is managed best by the trainer, physical therapist, physician, or chiropractor. In simple situations, joint play and indirect functional methods may help. The body area is placed in an ease position, and the client exerts muscle force to pull the body back into the neutral position (described in Unit Two). The pull of the muscle on the bone can help the structure to reposition and reduce nerve compression.

The location of the nerve entrapment is identified with palpation. When the area is located, the symptoms will be reproduced. If the nerve is irritated in this location, then sustained compression or intense stretching only increases the irritation. Once the impingement is located, next identify the nature of the impingement—muscle tension, connective tissue bind, fluid buildup, or structural misalignment—and then treat accordingly. When in doubt, apply all methods but do not overwork the area. Begin with general massage around the area before targeting the actual impingement site.

In athletes with muscle bulk and dense tissues, actually reaching the area of impingement is often difficult. In this case, use muscle energy methods, especially positional release. Normalization of firing patterns and gait reflexes is usually necessary. If the impingement is from muscle spasm, short-term use of muscle relaxing medication is effective.

SUMMARY

This chapter categorized injury types and explained the commonalities of these injuries.

The strategies were described for beneficial and safe therapeutic massage application. These conditions use treatment assessment procedures described in Unit Two and usually are treated in the context of full-body massage, which also is described in Unit Two.

1 List the general injury category(ies) that have lymphatic drainage as the major intervention.

_____
_____
_____
_____.

4 List the common injuries that usually are caused by a traumatic event.

_____
_____
_____
_____.

2 List the general injury category(ies) that have scar tissue management as a portion of the recommended treatment strategies.

_____
_____
_____
_____.

5 List the common injuries that have repetitive strain as the major causal factor.

_____
_____
_____
_____.

3 List the general injury category(ies) that would indicate appropriate application of muscle energy methods and lengthening.

_____
_____
_____
_____.

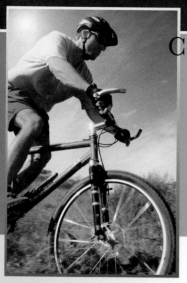

19

MEDICAL TREATMENT FOR INJURY

OBJECTIVES

Upon completion of this chapter, the reader will have the information necessary to do the following:

1 Explain the importance of appropriate use of surgery and medication to treat injury.

2 List indications and contraindications for massage.

3 Perform appropriate presurgical and postsurgical massage application.

4 Alter massage to interact appropriately with medication use.

Advances in surgical procedures, rehabilitation, treatment, and medication have prolonged the careers of many athletes and the general public. Sport medicine and orthopedic specialists now can repair, rehabilitate, and medicate injuries and illnesses that previously were destined at the least to end a career and at the most to result in permanent disability. This chapter describes some of those medical treatments and how massage can support successful outcomes.

SURGERY

ARTHROSCOPY

Arthroscopic surgery involves the use of fiberoptic cameras and small surgical instruments to visualize the intraarticular structures of the joint and to treat many abnormalities or injuries (Figure 19-1). This surgery includes trimming of meniscal tears, which is the most common abnormality treated, removal of loose bodies, trimming of articular cartilage flaps, débridement of scar tissue, and other abnormalities of the joint. In addition, the arthroscopic instruments can be used to obtain a more accurate diagnosis of abnormalities of the joint. Although many of today's magnetic resonance images are very

Arthroscopic surgery
Pre-surgery
Post-surgery

Steroid injections
Medication
Nonsteroidal anti-inflammatory drugs (NSAIDS)

Muscle relaxers

high quality, there are still times when a specific diagnosis may be in doubt, especially concerning articular cartilage lesions, and arthroscopy can be used to diagnose the size, depth, and condition of these articular cartilage lesions.

The technique of arthroscopic surgery involves the placement of small incisions (portals) around the joint. The standard arthroscopic incisions are a small fluid outflow (or in some cases inflow) portal. Fluid is introduced in the joint to allow for better visualization and separation of structures and to remove any blood that might be present from the surgical incisions or injuries.

The next standard arthroscopy portal is used for placement of the arthroscopic camera for the majority of work inside the joint.

The arthroscope is inserted through a small incision made in the side of the joint. A beam of light and a small camera project an enlarged image of the interior of the joint onto a television monitor.

The doctor inserts sterile fluid to expand the joint for easier viewing and inserts a probe to help investigate the joint structures. Repairs are made through portal incisions that are so small that stitches usually are not required to close them (Figure 19-2).

Arthroscopy can be used to examine and repair the joint problems in one operation. First used primarily on the knee joint, arthroscopy now can diagnose and treat problems in the shoulder, elbow, wrist, hip, and ankle. Whether the joint problems are the result of an acute event, such as a sports injury, or a chronic condition, such as arthritis, arthroscopy may help. Arthroscopy can be performed on individuals of all ages.

Arthroscopy not only makes joint surgery less invasive but also reduces the recovery time. Because less pain and swelling results, less disruption of other structures around the joint occurs. This allows weight bearing, range of motion, and strengthening exercises to begin earlier. The rehabilitation process should be easier, and the return to activity is accelerated as well.

Though some complex procedures still require traditional open surgery, many procedures can be enhanced by using an arthroscope.

Risks associated with arthroscopy are as follows:
- Nerve injury
- Infection
- Bleeding
- Stiffness

Almost all arthroscopic surgeries now are performed on an outpatient basis. Primarily used are Steri-strips over the arthroscopic portals to allow the skin incisions to heal and to minimize scarring. A loose, sterile dressing then is applied that can be removed in 3 to 4 days. Patients are allowed to bear weight as tolerated with the use of crutches and may wean off the crutches when they can walk without a limp. Rehabilitation should begin as soon as the surgeon permits so that the joint does not become stiff or muscles atrophy. Showers generally are allowed at 3 or 4 days after surgery. Most patients recover fully.

MASSAGE APPLICATION

BEFORE SURGERY (24 TO 48 HOURS)

The massage outcomes are to reduce anxiety and support restorative sleep. A rested, calm person requires less anesthesia and copes better with the stress of the surgical procedure. Do not work directly on the targeted surgical areas with deep pressure, intense drag, or any methods with the potential for tissue damage. Use a palliative approach. Target breathing function, parasympathetic dominance, and neurochemical balance.

AFTER SURGERY (24 TO 48 HOURS)

Postsurgical massage follows a combined sequence for wounds, pain management, and lymphatic drain. Depending on the extent of the procedure,

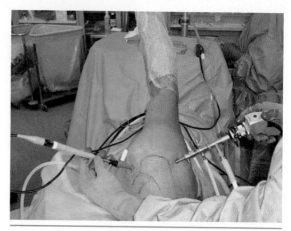

FIGURE 19-2 ■ Arthroscopy. (From Miller MD, Cole BJ: *Textbook of arthroscopy*, Philadelphia, 2004, Saunders.)

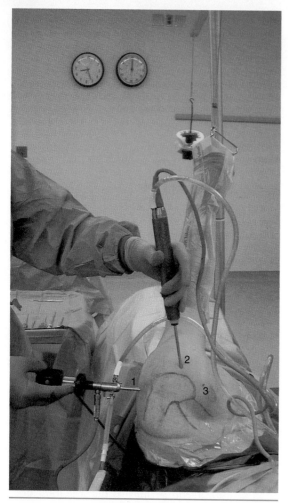

FIGURE 19-1 ■ Arthroscopic portals. Posterior (*1*), anterior (*2*), and lateral (*3*). (From Miller MD, Cole BJ: *Textbook of arthroscopy*, Philadelphia, 2004, Saunders.)

massage can begin within 24 to 48 hours. The focus is pain control, reduction of anxiety, and restoration of sleep. The duration is short and more frequent, such as 2 times per day. Target areas that are achy other than the surgical site. Often the neck, shoulders, and low back are sore from the bed rest or positioning during surgery. Massage of the head, face, hands, and feet is usually effective in calming the client. Do not use methods that cause pain. Do not work near the surgery site. For noncomplicated surgery, especially arthroscopic procedures, the client is home the day of the surgery or the next day. Infection control is important; therefore maintain meticulus sanitation.

3 DAYS AFTER SURGERY

For most surgery, especially arthroscopic procedures, the client is home and ambulatory. Massage

remains palliative with targeted lymphatic drain to manage postsurgical edema. Do not work on the surgical site, but careful and gentle work around the area is appropriate. (See the discussion of wounds in Chapter 18.) This is considered acute care, and the surgical sites are wounds. Sanitation and infection control are top priority. If the client has been instructed to do range-of-motion exercises, massage supports the movement pattern. Work with reflex patterns. Paired functional areas are the following:

- Right shoulder, left hip, and vice versa
- Right elbow, left knee, and vice versa
- Right wrist, left ankle, and vice versa
- Right hand, left foot, and vice versa
  Functional muscle units are as follows:
- Flexors with opposite side flexors and same side extensors
- Extensors with opposite side extensors and same side flexors
- Internal rotators with opposite side internal rotators and same side external rotators
- External rotators with opposite side external rotators and same side internal rotators
- Adductors with adductors and abductors with abductors
  Trunk paired patterns are as follows:
- Neck flexors with trunk flexors
- Neck extensors with trunk extensors
- Neck lateral flexors with trunk lateral flexors
  These relationships are especially helpful in the treatment of acute injury such as surgery. Because massage on the surgical area is contraindicated,

paired areas can be addressed to create beneficial reflex responses (Box 19-1).

If the client is able to move the surgical area, the effect is increased if the client moves the area gently while the targeted reflex areas are massaged. Intentional and deliberate focus is important. For the first example, in Box 19-1, when massaging the right biceps, be thinking about the left hamstring. Using these reflexes does not mean you are massaging the arm for the benefit of the arm. The arm is massaged to influence the leg. Continue to promote lymphatic drainage, and massage daily if possible.

SUBACUTE PHASE: 7 DAYS AFTER SURGERY

The stitches (if there are any) should be out, and gentle scar tissue work can begin in the surgical area. Use strategies for wounds. Do not pull on the incision. Use gentle bending and shear force to increase tissue pliability. The intensity increases each day, and by 14 days, if the incision is fully healed, tension force is added. At 18 to 20 days, add torsion force and work directly on the incision unless contraindication exists.

Continue to promote lymphatic drainage of the area and reset all firing patterns and gait reflexes. Support all rehabilitation exercises. Massage the client 3 to 4 times per week if possible.

REMODELING STAGE: 3 TO 4 WEEKS AFTER SURGERY

Resume use of full-body general protocol as presented in Unit Two. Continue to manage edema and muscle activation patterns and reflex patterns. Address scar tissue each massage. Normalize all residual muscle guarding. Continue this focus for at least 6 months. Massage 2 times per week if possible.

Total joint replacement surgery follows the same postsurgical patterns, but each healing phase will take longer, especially in the elderly.

STEROID INJECTIONS (CORTISONE)

Steroid injections are a common and effective treatment for a variety of conditions in which inflammation causes pain, swelling, and other problems. Glucocorticoids, particularly prednisone and cortisone, are used in injections for inflammation and pain. These hormones help reduce inflammation and pain in the body. Cortisone is the most well-known injected steroid, and it has a dramatic anti-inflammatory effect on tissues, particularly joints and tendons. This family of steroids is not the same as anabolic steroids, which are used to enhance muscular development and are largely illegal in international athletic competition.

Glucocorticoids are thought to interfere with immune system processes that result in inflammation, but the exact method by which they do this is not known. Injections of glucocorticoids are known to target the area of pain and inflammation better and faster than pill form. Cortisone injections typically result in pain relief in a matter of days and may last up to a month.

Conditions treated by steroid injections include the following:
- Tennis elbow (lateral epicondylitis)
- Golfer's elbow (medial epicondylitis)
- Joint pain of varying nature (osteoarthritis)
- Bursitis of the shoulder, hip, or knee
- Frozen shoulder
- Plantar fasciitis
- Carpal tunnel syndrome
- Herniated disk and other back pain

Steroid injections cannot cure any of these conditions and are targeted to symptom management. They generally are used as a last resort after antiinflammatory drugs and physical therapy have been tried and have failed to provide relief. Steroid injections may help with chronic, painful inflammation

---

Box 19-1	EXAMPLES OF MASSAGE AFTER SURGERY

Example 1: Arthroscopic Knee Surgery on the Left Knee
Reflexive massage would be targeted to the right elbow to include the biceps to influence the hamstring reflexively, the triceps to influence the quadriceps, and the wrist and finger flexors at the elbow to influence the calf. Lymphatic drainage is promoted and circulation is supported for the entire arm. Then massage application moves to the left elbow and is targeted to influence the right hamstring and the left quadriceps reflexively. The wrist extensors at the elbow target the calf. Then move to the right leg. The hamstrings on the left are influenced reflexively by the massage of quadriceps on the right. The quadriceps on the left is influenced by massage of the hamstring on the right.

Example 2: Sports Hernia in the Right Groin
Reflexive massage is applied to the left anterior and lateral neck, pectoralis major and pectoralis minor on the left, scapula region on the right, and neck extensor on the right.

and reduce recovery times, but unless the underlying cause is determined and treated, injections will provide only temporary relief. More than three to four injections in a year in the same area of the body are not recommended because glucocorticoids can result in the following potentially serious side effects:

- Weight gain
- High blood pressure
- Cataracts
- Diabetes
- Puffy face
- Osteoporosis (thinning of the bones)
- Reduced immunity and increased risk of infection
- Long-term joint and tendon damage
- Ulcers

Side effects are more likely to occur with steroid pills than injections, but research indicates that as few as six injections per year can damage a joint permanently or cause risk of tendon rupture.

MEDICATION

The main medications used for sport injuries are nonsteroidal antiinflammatory drugs (NSAIDs) and steroidal antiinflammatory drugs, muscle relaxers, and pain control medication. Antibiotics are used to prevent and treat infection.

Massage application needs to be altered to support the effect of the medications and not cause tissue damage because pain perception is altered. Massage may be substituted for muscle relaxers and pain medication, but this must be a medical decision with supervision by the medical team.

Nonsteroidal antiinflammatory drugs are used by competitive athletes and recreational exercisers because of their analgesic (pain reduction) and antiinflammatory benefits. Common NSAIDs and other analgesics available over the counter are the following: ibuprofen (Advil, Motrin IB), ketoprofen (Actron, Orudis-KT), and naproxen (Aleve). Related drug classes include aspirin (Genuine Bayer Aspirin, Bufferin, Ecotrin). Acetaminophen (Tylenol), is an analgesic but will not affect inflammation. It is very toxic to the liver. Common prescription antiinflammatory drugs include the following: rofecoxib (Vioxx), celecoxib (Celebrex), and valdecoxib (Bextra), which are all under scrutiny due to cardiovascular side effects.

In general, most NSAIDS increase potential for bruising, so the massage therapist needs to monitor pressure during the massage. Maintain a broad-based contact and do not poke, probe, or dig on the tissues.

Nonsteroidal antiinflammatory drugs act therapeutically by inhibiting prostaglandin synthesis and thereby reducing pain and inflammation. Excessive NSAID use may increase the potential for renal problems. This potential is magnified if prolonged exercise is combined with severe heat stress and/or dehydration. Proper hydration before and throughout exercise can minimize any risk that NSAIDs may pose to the kidney.

Muscle relaxers reduce motor tone in muscle and normal protective mechanisms against overstretching and overcontracting are altered. Massage and various muscle energy lengthening and stretching methods cannot be aggressive. Tissue may be damaged.

Common muscle relaxers include the following:

Cyclobenzaprine (Flexeril)
Metaxalone (Skelaxin)
Carisoprodel and aspirin (Soma)
Tizanidine (Zanaflex)

SUMMARY

Advances in surgical and medical treatment of physical exercise–related injuries have allowed persons to compete and perform daily life activities pain free or with significantly reduced pain. These advances will continue.

Athletic clients and those in physical rehabilitation may be taking medication for non–exercise-related conditions. A thorough clinical history including all medication supplements and herbs is necessary. Massage needs to be altered on an individual basis to support medication use. Refer to the Evolve web site accompanying this book for a list of medications for massage.

1 Develop a letter to an orthopedic surgeon explaining the benefit of massage before and after surgery.

_____

_____

_____

_____

_____

_____

_____

_____

_____

2 List and explain at least 10 adaptations for massage application if surgery and medication are used. Example: Client not comfortable on massage table at massage office. Will need to work with client in a reclining chair or at client's home.

_____

_____

_____

_____

_____

_____

_____

_____

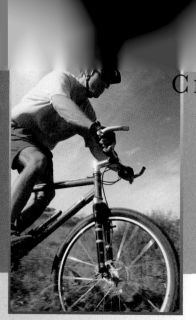

20

SYSTEMIC ILLNESS IMMUNITY AND DISORDERS

OBJECTIVES

Upon completion of this chapter, the reader will have the information necessary to:

1 Apply appropriate massage interventions for clients with infections, cardiovascular/respiratory disease, thermoregulating disorders and heat-related illnesses, and breathing pattern disorder.

Illness is different than injury. Illness involves the whole body; injury is more local. Various illnesses can target a body system. For example, a cold is an upper respiratory inflection. This is different than a localized bruise on the quadriceps. Illness occurs as a dysfunction in the immune response. Illness can be the result of infection by a pathogen–bacteria, viruses, or fungi–in which the immune system is unable to stop the progression of invasion. Illness can also be autoimmune, such as systemic lupus erythematosus (SLE), or an overreaction of the immune response such as occurs in allergies and multiple sclerosis. Illness can also be caused by a body system failure such as occurs in cardiovascular disease, kidney failure, and diabetes.

Athletes, just like other people, have allergies and systemic disease, and these conditions must be factored into the focused treatment plan. Cardiovascular/respiratory disease rehabilitation is a major reason for therapeutic exercise.

Disorders occur when the body is not able to adapt to homeostatic regulation in reponse to internal or external influences. Examples are thermoregulating disorders and breathing pattern disorder, which is extremely common and is discussed extensively in this chapter.

IMMUNE FUNCTION

Overtraining and aggressive physical activity can suppress the immune system, predisposing to infection. The main target of massage intervention is **immune function** support. The basic treatment plan is to reduce the stress response, support parasympathetic dominance, manage pain, and promote sleep.

When an athlete is ill, DO NOT overmassage. Regardless of the ongoing treatment plan, back off and apply general, nonspecific massage for no more than 45 to 60 minutes, with a relaxation/palliative outcome and encourage rest, sleep, proper fluid intake, and nutritional support.

Illness should be diagnosed and treated by the physician. If bacterial infection is detected, antibacterial medication may be prescribed. Digestive upset including diarrhea is common. Fever below 102 degrees is usually productive (often referred to as a low-grade inflammatory response) during infection and should not be reduced unless complicating factors exist. Sanitation is always important, but even more so during illness.

IMMUNITY IN ATHLETES

In the resting state, the adaptive immune system appears to be largely unaffected by intensive and prolonged exercise training. However, the innate immune system, those immune cells that act as a first line of defense against infectious agents, appears to respond differentially to the chronic stress of intensive exercise. Natural killer cell activity tends to be enhanced and neutrophil function suppressed.

In general, when analyzed in resting subjects, the immune systems of athletes and nonathletes appear to be more similar than different. Of the various immune function tests that show some change with athletic activity, only salivary IgA has emerged as a potential marker of infection risk. It is possible that each bout of prolonged exercise leads to short-term but clinically significant changes in immune function. Altered immunity may last between 3 and 72 hours. During this time, viruses and bacteria may gain a foothold, increasing the risk for both subclinical and clinical infection.

Taken together, the data suggest, but do not prove, that the immune system is suppressed and stressed for a short time, following prolonged endurance exercise. If this is so, infection risk may be increased when the endurance athlete goes through repeated cycles of heavy exertion, especially if the athlete is experiencing other stressors of the immune system such as lack of sleep, mental stress, malnutrition, and weight loss.

Athletes resist reducing training workloads. They are more receptive to taking nutritional supplements and using other stress-reducing, and therefore immune-enhancing, behaviors such as massage. Parasympathetic dominance is a very important area of therapeutic massage intervention for stress management and immune system function.

Investigators have measured the influence of nutritional supplements (primarily zinc, vitamin C, glutamine, and carbohydrate) on the immune response to intense and prolonged exercise (Figure 20-1).

The most impressive results have been reported in carbohydrate supplementation studies, which suggest that carbohydrate supplementation during prolonged and intensive exercise maintains or elevates plasma glucose levels, an effect that counterbalances the normal rise in stress hormones, thereby balancing negative immune changes. Research has established that a reduction in blood glucose levels is linked to hypothalamic-pituitary-adrenal axis activation, increased release of adrenocorticotrophic hormone and cortisol, increased plasma growth hormone, decreased insulin levels, and a variable effect on blood epinephrine levels. Given the link between stress hormones and

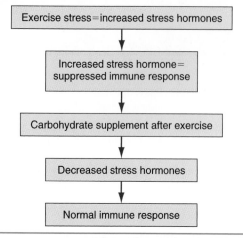

FIGURE 20-1 ■ Influence of nutritional supplements on the immune response to intense and prolonged exercise.

immune responses to prolonged and intensive exercise, carbohydrate ingestion should maintain plasma glucose levels, which modulate increases in stress hormones, and thereby diminish changes in immunity.

Data indicate that athletes ingesting carbohydrate beverages before, during, and after prolonged and intensive exercise experience lowered physiologic stress.

In addition, several lifetyle practices may be beneficial. Improper nutrition and psychological stress can compound the negative influence that heavy exertion has on the immune system. Indicators of overtraining include immunosuppression, loss of motivation for training and competition, depression, poor performance, and muscle soreness. The athlete needs to eat a well-balanced diet, keep other life stresses to a minimum, avoid overtraining and chronic fatigue, obtain adequate sleep, and space vigorous workouts and competitive events as far apart as possible. Immune system function appears to be suppressed during periods of low caloric intake and weight reduction; therefore, when this is necessary, the athlete is advised to lose weight slowly during noncompetitive training phases.

Mononucleosis

Significant complications of mononucleosis include enlargement of the spleen. In extreme cases, the spleen may rupture, causing sharp, sudden pain in the left side of the upper abdomen. Occasionally, a streptococcal (strep) infection accompanies the sore throat of mononucleosis and antibiotics are prescribed for these infections.

Colds

Cold viruses are spread by personal contact and by breathing the air near people with colds. Therefore, if at all possible, athletes should avoid being around sick people before and after important events.

MASSAGE APPLICATION DURING INFECTION

If massage is indicated, it would be palliative and targeted to support parasympathetic dominance, sleep, and reduction of general aching. Do not massage if fever is above 100° or if the client is fatigued. In general, if symptoms are primarily manifested above the shoulders, it is acceptable to massage the client. If symptoms involve the whole body, then massage could strain adaptive capacity. Energy-based modalities may be used if the client finds them soothing.

CARDIOVASCULAR/RESPIRATORY ILLNESSES

The most common reason for mature people to be in rehabilitation is cardiovascular/respiratory disease. Exercise is a necessary part of the rehabilitation and treatment plan for these conditions.

Cardiovascular disease is the number-one cause of death in the United States; coronary artery disease (CAD) is the number-one cause of death due to cardiovascular disease. CAD is caused by the collection of plaque (i.e., buildup of cholesterol, calcium, fibrous tissue) inside a coronary vessel, resulting in a narrowing of coronary arteries (stenosis) that decreases the delivery of oxygen to the heart owing to reduced coronary blood flow.

The events leading to cardiac injury during a heart attack begin with a transient blockage of coronary blood vessels that is usually caused by a blood clot that has broken loose from an area of coronary stenosis. This reduction in blood flow to the heart is called *ischemia* and is typically followed by a restoration of blood flow (*reperfusion*) when the clot dissolves. Commonly known as a heart attack, the overall process of ischemia followed by reperfusion results in cardiac injury and is technically referred to as **ischemia-reperfusion (I-R) injury.**

The magnitude of cardiac injury that occurs during an I-R insult is a function of the duration of ischemia—that is, a longer period of ischemia results in greater cardiac injury. For example, a relatively short duration of ischemia (e.g., 5 minutes) does not result in permanent cardiac damage but may depress cardiac function for 24 to 48 hours following the event. In contrast, a long duration of ischemia (20 minutes or more) promotes permanent cardiac injury (muscle cell death), resulting in a myocardial infarction. The severity of a myocardial infarction is significant because cardiac muscle cells are not easily capable of regeneration; therefore, following myocardial infarction, the pumping capacity of the heart is permanently diminished.

Regular exercise lowers the risk of developing CAD and reduces the risk of cardiac injury during a heart attack. The mechanism of exercise-induced protection against cardiac injury (called **cardioprotection**) is unknown but may be linked to increases of "heat-shock" proteins (discussed later) and antioxidants in the heart. Animal research suggests that supplementation with nutritional antioxidants reduces I-R–induced cardiac injury and disease. Additional research is required to determine if dietary antioxidants can provide myocardial protection in humans.

Finding ways to reduce the mortality of cardiovascular disease remains an important public health goal. In this regard, numerous studies reveal that regular exercise is cardioprotective. For example, epidemiologic studies indicate that compared to sedentary individuals, physically active people have a lower incidence of heart attacks. These investigations also demonstrate that the survival rate of heart attack victims is greater in physically active individuals compared to their sedentary counterparts.

Numerous epidemiologic studies indicate that regular physical activity reduces the risk of cardiovascular mortality independent of other lifestyle modifications such as diet or smoking.

The biologic mechanism responsible for exercise-induced protection against cardiovascular disease continues to be investigated. In this regard, it is clear that regular exercise reduces several cardiovascular risk factors, including hypertension, diabetes mellitus, obesity, blood lipids, risk of thrombosis (blood clotting), and endothelial (blood vessel) dysfunction. Therefore, it appears that the relationship between exercise and reduced cardiovascular mortality rates is due to the reduction of one or more risk factors.

Although it is clear that regular exercise reduces the risk of developing cardiovascular disease, it is also well established that exercise training improves myocardial tolerance to I-R injury. Endurance exercise training reduces myocardial injury resulting from an I-R insult.

At present, the mechanisms behind the exercise-induced myocardial protection against I-R injury are unknown. However, at least three primary mechanisms may explain this effect: (1) improved collateral circulation; (2) induction of myocardial heat-shock proteins; and (3) improved myocardial antioxidant capacity.

Proteins play an important role in maintaining homeostasis in cardiac and other cells. Damage to existing proteins or impaired protein synthesis during I-R injury results in disturbance of cellular homeostasis. To combat this type of disturbance, cells respond by synthesizing a group of proteins termed *heat-shock proteins*. These proteins are induced by a variety of stressful conditions, including elevated body temperature and prolonged exercise.

Improved protection against free radical–mediated cardiac injury is another possible mechanism of exercise-induced cardioprotection during an I-R insult. Free radicals are highly reactive molecules with available incomplete bonds on their surface that are produced during myocardial I-R injury. Antioxidants are molecules that can remove free radicals by filling their incomplete bonds and forming a new, less reactive molecule and therefore preventing free radical–mediated cellular injury. One can make this analogy: rust is the free radical and Rustoleum is the antioxidant that stops the spread of rust when applied to it.

Cells contain several naturally occurring enzymatic and nonenzymatic antioxidants. Primary enzymatic antioxidant defenses include superoxide dismutase, glutathione peroxidase, and catalase. Important non-enzymatic defenses are compounds such as glutathione, the trace mineral selenium, and vitamins A, E and C. Each of these antioxidants is capable of quenching radicals and preventing cellular injury.

Massage supports the necessary exercise program involved with cardiofitness and rehabilitation by managing muscle soreness and joint aching. Massage contributes to increased compliance with exercise programs. Procedures need to be altered to account for medications being taken by the client, as well as the client's age and general adaptive capacity. Otherwise, the methods discussed in Unit Two are appropriate.

HYPERTHERMIA AND HEAT-RELATED ILLNESSES

The body's ability to maintain a constant internal temperature is called *thermoregulation*. If the internal temperature drops significantly below normal, this is called *hypothermia*. If the internal temperature rises significantly above normal, this is called *hyperthermia*. The body's inability to maintain a steady temperature is a thermoregulating disorder that can result in various illnesses. The most common problems are heat-related.

Exercising in a hot, humid environment can cause various forms of heat-related illnesses, including heat rash, heat syncope, heat cramps, heat exhaustion, and heat stroke. Athletes cannot safely exercise at full capacity in the heat (Figure 20-2).

Heat Rash

Heat rash, also called *prickly heat,* is a benign condition associated with a red, raised rash accompanied by sensations of prickling and tingling during sweating. It usually occurs when the skin is continuously wet with unevaporated sweat. The rash is generally localized to areas of the body covered with clothing. Massage is regionally contraindicated.

Heat Syncope (Heat Collapse)

Heat syncope, or **heat collapse,** is associated with rapid physical fatigue during overexposure to heat. It is usually occurs after standing in heat for long periods or in persons not accustomed to exercising in the heat. It is caused by peripheral vasodilation of superficial vessels, hypotension, and/or a pooling of blood in the extremities, which result in dizziness, fainting, and nausea. Heat syncope is quickly relieved by lying the individual down in a cool environment and replacing fluids.

Heat Cramps

Heat cramps are extremely painful muscle spasms that occur most commonly in the calf and abdomen, although any muscle can be involved. The occurrence of heat cramps is related to electrolyte balance. Profuse sweating results in loss of water and small quantities of electrolytes, which upsets the balance in concentration of these elements in the body. This imbalance will ultimately result in painful muscle contractions and cramps.

The person most likely to get heat cramps is someone in fairly good condition who simply overexerts in the heat. An athlete who experiences heat cramps will generally not be able to return to practice or competition that day because cramping is likely to recur.

Although there are many causes of muscle cramps, large losses of sodium and fluid can be key factors that predispose athletes to run-of-the-mill muscle cramps. Sodium is an important mineral in initiating signals from nerves and actions that lead to movement in the muscles, so a deficit of this element and fluid may make muscles "irritable." Under such conditions, a slight stress such as a tensing movement may cause the muscle to contract and twitch uncontrollably. Massage does not help these cramps and may actually cause them. Only fluids and electrolytes will stop the cramping.

Diabetes, neurologic disorders, or vascular problems may be a factor in cramping episodes. Also, anecdotal reports indicate that the use of certain dietary supplements such as creatine may increase the risk of muscle cramps. If cramps suddenly occur in a client without a prior history, referral to a physician should be made to rule out more serious causes.

Preventing and Managing Cramping

1. Drink plenty of fluids to stay hydrated during exercise.

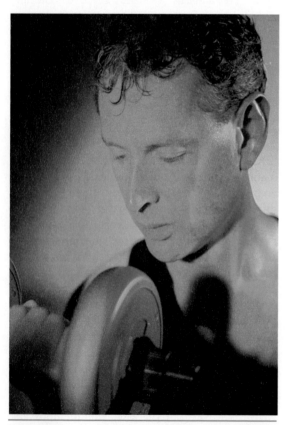

FIGURE 20-2 ■ Athletes cannot safely exercise at full capacity in the heat.

2. Replenish sodium levels during times of heavy exercise and profuse sweating with a diluted sports drink or other electrolyte solutions. Dilute 50% sports drink to 50% water.

3. Ensure adequate nutritional recovery (particularly for salt) and rest of muscles after hard training. Salt pills are not necessary; eating salty pickles is a good alternative.

When cramps strike an athlete during a workout or competition, take immediate action with the following:

1. Stretch. Because cramps are often related to a change in weight bearing, stretching and non–weight-bearing exercises are effective treatments.

2. Massage the area. Rubbing the cramped muscle may help alleviate pain as well as help stimulate blood flow and fluid movement into the area. Ice massage can also be used.

3. Stimulate recovery. Rest and adequate rehydration with fluids containing electrolytes, particularly sodium, will quickly bring improvement.

Heat Exhaustion

Heat exhaustion results from inadequate replacement of fluids lost through sweating. Clinical symptoms include collapse, profuse sweating, pale skin, mildly elevated temperature (102°F [39°C]), dizziness, hyperventilation, and rapid pulse.

It is sometimes possible to spot athletes who are having problems with heat exhaustion. They may begin to develop heat cramps and become disoriented and light-headed, and their physical performance will not be up to their usual standards. In general, persons in poor physical condition who attempt to exercise in the heat are most likely to suffer from heat exhaustion.

Immediate treatment of heat exhaustion requires ingestion or intravenous replacement of large quantities of water.

Heat Stroke

Unlike heat cramps and heat exhaustion, **heat stroke** is a serious, life-threatening medical emergency. The specific cause of heat stroke is unknown. Heat stroke can occur where there is a combination of hot environment, strenuous exercise, clothing that limits evaporation of sweat, inadequate adaptation to the heat, too much body fat, and/or lack of fitness.

During exercise, body heat is generated primarily in the active muscles. Transport mechanisms, which include the circulating blood and conduc-

tion between body tissues, bring the heat to the skin. At the skin, evaporation, convection, radiation, and–far less important–conduction, can transfer the heat from the skin to the environment. Certain situations can impede heat release. When, for example, the air temperature is higher than the skin temperature, convection, radiation, and conduction will result in the transfer of heat from the air to the body.

The evaporation of sweat decreases when the humidity of the air is high. To maintain a body temperature that is within a safe range, the following factors are important:

1. The intensity and the duration of the exercise and the body's efficiency for the effort being performed. This ratio establishes the amount of heat released by the body.

2. The blood circulation and blood volume determine the transport of heat from the muscles to the skin.

3. The amount of sweat produced and the temperature and humidity of the environment determine how much heat can be given off to the environment.

4. The capability of the body to make other physiologic adjustments in order to continue regulating the temperature.

Heat stroke is always a risk in summer sports. Victims of heat stroke are described as "the hardest worker" or "determined to prove himself." During a hard practice on a hot day, the never-quit mentality can work against a player.

In summer sports, it's not the heat but the heat *and* humidity that combine to predispose to heat illness. Getting heat-fit takes time. Lack of acclimation is a predictor of heat stroke in football. Triathletes unacclimated to tropical heat also suffer. Acclimation, much of which occurs in a week or two, leads to drinking more fluids, and the body holds onto water and salt, increasing blood volume so the heart pumps more blood at a lower rate. Heat-fit athletes also sweat sooner, in greater volume, and over a wider body area, so they stay cooler.

During physical training, the athlete who is disabled with a spinal cord injury faces the same risks of heat stress as the able-bodied athlete. However, the spinal cord injury also affects the disabled athlete's circulating blood volume, sweat production, and temperature regulation, and therefore can adversely influence thermoregulatory capabilities.

Opportunities to compete in the Paralympics, advances in medical treatment and therapies for functional recovery of the disabled, and the recognition that physical activity is beneficial for the health of everyone, abled or disabled, have contributed to increased participation of disabled individuals in regular physical exercise. Like able-bodied athletes, disabled athletes face limitations to performance–fatigue, nutrition and fluid needs, and the possibility of heat exhaustion. The greatest risk for heat stress appears to exist in individuals with spinal cord injury above the sixth thoracic vertebra because they are unable to increase heart rate to sustain cardiac output when blood must flow to both the muscle and the skin and because they have a reduced sweating capacity.

Preventing heat stroke hinges on heat acclimation, hydration, pacing, cooling, and vigilance. Physical fitness, especially aerobic fitness, provides some of the same physiologic benefits as heat acclimation. Fitness also makes workouts less taxing. In contrast, lack of fitness increases risk of heat illness.

The prime time for heat stroke is the day *after* an exhausting and dehydrating day in the heat. The misconception is that hydration prevents heat stroke. The truth is that hydration is critical, but not sufficient to prevent heat stroke.

Heat stroke symptoms include:

Sudden collapse with loss of consciousness
Flushed, hot skin with less sweating than would
 be seen with heat exhaustion
Shallow breathing
A rapid, strong pulse and a core temperature of
 106° F (41° C) or higher

The heat stroke victim experiences a breakdown of the thermoregulatory mechanism caused by excessively high body temperature, and the body loses the ability to dissipate heat through sweating.

Stimulants speed heat buildup, so products that speed players up heat them up. Amphetamine and cocaine are the most dangerous, but ephedra is the most prevalent. Many dietary supplements claim ephedra benefits of weight loss or quick energy. However, ephedra poses many health risks, including heat stroke, and should not be used. Excessive caffeine use can also pose a problem. Heat stroke risk is compounded by drugs that impair sweating, such as some antihistamines, antispasmodics, and certain medications for depression.

Heat stroke is often slow to evolve, and the vigilant observer can detect early warning signs. Heat stroke is always a threat during hard drills on hot days, especially in hefty players in full gear. Heat stroke can occur suddenly and without warning. The athlete will not usually experience signs of heat cramps or heat exhaustion. Athletes

sleeping poorly or those who are ill, especially with vomiting, diarrhea, or fever, are more prone to heat stroke. The same applies to athletes taking diuretics or drinking alcohol.

Early warning signs of impending heat stroke may include irritability, confusion, apathy, belligerence, emotional instability, and irrational behavior. The coach may be the first to notice a player who is heating up and can no longer think clearly. Giddiness, undue fatigue, and vomiting can also be early signs. Paradoxical chills and goose bumps signal shutdown of skin circulation, resulting in a faster rise in temperature. The player may hyperventilate–just as a dog pants–to shed heat; this can cause tingling fingers and face prior to collapse. Incoordination and staggering–"running like a puppet on a string"–are late signs, followed by collapse with seizure and/or coma. At this stage, core body temperature can be 108° F (42.2° C) or higher.

The possibility of death from heat stroke can be significantly reduced if body temperature is lowered to normal within 45 minutes. The longer the body temperature is elevated to 106° F (41° C) or higher, the higher the mortality rate.

Dehydration

Athletes in the heat can lose 1 to 2 liters of water in an hour through sweating, and most athletes drink fewer fluids than they lose in sweat. The result is dehydration. Dehydrating only 2% of body weigh–that's just five pounds in a 250-pound athlete–can impair physical performance. Dehydration increases heart rate and decreases cardiac output. Dehydration drains mental sharpness and willpower along with muscle power and endurance, so that the same level of activity seems as if it requires more effort.

Hydration helps prevent heat stroke, but there is no advantage in consuming fluid in excess of sweat loss. Likewise it's not necessary to overhydrate the night before or during the hours prior to a long run or practice. During training, the athlete should weigh in before and after a workout and learn to adjust fluid intake to minimize weight loss. If weight loss does occur, rehydration after activity is critical. The athlete should drink 20 to 24 ounces of fluid for every pound of weight loss and should eat foods with high water content (fruits and vegetables).

Treatment

Cool First   No faster way to cool exists than placing the athlete in an that ice-water tub. Submerge the trunk–shoulders to hip joints. Research suggests that ice-water immersion cools runners twice as fast as air exposure with the runner wrapped in wet towels. The U.S. Marines use ice-water cooling, and recent field research with volunteer runners suggests that cold water may cool as fast as ice water.

Transport Second

This is a medical emergency.

Some research suggests heat stroke patients may have brief or lasting heat intolerance, but whether this is innate or a result of the heat stroke is unclear. Most heat stroke sufferers have normal heat tolerance within 2 months. It seems likely that most athletes treated early for heat stroke and educated about prevention can return safely to their sport within weeks (Box 20-1).

After an episode of major heat exhaustion, an athlete is allowed to return to play when his or her weight has normalized and symptoms are gone, usually within 48 hours.

Massage is not applicable for heat-related illnesses except for temporary management of muscle cramps. Refer all clients with suspected heat-related illness to the trainer or appropriate medical personnel.

Box 20-1	WHAT TO WATCH FOR: SIGNS OF HEAT STROKE

Fuzzy Thinking
Can't follow the plays
Seems confused
Suddenly forgetful

Bizarre Behavior
Runs the wrong way
Talks nonsense
Blank stare
Laughs or cries at wrong time
Yells in rage at coach or peers
Wants to fight for no good reason

Physical Decline
Begins to lose coordination
Sudden or unusual fatigue
Nausea and vomiting
Chills and goose bumps
Overbreathing, tingly fingers
Wobbles or staggers, collapses
Seizure or coma

HYPOTHERMIA

Cold weather is a frequent adjunct to many outdoor sports in which the sport itself does not require heavy protective clothing: consequently, the weather becomes a pertinent factor in injury susceptibility (Figure 20-3). In most instances, the activity itself enables the athlete to increase the metabolic rate sufficiently to function normally and dissipate the resulting heat and perspiration through the usual physiological mechanisms. If an athlete fails to warm up sufficiently or becomes chilled because of relative inactivity for varying periods of time, he or she is more prone to injury.

Dampness or wetness further increases the risk of hypothermia. Air at a temperature of 50° F is relatively comfortable, but water at the same temperature is intolerable. The combination of cold, wind, and dampness creates an environment that easily predisposes the athlete to hypothermia.

A relatively small drop in body core temperature can induce shivering sufficient to materially affect an athlete's neuromuscular coordination and perform-

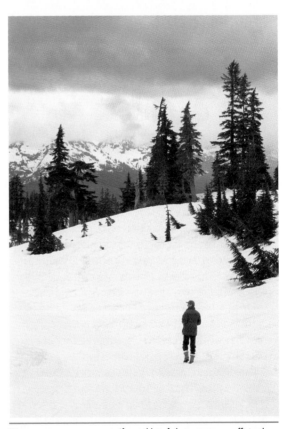

FIGURE 20-3 ■ If an athlete fails to warm up sufficiently or becomes chilled because of relative inactivity for varying periods of time, he or she is more prone to injury.

ance. Shivering ceases when the body temperature is 85° F to 90° F (29.4° C to 32.2° C). Death is imminent if the core temperature rises to 107° F (41.6° C) or falls to between 77° and 85° (25° C and 29° C).

Treatment consists of warming and drying the athlete.

Frostbite

Frostbite is local tissue destruction resulting from exposure to extreme cold; in mild cases, it results in superficial, reversible freezing followed by erythema and slight pain. In severe cases, it can be painless or paresthetic and result in blistering, persistent edema, and gangrene.

Do not massage any areas with frostbite.

BREATHING PATTERN DISORDER

The massage therapist working with athletes as well as with other clients involved in physical exercise

---

IN MY EXPERIENCE...

Breathing

Breathing pattern disorder is extremely common in competing athletes. This tendency occurs because of extremes in activity level. Running around and breathing heavily is perfectly normal during many sports activities. Yet this same breathing pattern at home with the family can lead to disrupted interaction.

I recall an athlete with multiple stressors as the result of a nagging injury that was compromising performance, who would go home to a young family with a 3-year-old son and 1-year-old twin girls. His breathing was just stuck in the upper chest, perpetuating sympathetic arousal patterns. On the playing field the result was too much "fight." At home it seemed that everything irritated him. Obviously this athlete needed help that went beyond massage strategies and that targeted normal relaxed breathing. As is often the case, the massage therapist may be the first to notice the cumulative strain. Sensitivity to noise is a common symptom of sympathetic dominance, either caused by, or perpetuated by, upper chest breathing.

I asked this client if he was having trouble with the "kid" noise. He looked at me and began to tear up. Then I asked if he was yelling at the kids, and he just hung his head and began to sob. The head coach, a great guy, was able to intervene, and the athlete was given help on multiple levels. Massage to manage breathing dysfunction and help for the nagging injury were both part of the intervention plan. I often wonder what might have happened to this young family if the coach had not been so supportive.

---

needs to be able to address the mechanism of breathing both to help correct dysfunction and to support optimal function. Persons in pain, including athletes, are prone to **breathing pattern disorder.** Those with any sort of respiratory disease are especially susceptible to breathing dysfunction. Increased upper chest breathing results in biochemical changes that may temporarily reduce pain but in the long run may make the situation worse. Respiratory illness such as a cold can shift the breathing function to an upper chest pattern, and then it may not reverse. Chronic respiratory disease such as asthma perpetuates breathing dysfunction. Persons with anxiety and depression often display breathing difficulties.

Athletes can get "stuck" in the breathing rate required for practice and competition and are not able to reverse the breathing to a resting phase. This interferes with mood, recovery, and further performance.

Breathing pattern disorder is a complex set of behaviors that leads to over-breathing without evident pathology. Because there is no specific pathology and the anatomy and physiology are normal, it is considered a functional syndrome. The breathing pattern is inappropriate, a situation resulting in confused signals to the central nervous system, which sets up a whole chain of events.

SIGNS AND SYMPTOMS

Increased ventilation is a common component of fight-or-flight responses, but when our breathing increases and our actions and movements are restricted or do not increase accordingly, we are breathing in excess of our metabolic requirements. Blood levels of carbon dioxide fall, and many of the following signs and symptoms can occur.

Cardiovascular

Cardiovascular symptoms include palpitations, missed beats, tachycardia, sharp or dull atypical chest pain, "angina," vasomotor instability, and cold extremities. Raynaud's phenomenon, blotchy flushing of blush area, and capillary vasoconstriction (face, arms, hands) may also be seen.

Neurologic

Neurologic symptoms include dizziness, unsteadiness or instability, sensation of giddiness, feelings of faintness (rarely actual fainting), visual disturbances (blurred or tunnel vision), headache (muscle tension and vascular migraine), paresthesia (numbness, uselessness, heaviness, pins and needles, burning) commonly of hands, feet, or face, but sometimes of the scalp or whole body. Limbs may feel "out of proportion"or as if they "don't belong." There may be hypersensitivity to noise or light, and pupils may be dilated (wearing dark glasses on a dull day).

Respiratory

Respiratory symptoms include shortness of breath (typically after exertion), irritable cough, tightness or oppression of chest, difficulty breathing, "asthma," air hunger (inability to take a satisfying breath), and excessive sighing, yawning, and sniffing.

Gastrointestinal

Gastrointestinal symptoms include difficulty in swallowing, dry mouth and throat, acid reflux (heart burn), exaggeration of symptoms of hiatal hernia due to aerophagia (air swallowing), nausea, flatulence, belching, abdominal discomfort, and bloating.

Muscular

Muscular symptoms include cramps, and pain, particularly in the occipitals, neck, shoulders, and between scapulae, and less commonly in the lower back and limbs. Tremors, twitching, weakness, stiffness or tetany (seizing up) may also occur.

Psychological

Individuals with breathing pattern disorder may complain of tension, anxiety, "unreal feelings," and "out of body" feelings. Other psychic symptoms include depersonalization, panic, phobias, and agoraphobia (fear of being in open spaces).

General

Other symptoms include feelings of weakness; exhaustion; impaired concentration, memory and performance; disturbed sleep, including nightmares; emotional sweating (axillae, palms, sometimes whole body); and a "thick-headed" sensation.

Cerebrovascular constriction, a primary response to disordered breathing, can reduce the oxygen available to the brain by about one half. Among the resulting symptoms are dizziness, blurring of consciousness, and possibly because of a decrease in cortical inhibition, tearfulness and emotional instability.

Other effects that therapists should watch for are generalized body tension and chronic inability to relax. Persons with breathing pattern disorder are particularly prone to spasm (tetany) of muscles involved in the "attack posture"—they hunch the shoulders, thrust the head and neck forward, scowl, and clench the teeth.

THERAPEUTIC MASSAGE

If the accessory muscles of respiration, such as the scalenes, sternocleidomastoid, serratus posterior superior, pectoralis minor, levator scapulae, rhomboids, abdominals, and quadratus lumborum, are constantly being activated for breathing when forced inhalation and expiration are not called for, dysfunctional muscle patterns will result.

Therapeutic massage can assist in normalizing these conditions and support more effective breathing. It is very difficult to breathe well if the mechanical mechanisms are not working efficiently. Many who have attempted breathing retraining have become frustrated with their inability to accomplish the change in breathing pattern because these muscle patterns are not changed. They may find more success once the muscles of the body and mechanism of breathing are normalized.

The massage therapist influences breathing in two distinct ways:
1. Supporting balance between sympathetic and parasympathetic autonomic nervous systems function. (This is generally accomplished with a relaxation focus in the general protocol.
2. Normalizing and then maintaining effective thoracic and respiratory muscle function.

The following protocol specifically targets these areas. The applications should be integrated into the general protocol to work more specifically with breathing function if assessment indicates a tendency toward breathing pattern dysfunction. Again, it is strongly recommended that the reader study *Multidisciplinary Approaches to Breathing Pattern Disorders.**

ASSESSMENT PROCEDURES

The client should be continually monitored for symptoms relating to breathing pattern disorder during each massage session (Figure 20-4).

---

*Chaitow L, Bradley D, and Gilbert C: *Multidisciplinary approaches to breathing pattern disorders*, Philadelphia, 2002, Churchill Livingstone.

FIGURE 20-4

ASSESSMENT AND TREATMENT OF BREATHING FUNCTION

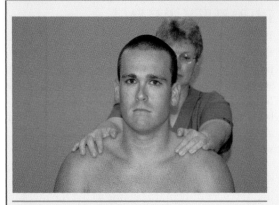

A Assess shoulder movement.

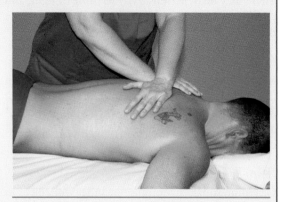

B Assess rib mobility, posterior.

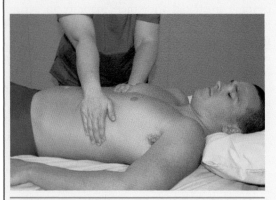

C Assess rib mobility, anterior.

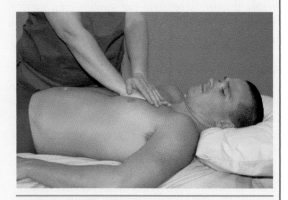

D Assess rib mobility, anterior.

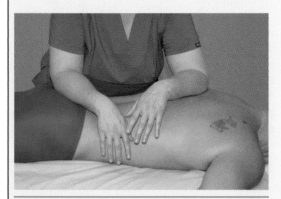

E General massage accesses posterior thorax.

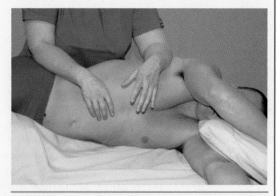

F General massage accesses lateral thorax.

FIGURE 20-4 CONT'D

ASSESSMENT AND TREATMENT OF BREATHING FUNCTION

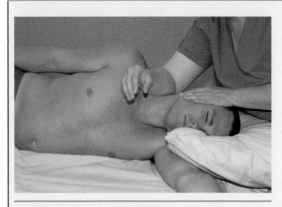

G General massage accesses shoulder.

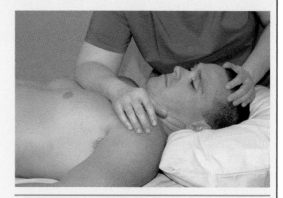

H Compression/mobilization treatment, rib mobility, anterior.

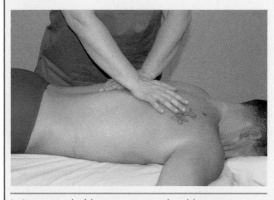

I Compression/mobilization treatment, rib mobility, posterior.

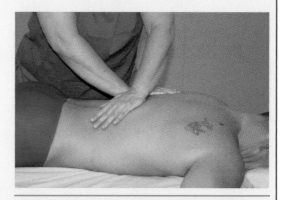

J Compression/mobilization treatment, rib mobility, posterior.

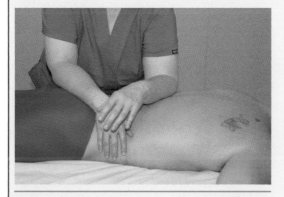

K Compression/direct pressure, target posterior serratus inferior.

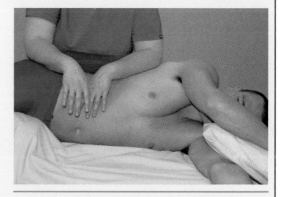

L Compression/mobilization treatment, rib mobility, lateral.

Continued

FIGURE 20-4 CONT'D

ASSESSMENT AND TREATMENT OF BREATHING FUNCTION

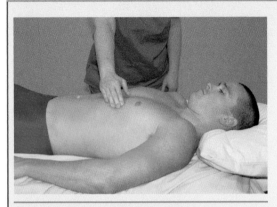

M Identify trigger/tender point (drag palpation).

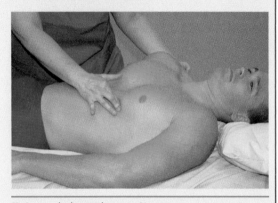

N Positional release (alternative 1).

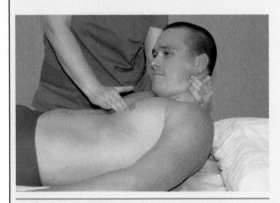

O Positional release (alternative 2).

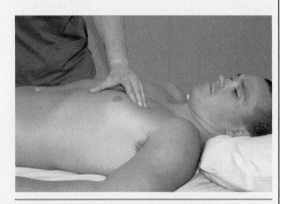

P Identify trigger/tender point.

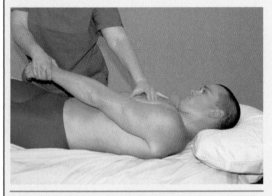

Q Positional release.

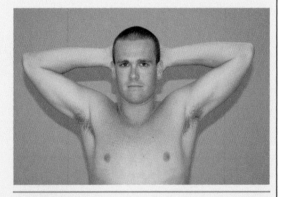

R Relief position 1.

FIGURE 20-4 CONT'D

ASSESSMENT AND TREATMENT OF BREATHING FUNCTION

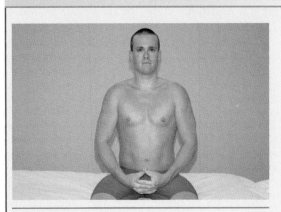

S Relief position 2.

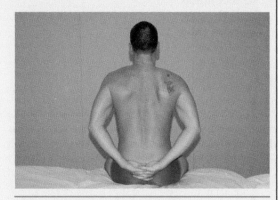

T Relief position 3.

- Observe and palpate for overuse of upper chest breathing muscles during normal relaxed breathing.
- Stand behind the client and place yours or the client's hands over the upper trapezius area so that the tips of the fingers rest on the top of the clavicles. As the client breathes, determine if he or she is using the accessory muscles during relaxed breathing.

If the shoulders move up and down as the client breathes it is likely that accessory muscles are being recruited. In normal relaxed breathing, the shoulders should not move up and down. The client is using accessory muscles to breathe if the chest movement is concentrated in the upper chest instead of the lower ribs and abdomen. Use of any of the accessory muscles for breathing results in an increase in tension and tendency for the development of trigger points. These situations can be identified by palpation. Connective tissue changes are common since this condition is often chronic. The connective tissues are palpated as thick, dense, and shortened in this area.

- Have client naturally inhale and exhale and observe for a consistent exhale that is longer than the inhale. Normal relaxed breathing consists of a shorter inhalation phase in relationship to a longer exhalation phase. The ratio of inhalation time to exhalation is one count inhale to four counts exhale. The reverse of this pattern is the basis for breathing pattern disorder.

The ideal pattern ranges from 2 to 4 counts during the inhale and from 8 to 16 counts for the exhale. Targeted massage and breathing retraining methods can be used to restore normal relaxed breathing.

- Have the client hold the breath without strain to assess for tolerance to carbon dioxide levels. The client should be able to comfortably hold the breath for at least 15 seconds, with 30 seconds being much better.
- Palpate and gently mobilize the thorax to assess for rib mobility. This is done with the client in the supine, prone, side-lying, and seated positions. The ribs should have a springy feel, and be a bit more mobile from the 6th to the 10th ribs.

TREATMENT PROCEDURES

The following muscles are specifically targeted by massage because they tend to shorten during breathing dysfunction.

Scalenes
Sternocleidomastoid
Serratus anterior
Serratus posterior superior and inferior
Levator scapulae
Rhomboids
Upper trapezius
Pectoralis major and minor

Latissimus dorsi
Psoas
Quadratus lumborum
All abdominals
Pelvic floor muscles
Calf muscles

The intercostals and diaphragm, which are the main breathing muscles, also will be addressed.

All of these muscles should be assessed for shortening, weakness, and agonist/antagonist interaction. Muscles that orient mostly transverse, such as the serratus anterior, serratus posterior superior and inferior, are rhomboids and are difficult to assess with movement and strength testing. Palpation will be more accurate. The typical patterns of the upper and lower crossed syndromes are often involved (Figure 20-5).

Muscles assessed as short need to be lengthened. If the primary cause of the shortening is neuromuscular, then use inhibitory pressure at the muscle belly and lengthen either by moving the adjacent joints, or more likely, by introducing tension, bend, or torsion force directly on the muscle tissues. For the scalenes, sternocleidomas-

toid, serratus anterior, pectoralis minor, latissimus dorsi, psoas, quadratus lumborum, diaphragm, rectus abdominis, and pelvic floor muscles, follow recommendations in the specific release section in Unit Two.

Work with each area as needed, as it becomes convenient during the general massage session. Use the least invasive measure possible to restore a more normal muscle resting length.

If the breathing has been dysfunctional for an extended period of time (more than 3 months) connective tissue changes are common. Focused connective tissue massage application is effective (see Unit Two).

Once the soft tissue is more normal, gentle mobilization of the thorax is appropriate. If the thoracic vertebrae and ribs are restricted, chiropractic or other joint manipulation methods may be appropriate and referral is indicated. The massage therapist can use indirect functional techniques to increase the mobility of the area as well. These methods are described in Unit Two.

Methods and sequences used to address the breathing function need to be integrated into a full-

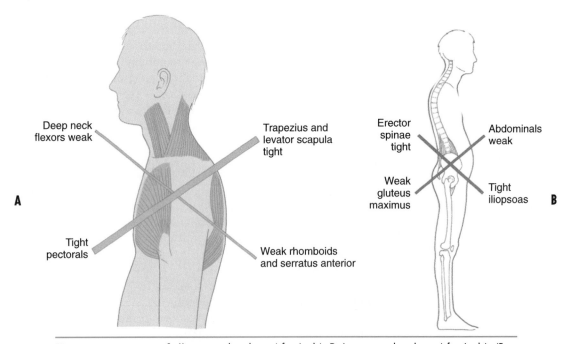

Deep neck flexors weak

Trapezius and levator scapula tight

Erector spinae tight

Abdominals weak

Weak gluteus maximus

Tight iliopsoas

A

Tight pectorals

Weak rhomboids and serratus anterior

B

FIGURE 20-5 ■ **A,** Upper crossed syndrome (after Janda). **B,** Lower crossed syndrome (after Janda). (From Chaitow L, DeLany J: *Clinical applications of neuromuscular techniques, vol 1, The upper body.* Edinburgh, 2001, Churchill Livingstone.)

body approach because breathing is a whole-body function. A possible protocol to add to the general massage session would be as follows:

- Give increased attention to general massage of the thorax; posterior, anterior, and lateral access to the thorax is used to primarily address the general tension or dysfunctional patterns in the respiratory muscles of this area. Address the scalenes, psoas, quadratus lumborum, and legs, especially the calves.
- Use appropriate muscle energy techniques to lengthen and stretch the shortened muscles of the cervical, thoracic, and lumbar regions, and legs.
- Gently move the rib cage with broad-based compression. Assess for areas that move easily and those that are restricted. Assess the anterior, lateral, and posterior areas.
- Identify the amount of rigidity in the ribs with the client supine by applying bilateral compression to the thorax, beginning near the clavicles and moving down toward the lower ribs, maintaining compressive force near the costal cartilage.
- Identify rigidity in the ribs with the client prone bilaterally (on both sides of the spine) at the facet joints, beginning near the seventh cervical vertebrae and moving down toward the lower ribs, maintaining compressive force near the facet joints.
- Use compression against the lateral aspect of the thorax with the client in a side-lying position to assess rib mobility in both facet and costal joints. Begin by applying compression near the axilla and then moving down toward the lower ribs. Sufficient force needs to be used while applying compression to feel the ribs spring but not so much to cause discomfort. Normal response is a feeling of equal mobility bilaterally. A feeling of stiffness or rigidity indicates immobility.

Identify the area of most mobility and the area of most restriction.

- Position the client so that a broad-based compressive force can be applied to the areas of ease—the most mobile
- Gently and slowly apply compression until the area begins to bind. Hold this position and have the client cough. Coughing will act as a muscle energy method and also support mobility of the joint through activation of the muscles. Repeat three or four times.

If areas of rigidity remain, the following intervention may be useful.

- Apply broad-based compression to the area of immobility, using the whole hand or forearm.
- Have the client exhale, and then increase the intensity of the compressive force while following the exhale.
- Hold the ribs in this position.
- Have the client push out against the compressive pressure.
- Instruct the client to inhale while continuing to hold the compressive focus against the ribs.
- Have the client exhale while following the action of the ribs. There should be an increase in mobility.
- Gently mobilize the entire thorax with rhythmic compression.

Reassess the area of most bind/restriction. If the area treated has improved, locate a different area and repeat the sequence. It is appropriate to do three or four areas in a session.

Next, palpate for tender points in the intercostals, pectoralis minor, and anterior serratus. (Clients are not very tolerant of this, so be direct and precise). Use positional release to treat these points by moving the client or having the client move into various positions until pain in the tender point decreases.

As a reminder, the procedure for positional release is as follows.

- Locate the tender point.
- Gently initiate the pain response with direct pressure. (Remember, the sensation of pain is a guide only.) The pain point is not the point of intervention.
- Slowly position the client's body, actively or passively, until the pain subsides. This position can be focal and accomplished by moving the client's ribs, arm, or head, or can be a whole-body process involving many different areas to achieve the position where there is a decrease in the pain.
- Have the client maintain the position for up to 30 seconds or until the client feels the release; while encouraging the client to breathe from the diaphragm, lightly monitoring the tender point with palpation.
- Slowly reposition the client to neutral, and then into a stretch, position for the tender point. Direct tissue stretching is usually most effective.

BREATHING RETRAINING PROGRAM

Once the thorax and breathing function begins to normalize–usually after four to six focused sessions–a breathing retraining program can be taught to clients. The main focus of a breathing retraining program is the exhale process. Do not even address the inhale. When the exhale pattern normalizes, the inhale pattern will as well. Three common activities can normalize a breathing pattern: yelling, crying, and laughing. Each of these activities sustained for 3 to 5 minutes can be valuable in any breathing retraining program.

Pursed lip exhale is helpful. The client inhales normally, holds the breath for 1 or 2 seconds, and then slowly exhales (as if gently trying to make a candle flame flicker about 1 foot away) by blowing the air through pursed lips.

Blowing up balloons can also be a good exercise supporting exhale function, as is playing a horn, flute, or similar musical instrument. Singing or chanting or simply toning the vowel sounds (a, e, i, o, u) are variations that support exhale function.

It is helpful for the client to combine a slow breathing pattern with a stretching/flexibility program that targets the short muscle areas. The client can also practice breath holding until the breath can be held comfortably for 30 seconds. Relief positions place the thorax in such a way to support normal, relaxed breathing or inhibit muscle function (see Figure 20-4).

SUMMARY

Illnesses and disorders are typically systemic and affect multiple body systems. Injury is more local. Injury, illness, and disorders interact. Clients that are injured are more apt to become ill. Those who have been or are ill are more susceptible to injury and thermoregulation problems. Those with disordered breathing are more prone to both injury and illness. Strain on adaptive capacity is the common thread here, and effective massage can at least temporarily reduce adaptive strain. Caution is necessary, however. Massage that is excessive for an individual client with a specific condition can add to adaptive strain. The skilled massage therapist should be able to balance the dynamics of appropriate or inappropriate massage application.

1 Describe a massage treatment plan that would be appropriate if the client had a viral respiratory infection.

_____
_____
_____
_____
_____

2 Describe a massage treatment plan that would NOT be appropriate if a client had suppressed immunity.

_____
_____
_____
_____
_____

3 Write a treatment plan for the following clients:

a. 23-year-old basketball player with a sinus infection.

_____
_____
_____
_____

b. 67-year-old male who has recently had a mild heart attack.

_____
_____
_____
_____

c. 19-year-old cheerleader with mononucleosis.

_____
_____
_____
_____

d. 27-year-old marathon runner, 24 hours post-event.

_____
_____
_____
_____
_____

e. 38-year-old deconditioned client playing tennis in heat and humidity.

_____
_____
_____
_____
_____

f. 44-year-old client with generalized anxiety and disrupted breathing, using exercise for both weight management and anxiety management.

_____
_____
_____
_____
_____

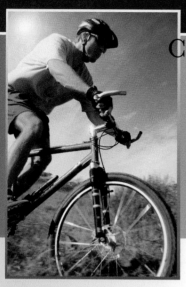

OBJECTIVES

Upon completion of this chapter, the reader will have the information necessary to:

1 Identify specific injuries based on location.

2 Develop and implement appropriate treatment plans for massage application for a specific injury.

Achilles bursitis
Achilles tendon rupture
Achilles tendinitis
Arthritis of the shoulder
Baker's cyst (popliteal cyst)
Biceps tendinitis
Black toenails
Blisters
Blowout fracture
Bo Jackson injury (avascular necrosis)
Bone chips
Boxer's wrist
Broken ankle
Broken cheekbone
Broken collarbone
Broken finger
Broken hand
Broken hip
Broken jaw
Broken neck
Broken nose
Broken patella
Broken rib
Broken toe
Bruised collarbone
Bruised quadriceps
Bruised ribs
Bulging disk
Bunion hallux valgus
"Burner" (stinger)
Bursitis
Buttock pull
Calf cramps
Calluses
Carpal tunnel syndrome
Cauliflower ear
Cervical stenosis
Cluster headaches
Compartment syndrome
Concussion
Cracked back
Cracked wing
Cruciate ligament injury
Short-leg syndrome
Dislocated finger
Dislocated knee
Dislocated patella
Dislocated shoulder

Dislocation of the peroneal tendons
Femur fracture
Fracture of the shoulder
Frozen shoulder (adhesive capsulitis)
Ganglion
Golfer's wrist
Groin pull
Hamstring pull
Headache
Heel spur
Heel stress syndrome
Hip pointer
Hyperextended elbow
Iliotibial band syndrome
Impingement syndrome
Jammed finger
Jumper's knee
Leg muscle pulls and tears
Little League elbow
Loose body
Metatarsal stress fracture
Metatarsalgia
Morton's foot
Morton's syndrome
Osgood-schlatter disease
Osteitis pubis
Osteoarthritis/arthrosis
Pain on the outside of the leg
Partial dislocation of the shoulder
Patellofemoral syndrome
Pes cavus (claw foot)
Pinched nerve
Pitcher's elbow
Plantar fasciitis
Pre-patellar bursitis
Pro's rotator cuff injury
Pronating foot
Psoas low-back pain
Quadriceps pull or tear
Quadratus lumborum pain
Quadriplasia
Midback pain
Lumbar pain
Mass reflex
Migraine headache
Paraplasia
Racquet wrist
Rib muscle pull or tear

Rib separation
Rotator cuff tear
Ruptured disk
Scaphoid fracture
Sciatica
Scratched cornea
Stretched nerve
Quadriplegia
Shin splints
Shoulder muscle pulls (strains)
Shoulder separation
Shoulder sprains
Ski pole thumb
Skull fractures
Spastic torticollis
Spinal cord injuries
Spondylolysis
Sports hernia/athletic pubalgia
Sprained finger
Sprained knee
Sprained neck
Sprained thumb
Sprained wrist
"Stinger" ("burner")
Stress fracture
Supinating foot
Tendinitis of the shoulder
Tendinitis of the wrist
Tennis elbow
Tennis leg
Tension headache
Terrible Triad of O'Donohue
Tibialis anterior tendon sheath inflammation
Tibialis posterior syndrome
Tibial stress syndrome
TMJ injury
Toe tendinitis
Torn biceps
Torn cartilage (in the knee)
Torn tendon
Trapezius triggers
Triceps tendinitis
Trigger finger
Turf toe
Weight lifter's shoulder
Whiplash

The previous chapters have prepared the reader to assess the indication (or contraindication) for massage therapy in cases of injury, illness, and disorders and to provide appropriate intervention. Typically the client will come to the massage therapist with an injury diagnosis. A massage treatment plan is then developed as part of a multidisciplinary care approach. This chapter enables the massage therapist to understand the physician's diagnosis, provides guidance for effective treatment, and discusses the injury in relation to its body region.

If massage therapy is appropriate as treatment or as an adjunct to treatment, the reader is referred to a section in a previous chapter outlining appropriate procedures. Occasionally a more expansive discussion is presented here, with specific strategies for the particular injury.

It is the responsibility of the massage therapist treating a client with an injury to thoroughly research the specific injury, understand the treatments being used by the medical team, and provide appropriate supportive care during the healing and rehabilitation process.

The massage applications recommended for a specific condition can be incorporated into the general massage session protocol described in Unit Two.

THE HEAD

Because the head houses all of the body's vital control centers, any injury to the head other than a mild bump or scrape should be seen by a physician. Head injuries should be monitored for at least 2 weeks because some conditions worsen slowly. Consider head injuries to be serious unti proven otherwise because they can be life-threatening.

CONCUSSION

A **concussion** is any disorientation or loss of consciousness, even for a moment, after a blow to the head. The brain floats within the skull surrounded by cerebrospinal fluid, which cushions it from the light bounces of everyday movement. However, the fluid is not able to absorb the force of a sudden blow or a quick stop, and it slides forcefully against the inner wall of the skull and becomes bruised. This can result in bleeding in or around the brain and tearing of nerve fibers. It is common for a person who suffered a concussion not to remember the events just before, during, and immediately after the injury. Memory of these events may return. Following recovery, however, cognitive function almost always returns to normal, although repeated concussions (even if mild) can result in minimal brain damage.

A serious aftermath of a concussion is a condition known as *second impact syndrome*. This can occur when a person who is still recovering from a concussion returns to a contact sport or activity or has recurrent head trauma. A seemingly minor trauma or bump on the head in these individuals can lead to devastating swelling of the brain, which may prove fatal.

Head trauma can result in various types of closed head injuries. The impaired functions depend on the area of brain injury. Any change in typical behavior or ability in a person who has suffered head trauma should be closely monitored.

More than 300,000 athletes suffer concussions each year. There is no way to predict which athletes are likely to suffer concussions. The severity of a concussion depends on how much force is applied to the head and whether the blow is head-on or glancing.

People who wear helmets, which absorb shock, will probably have milder concussions than those who do not. Advances in the design of protective headgear are helping to prevent head trauma and reduce the severity of a concussion. Although protective equipment continues to improve in quality, many athletes participate in high-impact sports activities, such as soccer, or sports in which head trauma can result from falling, such gymnastics, or the many sports in which head protection is not required. Therefore, concussions are an ongoing concern and repeated head trauma can have cumulative effects. Previous head trauma seems to make a person more predisposed to future problems.

The signs and symptoms of concussions can be subtle and may not immediately appear. Once present, symptoms can last for days, weeks, or longer. The severity and side effects of a head injury depend greatly on which area of the brain was most affected.

Immediate signs and symptoms of a concussion may include:

Confusion
Amnesia
Headache
Loss of consciousness after injury
Ringing in the ears (tinnitus)
Drowsiness
Nausea
Vomiting
Unequal pupil size
Unusual eye movements
Convulsions
Slurred speech

Delayed signs and symptoms may include:

Irritability
Headaches
Depression
Sleep disturbances
Fatigue
Personality changes
Poor concentration
Trouble with memory
Getting lost or becoming easily confused
Increased sensitivity to sounds, lights, and distractions
Loss of sense of taste or smell
Difficulty with gait or in coordination of the limbs

When diagnosing a concussion, the doctor may ask questions about the accident and may conduct a neurologic examination to assess memory, concentration, vision, hearing, balance, coordination, and reflexes. Depending on the results of the neurological examination, the doctor may request a computed tomography (CT) scan or a magnetic resonance imaging (MRI) scan.

Rest is the best recovery technique. Some over-the-counter and prescription drugs may be taken for headache pain. Aspirin and other non-steroidal antiinflammatory drugs (NSAIDs) are usually not recommended because they could contribute to bleeding. The healing process takes time—sometimes several months—and includes:

- Plenty of sleep at night, and rest during the day.
- Gradual return to normal activities.
- Avoiding activities that could result in a second head injury.

After a concussion, some symptoms may persist, including headache, dizziness, loss of memory of the event, fatigue, and general weakness. This is called *postconcussion syndrome.* In some people, these symptoms clear up and they feel fine, but the symptoms recur when they become active again. If these symptoms persist, the athlete should be reevaluated by the physician. No athlete should return to heavy physical activity until the symptoms clear completely.

Returning to athletic activity depends on the cumulative effects of the concussions. The following time frames are typical:

First concussion—7 days or until all postconcussion symptoms clear, whichever is longer.
Second concussion—3 weeks or until symptoms cease.
Third concussion—up to 6 months.

Massage Strategies

Massage, if approved by the physician, should be general and nonspecific. Avoid any abrupt movements of the head. The focus of the massage should be sleep support and recovery (parasympathetic dominance). Once the athlete is allowed to practice, gait patterns and ocular reflexes need to be reset. The massage therapist should maintain vigilant observation for any post-concussion symptoms and should urge the athlete to see the physician for even minor symptoms.

SKULL FRACTURES

A hard blow to the head can fracture the bones of the skull. Although not common, **skull fractures**

do occur, and a severe blow to the head can cause a fracture. Blood or clear fluid leaking from the ear or nose may be a sign of a skull fracture. This is a medical emergency— refer the client to a physician immediately.

A depressed skull bone from a fracture may put pressure on the brain or tear blood vessels in the lining of the skull, causing bleeding on the brain. The pressure and bleeding can cause coma and even death if not relieved.

Massage Strategies

Massage is not applicable in these cases.

BROKEN NOSE

A blow to the nose can fracture the nasal bones or the cartilage of the septum. A **broken nose** appears flattened or crooked, there is copious bleeding from the nose, and breathing is difficult.

If a broken nose is suspected, it should be iced down to limit swelling and bruising. The nose needs to be examined and x-rayed by a physician. If the broken bone has been displaced, it can cause later breathing problems if not repaired. Following treatment, the nose should be protected with a splint and/or a face guard until it heals completely, which can take 4 to 6 weeks.

Massage Strategies

Massage is general and nonspecific, avoids injured areas, manages pain, and promotes healing. The prone position may need to be avoided. Because of disrupted breathing, auxiliary breathing muscles may become strained. Include focus on normalized breathing in the general massage protocol. Use general procedures for fractures, broken bones, breathing support, and pain management.

BROKEN CHEEKBONE

A hard blow to the cheek can fracture the bone. The same athletes who are prone to broken nose may also be prone to a **broken cheekbone.** Treatment includes icing the cheek and possibly surgery. Healing may take several weeks.

Massage Strategies

Do NOT massage the area. Focus on pain management and support healing by encouraging parasympathetic dominance. The prone position should be avoided. See general procedures for fractures (see page 472).

BLOWOUT FRACTURE

A blow to the eye or cheek can fracture the bones surrounding the eyeball. A **blowout fracture** is easy to spot, as the orbit connects to one of the sinuses. When the client blows hard through the nose, the eye will suddenly swell shut as air gets into the tissues right under the eye. As with any fracture, the victim of a blowout fracture must see a doctor for treatment, which may include surgery. If the fractured orbit is displaced, as often happens, it can trap one of the eye muscles, and the eye won't move properly, causing double vision unless surgically corrected.

Massage Strategies

Massage avoids the area, and the prone position is not used. See general procedure for broken bones and pain management. Once the athlete has recovered, eye reflexes may need to be addressed.

SCRATCHED CORNEA

A **scratched cornea** commonly occurs when a person gets poked in the eye. Direct blows to the eye from a ball in sports such as racquetball can cause a scratched cornea as well as a variety of other injuries. This is an extremely painful injury. If severe, it can lead to loss of vision. Every eye injury must be considered serious. Treatment includes covering the eye with a patch and examination by a physician as soon as possible.

To guard their eyes, many athletes now wear protective gear, especially if they have already had an eye injury.

Massage Strategies

Massage supports pain management and healing by encouraging parasympathetic dominance.

CAULIFLOWER EAR

If an unprotected ear is bent over, punched, or caught in a wrestling hold, the cartilage in the ear can break. Bleeding occurs under the skin, and if the blood is not drained, scar tissue will form and the ear will look somewhat like a cauliflower—hence the name **cauliflower ear.**

Medical treatment includes ice and compression to the ear to limit bleeding, and having the excess blood drained from the ear by a physician.

Massage Strategies

Massage supports healing and avoids the area. Once healing is in the subacute phase, scar tissue management can begin.

BROKEN JAW

Symptoms of a **broken jaw** include pain on one side of the jaw and pain inhibiting the ability to clench the jaw. If the jaw can be closed, the teeth will not meet properly.

A broken jaw must be wired shut by a dental surgeon to allow it to heal, which typically takes about 6 weeks. Many athletes can compete with their jaws wired shut, but their diet is limited to liquids taken through a straw, which can result in weight and strength loss.

Massage Strategies

Use massage strategies for fractures.

TMJ INJURY AND PAIN

A blow to the jaw can injure the temporomandibular joint (TMJ). The ligaments may become torn, causing the joint to slide in and out of place. The jaw may become stuck in an open position, requiring manipulation by an oral surgeon to close it. This injury usually heals within 6 to 8 weeks, but a mouthpiece may be necessary to hold the jaw in position until the ligaments heal.

Preventing **TMJ injury** is one of the reasons athletes wear mouthpieces. The mouthpiece protects the jaw and teeth and disperses the shock from a blow. However, sustained biting down on the mouthpiece can cause pain and shortening in the muscles of mastication, causing TMJ pain.

Massage Strategies

Massage for TMJ pain targets the muscles of mastication. The muscles most effectively massaged for TMJ pain are the masseter, temporalis, and sternocleidomastoid. Muscle shortening, trigger point activity, and connective tissue bind can all occur. Intraoral muscles are not easily accessed for massage application but can be worked if necessary.

Wearing a glove, access the pterygoids and masseter, using a pinching technique. Instruct the client to exhale slowly through the open mouth immediately beforehand, which can reduce the gag reflex. Referral to a TMJ specialist may be required.

The general protocol used on the head, neck, and face is usually effective for addressing simple TMJ pain.

HEADACHE

Headache is a common symptom with a multitude of causes. Headaches can be caused by stress, muscle tension, biochemical imbalance, circulatory and sinus disorders, and tumors. Because the brain has no sensory innervation, headaches do not originate in the brain. The pain of a headache is produced by pressure on the sensory nerves, vessels, meninges, or muscle-tendon-bone unit. All headaches should be evaluated by a physician to rule out serious underlying conditions.

Migraine headache is believed to be caused by dilation of the cranial vessels. The pain is knifelike, throbbing, and unilateral. Any visual distortion (e.g., flashing lights) is believed to be caused by vasoconstriction preceding the vasodilation and pain.

Medications used to treat headaches are usually NSAIDs such as aspirin, but migraines may not respond to medication after the headache begins. Migraines sometimes may be prevented by the medication ergotamine (a vasoconstrictor) or other vasoconstricting medication. The judicious use of caffeine may reduce migraine symptoms. On the other hand, caffeine withdrawal also causes a vascular type headache.

Cluster headaches occur on one side of the head, with remissions and recurrence lasting for long periods. They usually occur at night and are associated with other symptoms, such as red eyes and sinus drainage.

A tension or muscle contraction headache is the most common headache type. **Tension headache** is believed to be caused by a muscle-tendon strain at the origin of the trapezius and deep neck muscles at the occipital bone or at the origin of the frontalis muscle on the frontal bone (*occipital* or *frontal headaches*). Tension headache also can originate in the TMJ muscle complex. Connective tissue structures that support the head may be implicated in headache if they are shortened and pull the head or scalp into nerves, creating pain. Conversely, if connective tissue support structures are lax and fail to support the neck and head, nerve structures may be compressed as well.

The treatment for most headaches is NSAIDs such as aspirin and ibuprofen. Frequent use of headache medications can cause a rebound headache pattern and should be used only if other methods fail.

Headaches are common in all people; however predisposing factors for headaches in athletes include:

- Head gear that puts pressure on pain-sensitive structures
- Squinting under bright lights or in the sun
- Dehydration
- Blood flow changes
- Competition stress and let-down
- Overbreathing tendency
- Blood sugar changes
- Impact trauma that increases neck muscle tension

Symptoms of Vascular or Fluid Pressure Headache

This headache type includes sinus, migraine, cluster, caffeine withdrawal, and toxic headaches. Pain is experienced as ache/pressure from the inside of the head pushing out. The head may feel like it will blow up. This headache type is difficult to manage with massage.

Symptoms of Muscle/Connective Tissue/Tension Headache

This headache type includes referred pain headache from trigger point activity or nerve impingement, muscle tension, and muscle guarding. Pain is experienced as pressure from the outside of the head pushing in and may feel like a tight band around the head. This headache type is effectively managed with massage.

Massage Strategies

21-1   Massage and other forms of soft tissue therapy are effective in treating muscle tension headaches but much less effective for migraine headaches and cluster headaches. Soft tissue therapy can relieve secondary muscle tension headache caused by the pain of the primary headache. Headache is often stress-induced. Stress management in all forms usually is indicated for chronic headache conditions. Massage and other forms of soft tissue therapy are effective in treating muscle tension headaches (Figure 21-1).

The following two massage strategies are effective for headaches.

Vascular/Fluid Pressure Headaches   Approach the massage as if there is excessive fluid in the skull and the goal of the massage is to help get the fluid out of the skull. Rhythmic compression on the head and face can act like a pump to move the fluid.

- Use broad-based compressive force on the head. The sensation felt by the client should be a pleasant relief from the pressure inside the head.
- Place your flat hands or forearm on the occipital bone/frontal bone and press firmly together. Then release. Rhythmically and slowly repeat up to 50 repetitions.

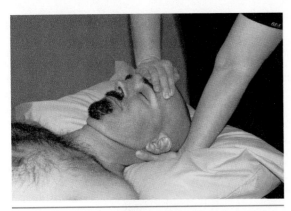

FIGURE 21-1 ■ Massage is effective in treating headaches.

• Repeat again, but with pressure applied at the temporal bones.

If the pain is more in the face, as in a sinus headache, the location of the rhythmic compression is also applied at the temples (sphenoid), cheeks (zygmatic), and side of the nose and over the eyes.

• Use either the palm of the hand or pads of the fingers.
• When applying pressure over the eyes, do not actually press the eyeball but cup it in the palm and apply pressure around it.

Often a tension headache accompanies a vascular headache.

Muscle/Connective Tissue/Tension Headache To treat tension headache, use inhibitory pressure on the muscles of the scalp—the occipital/frontalis, temporalis, and auricular (ear) muscles. Muscle energy and positional release methods are effective.

• Instruct the client to move the eyebrows, clench the teeth, and move the ears.
• Massage the entire muscle area, with special attention to both the belly and attachments. Pressure levels should be intense enough to recreate the headache symptoms. This is significantly more pressure than is typically used during general relaxation massage. The intensity should not cause guarding, and, while painful, it should be a "good" hurt.
• Nerve impingement by the suboccipital, scalene, sternocleidomastoid, and trapezius muscles can cause referred pain. Use inhibiting pressure with muscle energy and lengthening procedures on the muscles that create the headache symptoms.

Headaches more in the area of the face can arise from the muscles of mastication or those that control eyebrow movement. They are addressed as previously described.

The scalp has a significant amount of connective tissue structures. The tendons and fascial anchoring bands of the scalp (Figure 21-2) can shorten. Usually the forces applied during massage on these structures are shear and bend with localized tension force. As in any connective tissue application, the forces are applied slowly and rhythmically, into and out of bind. Again, this level of intensity is more than typically used during general massage, and both pressure and location should feel "right" to the client (Figure 21-3).

If possible, stretch muscles and connective tissue by pulling the hair.

• Grasp a large bundle of hair near the scalp and exert an even, firm pull.
• At the point of resistance, shift the direction into and out of bind.
• Repeat the process sequentially all over the scalp. This should feel intense but good to the client.
• If the client has no hair or very short hair, roll and twist the scalp around the skull, into and out of bind. Next, firmly massage along all cranial sutures with circular type friction.

Eye muscles can be a factor in headache pain.

• Have the client place his or her finger pads over the closed eyelids, and with the massage therapist's fingers on top of the client's fingers, exert gentle pressure on the eyeballs.
• While maintaining the compression, the client moves the eyes in alternating circles and a figure-of-eight pattern.

Thoroughly massage the neck and shoulder muscles, addressing any areas responsible for the headache symptoms.

The connective tissue structures from the skull to the sacrum, if short, can create headache. These structures need to be addressed to increase tissue pliability and reduce bind. Connective tissue methods generating mechanical forces and skin rolling approaches with sufficient drag from the scalp down the midline of the back to the sacrum are effective. Begin at the head and end at the sacrum, then reverse direction and begin at the sacrum and end at the head.

Additional approaches for treatment of headache of both types include reflexology, especially at the big toe, and acupressure.

Headaches may be caused by constipation. Abdominal massage is an option. A toxic headache

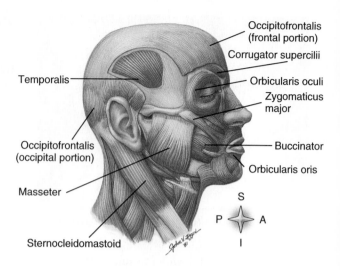

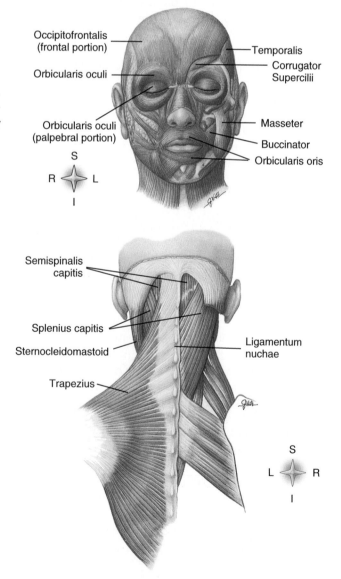

FIGURE 21-2 ■ Connective tissue: Tendon and anchoring bands of the scalp. (From Thibodeau GA, Patton KT: *Anatomy and physiology*, ed 5. St. Louis, 2003, Mosby.)

FIGURE 21-3

EXAMPLES OF MASSAGE FOR HEADACHE

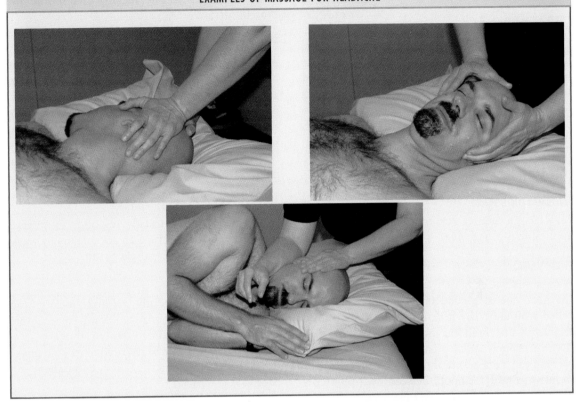

from chemicals such as monosodium glutamate (MSG) or from excessive alcohol consumption will often respond to hydration and the strategy for vascular headache. However, until the liver detoxifies the substance and it is cleared from the body, the headache will persist.

A menthol- or peppermint-based cooling counterirritant ointment applied to the base of the neck and temples and forehead is effective for all headache types. Essential oils can be placed on cotton balls and put in plastic bags for the client to smell. Sinus headaches tend to respond to eucalyptus. Tension headaches respond to peppermint and lavender, and toxic headaches to citrus (lemons, orange, limes). If the headache is a migraine type, using various aromas may make the headache better or may make it worse. Their use should be guided by the client's reaction.

The massage therapist needs to know if the client has been taking medications for headaches and adjust massage accordingly.

Self-Help for Headaches

Vascular (inside the head) type headache responds to external compression, such as wrapping a towel or Ace bandage tightly around the head, wearing a tight hat, or a placing a weight on the top of the head, such as rice bag.

Muscle tension headache responds to compression of the muscles. As silly as this may sound and look, putting a plastic clothes hanger over the head on the muscles that are creating the symptoms relieves the pain somewhat. Areas of the hanger that poke should be padded. A sand or rice bag also works.

THE NECK

Neck injuries are serious. The neck is much less stable and much more prone to injury than the rest of the spine. Because the neck must be tremendously mobile to allow the head to swivel, the range of motion between the vertebrae in the neck is much greater than in the lower spine. Also, neck muscles are smaller and weaker than those in the lower back, where the strongest muscles in the body support the spine.

Do NOT move a person with a neck injury. An injury can turn into a disaster if the neck isn't properly stabilized. Moving a fractured neck can cut the spinal cord. Call emergency medical personnel for help immediately.

SPRAINED NECK

Ligaments hold the vertebrae together, and those ligaments can be stretched or ruptured, often by the head snapping backward. The result is a **sprained neck.** If the injury is severe, a vertebra may slide forward out of place and compress the spinal cord—the same injury as a fracture. If the sprain is mild, there will be pain and stiffness in the neck area. Anything more severe than a mild sprain should be seen by a physician.

Massage Strategies

Massage procedures for sprains and strains are applicable (see page 458).

WHIPLASH

A combination of muscle and ligament strains on the neck due to a sudden, violent movement is called **whiplash.** The neck muscles, as well as the ligaments that hold the bones of the neck, can become severely strained and sprained.

This can be a severe injury that takes up to 6 months to heal. It should be seen by a physician and x-rayed to make sure that the vertebrae in the neck have not slipped out of alignment or become fractured.

The treatment for whiplash is rest for 2or 3 days, followed by physical rehabilitation. Antiinflammatory drugs can help to ease the discomfort. The client may need to wear a cervical collar, which supports the weight of the head and takes the strain off the ligaments.

Massage Strategies

Massage therapy is beneficial following acute, subacute, and remodeling healing stages. Common errors when treating these cases include (1) being overly aggressive with the neck during the acute/subacute healing phase and (2) failing to realize that this phase may last for up to 2 weeks.

In addition to the general massage application during the subacute and remodeling stages, it is appropriate to work with the oculopelvic reflexes, firing patterns, and gait reflexes. During whiplash, as with concussion, the eye muscles are affected during the impact.

Pain management is an important goal, and energy-based applications are very comforting. Cradling the neck in the hands and applying a gentle compression with the intention of supporting circulation and healing feels very good to the client. Gentle rhythmic rocking can soothe the muscle spasms.

PINCHED NERVE

An injury that seems like a sprain but is more complex is a **pinched nerve.** This can happen when a cervical disk ruptures or degenerates. Commonly, when a disk ruptures, gel-like material from inside the disk presses on a nearby nerve and causes sharp pain that extends down into the arm. There may be a sudden onset of severe pain in the neck, or the pain may develop gradually.

Any athlete who makes fairly violent neck motions is prone to this injury.

A pinched nerve usually responds to cervical traction for 2 to 6 weeks, with accompanying physical therapy to reduce muscle spasm.

Massage Strategies

Gentle massage, especially rhythmic rocking, can help reduce muscle spasm. However, if severe symptoms persist, particularly in the arm and the hand, surgery may be required to repair damage to the disk. See massage for entrapment on page 477.

BROKEN NECK

The most serious neck injury is damage to the cervical vertebrae in the neck; this is commonly called a **broken neck.** Each year a few football players, from the high school level on up to the professionals, suffer spinal cord injuries, such as a broken neck, that leave them quadriplegics. However, the most common cause of a broken neck is diving. Skiers, gymnasts, and skaters are also prone to this type of neck injury.

A head-on blow may cause a compression fracture of the neck, in which the force to the top of the head compresses and shatters some of the cervical vertebrae. This injury may be as mild as a simple chipping of the vertebrae or it may cause compression or severing of the spinal cord.

An equally severe injury can occur from a blow when the neck is bent down. This is more common in football, where a tackler ducks his head as he makes contact.

Massage Strategies

See the section entitled Spinal Cord Injuries for massage strategies applicable to treatment of a broken neck.

CERVICAL STENOSIS

Athletes who have recurrent, short episodes of numbness or weakness in the arms and hands may have a narrowed spinal canal. This condition is called **cervical stenosis.** An MRI scan will show a narrowing of the cervical canal, which is the area from the base of the skull to the shoulder. The symptoms of numbness or weakness may occur after relatively mild trauma to the neck, because the spinal cord does not have adequate room in the canal to begin with.

Massage Strategies

Focus massage on maintaining as much soft tissue pliability as possible without reducing stability. Do not move the neck to the ends of range of motion. Stay in midrange.

"BURNER," "STINGER," AND STRETCHED NERVES

Two nerve injuries to the neck feel the same at first. Both are caused by a blow to the head or neck, and both cause burning pain down the arm and weakness in the arm and hand. One, a **"burner"** or **"stinger,"** is a simple injury, but the other, a **stretched nerve,** is a serious injury that requires rehabilitation.

A "burner", or "stinger," is characterized by sudden burning pain down one arm, which feels weak. This is due to a pinched nerve in the neck. Usually the pain disappears, and full strength in the arm returns within 5 minutes. It is very important to know which side of the head was hit and on which side the pain is felt. If a blow is received to the left side of the head, the head will be knocked toward the right shoulder (and vice versa), and a burning pain will be felt down the right arm. The pain results from the nerve being pinched as vertebrae in the neck flex sharply to the right. When the athlete's arm strength recovers, he or she can return to full activity. There will usually be muscle guarding in the area, which presents as a stiff neck. Massage should be cautious, allowing the guarding to reduce slowly over a few days.

A similar but more dangerous injury, a stretched nerve in the brachial plexus, has almost the same symptoms. If the blow is to the left side of the head, the head is knocked toward the right shoulder, and the pain is felt down the left arm. This is because the nerve is being stretched on the left side of the neck as the head is pushed to the right. In this injury, however, the pain and weakness persist. This is a serious injury that must be treated by the medical team. Recovery of full strength may take weeks.

Strong neck muscles may help prevent these types of injuries. Protective equipment is sometimes used to prevent excessive neck motion.

The athlete should not return to action without the doctor's approval. An early return may reinjure the nerves and cause permanent damage.

Massage Strategies

Be cautious when applying massage around the injured area. Pressure on nerves, especially the injured nerves, is contraindicated and tends to further irritate the area. Do not use any methods that increase pain. Massage is focused on assisting the return to normal of the protective muscle guarding while avoiding the injured nerves.

SPASTIC TORTICOLLIS

Wryneck, or **spastic torticollis,** is caused by a pulled muscle or muscle spasm. The neck will not turn equally in both directions (left and right). When turning the neck in one direction, the movement is restricted and painful. Pain occurs on one side of the neck, and the neck may be pulled over slightly to that side. It's particularly painful to turn the head in the direction of the pain. That is, if the pain is on the left side of the neck, the client can turn to the right but not to the left. This type of injury can happen in sports such as tennis, when the player looks up while serving the ball or hits an overhead smash.

Treatment consists of an ice application for 20 minutes at a time, with gentle stretching of the neck. If the pain is severe, medications such as a muscle relaxer or NSAID may be prescribed.

Massage Strategies

Massage application, in addition to the general protocol, typically focuses on the sternocleidomastoid muscle that is spasmodic, with one overpowering the other (the one that is shorter is the stronger). Treat as for spasm. If the condition persists longer than 2 to 4 days, more aggressive work is appropriate. See sternocleidomastoid release in Unit Two.

TRAPEZIUS TRIGGERS

Severe muscle spasm in a localized area of the neck can cause **trapezius triggers.** Symptoms include a very painful area at the base of the neck or extending out above the collarbone. Any athlete can suffer this injury by pulling fibers in the trapezius muscle or as a result of a direct blow to the muscle fibers in the neck.

The muscle spasm sets up the pain-spasm-pain cycle: the spasm causes nerves to fire and gives the sensation of pain; this electrical impulse causes other nerve fibers to fire and the muscle to contract further.

Very severe pain may require injection of cortisone and Novocain into the area.

Massage Strategies

Treatment includes icing the neck for 20 minutes followed by massage and gentle stretching. Use the muscle spasm procedure beginning on p. 447.

Very severe pain may require an injection of cortisone and Novocain into the area.

SPINAL CORD INJURIES

Spinal cord injuries can result in a number of neurologic problems. Studies of blood flow and metabolism indicate that spinal cord injury involves not only direct neuronal trauma but also direct and delayed vascular trauma. The most frequently injured sites are at the most mobile segments of the spine, such as the cervicothoracic (C7 to T1) and the thoracolumbar (T12 to L1–L4) junctions. About 40% of spinal cord injuries result in complete function interruption. The remaining 60% result in the impairment or destruction of certain sensory and motor functions.

Injury to the spinal cord is followed by a 2- to 3-week period of spinal shock in which all spinal reflex responses are depressed. The spinal reflexes below the cut become exaggerated and hyperactive. The neurons become hypersensitive to the excitatory neurotransmitters, and the spinal neurons may grow collaterals that synapse with excitatory input. The stretch reflexes are exaggerated and the tone of the muscle increases.

If spinal cord injury occurs above the third cervical spinal nerve, loss of voluntary movements of all four limbs occurs, This is known as **quadriplegia.** If the lesion is lower, and only the lower limbs are affected, the condition is called **paraplegia.** Should the nerves to only one limb be affected, the condition is referred to as **monoplegia.**

Respiratory movements are affected if the phrenic nerve arising from the 3rd, 4th, or 5th cervical nerve to supply the diaphragm is affected.

One of the complications common among persons with spinal cord injuries is decubitus ulcer. Because voluntary shifting of weight does not occur, the weight of the body compresses the circulation to the skin over bony prominences and produces ulcers.

Fluctuations in blood pressure can occur. Because of disuse, calcium from bones is reabsorbed and excreted in the urine, increasing the incidence of calcium stones in the urinary tract.

Paralysis of the muscles of the urinary bladder results in stagnation of urine and urinary tract infection.

Connective tissue changes occur in the muscles and joints. The function of the autonomic nervous system below the level of the lesion is affected. Voluntary control of the bladder and rectum is lost if the lesion is above the sacral segments; reflex contractions of the bladder and rectum occur as soon as they become full, resulting in incontinence.

In the **mass reflex,** which occurs with severe spinal cord injury, a slight stimulus to the skin triggers emptying of the bladder and rectum, sweating below the level of the lesion, and blood pressure changes. Persons with chronic spinal injuries can be trained to initiate these reflexes by stroking or pinching the thigh to trigger the mass reflex, thereby giving them some control over urination and defecation.

Circulating blood volume, sweat production, and skin surface area—all factors necessary for effective heat transfer to the environment—are affected in spinal cord injuries, and this can impair the ability to stay cool during sustained exercise training. The physiologic responses to exercise, especially in the heat, of people with spinal cord injury differ from normal responses and depend on the level and completeness of the lesion.

The extent to which the circulation is affected depends on the level and severity (incomplete or complete) of the spinal cord lesion. Figure 21-4 identifies the levels of spinal cord injury. In a complete lesion above the 6th thoracic vertebra (T6), the sympathetic regulation of the heart is affected; the heart rate remains low, and the myocardial contractile force is impaired. The distribution of blood below the level of the lesion is impaired because of lack of vasoconstriction in the internal organs of the abdomen and the pelvis; this diminishes the redistribution of blood during exercise. In addition, blood flow in muscles and skin, as well as sweat gland activity in the affected skin, below the lesion is impaired.

A complete lesion between T6 and T10 will not affect cardiac function. However, sympathetic vasoconstriction in the abdominal and pelvic

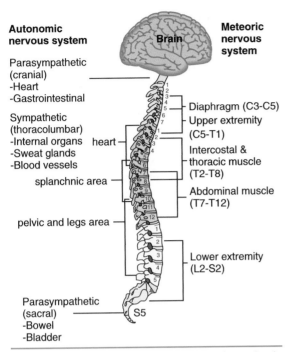

Autonomic nervous system

Parasympathetic
(cranial)
-Heart
-Gastrointestinal

Sympathetic
(thoracolumbar)
-Internal organs
-Sweat glands
-Blood vessels

splanchnic area

pelvic and legs area

Parasympathetic
(sacral)
-Bowel
-Bladder

Brain

heart

S5

Meteoric nervous system

Diaphragm (C3-C5)
Upper extremity
(C5-T1)
Intercostal & thoracic muscle
(T2-T8)
Abdominal muscle
(T7-T12)

Lower extremity
(L2-S2)

FIGURE 21-4 ■ Levels of possible injury to the spinal cord.

organs is absent below such a lesion. The regulation of the sweat glands and blood flow to the muscles and skin below the lesion is impaired.

With a complete lesion at or below T10, there is a loss of the central regulation of vasoconstriction in the pelvic area, diminished blood flow in the legs (muscles and skin), and reduced activity of the sweat glands below the lesion.

Massage Strategies

Therapy following spinal cord injuries is managed by the medical team. If massage is used, the massage for fractures sequence is appropriate, combined with general full-body massage. However, caution is advisable concerning pressure levels and intensity.

Massage is an effective part of a comprehensive, supervised rehabilitation and long-term care program. Massage can help manage secondary muscle tension resulting from the alteration of posture and the use of equipment such as wheelchairs, braces, and crutches. Specifically focused massage on the abdomen can help manage difficulties with bowel paralysis. Circulation enhancement by massage can assist in the management of a decubitus ulcer.

The functioning areas of the body can become stressed by compensating for areas that have reduced function. Do NOT assume that paralysis equals no feeling in the area. This totally depends on the area of the break, the type of break, the extent of damage to the spinal cord, and the body's adaptive capacity, as well as the type of medical treatment and rehabilitation received following injury. Because there are so many variables, it is imperative for the massage therapist to communicate effectively with the client and medical team in order to understand the effects of the injury and then adjust the general protocol to meet the needs of the client.

THE ANTERIOR TORSO

The thorax, or chest, includes the area between the neck and thoracic diaphragm. The primary function is breathing and protection of vital organs. Core stability influences torso stability and protects abdominal contents.

The ribs act like the bars of a cage to protect the lungs and heart from blows, and they help the chest wall expand and collapse so that air can move through the lungs.

The ribs do not attach directly to the breastbone in the front. If they did, the rib cage would be so rigid that breathing would be restricted. Flexible cartilage connects the end of each rib to the breastbone.

BRUISED RIBS

A blow to an unprotected rib cage can bruise the ribs. The treatment for **bruised ribs** is to rest them and apply ice until the pain is gone. Athletes can wear a protective pad made of strong plastic with an absorbent material underneath. It hangs on the shoulders and wraps around the rib cage.

Massage Strategies

Massage is contraindicated in the area of the bruise. Lymphatic drain methods are appropriate. See massage strategies for separated ribs in the following section.

SEPARATED RIBS

A severe blow can cause a **rib separation,** in which the rib tears loose from the cartilage.

There is severe pain, usually toward the front of the rib cage, and it "hurts to breathe." When the person bends over or rotates the body, there may be the feeling of a "pop." It is particularly painful to go from a lying to a sitting position, such as when getting out of bed in the morning. If you place one hand on the back and the other on the breastbone, and then squeeze, the client will feel tremendous pain.

The treatment is to use a rib belt. This is a strap of elastic, about 8 inches wide, that goes around the rib cage. It stretches tight and closes in front with Velcro. This compresses the rib cage so that it cannot overexpand. The belt holds the rib ends in place until the separation heals and the pain of everyday movements is lessened.

Participating in sports activity is usually not feasible because of extreme pain; however, some athletes manage.

Massage Strategies

These methods are suitable for treating bruised as well as separated ribs.

Full-body massage is applied. The goal is pain management, incorporating counterirritation and hyperstimulation analgesia with support of parasympathetic dominance. Various essential oils that are relaxing and have analgesic action may be incorporated into the massage.

Because it is painful for the client to contract the muscles, direct work on the ribs is limited to positional release. Positioning the client is very difficult and requires creative bolstering until a comfortable position with reduced pain is found. In effect, the bolstered position becomes a treatment using positional release concepts. Direct manipulation of the spindle cells and Golgi tendon apparatus may work with gentle passive lengthening to reduce muscle spasms.

The breathing pattern is disturbed, and muscles used during upper chest breathing can become short and tense. Massage can reduce the shortening somewhat, but it will return until the ribs are healed.

The application of positional release is somewhat different than the typical method (use of a painful point), and because movement is so painful.

- Instruct the client to locate the painful area with the fingers.
- Place one hand above or below the painful point and the other hand on the opposite side. Then gently move the hands toward each other, slowly applying gentle compression to the rib cage in various directions, until the client indicates that the pain is reduced.
- Hold this position for as long as the client indicates that it is comfortable.

This procedure is very experimental, and it may be necessary to keep changing the hand position until the correct position is found. If no relief is obtained or if pain increases after three or four attempts, stop.

The pain is primarily caused by protective spasm (*guarding*) of the intercostals, anterior serratus, transversus thoracis, pectoralis minor, and other muscles that can stabilize rib movement. Guarding muscle spasms is a resourceful function and may not respond to the positional release method. Even if the method is successful, use no more than two to three positions to protect rib stability. The goal is pain reduction and easier breathing without interfering with the body's protective mechanisms.

Gentle repetitive stroking and slow rhythmic rocking over the injured area can be soothing. However these methods may also cause irritation. Avoid any procedure that increases the client's pain or discomfort.

BROKEN RIBS

A blow to the rib cage may cause a **broken rib.** The resulting pain may occur anywhere in the rib cage, depending on where the rib or ribs are broken.

The pain from broken ribs is similar to that from bruised or separated ribs, only more severe. Any excessive strain or movement, or another blow, can cause the sharp ends of broken ribs to puncture a lung. This is a medical emergency.

Treatment includes rest (for about 6 weeks) and use of a rib belt until the pain is gone. An x-ray must show that the ribs have healed before the athlete can return to activity.

Massage Strategies

Apply full-body massage for pain management and healing. Do not massage the thorax until the ribs are stable; then use the procedure given for bruised and separated ribs.

RIB MUSCLE PULLS AND TEARS

The muscle between each pair of ribs, the intercostal muscle, which is the muscle used in respiration, may pull or tear as a result of overstress. A **rib muscle pull or tear** can happen when a tennis or football player makes a sudden, violent lateral motion or suddenly rotates the trunk.

Tenderness is felt in the area between the ribs, not in the ribs themselves. Treatment consists of rest and ice application until the pain disappears. A rib belt provides stability and eases pain.

Massage Strategies

It is difficult to use the massage strategies for muscle tears in this area.

See suggestions for separated ribs.

THE BACK

General massage protocols for back dysfunction and pain are discussed beginning on page 525. See also massage strategies for individual back disorders in the following sections.

BACK PAIN

The best way to prevent back problems is to develop a strong back. Because most muscle injuries are due to muscle weakness, increased strength can correct almost every back problem. Strengthening the core is essential.

Nearly all injuries to the back are muscular in nature. About 95% of cases of low-back pain are the result of muscular problems caused by lack of exercise, weak muscles, or overweight. Back problems can also be caused by tense muscles or strain from suddenly overloading muscles during activity. Muscle fibers may pull or tear, sending the back muscles into spasm and causing pain.

Fortunately, most simple backaches go away within a few days or weeks, with or without treatment, and 90% disappear within 2 months. A workout that strengthens the back muscles and abdominal muscles (the core) and stretches the pectoralis major and other anterior thorax muscles can prevent back pain, provide relief, and help prevent pain from recurring.

Bed rest for more than a couple of days only weakens muscles and can be disabling. The client needs to get out of bed as soon as possible. Alternating applications of heat and cold (ice) may be helpful. Surgery should be considered only as a last resort.

Orthopedists often advise people with back pain to avoid sports that put stress on the back. Recommended activities include swimming, walking, cross-country skiing, and stationary cycling. These can all be done without sharp, sudden movements such as severe arching of the back and twisting or rotating of the trunk. Low-impact, not high-impact, aerobics, or water aerobics are appropriate activities for those with back pain.

Sports that require arching and twisting of the body and sudden starts and stops can strain the back. Examples are basketball, volleyball, downhill skiing, dancing, bowling, football, and baseball. Sports-related back pain is common in football players, wrestlers, ice hockey players, gymnasts, figure skaters, and skateboarders. Bike riders, including motorcyclists, and horseback riders can experience compression of the sacroiliac (SI) joint and lower lumbar vertebrae as well as muscle strain. Gymnasts and divers tend to experience sprains and strains during athletic activity.

The incidence of low-back pain in collegiate athletes is increasing, mostly as the result of improper form and overtraining in strength development and conditioning activities.

Improper posture and overstressing of the immature spine may also cause low-back pain (Figure 21-5). Back pain often results from an excessive load on the normal back or a normal load on a weak or unprepared back.

Golfers should beware of the torsion placed on the back during the swing. Tennis and golf can be challenging for anyone with back pain, with

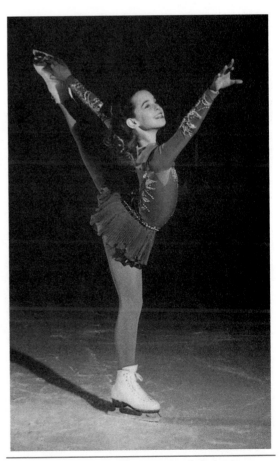

FIGURE 21-5 ■ Predisposing activity for back pain.

its twisting, flexing, and extending motions (Figure 21-6).

Golfing, baseball, and bowling are the three activities most likely to cause lumbar disk problems, including herniation.

Running can lead to back problems because of the impact of the foot strike, abnormal foot mechanics, the necessity for of imbalanced muscles to work harder, and running too fast, or if one leg is slightly longer than the other.

Back pain is a common symptom and cause of injury, regardless of an individual's health or fitness status. Almost everyone will complain at some time of back pain, and 50% of working-age adults experiencing back pain symptoms.

Common causes of back pain in athletes include spondylolysis, stress fractures, discogenic defects in intervertebral disks, strains of the musculature of the back, hyperlordotic mechanical back pain, and back pain from other causes, including infections and tumors that become symptomatic in the course of sports participation.

The causes of back pain are different in young versus older athletes. The young athlete generally does not have degenerative changes in the spine, and back pain is usually the result of a specific injury or event. The incidence of spondylolysis is statistically higher in the young athlete than in the older athlete. The older athlete often has back pain related to disk degeneration, other pathology, and weight-control problems.

The majority of back pain in athletes is the result of a combination of mechanical factors, including improper weight-lifting techniques, overstretching, torsion, impact trauma, static positioning, repetitive loading, hard repetitive contact, sudden violent muscle contraction, musculotendinous strains, ligament-vertebrae sprains, irregular anatomic positioning, and spondylolysis or spondylolisthesis. Impact trauma is caused by contact with hard or

FIGURE 21-6

COMMON PAIN AREAS FOR GOLFERS

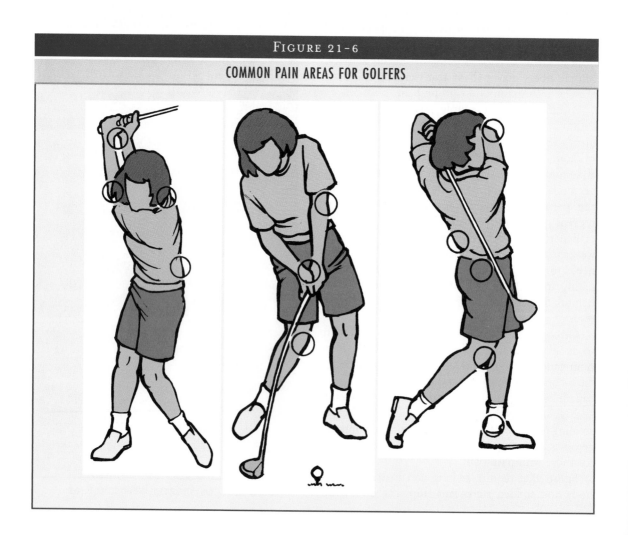

nonmovable objects such as playing surfaces, walls, and other people.

The possibility of a disk condition and related nerve irritation must be considered in any long-lasting episode of back discomfort, especially if there is any radiating pain into the leg.

Diagnostic testing includes a thorough physical examination with attention to range-of-motion/flexibility testing and neurologic testing for motor, sensory, and deep-tendon reflex loss, straight-leg raising, and other signs of disk disease. X-rays, MRI and CT scans, electromyography (EMG), myelography, fluoroscopy, and bone scan are all viable diagnostic tests. Blood work can help to identify Paget's disease, tuberculosis, cancer, and infection. Urinalysis can aid in the diagnosis of kidney or other urologic involvement.

A quick assessment for serious back injuries is the forward trunk flexion and the backward trunk extension. Increased pain during flexion indicates possible disk involvement. If extension increases pain, then there may be a stress fracture of a vertebra or vertebrae (Figure 21-7).

The success rate for surgical treatment of low-back pain is questionable, and it is the final option only after more conservative treatment has failed. However, new microscopic surgical procedures are less invasive and show promising results.

The treatment plan for back pain often varies among health care professional groups. It is important to realize that neurosurgeons, orthopedists, osteopaths, chiropractors, and massage therapists bring different approaches, training, and philosophies to the treatment of back pain.

Back pain is usually muscular in origin. Once a thorough assessment has ruled out all other possible causes, use ice for inflammation, massage for muscle spasm, and pain control and counterirritants such as heat, ice, and ointments for pain. Electrical stimulation modalities for pain and spasm are helpful. A comprehensive rehabilitation program is necessary and should include core

FIGURE 21-7

ASSESSING FOR CAUSES OF BACK PAIN

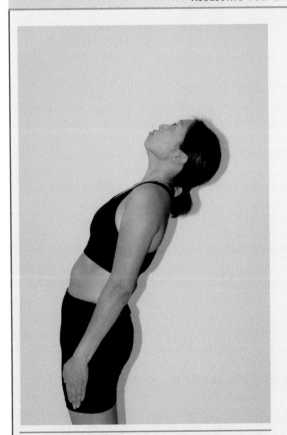

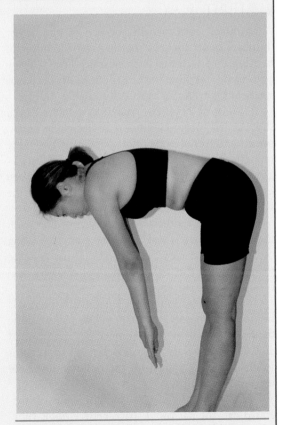

A Pain that increases during extension indicates a possible bone fracture.

B Pain that increases during flexion may indicate a disk injury.

stability training and a flexibility program especially for the pectoralis major, latissimus dorsi,
hamstrings, piriformis and external rotators of the
hip, and hip flexors, including the psoas and gluteal
muscles. Patients in rehabilitation programs should
progress from single-plane to multi-plane exercises,
and dynamic stabilization should be emphasized.
Chiropractic or osteopathic mobilization for
abnormal facet function can be helpful. Muscle
activator sequences for the trunk, hip extension,
and knee flexion are usually dysfunctional and
need treatment (Figure 21-8).

BULGING DISK

One of the most common back problems is a
bulging disk. The wall of the disk bulges out into
the spinal column. The disk, however, is not ruptured completely. The disk bulge can impinge on a
nerve, resulting in pain and muscle spasm. A
bulging disk cannot be seen on an x-ray but can be
seen on a CT or MRI scan.

Massage Strategies

Conservative treatment is used and massage is
appropriate with caution.

RUPTURED DISK

A **ruptured disk** usually occurs in the lower
(lumbar) spine, the area that receives the brunt of
twisting and turning. Poor posture, lifting heavy
objects, or repetitive twisting motions in sports can
weaken the disks and eventually cause a rupture.

A ruptured disk, also called a herniated or a
slipped disk, occurs when the disk capsule breaks
open and protrudes into the spinal canal, pressing
on nerve roots. Gel oozes out of the disk and causes
more pressure on the spinal cord or the nerve roots.
Over time, the gel usually disintegrates, and the
symptoms may be relieved.

When a disk ruptures, however, the pad between
the two vertebrae is gone, and the gradual wearing
of bone on bone leads to arthritis. This can cause
serious pain if the arthritic spurs of the vertebrae
press on the nerve root.

The pain of a ruptured disk is usually sharp and
sudden. Commonly, the pain will be passed along
the course of the nerve impinged by the ruptured
disk. A disk pressing on the sciatic nerve root causes
sciatica, sending pain from the buttock down the
leg and into the foot.

Only when the disk has completely disinte-
grated can the narrowed space between two vertebrae be seen on a radiography.

If the symptoms do not subside, surgery may be
needed to remove some or all of the disk. What used
to be a crude, major operation requiring a long
recuperation time has become a much more
sophisticated endoscopic and microscopic surgical
procedure. The classic back operation, called a
diskectomy, involves an incision in the back and
removal of a small piece of the vertebra to expose
the injured disk. Then the damaged part of the disk
is cut out. Surgery now usually involves insertion of
an arthroscope into the ruptured disk to suck out
the gel and relieve pressure on the nerve.

A nonsurgical procedure popular in Europe is
the injection of a papaya derivative called chy-
mopapain into the center of the ruptured disk. This
natural enzyme dissolves the gel to relieve the pain.
However, this treatment has hazards and is not
widely used in the United States.

The majority of people get better without
surgery, even those with acutely ruptured disks.
Surgery is prescribed for the 10% to 15% of
patients who fail to respond to conservative treatment or who develop weakness or numbness in the
limbs, which is a sign of neurologic problems. The
problem for competing athletes is the time needed
for the condition to heal without surgical intervention. Athletes must compete or lose their jobs.
Therefore, many more athletes opt for surgery than
the general population.

Massage Strategies

If conservative therapy is the option, massage is
an important component of the treatment plan
(see page 525). Massage targets muscle spasm and
manages pain. If the condition is surgically corrected, often preoperative and postoperative
massage strategies are used.

CRACKED BACK

Abnormal separation of a vertebra into front and
rear portions is called **spondylolysis.** It is also
known as **cracked back.** Originally, this was
thought to be a congenital failure of the two halves
of the vertebra to fuse, but it is now believed that
this condition is due to acute fracture caused by
back trauma. A quick assessment for a cracked back
is to compare lumbar flexion and extension. If
extension increases the pain, especially in an isolated area, it may be a small fracture.

Spondylolysis is most common in young
people who have chronic back pain with no obvious
cause. Often, they have taken a fall before feeling
any pain.

FIGURE 21-8

ASSESSMENT FOR BACK PAIN

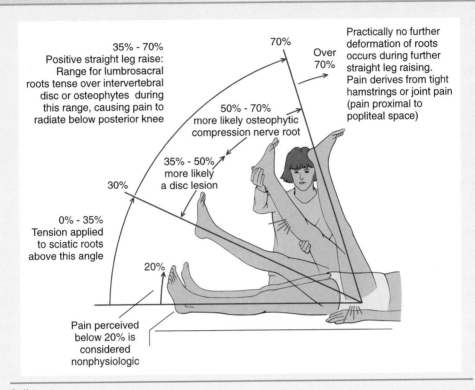

35% - 70%
Positive straight leg raise:
Range for lumbrosacral
roots tense over intervertebral
disc or osteophytes during
this range, causing pain to
radiate below posterior knee

70%

Over
70%

Practically no further
deformation of roots
occurs during further
straight leg raising.
Pain derives from tight
hamstrings or joint pain
(pain proximal to
popliteal space)

50% - 70%
more likely osteophytic
compression nerve root

35% - 50%
more likely
a disc lesion

30%

0% - 35%
Tension applied
to sciatic roots
above this angle

20%

Pain perceived
below 20% is
considered
nonphysiologic

A Hamstring test.

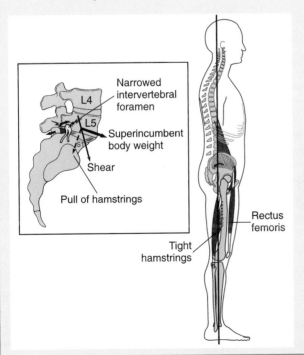

Narrowed
intervertebral
foramen

L4

L5

S1

Superincumbent
body weight

Shear

Pull of hamstrings

Tight
hamstrings

Rectus
femoris

B Tight hamstrings cause a pull on the pelvis that rotates it backward about the common hip axis as a posterior pelvic tilt and therefore increases shear of the L5 on the S1 and predisposes to accelerated disk and facet degeneration.

(From Saidoff DC, McDonough A: *Critical pathways in therapeutic intervention—extremities and spine.* St. Louis, 2002, Mosby.)

If the fracture is old or congenital, the treatment of choice is a strengthening program with reduced physical activity until the symptoms cease. If the fracture is fresh, all sports and and similar athletic activities should be avoided for about 6 months to allow the fracture to heal. Usually, rest alone is not enough to relieve all the symptoms, and a program to strengthen the back muscles is required.

A back brace may be helpful during this time. However, a brace should be used only in the presence of acute pain. Back braces are not useful in the long run because they further weaken the back muscles.

If the fracture fails to heal, it may lead to another condition called spondylolisthesis, in which the front portion of a vertebra slips forward out of line with the other vertebrae. Most of the stabilizing ligaments of the spinal column are located on the anterior surface of the vertebral column. If the connecting bone does not heal, then almost any activity can cause the front part of the vertebra to slip forward.

Normal activity can be resumed after an initial period of rest and when the bone heals. If the vertebra remains unstable, activities such as diving and gymnastics, which requires arching of the back, and contact sports such as soccer, football, and basketball, in which a person might take a heavy blow to the back, need to be avoided. If a slipped vertebra progresses despite conservative treatments, the vertebra will need to be fused surgically.

Massage Strategies

Massage is focused on management of protective muscle guarding that develops to stabilize the back. This muscle guarding is persistent, and best results are achieved when the goal is to reduce but not eliminate the muscle tightening in the area. Trigger points should not be treated. Instead, apply broad-based compression, gliding in the general area to gently inhibit some of the muscle tension (see page 525 for specific procedure).

CRACKED WING

A **cracked wing** is a fracture of the protuberance at the lower side of each vertebra, known as a wing but properly called the *transverse process*. It can be cracked from a blow to the back. The back muscles and ligaments attach to the spine at the wing. In football, a wing fracture commonly occurs in running backs hit with a helmet from behind.

Although very painful, this is not a serious injury. Once the pain disappears, extra padding around the wing protects it.

Massage Strategies

Do NOT reduce muscle guarding in the area of the fracture. Avoid the area and any positioning that causes the back to be extended. Follow bone fracture strategies.

SHORT-LEG SYNDROME

A common cause of lower-back pain is a difference in the lengths of the legs, or **short leg syndrome.** A difference of one-fourth of an inch can be significant in an athlete, whereas a nonathlete may get away with a difference of up to a half an inch. The back pain is usually felt on the side of the longer leg. This leg pounds into the ground during walking, running, jumping, and so forth, throwing that side of the body out of alignment. The stress works its way all the way up to the back.

Short-leg syndrome may be caused by displacement of the pelvis and muscle imbalance. Usually the condition is functional and can be corrected by mobilization of the pelvis and targeted lengthening and strengthening exercises.

Massage Strategies

Massage is supportive. Use the indirect function technique for the pelvis, along with quadratus lumborum and psoas release if indicated. Treatment is focused on lengthening the soft tissue of the *short leg* (see Unit Two).

SCIATICA

Sciatica is not a true back problem; it refers to pain along the course of the sciatic nerve. This nerve runs from the buttock down the back of the leg to the foot. Pressure on the sciatic nerve root at the spine causes the pain. It is necessary to determine the cause of the pressure and then treat the cause. Possible causes include nerve impingement from a disk, an arthritic spur of a vertebra, a muscle spasm, or neurologic problems in the spinal cord. Treatment for sciatica itself is not the answer, as sciatica is only a symptom of the underlying problem.

Sciatica may be very easy or very difficult to diagnose. If pain occurs only in the posterior thigh, it can be easily confused with a hamstring pull. If the pain is more in the lateral thigh, the lumbar plexus may be the issue. If the pain goes all the way down the leg to the foot, it is more likely sciatica.

Increased pain when bending over or while doing a straight leg raise indicates possible sciatica. Other indications of sciatica are a weak big toe, trouble in raising the front of the foot, and a diminished ankle reflex. Entrapment of the sciatic nerve by the piriformis muscle is called *piriformis syndrome.* Lengthening this muscle may help decrease symptoms.

MASSAGE PROTOCOLS FOR TREATMENT OF PAIN ASSOCIATED WITH BACK DISORDERS

The massage therapist targeting the athletic population must be able to effectively work with back pain because it is so common. Athletes are prone to this condition at the beginning of a training period, when fatigued, and when compensating for an existing injury.

Therapeutic massage best addresses back pain of muscular origin such as simple back strain and overuse without joint or disk involvement. Low-back pain is the most common complaint (Figure 21-9).

Massage is useful as part of a comprehensive treatment program for more complicated conditions such as disk dysfunction. Joint dysfunction usually requires manipulation by a physician, physical therapist, chiropractor, or trainer. Massage is preadjustment and postadjustment adjunct treatment. More complex back pain often results in muscle tension and spasm that is guarding and therefore stabilizing. If the muscles are excessively tense, there is stiffness, pain, and possible increased irritation of the joint structure, because the muscles pull on the structure and cause compression. Unequal forces are being applied to the joint structure because flexors, adductors, and internal rotators exert more pull than extensors, abductors, and external rotators.

Massage can reduce muscle tension from guarding but should not seek to eliminate it. The guarding response is appropriate. Pain control methods are appropriate as well. These two strategies combined should support more normal movement and allow other treatments to be more effective. Manipulation of joints is easier if massage is applied to surrounding soft tissue. Massage after joint manipulation can reduce any spasm that may result. Complex back pain that is more than muscle related needs multidisciplinary treatment, with massage in the supporting role.

Massage for simple back pain is best combined with hot and cold hydrotherapy, and counterirri-

tant ointment. Rest with ongoing gentle range of motion with stretching activities is recommended. It is not advisable to rest without movement because that can make the situation worse.

Massage is targeted at the following muscles: abdominals, psoas, quadratus lumborum, hamstrings, and gluteal group. Firing pattern dysfunction is almost always present. Gait reflexes are usually disrupted.

Midback Pain

The cause of **midback pain** is usually short anterior serratus, pectoralis minor, and pectoralis major muscles and weak core muscles. The rhomboids and trapezius are usually long, with protective spasms and trigger point activity at the attachments. The biggest massage error is to massage the long areas in the area of the pain, which only makes them longer. Massage targeted at the long structures consists of local pain control only, using surface rubbing with a counterirritant ointment and hyperstimulation analgesia. Use all muscle energy methods and inhibitory pressure on the muscle belly and lengthen the short tissues in the anterior chest. See anterior serratus and pectoralis minor release in Unit Two.

If connective tissue bind exists in the pectoralis region, use appropriate mechanical forces by kneading, compressing, or stretching the tissues. Therapeutic exercise can strengthen the inhibited muscles, such as the rhomboids. The scalene muscles can impinge on a portion of the brachial plexus, resulting in a pain pattern to the midscapular region. Massage addresses the impinging tissue in the neck that recreates the symptoms.

If the client feels as if he or she wants to "crack" the back, the paraspinal muscles are usually the problem. See release of paraspinal muscles, multifidi, and rotators in Unit Two.

If the client is sniffling, coughing, or sneezing or has been laughing excessively, the posterior serratus inferior is often the cause. This muscle can shorten and because of its fiber direction is very difficult to stretch. The symptoms include an aching sensation just below the scapula at the location of the muscle. Compression into the muscle belly with local tissue stretching usually relieves the symptoms.

Lumbar Pain

There are various types of **lumbar pain.** The most serious is referred pain from kidney or bladder injury or infection or a ruptured disk. These conditions need medical treatment.

FIGURE 21-9

MAJOR MUSCLES INVOLVED IN LOW-BACK PAIN

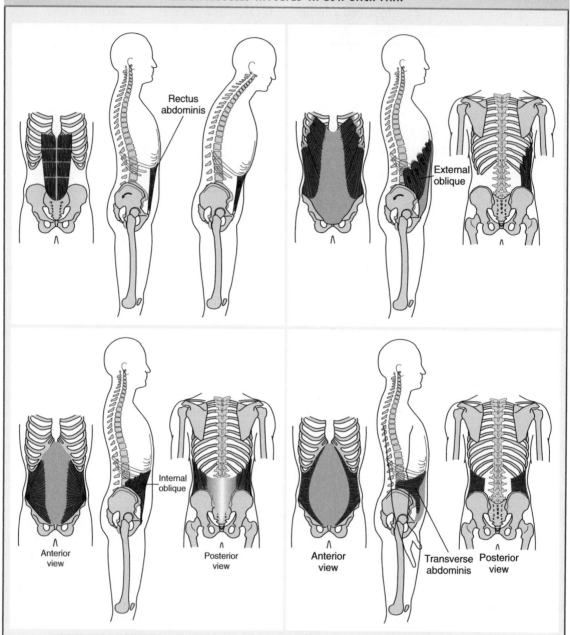

Rectus abdominis

External oblique

Internal oblique

Transverse abdominis

Anterior view

Posterior view

Anterior view

Posterior view

(From Saidoff DC, McDonough A: *Critical pathways in therapeutic intervention—extremities and spine.* St. Louis, 2002, Mosby.)

FIGURE 21-9 CONT'D

MAJOR MUSCLES INVOLVED IN LOW-BACK PAIN

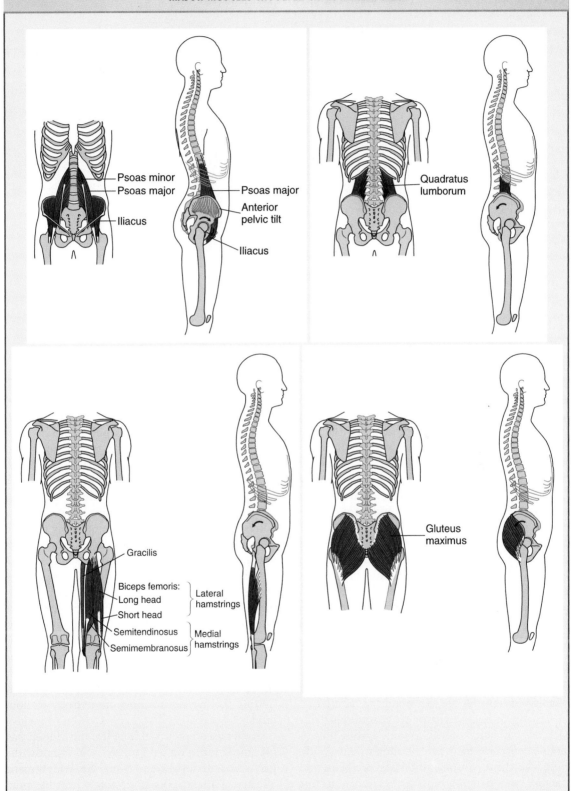

Continued

FIGURE 21-9 CONT'D

MAJOR MUSCLES INVOLVED IN LOW-BACK PAIN

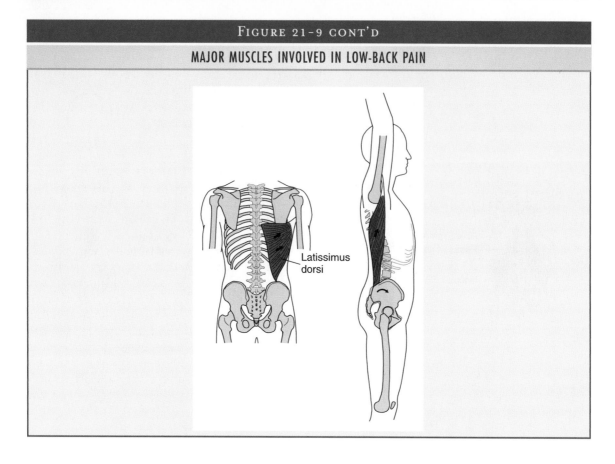

Latissimus
dorsi

SI joint dysfunction is a major cause of pain that requires a multidisciplinary approach. The joint can be jammed or fused, interfering with pelvis movement during gait (Figure 21-10). The restricted pelvic movement creates increased movement at L 4-5 to S-I area or at the hip, or both. Pain occurs in the hip abductors and around the coccyx/sacrum area on the affected side. Proper mobilization of the joint by the trainer, physical therapist, physician, or chiropractor is necessary. Massage supports the mobilization process by reducing muscle guarding and increasing tissue pliability. Once the joint is adjusted, the mobilization sequence for the SI joint (see Unit Two) can be incorporated into the general massage. The latissimus dorsi muscle opposite the symptomatic SI joint is part of the force couple that stabilizes the SI joint. The lumbar dorsal fascia needs to be pliable but not so loose that stability is affected.

Usually the symphysis pubis is somewhat displaced in conjunction with SI joint dysfunction. A simple resistance method can address this condition. The client is supine, the knees are bent, and the massage therapist provides resistance against the action of the client's attempt to push the knees

together. The action activates the adductors, which can then pull the symphysis pubis into a better alignment. Sometimes there is a popping sound when the symphysis resets, but that is not necessary or desirable for effective results.

Reflexively and functionally, the sternoclavicular (SC) joint is a factor in SI joint pain. Assess for corresponding pain in the SC joint, apply massage to inhibit muscle tension, increase tissue pliability, and use the SC joint technique shown in Unit Two.

Often the sacrotuberous and sacrospinous ligaments are short, or the hamstring and gluteus maximus attachments near these ligaments are binding. These ligament structures are difficult to reach, and when located, a compressive force is applied to the ligament while the client activates the hamstrings and gluteus maximus. The results should be increased pliability of the ligament, permitting the muscles to move more freely without bind.

If there is a functional long leg, the SI joint can become jammed on the long leg side. Typically the pelvis is anteriorly rotated on the symptomatic affected side and posteriorly rotated on the nonsymptomatic side, with quadratus lumborum short

FIGURE 21-10

ASSESSMENTS FOR THE SI JOINT

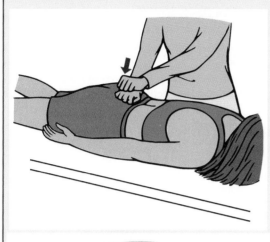

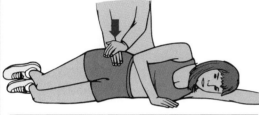

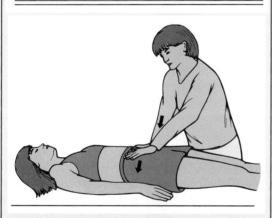

Pain in response to compression indicates SI joint dysfunction. (From Saidoff DC, McDonough A: *Critical pathways in therapeutic intervention— extremities and spine.* St. Louis, 2002, Mosby.)

on that side. The indirect function techniques for anterior rotation combined with quadratus lumborum release are effective (see Unit Two). The physical trainer or chiropractor rotates the pelvis and the massage therapist deals with the soft tissue compensation. Gait patterns and firing patterns need to be assessed and normalized.

Quadratus Lumborum Pain

Quadratus lumborum pain is felt in the lumbar region just above the iliac crest. Usually pain is more on one side than the other combined with a rotated pelvis and functionally uneven legs. Coughing and sneezing increase pain. SI joint pain is a common aspect of quadratus lumborum pain. There is often a history of short-leg syndrome, stepping in a hole, or one leg coming down hard on an uneven surface during running, any of which can cause the leg to be driven up into the joint, resulting in muscle spasms as the SI joint jams. The paired muscle group is the scalenes, which need to be addressed in conjunction with the quadratus lumborum. Apply both the scalene and the quadratus lumborum releases (see Unit Two) in the general massage.

Psoas Low-Back Pain

The main symptoms of low-back pain related to psoas dysfunction are a deep aching in the lumbar area, difficulty moving from a seated to standing position and vice versa, and difficulty rolling over when lying down. **Psoas low-back pain** is often the end result of a series of events that begin at the core muscles. The most common pattern is that the transverse abdominis and oblique muscles are weak, and therefore trunk muscle activation patterns are ineffective. The rectus abdominis becomes dominant and the psoas shortens. The gluteus maximus muscle becomes inhibited, and hip extension function is assumed by the erector spinae and hamstrings. As a result, hip extension firing patterns are abnormal. Hamstrings shorten and become prone to injury. The gastrocnemius begins to function as a knee flexor and shortens. This interferes with ankle mobility. Uneven forces are placed on the knees, and the calf muscles usually stick together and pull at the Achilles tendon. Eventually, Achilles tendon and plantar fascia problems can occur.

The massage strategy is to normalize the muscle activation firing pattern sequences and reduce tone in the shortened muscles (i.e., the psoas, hamstrings, and calves) (see psoas and hamstring treatment in Unit Two). However, this sequence only treats the symptom. The problem is core instability. A proper strength and conditioning sequence must deal with core strength. However, the target muscles of the strengthening program will be inhibited by the short tense erector spinae, psoas, hamstring, and calves and a vicious cycle is created. The short muscles need to be treated and normal resting length restored as much as possible before core training takes place. This can take up to a month of concentrated effort with massage two to three times a week combined with a sequential stretching program. Then core training begins. Massage sessions are reduced to twice a week, and daily stretching continues.

The full-body protocol is necessary, with attention to reflex paired body areas—the hamstrings/biceps, quadriceps/triceps, calf/forearm, quadratus lumborum/scalenes, psoas/sternocleidomastoid and longus colli. The rectus abdominis needs to be inhibited, and the psoas released. Also include thorough massage of the feet and connective tissue strategies on binding structures.

Assess and address breathing dysfunction, using the strategies shown in Chapter 19.

Connective tissue muscle stabilizing patterns become strained. The latissimus dorsi lumbar dorsal fascia, with the gluteus maximus and the IT band on the opposite side, is a common pattern. Massage inhibits the latissimus dorsi and gluteus maximus and increases pliability in the lumbar fascia and IT band.

To further complicate the treatment of back pain, there may be underlying joint instability in the lumbar and SI joints. If too much mobility is restored, joint pain may result. Slowly introducing change allows the body to adapt. If symptoms are improving and then suddenly return, too much soft tissue stability was released, and joint stability is compromised. Back off and return to general massage until the condition improves.

ACUTE TREATMENT USING MASSAGE

The side-lying position is recommended.

- If the client is prone, support with pillows under the abdomen and ankles. Do NOT keep client in the prone position for an extended time—15 minutes is maximum.
- When moving client from the prone to the side-lying position, have the client slowly assume a position on the hands and knees and then slowly arch and hunch the back (cat/camel move, valley/hill). Next, have the client stretch back toward the heels with arms extended.
- Then slowly have the client move to the side position; bolster for stability.

Target pain control mechanisms:

- Do NOT do deep work or any method that causes guarding, flinching, or breath holding. Use rocking, gentle shaking combined with gliding and kneading of the area of the most severe pain and symptomatic muscle tension. This will most likely be on the back, even though the causal muscle tension and soft tissue problem are usually in the anterior torso.
- Massage the hamstrings, adductors, gluteals, and calves. These muscles are usually short and tight and the firing is out of sequence.
- Do not attempt to reset firing patterns during acute symptoms. Include massage of the reflex points of the feet relating to the back.
- Turn client supine after working with both left and right sides; bolster the knees.
- The rectus abdominis and pectoralis muscles are likely short and tense. Massage as indicated in general protocol. Psoas muscles and adductors are likely short and spasmodic, but it is best to wait 24 to 48 hours before addressing these muscles. Continue rocking and shaking.

SUBACUTE TREATMENT USING MASSAGE

24 to 48 Hours After Onset

- In the context of the general massage protocol, repeat acute massage application, but begin to address second- and third-layer muscle shortening, connective tissue pliability, and firing patterns.
- Use direct inhibition pressure on the psoas, quadratus lumborum, and paraspinals, especially the multifidi, always monitoring for guarding response. Do NOT cause guarding or changes in breathing.
- It is likely that the hip abductors will have tender areas of shortening, but lengthen the adductors first.
- Gently begin to correct the trunk, gluteal, hamstring, and calf firing patterns. Include massage application for breathing

dysfunction, as it is commonly associated with low-back problems. Do not overdo.

3 to 7 Days After Onset

- Continue with subacute massage application in the context of the general massage protocol, increasing intensity of the massage as tolerated.
- In addition, normalize the gait and eye reflexes.
- Gently mobilize the pelvis for low-back pain and the ribs for upper back pain. No pain should be felt during any active or passive movements.
- Positional release methods and specific inhibiting pressure can be applied to tender points. The pressure recreates the symptoms but does not increase the symptoms. Work with trigger points that are most medial, proximal, and painful. Do not address latent trigger points or work with more than three to five areas at a time.
- Continue to address breathing function.
- The client should be doing gentle stretches and appropriate therapeutic exercises.

POSTSUBACUTE TREATMENT USING MASSAGE

- Continue with general massage and address muscles that remain symptomatic.
- Assess for body-wide instability and compensation patterns that are commonly associated with an acute back pain event. Usually the core muscle firing is weak, with synergistic dominance of the rectus abdominis and psoas.
- If breathing is dysfunctional, there can be midback pain as well. Continue to normalize breathing muscles.
- If the client has chronic back pain, continue with postsubacute treatment and encourage rehabilitative exercises, including breathing retraining.

THE SHOULDER

The shoulder is prone to a number of sports injuries. It is a very shallow ball-and-socket joint, which means that it is not very stable.

The shoulder is the only joint in the body not really held together by ligaments. The few ligaments in the shoulder serve only to keep the shoulder from moving too far in any one direction. The ligaments have little to do with holding the joint in place. Muscles provide most of the joint stability.

The shoulder socket contains the tendons of the long and short heads of the biceps muscle and the supraspinatus tendon. Directly below the socket is the brachial plexus, which contains all of the nerves that supply the arm.

The shoulder bones are held together by the rotator cuff muscles. These muscles are also responsible for the shoulder's fine movements, such as throwing a ball. Because of the shoulder's shallow socket and lack of ligaments, any weakness of the small rotator cuff muscles makes it easy for the head of the shoulder to slide part way out of the socket, which is a partial dislocation, or subluxation. Or it may slide all the way out, which is a full dislocation.

The shoulder joint is composed of three bones: the clavicle, the scapula, and the humerus. Three joints facilitate shoulder movement. The acromioclavicular (AC) joint is located between the acromion and the clavicle. The sternoclavicular (SC) joint formed by the clavicle and sternum must function to allow proper range of motion in the AC joint. The glenohumeral joint, commonly called the shoulder joint, is a ball-and-socket type joint that helps move the shoulder forward and backward and allows the arm to rotate in a circular fashion or hinge out and up away from the body. The capsule is a soft tissue envelope that encircles the glenohumeral joint and is lined by a thin, smooth synovial membrane.

The front of the joint capsule is anchored by three glenohumeral ligaments.

The rotator cuff is composed of tendons that, with associated muscles, hold the ball at the top of the humerus in the glenoid socket and provide mobility and strength to the shoulder joint. Bursae permit smooth gliding between bone, muscles, and tendons and cushion and protect the rotator cuff from the bony arch of the acromion.

Some shoulder problems develop from the disturbance of soft tissues as a result of an injury or from overuse or underuse of the shoulder. Other problems arise from a degenerative process in which tissues break down and no longer function well.

Shoulder pain may be localized or may be referred to areas around the shoulder or down the arm. Diseases within the body (such as gallbladder, liver, and heart disease and disease of the cervical spine of the neck) also may generate pain that travels along nerves to the shoulder. Referral is necessary for proper diagnosis.

DISLOCATED SHOULDER

The shoulder is the most frequently dislocated joint of the body. A dislocation may stretch or tear the rotator cuff muscles. Usually these muscles are only stretched, particularly in younger athletes. In older athletes, who have more brittle rotator cuffs, the muscles are more likely to be torn.

In a typical case of a **dislocated shoulder,** a strong force that pulls the shoulder outward (abduction) or extreme rotation of the joint pops the ball of the humerus out of the shoulder socket. The shoulder can dislocate forward, backward, or downward. Dislocation commonly occurs when there is an intense unexpected backward pull on the arm. A partial dislocation, in which the upper arm bone is partially in and partially out of the socket, is called a *subluxation.*

Shoulder instability occurs when a shoulder dislocates frequently. The arm appears out of position when the shoulder dislocates, and there is pain. Muscle spasms may increase the intensity of pain. Swelling, numbness, weakness, and bruising are likely to develop. Problems seen with a dislocated shoulder are tearing of the ligaments or tendons reinforcing the joint capsule and, less commonly, nerve damage.

Diagnosis of a dislocation is made by a physical examination. X-rays may be taken to confirm the diagnosis and to rule out a related fracture.

Medical treatment for dislocation consists of putting the ball of the humerus back into the joint socket–a procedure called *reduction.* The arm is then immobilized in a sling or a device called a shoulder immobilizer for several weeks. The shoulder is rested and iced three or four times a day. After pain and swelling have been controlled, a rehabilitation program that includes exercises to restore the range of motion of the shoulder and strengthen the muscles to prevent future dislocations begins. These exercises progress from simple movements to the use of weights.

After treatment and recovery, a previously dislocated shoulder may remain more susceptible to reinjury, especially in young, active individuals. A shoulder that dislocates severely or often, injuring surrounding tissues or nerves, usually requires surgical repair to tighten stretched ligaments or reattach torn ones.

If surgery is necessary, arthroscopic surgery is used if possible. Following surgery, the shoulder is generally immobilized for about 6 weeks, and full recovery takes several months. Many surgeons prefer to repair a recurring dislocated shoulder by the open surgery procedure. There are usually fewer repeat dislocations and improved movement following open surgery, but it may take a little longer to regain motion.

Massage Strategies

Massage is focused on pain management, reducing edema, and supporting rehabilitation. The muscles of the shoulder need to be somewhat short for stability. Do not over-massage. If massage is required following surgery, use the postsurgery sequence in Chapter 19.

SPRAINS

As with all sprains, there are three degrees of severity of shoulder sprains. A mild, or first-degree, **shoulder sprain** causes a minimal stretching of the ligaments without much tearing of fibers, and the joint remains stable. There will be pain and swelling around the joint.

In a moderate, or second-degree, sprain, the ligaments are stretched more and partially torn, and the outer end of the collarbone will partially snap in and out of the joint.

It's much easier to diagnose a severe, or third-degree, sprain. The complete disruption of all of the ligaments around the joint causes the collarbone to displace.

The treatment for first- and second-degree shoulder sprains is rest. The shoulder is placed in a sling to bring the damaged tissue together and encourage healing. The sling is worn for 1 to 3 weeks, depending on the severity of the injury. Also, in addition to resting the shoulder, ice is applied for 20 to 30 minutes a few times each day to ease the pain. These are particularly frustrating injuries because they can take 6 to 8 weeks to heal.

For a third-degree shoulder sprain, surgical repair of the ligaments is necessary to stabilize the joint. Up to 6 weeks of recovery from surgery is necessary before a rehabilitation program begins. This program consists of range of motion and strengthening exercises.

Massage Strategies

Use the strategies for sprains and strains shown on page 456.

SHOULDER SEPARATION

A **shoulder separation,** which technically is a sprain, occurs where the clavicle meets the scapula. When ligaments that hold the joint together are partially or completely torn, the outer end of the clavicle may slip out of place, preventing it from properly meeting the scapula. Most often the injury is caused by a blow to the shoulder or by falling on an outstretched hand.

Shoulder pain and/or tenderness and, occasionally, a bump over the AC joint are signs that a separation may have previously occurred. Sometimes the severity of a separation can be detected on x-rays taken while the athlete holds a light weight that pulls on the muscles, making a separation more pronounced.

Risk factors for shoulder separation include athletic activities, especially:

baseball (pitching)
football (blocking, throwing)
gymnastics
weight lifting
tennis
volleyball
swimming (especially backstroke and butterfly swimming techniques)

Congenital collagen disorders may also play a role, including Marfan syndrome and Ehlers-Danlos syndrome. Marfan syndrome is a connective tissue multisystemic disorder affecting the skeleton and ligaments (joint laxity) and producing substantial cardiovascular defects. People with Ehlers-Danlos syndrome have fragile skin and loose (hypermobile and frequently dislocated) joints due to faulty collagen synthesis.

Another risk factor for shoulder dislocation is a history of family members with shoulder instability.

Shoulder separations are classified according to the severity of the injury as follows:

Type (grade) I: A sprain (without a complete tear) of the ligaments holding the joint together.
Type (grade) II: A tear of the acromioclavicular ligament.
Type (grade) III: A tear of the acromioclavicular and coracoclavicular ligaments.
Type (grade) IV: Both ligaments are torn, and the clavicle is pushed forward and sideways into soft tissue.

With proper treatment of a Type I separation, the client should be pain-free, with full range of motion, in about 2 to 3weeks. It may take 3 to 5 weeks for Type II separations to reach this stage of recovery. Complete healing of Type III separations, when surgery is not necessary, may take 6 weeks to 2 months. Should a type III acromioclavicular separation need surgery, full recovery may take 3 to 6 months.

Type IV separations are surgically treated. Even with proper rehabilitation, full recovery may not be achieved for 6 months to a year, and recurrences are common.

Type I, II, and III shoulder separations are usually treated conservatively with rest, and the affected shoulder/arm is placed in a sling. Soon after injury, an ice bag may be applied to relieve pain and swelling. After a period of rest, treatment consists of exercises that put the shoulder through a range of motion and increase muscle strength. Most shoulder separations heal within 2 or 3 months without further intervention. However, if ligaments are severely torn, as in type IV separations, surgical repair may be required to hold the clavicle in place. The physician may wait to see if conservative treatment works before deciding whether surgery is required.

Massage Strategies

It is important that the stability of the shoulder not be compromised. Most of the pain is caused by protective guarding from the surrounding muscles. The guarding should not be eliminated, because to do so would destabilize the shoulder and interfere with the progressive healing process.

The following sequence is appropriate for nonsurgical treatment of shoulder separations, especially types I and II. It should be added to a general massage session with outcome goals of parasympathetic dominance, hyperstimulation analgesia, and increased pain-modulating neurochemicals for pain management and supporting restorative sleep.

- Place the injured shoulder in the loose-packed position and in the direction of ease to avoid any strain on the healing tissue and reduce the tendency for increased muscle guarding. The client's arm should be resting by the side with the shoulder abducted approximately 50 degrees and horizontally adducted 30 degrees.
- With the client in the prone position, place a pillow under the chest with additional bolsters in the axilla area if necessary. Side-lying position is best avoided on the injured side but can be effective if the client is placed on the noninjured side with a pillow supporting the head with another pillow placed on the chest for the client to "hug." It is difficult to achieve abduction in this position.

- With the client in the supine position, place bolsters under the knees and head, with an additional pillow under the scapula and arm on the injured side. Place an additional small pillow or folded towel under the elbow, with the arm bent over the chest.

The shoulder itself in the area of the injury is not massaged, but the muscles of scapular stabilization need to have tension reduced approximately 50%. These include the trapezius, rhomboids, levator scapulae, pectoralis minor, and anterior serratus. Also address the latissimus dorsi, pectoralis major, and deltoids. Do not work with the rotator cuff muscles, because these are a major source of stability. Do not work specifically around the AC joint.

- Use gliding and broad-based compression with some kneading. Avoid ischemic compression and trigger point methods. Methods used should not cause flinching or exert pain but do need to be applied with enough depth of pressure and drag to affect the spindle cell and Golgi tendon mechanism so that the tension reduces in the muscles. *Do not stretch the area.*
- Work on the opposite hip and adductors, because reflexive muscle tightness will tend to occur in these areas, and massage in this area can reflexively reduce muscle tension in the injured shoulder.
- Also address the reflexology areas on the hands and feet for the shoulder, which are located on the plantar/palmar surface adjacent to the little finger and toe on each hand and foot.
- With the client in the supine position, apply gentle oscillation to reduce pain and tension in the area. Gently place one hand under the shoulder so that the scapula lies in the palm of the hand. Place the other hand gently on top of the cap of the shoulder so that the injured area is in the center of your palm. Then gently compress the two hands together to cradle the injured area. Begin moving the hands together in small, rocking circular movements. There should be no pain or guarding. Sustain this action for as long as it feels comfortable to the client.
- During subacute healing, do NOT reduce the increased tone in the rotator cuff muscles. This is a resourceful compensation pattern that creates some joint stability. Massage

needs to support strengthening exercises for the shoulder.

SHOULDER "POPS": PARTIAL DISLOCATION

Partial dislocation of the shoulder can occur when a sudden force is exerted against the shoulder, causing the head of the humerus to "pop," or slip momentarily out of the socket—that is, become partially dislocated, or subluxated. The shoulder's structures and shallow socket may allow the head to slip part way up onto the rim of the socket, and then the shoulder snaps back into place spontaneously. It feels as if the shoulder has popped out and then popped back in. If the shoulder were truly dislocated, this would not occur.

When the head of the humerus slides partially out and then snaps back in, it stretches the rotator cuff muscles, creating an overuse injury. The shoulder begins to slide around, causing impingement and tendinitis. Because the rotator cuff muscles are stretched, the next time the shoulder takes a blow, the head of the humerus is likely to slide out again. With each blow, the rotator cuff gets looser, until finally the shoulder is in danger of truly dislocating.

The standard treatment for a subluxated shoulder is rest and an exercise program to strengthen the rotator cuff muscles to prevent future slipping.

These muscles are slow healers. The strengthening program usually takes 6 to 12 weeks, and the shoulder may not be back to full strength for 6 months or more.

Massage Strategies

Massage must not destabilize the area. Use strategies for dislocation on page 470.

TENDINITIS, BURSITIS, AND IMPINGEMENT SYNDROME

Tendinitis of the shoulder is different from **bursitis,** although both can be very painful. Usually, the pain of tendinitis does not occur unless the tender body part is used. With bursitis, the body part is constantly painful. The tenderness of tendinitis occurs all along the length of the tendon, but pain is felt it in one specific spot with bursitis.

In **tendinitis of the shoulder,** the rotator cuff and/or biceps tendon become inflamed from repetitive strain or as a result of being pinched by surrounding structures. The injury may vary from mild inflammation to involvement of most of the rotator cuff. When a rotator cuff tendon becomes inflamed and thickened, it may get trapped under the acromion. Squeezing of the rotator cuff is called **impingement syndrome.**

Tendinitis and impingement syndrome are often accompanied by inflammation of the bursal sacs (bursitis) that protect the shoulder.

Signs of these conditions include the slow onset of discomfort and pain in the upper shoulder or upper third of the arm and/or difficulty sleeping on the shoulder. Tendinitis and bursitis also cause pain when the arm is lifted away from the body or raised overhead. If tendinitis involves the biceps tendon, pain will occur in the front or side of the shoulder and may travel down to the elbow and forearm.

Diagnosis of tendinitis and bursitis begins with a medical history and physical assessment. X–rays do not show the tendons or bursae, but they may be helpful in ruling out bony abnormalities and arthritis. The doctor may remove and test fluid from the inflamed area to rule out infection. Impingement syndrome may be confirmed if injection of a small amount of anesthetic (lidocaine hydrochloride) into the space under the acromion relieves pain.

The first step in treating these conditions is to reduce pain and inflammation with rest, ice pack applications, lymphatic drain massage, and NSAIDs. In some cases ultrasound (noninvasive sound-wave vibrations) may be used to warm deep tissues and improve blood flow. Gentle stretching and strengthening exercises are added gradually. These may be preceded or followed by use of an ice pack. If there is no improvement, the doctor may inject a corticosteroid medicine into the space under the acromion. Steroid injections are a common treatment, but they should be used with caution because their use may lead to tendon rupture. If there is still no improvement after 6 to 12 months, arthroscopic or open surgery may be necessary to repair damage and relieve pressure on the tendons and bursae.

The rotator cuff muscles are not meant to function under stress with the arm raised above a line parallel to the ground. If the shoulder joint is continually stressed with the arm in this overhead position, the rotator cuff muscles begin to stretch out. This allows the head of the joint to become loose within the shoulder socket. Extension of the arm backward over the shoulder will cause the head of the humerus to slide forward, catching the tendon of the short head of the biceps between the ball and the socket. The head of the humerus will drop in the socket, so that it impinges on the tendon of the long head of the biceps and, in some cases, on the supraspinatus muscle as well. Sports that require repeatedly raising the arm up over the head, such as baseball, tennis, volleyball, and swimming, are the main contributors to shoulder impingement injuries.

This impingement causes the tendons to become inflamed and painful. Baseball pitchers tend to feel the pain in both the long and short heads of the biceps, and tennis players feel the pain particularly in the long head of the biceps. Athletes such as freestyle and butterfly swimmers may feel pain deep in the shoulder because of impingement on the the supraspinatus tendon.

Tennis players may state that they can hit ground strokes without pain, but when they hit an overhead stroke or serve, the shoulder hurts. The same thing can happen to golfers in both the backswing and the follow-through, when the arms are higher than parallel to the ground.

The proper way to treat a shoulder impingement is through an exercise program that strengthens the rotator cuff muscles sufficiently so that the head of the humerus is held firmly in place and will not slip out of the socket. With no slipping, the tendons will no longer be inflamed or irritated.

Some people do not respond to rehabilitation, even with physical therapy, and surgery will be required to repair the shoulder joint.

Massage Strategies

Massage must not destabilize the joint. See sequence for tendinitis and bursitis on page 466.

THE PRO'S ROTATOR CUFF INJURY

In professional athletes, the rotator cuff muscles can become so overdeveloped that they no longer fit into the shoulder socket. As a consequence, they rub along the outside of the socket, and eventually some of the muscle fibers are sawed through as they ride back and forth against the rim of the socket. This condition is known as the **pro's rotator cuff injury.** The only way to correct this is through surgery to enlarge the socket and repair the damaged muscle fibers.

ROTATOR CUFF TEAR

One or more rotator cuff tendons may become inflamed as a result of overuse, aging, a fall on an outstretched hand, or a collision. Sports that require repeated overhead arm motion and occupations that require heavy lifting place a strain on rotator cuff tendons and muscles. Normally, the tendons are strong, but continued strain of this type may lead to a tear.

Typically, a person with a **rotator cuff tear** feels pain over the deltoid muscle at the top and outer side of the shoulder, especially when the arm is raised or extended out from the side of the body. Motions such as those involved in getting dressed can be painful. The shoulder may feel weak, especially when trying to lift the arm into a horizontal position. A person may also feel or hear a click or pop when the shoulder is moved.

Pain or weakness on outward or inward rotation of the arm may also indicate a tear in a rotator cuff tendon. There is pain when lowering the arm to the side after the shoulder is moved backward and the arm is raised. A doctor may detect weakness but may not be able to determine from a physical examination the location of the tear. X-rays may appear normal. An MRI scan can help detect a full tendon tear, but not partial tears. If the pain disappears after a small amount of anesthetic is injected into the area, impingement is likely to be present. If there is no response to treatment, arthrography may be used to inspect the injured area and confirm the diagnosis.

A torn rotator cuff receives the same initial treatment as a stretched one–a comprehensive rehabilitation program. Some tears will heal without surgery. The surgery is difficult and should be avoided if at all possible. Arthroscopic surgery is coming into more widespread use for the shoulder and is a less invasive approach to treat the injury.

Massage Strategies

Use strategies for a muscle strain described on page 455.

FROZEN SHOULDER (ADHESIVE CAPSULITIS)

In cases of **frozen shoulder,** movement of the shoulder is severely restricted. This condition, also called *adhesive capsulitis,* is frequently caused by injury that leads to lack of use due to pain. Intermittent periods of use may cause inflammation. Adhesions grow between the joint surfaces, restricting motion. There is also a lack of synovial fluid, which normally lubricates the gap between the humerus and socket to help the shoulder joint move. It is this restricted space between the capsule and head of the humerus that distinguishes adhesive capsulitis from a less complicated painful, stiff shoulder.

There are a number of risk factors for frozen shoulder, including rotator cuff injury, diabetes, stroke, accidents, lung disease, and heart disease. The condition seldom occurs in people less than 40 years of age.

With a frozen shoulder, the joint becomes so tight and stiff that it is nearly impossible to carry out simple movements, such as raising the arm. People complain that the stiffness and discomfort worsen at night. A doctor may suspect a frozen shoulder if a physical examination reveals limited shoulder movement. An arthrogram may confirm the diagnosis.

Treatment of this disorder focuses on restoring joint movement and reducing shoulder pain. Usually, treatment begins with NSAIDs and the application of heat, followed by gentle stretching exercises and massage. In some cases, transcutaneous electrical nerve stimulation (TENS) may be used to reduce pain by blocking nerve impulses. If these measures are unsuccessful, the doctor may recommend manipulation of the shoulder under general anesthesia. Surgery to release the adhesions is necessary only in severe cases.

Massage Strategies

Massage cannot access adhesion inside the joint capsule. Instead massage is focused on increasing range of motion and pliability of the muscles related to shoulder mobility. Often the latissimus dorsi is short and a major source of symptoms. The pectoralis major and minor fascial covering can be stuck together, and this needs to be corrected. Massage applied to the hip opposite the affected shoulder while the client actively moves the frozen shoulder may stimulate reflex responses supporting mobility.

The sequence for subscapularis release is often helpful. All rotator cuff muscles need to be thoroughly massaged, lengthened, and stretched.

FRACTURE

Fracture of the shoulder usually occurs as a result of an impact injury such as a fall or blow to the shoulder. The fracture, which can be either a partial or total crack of the bone, usually involves the clavicle or the neck of the humerus.

A shoulder fracture that occurs after a major injury is usually accompanied by severe pain. Within a short time, there may be redness and bruising around the area. Sometimes a fracture is obvious because the bones appear out of position. Both diagnosis and severity can be confirmed by x-rays.

Initially, the doctor attempts to bring the affected parts into a position that will promote healing and restore arm movement *(reduction)*. If the bones are out of position, surgery may be necessary to reset them.

Fracture of the clavicle or neck of the humerus is usually treated with a sling or shoulder immobilizer. Exercises restore shoulder strength and motion.

Massage Strategies

See massage for fractures on page 472.

ARTHRITIS

Arthritis/arthrosis is a degenerative joint disease caused by wear and tear. Arthritis not only affects joints; it may secondarily affect supporting structures such as muscles, tendons, and ligaments.

The usual signs of **arthritis of the shoulder** are pain, particularly over the AC joint, and a decrease in shoulder motion. Arthritis is suspected when there is both pain and swelling in the joint. The diagnosis is confirmed by a physical examination and x-rays. Analysis of synovial fluid from the shoulder joint may be helpful in diagnosing some types of arthritis. Although arthroscopy permits direct visualization of damage to cartilage, tendons, and ligaments and may confirm a diagnosis, it is usually only done if a repair procedure is to be performed.

Athletes are particularly prone to developing arthritis if they have repeatedly damaged the shoulder joints.

Usually, osteoarthritis of the shoulder is treated with NSAIDs. When conservative treatment fails to relieve pain or improve function, or when there is severe deterioration of the joint, shoulder joint replacement *(arthroplasty)* may provide better results. Success of this procedure requires participation in a physical rehabilitation program. In this operation, an artificial ball replaces the humerus, and a cap replaces the scapula. Passive shoulder range of motion is started soon after surgery. Eventually, stretching and strengthening exercises become a major part of the rehabilitation program.

The success of the operation often depends on the condition of rotator cuff muscles prior to surgery and the degree to which the person follows the rehabilitation program.

Massage Strategies

Treatment that incorporates the strategies for arthritis is found on page 468; if surgery was necessary, see procedures shown in Chapter 19.

WEIGHT LIFTER'S SHOULDER

Weight lifting can cause overuse injuries of the shoulder. In particular, bench press exercises often lead to shoulder pain in the AC joint. The small amount of cartilage between the two bones of this joint—the acromion and the clavicle—can tear or degenerate from the stress of weight lifting. When the cartilage is damaged, bone rubs on bone, causing pain.

This injury, known as **"weight lifter's shoulder,"** is not common among well-trained or world-class weight lifters; people who work out on their own are those most likely to develop weight lifter's shoulder.

Usually, rest for a few weeks and an injection of cortisone provide relief. If the pain becomes chronic, then a small piece of the outer end (acromion process) of the collarbone can be surgically removed. This widens the space between the two bones and relieves the pressure in the joint, enabling return to full, pain-free weight lifting.

Massage Strategies

Use the same strategies as for arthritis, shown on page 468.

SHOULDER MUSCLE PULLS (STRAINS)

Shoulder muscle pulls (strains) occur when the muscles contract excessively or are overstretched, causing muscle fibers to tear. This is common in wrestling and in sports requiring throwing, such as basketball and baseball.

Treatment includes rest for 3 to 7 days, followed by stretching and then strengthening exercises.

Because of the complexity and number of muscles around the shoulder that can be injured, the diagnosis should determine the particular muscles involved, and a program specifically focusing on for those muscles is necessary.

Massage Strategies

Use strategies for strains and sprains on pages 458.

THE COLLARBONE (CLAVICLE)

BRUISED COLLARBONE

A blow on the head of the collarbone can cause a painful bone bruise, or contusion but not actually sprain the AC joint. This injury usually heals without difficulty but may lead to a condition called osteolysis.

Osteolysis causes the bone to dissolve and deteriorate due to a loss of calcium. On an x-ray the collarbone has a mossy appearance, and bone loss is evident on the outer end of the bone.

Although a **bruised collarbone** can be quite painful, the bone usually heals and becomes healthy again in 6 to 12 months, and the pain decreases. If the pain persists, the outer edge of the collarbone can be shaved in a surgical procedure to relieve the pain.

Massage Strategies

Apply lymphatic drain massage over the bruised area.

BROKEN COLLARBONE

The collarbone heals easily. A **broken collarbone** does not need to be set perfectly. However, in severe cases sharp fragments can cause damage to the surrounding tissue. As long as the pieces of the bone are in close proximity, they will bridge any gaps, heal, and form a new collarbone even stronger than the old one.

A broken collarbone is usually a concern only because it prevents the client from functioning. Proper treatment for a broken collarbone is immobilization to allow it to heal. A brace is used to pull the shoulders back and hold the ends of the bone in line. This injury takes 6 to 8 weeks to heal completely, but there is usually enough early healing so that the brace can be removed in about 3 weeks. Because the shoulder joints are not involved in the bracing, there is full use of the arms and shoulders.

Massage Strategies

See procedures for fractures on page 472.

THE ELBOW

The elbow has three separate joints, consisting of the junction of the two bones of the forearm–the radius and ulna–and the junction of each of these bones with the humerus. These three joints allow the elbow to flex and extend and also to rotate, allowing *supination* and *pronation*. The elbow is a common source of injury, particularly in racquet and throwing sports.

Elbow pain can be caused by wrist problems. The muscles that control the wrist originate from the bones of the elbow, and many problems caused by excessive wrist strain cause pain in the elbow rather than in the wrist.

TENNIS ELBOW

Tennis elbow, a common elbow injury, is an inflammation of the muscles of the forearm and the tendon that connects the muscles to the bones in the elbow. These muscles are used in wrist extension and supination. When the muscles and tendons become inflamed from overuse, pain occurs on the outside of the elbow (lateral epicondyle). The pain is worse during lifting with the palm facing down (for example, when picking up a cup).

Tennis elbow also causes pain during rotation of the hand in a clockwise direction (the direction used to screw in a light bulb). During clenching or squeezing, pain will be felt such as when shaking hands or holding a racquet or golf club.

Golfers also suffer from tennis elbow, but on the nondominant side: a right-handed golfer will feel the pain in the left elbow. Pulling the club through the swing with the left wrist causes irritation in the left elbow.

Tennis players most often aggravate the elbow by hitting the ball late on a backhand swing, straining the forearm muscles and tendon.

Once the elbow becomes inflamed, everyday activities are enough to keep it irritated. Treatment includes rest and an exercise program to increase the strength and flexibility of the forearm muscles and tendons. Massage is very helpful in increasing flexibility and pliability in these muscles.

One treatment for tennis elbow is cortisone injections; however, this is not the best long-term strategy. Injecting an antiinflammatory agent such as cortisone around an inflamed tendon will reduce the inflammation and ease the pain, but this does not address the cause of the problem, which is overstressing the forearm tendons. When the cortisone begins to wear off (in 4 to 6 weeks), the forces that caused the tendinitis in the first place remain, causing the pain and stress to recur. Repeated cortisone injections can irreparably damage tendons.

In deep friction massage, pressure is applied back and forth across the tendon. The irritation causes increased blood flow to the tendon and promotes healing. Another way of increasing blood flow is electrotherapy, in which an electric current is passed through the tendon. Other modalities include iontophoresis, in which a cortisone solution is painted on the skin and then driven through the tendon using an electric current. This concentrates cortisone around the tendon without subjecting it to damage from an injection.

Persons with a history of tennis elbow, or who feel twinges of pain after playing tennis, should ice the elbow down. Icing is more effective once the elbow has returned to normal body temperature.

Another type of tennis elbow is characterized by pain on the inner side of elbow at the medial epicondyle. This pain involves inflammation of the muscles and tendons that allow pronation of the wrist.

Other sports that require a snap of the wrist, such as the throwing sports, can also lead to this type of elbow pain. Prevention and treatment are the same as for tennis elbow.

Massage Strategies

Use massage strategies for tendinitis shown on page 466. Deep friction massage does increase circulation, but it also creates inflammation. The benefit of friction massage needs to be evaluated on a case-by-case basis.

PITCHER'S ELBOW

Baseball pitchers may develop elbow pain that occurs on the inner (medial) side of the elbow or on both the inner and outer (lateral) sides. This is called **"pitcher's elbow."** Pitching requires a tremendous external rotational force on the elbow that stretches the ligaments that hold the inner bones together, causing pain, and compresses the outer side, causing the head of the radius to jam against the humerus.

The repeated trauma of this compression can cause an area of bone in the humerus to die. This disorder is called *osteochondritis dissecans*. The dead piece of bone can actually fall into the joint, leaving a crater. This causes continued pain and clicking in the elbow. If a fragment gets caught in the joint, it becomes a **loose body** and may cause the elbow to lock.

The treatment for this condition is rest, which allows the elbow ligament and bone to heal. It may take a full year for the bone to heal. If there are loose pieces of bone inside the elbow, arthroscopic surgery will be required to remove them.

Massage Strategies

Use the strategies for tendinitis shown on page 466. Apply lymphatic drain massage if edema is present. If friction massage is used, the location needs to be precisely at the specific area of pain in the tendons.

LITTLE LEAGUE ELBOW

A young baseball player who throws too often or too hard can irritate the growing part of the elbow bone, and the medial epicondyle enlarges. In the act of throwing, the flexor muscles of the wrist contract to propel the ball. These muscles are connected to the medial epicondyle, and the constant yanking pulls the soft growth center (epiphysis) apart, causing pain. Also, irritation of the growth center stimulates it and causes excessive growth of the medial epicondyle.

Treatment for this condition, called **"Little League elbow,"** is rest until the condition subsides. This usually takes from 6 weeks to 6 months, depending on the severity of the injury.

In severe cases, the medial epicondyle may be torn completely off the bone through the soft growth center. This injury is an emergency situation, and the epicondyle will need to be surgically reimplanted.

Rehabilitation, which includes immobilization followed by gradual range-of-motion exercises with an experienced physical therapist, may take 6 months or longer after surgery.

Sanctioned Little Leagues now restrict the number of innings that a pitcher can pitch in a week.

Massage Strategies

No specific massage is used. If the client has surgery, massage should follow the recommendations of the physical therapist or physician for presurgery and postsurgery care.

"FUNNY BONE" (CUBITAL TUNNEL) SYNDROME

Hitting the elbow in a certain way stimulates the ulnar nerve and causes the numbness, tingling, and pain characteristic of the **"funny bone" syndrome,** or cubital tunnel syndrome. The ulnar nerve traverses the back of the elbow in a groove behind the medial epicondyle.

Some athletes may feel as if they have hit their funny bone as a result of repeated trauma to the elbow. Scar tissue may form over the nerve and compress it into the canal, resulting in severe pain in the elbow. Numbness and tingling radiate down into the fourth and fifth fingers, with loss of strength in these fingers. This syndrome is similar to carpal tunnel syndrome in the wrist.

The treatment is surgery to remove the scar tissue formed over the nerve. The nerve may have to be transplanted outside of the canal to prevent scar tissue from building up around it again.

Massage Strategies

Massage is not appropriate to reduce the scar tissue because of the close proximity to the nerve and the potential for nerve damage. A skin rolling application over the adhered area may increase tissue pliability. Restoring normal resting length to all muscles in the area may reduce symptoms. Postsurgery massage can encourage more appropriate scar formation. See postsurgery strategies in Chapter 19.

HYPEREXTENDED ELBOW

When force applied to the elbow extends farther than normal, the result is hyperextension. This tears the fibers that hold the front of the elbow joint together and overextends the biceps muscle, which attaches just below the elbow.

A **hyperextended elbow** causes pain and swelling. Treatment consists of rest, ice application, and possibly splinting to keep the elbow bent until the pain subsides. Stretching is slowly introduced until pain-free range of motion returns. Total recovery time is usually 3 to 6 weeks, depending on the severity of the injury.

Massage Strategies

Agonist/antagonist balance is altered with hyperextension injury. The biceps muscles are pulled into a forced eccentric pattern and may also spasm in an attempt to decelerate the movement. Triceps shorten concentrically and can develop trigger points. Co-contraction of both muscles stabilizes the joint, but the joint can become jammed, interfering with range of motion. Massage targets all of these issues from the subacute phase on, into the remodeling phase of healing. Follow strategies for strains and sprains–acute, subacute, and remodeling.

BONE CHIPS

Bone chips are the result of many years of overuse of the elbow and usually afflict an older pitcher or tennis player. Football players, especially linemen, are also prone to this condition. Little pieces of bone break off the elbow due to long and repeated stress. Arthroscopic surgery is the usual treatment option if the pain cannot be tolerated.

Massage Strategies

Massage can reduce symptoms of compensatory muscle tension. All massage methods aimed at muscle length and connective tissue pliability are appropriate. If surgery is performed, follow pre- and post-surgical massage protocols in Chapter 19.

TRICEPS TENDINITIS

Throwing sports can cause pain in the back of the elbow at the olecranon process. **Triceps tendinitis** may also occur in basketball players, as the result of dribbling and throwing motions. The triceps muscle and tendon combine to straighten out the elbow. In the throwing motion, the elbow begins at a flexed position as the arm is cocked and extends as the throw is delivered, causing stress where the triceps tendon attaches to the elbow. The pain of triceps tendinitis can be severe, primarily for baseball pitchers.

Treatment includes rest, ice application, and a structured rehabilitation exercise program.

Massage Strategies

See general treatment for tendinitis on page 466.

BICEPS TENDINITIS

Biceps tendinitis, or inflammation, is characterized by pain in the lower portion of the biceps muscle where it attaches to the elbow. It is a common phenomenon in beginning weight lifters who overstress themselves, and among veteran weight lifters who make too big a step-up in the weights that they are lifting. The pain usually occurs the day after lifting. There will also be a limitation in the range of motion due to inflammation and spasm in the muscle fibers that have been overstressed.

Treatment consists of icing and rest in the acute phase. An adjustment in the training intensity and form is necessary, as well as rehabilitation exercise.

Massage Strategies

See massage treatment for tendinitis on page 466.

TORN BICEPS

A sudden, severe movement of the arm can tear the biceps muscle, as when a golfer unexpectedly hits the ground hard with a club, a tennis player hits a hard forehand smash, or a weight lifter makes a clean-and-jerk motion. The **torn biceps** results in pain, bleeding, loss of function, and muscle deformity. The biceps muscle may contract and ball up, creating a defect the size of a small orange on top of the muscle.

Cosmetic surgery can correct the muscle defect, but it cannot restore the strength of the muscle. The buildup of scar tissue weakens the muscle, and a torn biceps that has been repaired will likely tear again.

Medical treatment consists of rest for 2 or 3 weeks while the torn muscle heals, followed by a training program to strengthen the other head of the biceps so it can compensate for the loss of strength and function.

Massage Strategies

Use the muscle strain strategies shown on page 458. Scar tissue management is also appropriate.

THE WRIST

The wrist is one of the most complex structures in the body. There are 10 bones involved in moving the wrist joint in various directions. These small bones are extremely sensitive to excessive force or trauma, commonly occurring in racquet and throwing sports. In addition, tremendous head-on forces on the wrist are generated in boxing, football, and wrestling. Because of all of these forces, the wrist is one of the more frequently injured parts of the body.

Any severe wrist pain following a fall or blow should be seen by a physician and x-rayed because of the possibility of a fracture. The wrist is usually fractured because of a fall. However, a wrist can also fracture by being hit. A wrist fracture can be mis-diagnosed as a sprain or a bruise.

SPRAINS

The most common injury to the wrist is a sprain.

All but the most minor wrist sprains should be x-rayed, because a sprained ligament may pull off a little piece of bone, which changes the injury to an avulsion fracture. A sprained wrist may not need anything more than a soft splint. A fractured wrist, however, requires casting.

The treatment of a **sprained wrist,** as for any sprain, is PRICE (*p*rotection, *r*est, *i*ce, *c*ompression, and *e*levation) therapy, followed by range-of-motion exercises and then by strengthening exercises.

Subluxation of the wrist bones is a serious sprain. This happens when the ligaments connecting two or more of the small bones are torn completely, and the bones slide out of place.

This is a common injury among boxers, and usually results from hitting the heavy bag in training.

Massage Strategies

Use the sequences for sprains (see page 458).

TRAPEZIUM FRACTURE

The trapezium bone is the small bone in the wrist just behind the base of the thumb. This fracture is usually caused by stretching the hand out to break a fall or by hitting the hand against an opposing player's helmet. Healing is more difficult for this fracture than for most other fractures in the body because there may not be adequate blood supply to the broken bone. It can take 8 weeks to 8 months for this bone to heal.

New techniques, however, such as implanting an electromagnet in the cast, can speed bone healing. The magnet causes the underlying filaments of the bone matrix to line up with the same polarity. This method is commonly used when there is no evidence of healing after a reasonable amount of time (about 6 weeks). If the bone does not reknit, it probably will need to be repaired surgically with a bone graft.

If left untreated, trapezium fracture will lead to chronic pain in the wrist and the loss of ability to extend the wrist backward.

Massage Strategies

Use the sequences for contusions (page 447) and fractures (page 472).

SCAPHOID FRACTURE

Even slight tenderness in the anatomic snuffbox around the scaphoid, as well as swelling obliterating the space between the thumb's extensor tendons, suggests the presence of a **scaphoid fracture** that may not appear on an x-ray until 2 weeks following trauma. Percussion on the knuckle of the index finger when the fist is closed will usually elicit pain in the scaphoid if it is fractured. Scaphoid fracture is common in ice hockey players.

Massage Strategies

Use the strategies for contusions (page 447) and fractures (page 472).

GOLFER'S WRIST

If a golf club in full swing hits the ground or a hard object other than the ball, an isolated fracture of the wrist may result. This injury is called **golfer's wrist**. The mechanism seems to be violent contraction of the flexor carpi ulnaris insertion through the pisiform-hamate ligament. X-rays may show a fracture of the hamate.

Massage Strategies

Use the strategies for contusions (page 447) and fractures (page 472).

LUNATE INJURY

Carpal dislocations, especially lunate, are frequently missed during evaluation. These are often associated with a trans-scaphoid fracture and necrosis. Lunate dislocation and/or fracture, or **Boxer's wrist**, may be seen in any athlete as the result of a fall on the outstretched hand, but it is most common in boxers whose hands are carelessly wrapped. Damage to the median nerve is a complication. The symptoms include anterior wrist swelling, with stiff and semiflexed fingers.

The lunate usually dislodges posteriorly or anteriorly, disrupting its relationship with the neighboring carpals and the distal radius. Anterior displacement is the common direction, where the bone rests deep in the annular ligament and may affect the median nerve. The lunate is loosely stabilized by anterior and posterior ligaments that contain small nutritive blood vessels. A torn ligament thus interferes with the lunate's nutrition, resulting in necrosis.

Massage Strategies

Use the strategies for contusions (page 447) and fractures (page 472).

RACQUET WRIST

Tennis or racquetball players may develop pain at the base of the hand below the little finger. Every time the player hits a ball, the racquet butt bangs into and bruises one of the small bones of the wrist.

If the pain is severe, this indicates that the little hook of bone at this spot may be broken and will need to be treated as a fracture.

Sometimes a bone bruise is found deep in the proximal hypothenar eminence in the hamate-pisiform area. This condition, known as **racquet wrist**, is common in sports requiring a hand-held object such as a hockey stick, ski pole, baseball bat, or racket, because of the impact on the hamate prominence. It may also result from a fall when the outstretched hand strikes an irregular surface.

Chronic aggravation results in deep swelling, vascular symptoms similar to those of carpal tunnel syndrome, and distal neuralgia.

Massage Strategies

Use the strategies for contusions (page 447) and bone fractures (page 472).

TENDINITIS

The wrist is the passageway for tendons that begin in the forearm and extend into the fingers. The fingers are actually controlled by muscles in the forearm, not in the hand. Overuse of the wrist in sports causes inflammation of the finger tendons attached to these forearm muscles. This results in swelling, pain, and limited function in one or more of the fingers.

The extensor and flexor tendons in the thumb are particularly sensitive to overuse. The extensor tendon moves the thumb away from the second finger, and the flexor tendon moves it toward the second finger. Tendinitis limits the ability to grasp with the thumb. This condition is common in tennis players with pain and swelling on the thumb side of the wrist, which is caused by gripping the racket too tightly.

Treatment consists of rest and icing the tendon in the wrist, followed by administration of antiinflammatory medications and immobilization of the thumb and wrist to further reduce the inflammation.

Massage Strategies

Use treatment strategies for tendinitis on page 466.

GANGLION

A **ganglion** is a cyst that appears as a small lump on the wrist or hand, which can vary from the size of a kernel of corn to the size of a cherry. It can occur on the back or front of the wrist, depending on whether an extensor or flexor tendon is involved. Both of these tendons slide through a sheath that produces synovial fluid.

If a finger tendon and its sheath become inflamed from overuse or a blow to the wrist, part of the tendon sheath may seal off. A cyst forms because the liquid produced by the sheath is trapped. The cyst, or ganglion, swells inside the tendon sheath as the cells produce more fluid, and it can become quite painful.

The ganglion may open at one end if there is pressure from overproduction of fluid or from a sudden blow. The fluid runs out and the ganglion collapses. The problem is that the raw surfaces that have blown out may seal off again, causing the ganglion to re-form.

A ganglion is a problem when it becomes painful with activity. As long as it doesn't bother the athlete, there is no need to treat it. If the ganglion is problematic, medical treatment includes injecting it with cortisone, which causes it to disappear. If the ganglion continues to re-form after several injections, surgical removal may be necessary.

Massage Strategies

Do not irritate the area or attempt to massage the area. If cortisone is used, avoid the area. Follow presurgery and postsurgery strategies in Chapter 19, if surgery is performed.

CHRONIC OSTEOARTHRITIS/ ARTHROSIS

Chronic **osteoarthritis/arthrosis** of the wrist is a degenerative joint disease characterized by deterioration and abrasion of articular cartilage, with new bone formation at the borders of the joint. It is the most common form of arthritis. Wear from aging, trauma, and the abuse of weight bearing are typical causes. There is also disruption of collagen, decreased ground substance, many microscopic changes, and frequent increase in water content of the involved cartilage.

Morning stiffness that eases with activity, pain on prolonged exercise, slight joint swelling from fluid accumulation, crepitus on movement, disuse atrophy, and joint deformity are characteristic.

Massage Strategies

Use the sequences for arthritis and arthrosis (page 468).

CARPAL TUNNEL SYNDROME

The finger tendons pass through the wrist in a narrow, tunnel-like enclosure. With chronic overuse or excessive twisting of the wrist, fluid builds up in the sheaths of the tendons, causing the tendons to become inflamed and swollen. The carpal ligament can become thickened from overuse. Both of these conditions narrow the tunnel and pinch the main nerve that passes through the tunnel to the fingers.

The complex of symptoms resulting from this condition is called **carpal tunnel syndrome**. The pain extends up into the forearm and down into the hand, and there may be numbness, tingling, and even loss of strength in the middle and ring fingers.

Tightly gripping something while exercising can lead to carpal tunnel syndrome. People who use a walker and cane can be susceptible to this disorder.

The treatment is rest of the affected wrist and ice application. If the symptoms do not subside, then NSAIDs may be prescribed. A splint minimizes or prevents pressure on the nerve, and steroid injection into the ligament helps reduce swelling. If the pain persists, surgery to cut the ligament at the bottom of the wrist releases the pressure.

Brachial plexus impingement at the neck and shoulder can mimic carpal tunnel syndrome symptoms. This condition needs to be ruled out before invasive treatment of the wrist.

Massage Strategies

It is difficult for the massage therapist to differentiate between brachial plexus impingement, carpal tunnel impingement, or a combination of the two; and the choice of massage therapy should be based on diagnosis by a physician.

A simple assessment can provide some clues, however. If tapping the area of the carpal tunnel impingement increases symptoms more than applying pressure on the scalenes, pectoralis minor, or brachial plexus, the primary location of the impingement is at the wrist. If applying pressure at the brachial plexus increases the symptoms more than tapping the wrist, the brachial plexus impingement may be the primary causal factor. Unless specific diagnosis of carpal tunnel syndrome has been made, massage should address both the possible brachial plexus impingement and actual impingement at the wrist. See massage for impingement on page 477.

- Address the entire arm with the goal of reducing muscle tension and increasing connective tissue pliability.
- Fluid accumulation at the wrist can impinge the nerves, so lymphatic drain is appropriate.
- Specifically apply bend and shear force to the retinaculum and palmar fascia. Use enough intensity to increase pliability of these connective tissue structures but do not increase inflammation or irritation of the nerve.
- Also address reflex areas such as the opposite ankle and leg and reflex points for the arm and wrist or the foot.

THE HAND

Hand injuries can be so complex that a medical specialist in hand therapy may be necessary.

BROKEN HAND

The metacarpals are commonly fractured, almost always due to a head-on blow to the knuckle, as when a player smashes his hand into another player's helmet or is stepped on.

The treatment for a **broken hand** is to cast or splint it for 4 to 6 weeks. If the break is directly across the shaft of the bone and the ends are jammed together, an athlete may be able to return to activity in a much shorter time with a light plastic splint. If the bones have been twisted apart and there are sharp ends at the fracture, the hand will have to stay in a cast until the fracture heals.

The type of fracture depends mainly on the direction of the injuring force applied to the hand, not the particular sport.

Massage Strategies

Use the strategies for fractures (page 472). Also address compensation in the forearm resulting from supporting the weight of the cast and limited movement.

BROKEN FINGER

A **broken finger** is very common in sports and usually occurs when a ball hits the end of a finger. Finger fractures often are not serious, particularly those in the tip of the finger. "Buddy taping," or taping an injured finger to a healthy one next to it, usually allows the athlete to continue sports activity. If the fracture is in the second or third bone of the finger, it will need to be splinted for 4 to 6 weeks to allow healing.

Massage Strategies

Use the strategies for fractures (page 472).

DISLOCATED FINGER

If a finger is struck with a great deal of force, one of its joints may dislocate. This is common in football and basketball. It's usually simple for the team doctor or trainer to pop the joint back into place. Buddy taping the **dislocated finger** to a healthy one stabilizes the joint, and the player can return to the game.

However, the finger needs to be x-rayed later on. A piece of bone at the base of the dislocated finger may break off, causing a fracture that extends into the joint. If not taken care of, this can result in loss of function in the finger and future disability.

Massage Strategies

Apply massage to the forearm to manage guarding. Treat as described for fractures (see page 472) and use lymphatic drain methods.

JAMMED FINGER

A **jammed finger** occurs when the tip of the finger hits something head-on. One of the joints holding the bone in the finger may not be totally dislocated, but the bone may have snapped partway out of joint and then snapped back in. This injures the cartilage on the end of the bone, as well as the capsule around the joint, and stretches the ligaments that hold the joint together. The result is a swollen, painful finger that may appear normal on an x-ray.

A jammed finger heals very slowly. The finger should be immobilized for 7 to 10 days and then buddy taped to the finger next to it. It can take 6 months for the joint to return to normal size, or it may remain larger than it was and/or larger than the joint on the opposite hand. Flexibility in the finger is often lost, but usually not enough to cause any great difficulty in dexterity.

Massage Strategies

Initially address the swelling with lymphatic drain massage. Once the swelling is reduced, use joint play methods (see Unit Two). Do not force joint movement.

TENDON TEARS

A sudden, violent force applied to the fingers can cause tendons to tear. Any inability to move one of the joints in a finger may indicate a **torn tendon**, and the client should be referred to a trainer or physician immediately. A torn tendon must be repaired surgically to prevent permanent loss of finger function.

Baseball players often tear the tendon at the top of a finger from a blow to the end of the finger. As a result, the tip of the finger droops and cannot be straightened out at the fingertip. The tendon itself may be torn in half or a piece of bone where the tendon attaches to the tip may have been broken off.

This condition is known as baseball finger. It also occurs in basketball and volleyball players who are hit by the ball on the end of the finger.

Treatment consists of splinting the finger, the fingertip held in the extended position, for about 6 weeks. If the tendon doesn't heal, surgery is required to straighten out the fingertip.

Massage Strategies

Apply massage to manage compensation patterns in the forearm.

SKI POLE THUMB

The most common ligament tear in the hand occurs on the inner side of the thumb. This is the so-called **ski pole thumb** injury suffered by snow skiers when a thumb gets trapped in the loop of the pole during a fall. Occasionally, basketball players also suffer this injury. When the thumb ligaments are torn, the thumb cannot press sideways against the other fingers to grasp an object.

The immediate treatment is icing of the thumb and splinting. The thumb is immobilized for approximately 6 weeks. If it fails to heal, it will have to be surgically repaired.

Massage Strategies

Apply massage to manage compensation in the forearm.

TRIGGER FINGER

Trigger finger is the result of repeated trauma to the palm of the hand, such as occurs when a tennis racket jams into the palm or a baseball repeatedly hits a catcher's palm. The trauma causes injury and inflammation to the flexor tendon of a finger. The tendon's sheath thickens, narrowing the space around the tendon, and the tendon itself also thickens. It becomes difficult for the thickened tendon to move in the narrowed sheath.

The flexor muscles of the finger, which are stronger than the extensor muscles, are able to pull on the tendon and bend the finger. But the extensors are not strong enough to pull it back and straighten it. The finger ends up in a bent position, similar to the position of a finger that is pulling the trigger on a gun.

This injury sometimes responds to cortisone injection, which reduces inflammation in the tendon sheath. If not, the sheath will need to be split surgically to allow free motion of the finger.

Massage Strategies

Massage can reduce the muscle imbalance by inhibiting the finger flexors. This is a temporary solution, but massage can manage compensation

and help prevent the situation from getting worse.

BLISTERS

Athletes often suffer **blisters** and calluses on their hands and fingers from gripping balls, clubs, bars, and tennis rackets. Sweat makes the skin sticky, and the friction between the hands and the objected gripped can cause blisters. The feet are also a common location for blisters.

There are two theories on treating blisters. One is to leave the blisters alone and let them heal. New skin forms under the blister, and the fluid in the blister gradually becomes absorbed. Eventually, the outer layer of skin sloughs off. Simple table salt can be made into a paste with a bit of water. This salt paste is put on a gauze pad and taped over the blister. The salt will draw the fluid out, decreasing the time necessary for healing. Usually this is done at night while the person is sleeping. The process may need to be repeated for 3 or 4 days.

The other theory recommends opening up the blister and letting the fluid drain. The trainer should choose which method to use.

Massage Strategies

Massage therapy is not applicable in these cases.

CALLUSES

Calluses are areas of skin that have thickened because of constant pressure. The pressure causes the tissues underneath the callus to become tender. If the callus becomes bothersome, it can be softened with a cream or ointment. The dead skin is then rubbed away with a pumice stone. If this does not help, a physician may trim the callus surgically or chemically.

Massage Strategies

Massage therapy is not applicable in these cases.

SPRAINED THUMB

If the thumb is forced out of its normal range of movement (usually backward), the ligaments supporting the metacarpophalangeal joint at the bottom of the thumb are damaged.

Pain occurs in the web of the thumb when the thumb is bent backward, and there is swelling over the joint at the bottom of the thumb. If the resultant laxity and instability in the joint are severe, a total rupture may have occurred, and surgery is required.

Treatment for a **sprained thumb** includes rest and taping of the thumb to provide support and prevent further damage. Most athletes are able to return to sports activity within 4 to 6 weeks, depending on the severity of the injury. It is important that strengthening exercises are done to restore stability and prevent reinjury. If the injury is not treated properly, then there is a greater risk of reinjury and permanent instability, which will eventually require surgery.

Massage Strategies

Treat as a sprain (see page 458). Manage muscle guarding in the forearm.

SPRAINED FINGER

A **sprained finger** is common in games such as football, basketball, baseball, cricket, and handball. Usually the collateral ligaments at the side of the finger are damaged.

There is point pain over the joint in the finger where the damage has occurred, as well as pain when bending the finger and stressing the injured ligament. Swelling of the joint is possible, causing restricted mobility. Instability of the finger occurs if the injury is severe or if there is a complete rupture of the ligament.

Treatment involves taping the finger to protect it while healing. If the ligament is completely ruptured, surgery is necessary.

Massage Strategies

Treat as a sprain (see page 458) and manage guarding in the forearm.

LOWER ABDOMEN AND GROIN

The anatomy of the lower abdomen, groin, and pelvic girdle is quite complex. Because the pelvis is a ring, any change in anatomy or applied forces to one area will be compensated throughout the ring. This simple fact makes it easier to understand why a leg length discrepancy or SI joint dysfunction can greatly change the shear forces across the pubic symphysis. The hip adductors (gracilis, adductor longus, adductor brevis, adductor magnus) attach at the inferior pubic ramus. The pectineus and rectus abdominis muscles, along with the inguinal ligament, attach superiorly. The muscles of the pelvic floor attach posteriorly.

SPORTS HERNIA (ATHLETIC PUBALGIA)

Athletes who participate in sports that require rapid repetitive twisting and turning movements, such as soccer, ice hockey, field hockey, tennis, and football, may be at risk of developing a sports hernia, also called *athletic pubalgia*. A sports hernia is a disruption of the inguinal canal without a clinically detectable hernia. These injuries occur because adductor action during sporting activities creates shearing forces across the pubic symphysis that can stress the posterior inguinal wall. Ongoing repetitive stretching of, or a more intense sudden force on, the transverse fascia and the internal oblique muscles can lead to their separation from the inguinal ligament. This mechanism may also account for the common finding of coexisting osteitis pubis and adductor tenoperiostitis in these clients (Figure 21-11).

The inguinal canal carries the spermatic cord in males and the round ligament in females. The anterior wall of the canal consists of the external oblique aponeurosis and the internal oblique muscle. The posterior wall is formed by the fascia transversalis, which is reinforced in its medial third by the conjoined tendon, the common tendon of insertion of the internal oblique and transversus abdominis, which attaches to the pubic crest and pectineal line. The superficial inguinal ring lies anterior to the strong conjoined tendon.

Sports hernia typically consists of one or more of the following: a torn external oblique aponeurosis causing dilatation of the superficial inguinal ring; a torn conjoined tendon; a dehiscence (bursting open, splitting, or gaping along natural or sutured lines) between the torn conjoined tendon and the inguinal ligament; a weakening of the transversalis fascia with separation from the conjoined tendon; tears in the internal oblique muscles; and tears in the external oblique aponeurosis.

Insidious onset of unilateral groin pain is the most common symptom. The predominant complaint of athletes with a sports hernia is unilateral groin pain, though bilateral pain may also occur. The pain usually occurs during exercise, but may be experienced during other activities. The onset is typically insidious, but in a third of cases the athlete may describe a sudden tearing sensation. Insidious onset often occurs in runners, whereas

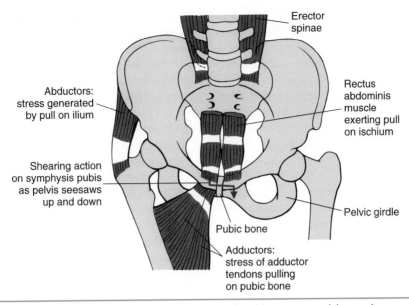

FIGURE 21-11 ■ Shearing action of symphysis pubis as the pelvis seesaws up and down predisposes to osteitis pubis and adductor tenoperiostitis. (From Saidoff DC, McDonough A: *Critical pathways in therapeutic intervention—extremities and spine.* St. Louis, 2002, Mosby.)

sudden onset is more common in ice hockey and soccer players.

Signs may be similar to those of osteitis pubis and adductor tendonopathy.

Symptoms include:

- Local tenderness over the conjoined tendon and inguinal canal.
- Tenderness increased by resisted sit-ups.
- Radiating pain to the adductor region and testicles.
- Pain aggravated by sudden movements.
- Pain increased by coughing or sneezing.
- Resistance to conservative treatment.

Surgery is the preferred treatment, although often a trial of conservative treatment is used. Specific rehabilitation that avoids sudden, sharp movements should enable athletes to return to sports participation 6 to 8 weeks after surgery. All aspects of pelvic flexibility, strength, and core stability should be addressed. Overlapping conditions should also be addressed, and coexisting osteitis pubis or adductor tendonopathy may indicate a more gradual return to athletic activity.

Massage Strategies

Therapeutic massage supports presurgery and postsurgery rehabilitation. Prevention is supported by addressing proper movement of the pelvis and SI joints, and appropriate tension/length relationships of the hip flexors and adductors. Massage can also maintain normal firing patterns of the involved muscles. The attachments of the rectus abdominis can become painful if trunk firing is synergistically dominant. Use inhibitory pressure on the attachment at the ribs and down the muscles to the pubic bone. Use direct stretching on the rectus abdominis. Do not apply deep pressure into the inguinal area.

OSTEITIS PUBIS

Osteitis pubis is an inflammation of the pubic symphysis and surrounding muscle insertions likely caused by muscle injury to the hip adductors or abdominal musculature causing muscle spasm, which in turn produces increased shearing forces across the pubic symphysis. SI joint dysfunction is often involved.

Osteitis pubis seems to be more prevalent in sports such as soccer, hockey, and football that involve running, sprinting, kicking, or rapid lateral movements and change of direction. These movements can lead to strain of the adductor muscles, which changes the forces directed on the pelvis. Other contributing factors are collisions that often cause minor injuries that are "played through," as well as back-pedaling (running backward), with rapid abduction of one hip to turn and run, causing hamstring or adductor strains, which change the muscle balance and forces across the pubic symphysis.

Signs and symptoms of osteitis pubis include:

- Pain in the lower abdominals, groin, hip, perineum, or testicles.
- Adductor pain or lower abdominal pain that then localizes to the pubic area.
- Unilateral pain that has been present for a few days to weeks. Tenderness over the superior pubic ramus.
- Pain over one or both SI joints.
- Piriformis spasm and resultant sciatic-type pain.

The pain increases with running, kicking, or pushing off to change direction. If the athlete complains of pubic pain of acute onset with fever and chills, a full workup for osteomyelitis must be performed.

When discrepancies of leg length are involved, the athlete may complain of hip pain in the longer limb. This also can be seen in runners and joggers who consistently run in the same direction along roadsides, with the result that one leg is shorter than the other.

Pelvic and hip inflexibility, instability, or imbalance may contribute to the development of osteitis pubis. Therapeutic exercises can increase the flexibility and strength of muscles attaching and acting across the pubic symphysis. Particular attention should be paid to the strength and flexibility of the hip flexors, abductors, adductors, abdominals, and pelvic stabilizing muscles. Care need to be taken that during core training the rectus abdominis does not become dominant. Chiropractic or other forms of joint manipulation may help with SI joint dysfunction and leg length discrepancy.

Massage Strategies

Therapeutic massage supports rehabilitation and maintains prevention by addressing proper movement of the pelvis and SI joints, as well as tension/length relationships of the hip flexors and adductors. Massage can also maintain normal muscle activation sequences (firing patterns) of the involved muscles and support proper function of the latissimus dorsi, lumbar dorsal fascia, gluteus maximus which act as a force couple of the SI joint. The gait reflexes are often disrupted, especially the adductor/abductor interaction. At each massage session, normalize all gait reflexes.

The attachments of the rectus abdominis can become painful if trunk firing is synergistically dominant. Use inhibitory pressure on the attachment at the ribs and down the muscles to the pubic bone. Use direct tissue stretching on the rectus abdominis. See rectus abdominis release in Unit Two.

Often there is reflexive tension in the sternoclavicular joints and surrounding muscles, because they are functionally paired with the SI joints. The integrated muscle energy technique is especially effective with leg length discrepancy:

- Increase the distortion by pulling on the long leg to make it longer or by pushing up on the heel of the short leg to make it shorter, and then have the client push or pull out of the distortion pattern. The quadratus lumborum will be short on the short leg side.
- Use quadratus lumborum release paired with scalene release. The psoas may also be involved and the pelvis will likely have some sort of rotational pattern.
- Use indirect functional techniques to balance the pelvis. Those methods are described in Unit Two.

GROIN PULL

Making a sudden lateral movement while rotating the leg when running or skating can pull a groin muscle. Several different groups of muscles attach to the groin area. The flexor muscles bend the hip, the adductor muscles bring one leg in against the other, and the rotator muscles bring the knee across the opposite leg. Muscle testing to identify which motion creates the pain can determine which muscle is involved. The rectus abdominis attachment at the symphysis pubis can mimic a **groin pull**.

Treatment includes rest for 3 or 4 days, followed by a gentle stretching program. Return to activity should be gradual.

Massage Strategies

See rectus abdominis release methods in Unit Two. Address compensation patterns and apply the massage sequence for strains (see page 458). Because the injury is located in the groin, massage in this area must be applied with specific permission and performed confidently.

THE HIP

The hip is a stable ball-and-socket joint. Because the ball of the hip fits so tightly into the socket, it doesn't dislocate as easily as the shallow shoulder joint and is much less prone to injury. Because a hip dislocation requires immense force, it is very rarely seen in athletics.

OSTEOARTHRITIS/ARTHROSIS

Osteoarthritis/arthrosis of the hip is a degenerative process in the hip caused by wear and tear or by an injury. The surfaces of the joint become rough, causing pain during hip movement. There is no apparent swelling because the tight hip joint has little room for fluid accumulation. Also, the joint is buried under large muscles, so any swelling is not apparent.

Treatment for osteoarthritis/arthrosis of the hip includes antiinflammatory medication and rehabilitative exercise. Hip replacement may be required later in life. Hip replacement is a major reason why people are in physical rehabilitation.

Massage Strategies

Use the sequence for arthritis (see page 468). If a hip replacement is done, follow sequences for presurgery and postsurgery massage.

BO JACKSON INJURY

Avascular necrosis, or **Bo Jackson injury**, was a little-known sports injury until super-athlete Bo Jackson developed it. It is usually caused by a blow to the knee or foot with the leg extended. During the injury, all of Bo Jackson's weight came down on one leg that was locked at the knee. The full impact of the blow was transmitted up to the hip. This caused the ball of the hip joint to hit the wall of the socket with great force, compromising the blood supply in the area and causing gradual deterioration of the surrounding cartilage and bone.

Diagnosis of avascular necrosis is confirmed by an MRI scan. Treatment typically consists of rest, with no weight bearing on the hip, for 6 to 12 months. Surgical procedures may hasten recovery. If the condition does not improve, the bone will eventually be destroyed and a hip replacement will be required.

Massage Strategies

Use the sequence for increasing arterial circulation and lymphatic drainage (see Unit Two).

BROKEN HIP

A **broken hip** causes severe pain and the inability to move the hip or walk. In the supine position, the leg with the broken hip may appear to be shortened, with the foot rolled to the outside while the other foot points up.

Usually, surgical repair is necessary. This injury is rare among young athletes, although a violent force can break even a young athlete's hip. A broken hip usually occurs in the elderly, who have more brittle bones. A broken hip is a major reason why older women, in particular, are in orthopedic rehabilitation.

Massage Strategies

Massage is targeted at compensation patterns. Use presurgery and postsurgery massage procedures (see Chapter 19). Older clients require more healing time and less aggressive massage application.

BUTTOCK PULL

A pull on the gluteal muscles, or **buttock pull**, will cause pain in the area, particularly in response to any physical effort. Performing a straight leg raise will be painful.

Massage Strategies

Focus on compensation patterns. Use the sequence for muscle strains (see page 458). Firing patterns will need to be normalized during the subacute phase.

ILIOTIBIAL BAND SYNDROME

The iliotibial (IT) band provides lateral stability to the hip so that it can't move too far to the outside. In some people, particularly runners, the band overdevelops, tightens, and saws across the hip bone. Each time the athlete flexes and bends the knee, the band rubs against bone, causing pain. Although this condition, known as the **iliotibial band syndrome**, often causes knee pain, it may also cause pain over the point of the hip.

A snapping pain in the hip is almost always due to the snapping back and forth of the IT band over the point of the hip.

Massage Strategies

The fascial sheath weaves into the hamstrings and quadriceps. Also, contraction of the gluteus maximus and tensor fasciae latae muscles increases tautness of the IT band. It may be necessary to reduce tension in the lattisimus dorsi muscle, because the fascial tension pattern runs from the left shoulder lattisimus attachment to the lumbar dorsal fascia and then crosses to the right gluteus maximus into the right IT band, and vice versa.

- To increase pliability of the IT band, massage and stretch the lumbar fascia.
- Then massage and lengthen the gluteus maximus. Muscle energy methods are appropriate.
- Address the tensor fasciae latae muscle, especially trigger point activity. This muscle is too small to be adequately lengthened and stretched using joint movement. Direct manual stretch is more effective.
- Massage and lengthen the calf muscles on the affected side. Make sure the gastrocnemius and soleus are not adhered. Use mechanical force at the fibula head to soften the connective tissue in this area.
- Massage and lengthen the hamstrings and quadriceps.

Finally, specifically address the IT band.

- Massage the IT band using a connective tissue approach across the direction of the fibers. Massage applied in the longitudinal direction to create tension force is not very effective and can irritate nerves under the IT band. Use bend, shear, and torsion forces instead, and continue until the band is warm and pliable. Do not over-massage or create any inflammation.

HIP POINTER

A **hip pointer** is a blow to the rim of the pelvis that causes bleeding where the muscles attach. Hockey and football players are susceptible to hip pointers. Treatment consists of ice application and rest until the pain subsides, which usually takes 1 to 2 weeks.

Massage Strategies

Use lymphatic drain methods (see Unit Two) in the injured area.

THE THIGH

The thigh muscles are often massive in athletes. These muscles are involved in all lower extremity activities and have dual functions of stability and mobility.

The thigh contains the major leg muscles. The hamstring muscles in the back of the thigh are the driving force in all running activity. Hamstring function helps determine how fast and how strong a runner is. The large quadriceps muscle in the front of the thigh straightens the knee. This is the main muscle used in jumping, and it also provides

the power to pedal a bicycle or to decelerate movement burst or start and stop actively, and it stretches rapidly during the long running stride as the foot moves forward.

HAMSTRING PULL/TEAR/STRAIN

Probably the most common injury in the thigh area, and the most common muscle pull, is the **hamstring pull**. The hamstrings are implicated in conditions ranging from low-back pain to jumper's knee. Many sport activitie subject the hamstring muscles to great force, and consequently they are prone to strain. A weak core increases susceptibility to hamstring injury.

Although a hamstring will sometimes tear as a sprinter drives out of the starting block, a hamstring usually pulls from overstretching, not overcontracting, the muscle. It is not the first part of the stride, when the muscles contract (concentric function), but the second part of the stride, as the leg muscles stretch (eccentric function) that causes the muscle strain injury.

A hamstring tear may feel as if the muscle has "popped," and there is sharp pain and swelling in the thigh, and maybe even bleeding, depending on the degree of muscle damage. Degrees of tears are one (mild), two (moderate), and three (severe). The back of the thigh may turn black and blue, usually right below the area of pain, because blood works its way down by gravity. Palpation of the back of the thigh may indicate a defect or gap in the muscle where the fibers have torn if the strain is second degree or higher. The athlete will not be able to raise the leg straight off the ground more than 30 to 40 degrees without feeling severe pain.

Rehabilitation begins with the combination of protection, rest, ice, and compression during the acute phase. The amount of rest depends on the severity of the pull or tear, and is typically 2 to 3 days. This should be followed by limited activity until pain-free range of motion is achieved. Icing the muscle for 20 minutes 3 or 4 times a day will reduce the chance of aggravating the condition. Care for subacute cases includes a gentle stretching program. As long as the stretch is gentle and steady and does not separate the healing ends of the injured hamstrings, this is beneficial. In the early phase of healing, passive stretching of the muscle by movement in a bend-and-shear pattern above and below the tear is preferable to tension stretching by straightening the leg.

The symptoms of sciatica can mimic a hamstring pull, with pain in the back of the thigh. If the thigh pain extends below the knee, if there is any numbness in the lower leg or foot, or if the pain in the back of the leg becomes worse with stretching, sciatica may be the culprit.

Massage Strategies

- Use sequence for muscle strains and passive stretching by bending the hamstring back and forth, above and below the injury.
- Do not use longitudinal tension to stretch during early healing (the first 5 to 7 days).
- Focus massage on the opposite biceps and same-side triceps and quadriceps for reflex action.
- Reset firing patterns during the second and third stage stages of healing.

Because hamstring injuries are so next common, specific applications are outlined next.

Prevention of Hamstring Strain and Treating Short Hamstrings

It is important to address the specific muscle group function to prevent or deal with an injury when it is minor (tweaked). The first protocol will describe these strategies. The second protocol will address the sequence for treating actual hamstring injury.

Understanding the importance of the kinetic chain influence is essential in order to effectively work with the hamstrings. This group of muscles functions as both postural (stabilizers) and phasic (movers) muscles. That is, they hold the body upright in gravity and also produce movement. The movement function affects both the hip as extensors and the knee as flexors. The quadriceps group is antagonist and often functions in co-contraction with the hamstrings to stabilize the knee if instability is present or if the knee has been injured.

The hamstrings cross two of the three joints in the kinetic chain in the lower limb. This interactive function is most apparent in closed chain functions. The hamstrings are also reflexively functional with the biceps brachii muscles, especially during gait activity such as walking and running.

If the core is weak, there is a predictable chain of events that can be described as an extended result of lower crossed syndrome or layer syndrome (Figure 21-12). The general pattern of dysfunction is as follows:

- Weak transverse abdominis and internal and external obliques
- Short psoas and rectus abdominis
- Inhibited gluteus maximus

- Short hamstrings
- Short gastrocnemius
- Synergistic dominance in trunk flexion, hip extension, and knee flexion firing patterns
- Short biceps brachii
- Short muscles (with increased tension) of the cervical area, especially the erector spinae in the cervical area, the upper trapezius and levator scapulae, and the thoracolumbar erector spinae
- Alteration of the kinetic chain gait reflexes (usually with flexors not inhibiting when they should)

As you can see, hamstring dysfunction influences are a full-body pattern, and all of these areas must be addressed to support optimal hamstring function, including healing of injury. Specific treatment of the hamstrings is an extension of the strategies found in the general protocol. If hamstring shortening is present, then begin working with the arms, trunk, and foot and work toward the

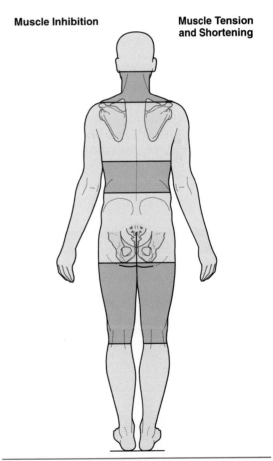

Muscle Inhibition   **Muscle Tension and Shortening**

FIGURE 21-12 ■ Areas of muscle inhibition (lighter shading) and muscle tension and shortening (darker shading).

hamstrings. Direct work with the hamstrings should be the very last aspect of treatment.

- Use general massage coupled with focused inhibitory pressure on the belly or attachments of all muscles that were assessed as short. While working on the short muscles (e.g., the biceps brachii), have the client flex and extend the knee.
- Correct all firing patterns.
- Correct all gait reflexes.
- Specifically address the hamstrings. An effective method is to have the therapist lower the leg to apply compression on the client's hamstrings while the client moves the knee. It is important that the compressive force applied is down and out to carry the muscle tissue away from the bone. Alternatively, the forearm can be used.
- Knead the hamstring muscles, making sure that all muscles slide over each other. If there is any binding, use shear force or compression with movement to separate the soft tissue layers.
- Next, use the position of the eyes and head to assist hamstring lengthening and stretching. Avoid direct application of contract-and-relax application, as the hamstring muscle tends to cramp. To address the hip portion of the hamstrings, use a straight leg raise; stop at the first indication of bind and have the client turn the eyes and head in large, slow circles. Slowly lengthen the muscle.

When there is no longer an increase in range, apply slight overpressure to stretch the connective tissue. Hold for 30 to 60 seconds. Slowly return the leg to a neutral position. Repeat.

- To address the hamstring portion at the knee, flex the hip to 90 degrees and then extend the knee to the first indication of bind (Figure 21-13).
- Again, have the client turn the eyes and neck in slow circles and add alternating flexion and extension of the client's elbows.
- Slowly increase the length until no further increase in range of motion is possible. Apply overpressure to stretch the area just past bind and hold 30 to 60 seconds. Slowly return the leg to a neutral position and repeat.

Do not apply this sequence 24 hours or less prior to competition, because the proproceptive functions will be altered and the legs may feel rubbery.

Injury Treatment

If there is a strain in the hamstrings, it is necessary to follow the massage recommendations for acute, subacute, and remodeling phases of healing. The sequence just described is used gently in the last two or three stages of the subacute healing phase and more aggressively as the third stage (remodeling) of healing progresses.

During the acute stage of healing, only approximate the tissue. Remember, a strain is a hole in the muscle tissue. It is important to keep the ends of the hole as close together as possible. The acute phase of healing can last up to 7 days and even longer in severe, second-degree strains and third-degree injuries.

FIGURE 21-13

HAMSTRING STRETCH FOR THE KNEE ATTACHMENTS

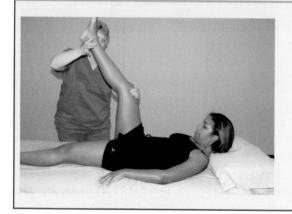
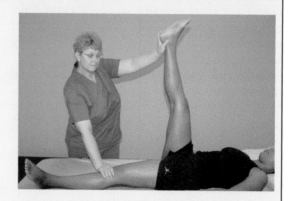

- Do not reduce muscle guarding or stretch the hamstrings. Do not use friction or compression.
- Work with lymphatic drain and gentle gliding to push the healing ends of the muscle together (approximate tissue).
- Massage all reflex areas. In the later stages of the acute phase, gentle shaking can be applied.

In the subacute phase, continue to follow the acute strategies but increase intensity and begin to knead the injured area. As the final healing stage begins, treat as short hamstrings with kneading.

Continue to address the scar tissue development for up to a year in hamstring strains. At every massage session, beginning in the later stages of the subacute phase, the area should be kneaded more aggressively as healing progresses. Occasionally, adhesions form, and shear forces (friction) are required. Areas of adhesion that have been frictioned need to be treated as if they are in the subacute phase for 3 days. Friction is applied every third day until the tissue normalizes.

It is absolutely necessary for the client to begin and maintain effective core-training, flexibility, and proprioceptive retraining programs. Although therapeutic exercise is the job of the physical therapist/athletic trainer, it is important for the massage therapist to encourage compliance and educate the client about effective exercise methods.

Unfortunately, athletes often begin to practice and compete before total healing has taken place. Typically, the athlete returns to training 2 to 3 weeks after the injury. This is usually right in the middle of the subacute healing phase, and muscle guarding still performs a useful purpose. Do not overstretch the area. Performance intensity will need to be reduced and reinjury is common. Those that begin performance-based activity too soon are prone to fibrotic tissue formation.

If the client has an old hamstring injury, especially one with scarring and fibrosis, knead the area thoroughly with each massage and use the short muscle prevention sequence. There should be noticeable improvement in 6 months if massage is applied at least once a week and the client follows core-training and flexibility programs. Clients who are not diligent with self-help will need massage at least twice a week.

BRUISED QUADRICEPS

A blow to the quadriceps muscles can crush the muscle fibers against the femur bone and cause bleeding into the muscle. This muscle is highly vascularized and therefore prone to heavy bleeding. The bleeding causes swelling and sometimes severe pain, as well as inability to fully flex the knee.

Immediate treatment of a **bruised quadriceps** is application of ice to the muscle for 20 to 30 minutes, with the knee flexed as far as it will go. Apply ice packs to the thigh and then wrap the leg with the knee fully flexed, using an elastic bandage to pull the leg back against the hamstring. This compresses the quadriceps muscle and puts enough pressure on the blood vessels to stop the bleeding.

The athlete should apply ice to the thigh several times a day as long as discomfort and/or swelling exists, and should stretch the muscle by flexing the knee as far as it will go.

Blood in the quadriceps can cause *myositis ossificans*. If this condition is not treated vigorously, bony deposits will prevent the fibers in the muscle from extending fully, limiting range of motion. This is a difficult condition to treat and can disable an athlete for up to a year.

Massage Strategies

- Apply repeated lymph drain massage to the entire leg.
- Address reflex patterns in opposite triceps and same-side biceps and hamstrings for pain control.
- During the subacute healing phase, use torsion forces to knead the area to prevent fibrosis.

QUADRICEPS PULL OR TEAR/STRAIN

A **quadriceps pull or tear** is usually a running or jumping injury. It is less common than a hamstring strain, but the treatment is the same. The muscle is iced and rested for a few days and then stretched.

Massage Strategies

Use the massage sequences for muscle strains (page 458) and lymphatic drain (see Unit Two). Address the opposite triceps and same-side biceps and hamstring for reflex stimulation pain control.

FEMUR FRACTURE

A **femur fracture** in sports is rare because the femur is so strong. Also, much of the rotary force of the leg is absorbed by the knee and is not transferred to the thigh bone.

This injury causes sharp pain in the leg and usually requires surgery to fixate the bone.

Massage Strategies
Use the procedures for fractures (see page 472).

THE KNEE

Note: Comprehensive massage treatment for the knee is found on page 561.

The knee is a complex joint that not only bends and straightens but also twists and rotates (Figure 21-14). It depends heavily on the soft tissues that surround it—the muscles, tendons, and ligaments—for stability. The knee joint is held together by four very strong ligaments. The medial and lateral collateral ligaments provide side-to-side stability. They are found on the inside and outside of the knee between the femur and the tibia. The anterior and posterior cruciate ligaments provide front-to-back stability. They are found inside the knee. The anterior cruciate runs from the front of the tibia to the back of the femur, and the posterior cruciate runs from the back of the tibia to the front of the femur. They cross in the middle.

Because the knee is a weight-bearing joint that is subjected to many different types of motion, it is vulnerable to tearing of its cushioning cartilage—the medial meniscus and the lateral meniscus—and of the supporting ligaments on both sides and inside the knee.

Because of its structure, the knee is extremely susceptible to blows from the side. It also can be severely damaged by rotating, twisting forces. It is the most poorly designed of all the joints in the body to withstand athletic activity. The knee is the most commonly injured joint in the body, accounting for about one fourth of all sports injuries. A knee injury is also the injury most likely to end an athlete's career. Nearly one million knee surgeries are performed each year.

PATELLOFEMORAL SYNDROME

Patellofemoral syndrome describes a variety of injuries affecting the patella and its groove on

---

FIGURE 21-14

KNEE INJURY

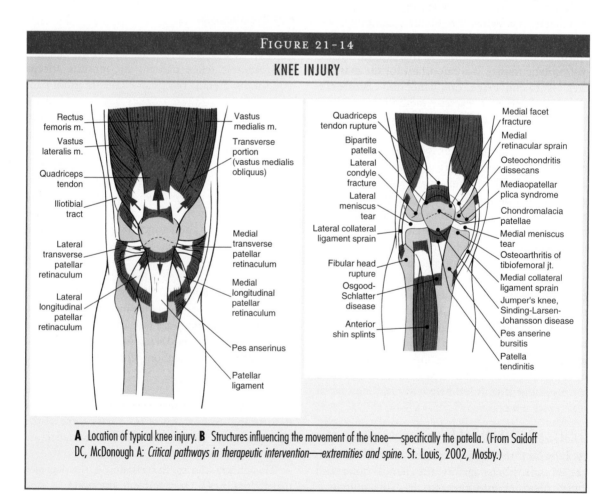

A Location of typical knee injury. **B** Structures influencing the movement of the knee—specifically the patella. (From Saidoff DC, McDonough A: *Critical pathways in therapeutic intervention—extremities and spine.* St. Louis, 2002, Mosby.)

the femur. Patellofemoral syndrome is the most common knee injury in athletes and other physically active people. Typically, women—especially adolescent females—experience more patellofemoral problems than men. Runner's knee, biker's knee, patellofemoral pain syndrome, patellofemoral stress syndrome, patellalgia and chondromalacia patella are just a few of the common terms used to identify this syndrome.

The precise cause of pain in this syndrome is not known. The cartilage that lines the undersurface of the kneecap has no nerve endings, and is not the likely cause of the pain. Some experts feel the pain is a result of wear on the bone underlying the cartilage, or possibly breakdown products of injured cartilage.

Injury is usually a result of repetitive running and jumping activity rather than a single traumatic event. Symptoms usually develop gradually, with initial pain consisting of a dull knee stiffness or ache present early in activity. During warm-up, the stiffness/pain may lessen or disappear and then return hours after a workout. As the injury progresses, pain may be present throughout activity. Symptoms may worsen when descending steps or hills. Squatting and kneeling may also aggravate the symptoms. *Crepitus* (a "crunching" sound under the patella with movement of the knee) can occur. Sitting for an extended time and then resuming activity may result in pain and stiffness until the muscles "loosen up." In advanced cases, the knee may "give way" when the person is walking or running.

The patella moves up and down in its groove when the knee is extended or flexed. If repetitive forces acting on the patella during this up-and-down motion are unbalanced, as during running and jumping, or if the patella moves side-to-side too much, painful symptoms may develop, caused by misalignment of the patella in its groove. The patella normally goes up and down (tracks) in the groove as the knee flexes and straightens. If the patella is misaligned, it will pull off to one side and rub on the side of the groove. This causes both the cartilage on the side of the groove and the cartilage on the back of the patella to wear out. Occasionally, fluid builds up and causes swelling in the knee.

As a result, of altered patella tracking, pain occurs on the back of the patella or in the back of the knee after running, going up and down stairs, and running hills. It will become painful to sit still for long periods with the knee bent. This is called the "theater sign," because people can't sit through an entire movie or play without having to get up and move around. One causal factor is an inward roll of the foot and ankle that causes the tibia to internally rotate, which turns the knee to the inside as well. The kneecap ends up sliding at an angle instead of straight up and down.

Muscle activation sequences are disrupted and are both the cause and the result of the condition. Inappropriate firing patterns of the quadriceps muscle (usually firing of the vastus lateralis initially and inhibition of the vastus medialis), especially the oblique pattern of the vastus medialis obliquus, are part of the problem. Trigger points develop that can refer pain into the knee.

Diagnosis depends on a history of symptoms and pain elicited during physical examination. There is no single test that confirms patellofemoral syndrome. In fact, some athletes with this injury may have normal exam results. X-rays or other medical imaging techniques of the patella joint may be helpful.

About 80% of all patellofemoral problems can be treated without surgery. Treatment is directed at correcting muscle imbalance, including weakness or alignment problems of the lower back, pelvis, hip, and lower extremity. Almost all studies of patellofemoral syndrome indicate weakness in the quadriceps, specifically the vastus medialis. Appropriate flexibility and strength exercises are required, and strengthening hip and abdominal muscles corrects abnormal alignment of the low back, hip, and pelvis, relieving patellofemoral strain. Persons who pronate excessively (flat feet) are believed to be at increased risk for patellofemoral injuries. Therefore, treatment may include orthotics to correct overpronation.

Braces and taping are commonly used to relieve symptoms. They are effective in reducing pain severity but do not cure the problem. Ice therapy after exercise may relieve symptoms. NSAIDs can reduce pain.

Massage Strategies

The vastus lateralis is usually dominant and needs to be inhibited with compressive gliding and kneading. Make sure to address all firing patterns and gait reflexes. Use bend, shear, and torsion forces to maintain pliability in the connective tissue structures surrounding the patella.

JUMPER'S KNEE

Inflammation of the tendons that hook into the upper and lower ends of the patella is called

jumper's knee. The quadriceps and patellar tendons help to straighten the leg. When these tendons are overstressed, they become inflamed. The sudden, violent vertical leap that occurs when jumping straightens out the knee and may cause tiny tears that irritate the tendons. It usually hurts more going up than coming down because a greater force is exerted to get up into the air. Any jumping exercises can aggravate the condition.

Treatment consists of rest and ice application. NSAIDs may reduce the pain.

Massage Strategies

Massage strategies for tendinitis are appropriate (see page 466).

SPRAINED KNEE

A **sprained knee** can result from twisting during a fall, by stepping in a hole while running, or by being hit from the side while playing sports.

A knee sprain, by definition, is an injury to a knee ligament. The sprain may vary in severity from a slight stretch to a complete tear of the ligament. A mild, or grade 1, sprain stretches the ligament and causes pain and swelling. A moderate, or grade 2, sprain partially tears the ligament and is much more disabling. A severe, or grade 3, sprain is a complete rupture and often needs surgical repair.

The most commonly sprained knee ligament is the medial collateral ligament (MCL). This ligament can be injured by a blow to the outside of the knee, particularly when the foot is planted in the ground when impact occurs. The blow causes the knee to move toward the inside of the body and stretches the ligament. Point tenderness and pain occur on the inside of the knee, and the knee will feel like it may buckle to the inside.

A sprain of the ligament on the outside of the knee, the lateral collateral ligament, is caused by a blow to the inside of the knee, which forces the knee to the outside. This is much less common than an MCL sprain because it is hard to get hit on the inside of the knee.

If an athlete receives a blow to the knee and the pain is on the same side of the knee that was hit, it's probably a bruise, and the pain will go away. Pain on the opposite side of the impact is considered a serious injury that needs careful treatment.

The immediate treatment for a sprain is standard PRICE therapy. Rest the knee while it aches and ice it intermittently several times a day. Wrap it in an elastic bandage in between icings and keep it elevated as much as possible.

The purpose of rehabilitation exercises is to strengthen the quadriceps muscles in the front of the thigh (leg extensions) and the hamstring muscles in the back of the thigh (leg curls). These muscles, particularly the quadriceps, begin to lose strength within 12 hours after a knee injury. These muscles control the knee and must be restrengthened.

Massage Strategies

Use the procedure for sprains (page 458) and the specific protocol for the knee (page 561). Massage supports appropriate firing patterns, making rehabilitation exercises more effective.

THE TERRIBLE TRIAD OF O'DONOHUE

A very severe injury to the knee, and one common among athletes, is called the **Terrible Triad of O'Donohue**, named after a long-time team physician at the University of Oklahoma and one of the deans of sports medicine. He was the first to describe this injury, which consists of an MCL sprain or tear, an anterior cruciate ligament (ACL) tear, and a medial cartilage tear, all due to a single blow to the knee.

This devastating injury requires complete surgical repair. It's impossible to rehabilitate all of these structures and have a functioning knee again without surgery.

Massage Strategies

Use presurgery and postsurgery protocols (see Chapter 19). Normalize firing and compensation patterns during the mid-subacute phase of healing and introduce strategies for the knee (see page 561).

ANTERIOR AND POSTERIOR CRUCIATE LIGAMENT INJURY

Cruciate ligament injury of the knee is a sprain. The anterior cruciate ligament (ACL) is most often stretched, torn, or both, by a sudden twisting motion when the feet are planted one way and the knees are turned another way. The posterior cruciate ligament (PCL) is most often injured by a direct impact, such as in an automobile accident or football tackle.

Injury to a cruciate ligament may not cause pain. Rather, the person may hear a popping sound, and the leg may buckle when he or she tries to stand on it. The anterior and posterior drawer test indicates whether the knee stays in proper position when pressure is applied in different directions. An MRI is very accurate in detecting a complete tear, but arthroscopy may be the only reliable means of detecting a partial tear.

Treatment for an incomplete tear includes an exercise program to strengthen surrounding muscles and possibly a protective knee brace for stability.

The most severe ruptures are usually caused when a heavy athlete, such as a football lineman, is running and then plants his foot and turns 90 degrees to go upfield. This twisting can cause a complete ACL rupture. If the ACL ruptures, there is a usually a loud pop and a sudden pain and instability in the knee. The knee will swell up rapidly because the ACL bleeds heavily when injured. Medical treatment is necessary.

An MRI scan may help determine whether the ligament is stretched or totally torn. If it is torn, it will need to be repaired surgically. Modern methods of repair, such as arthroscopic surgery, and new approaches to rehabilitation, such as beginning exercises immediately after surgery, support recovery, which may take as long as 6 to 7 months. Knee braces are available that will allow return to activity.

The surgeon may reattach the torn ends of the ligament or reconstruct the torn ligament by using a graft of healthy ligament from the client or from a cadaver. Although repair using synthetic ligaments has been tried experimentally, the procedure has not yielded as good results as use of human tissue.

One of the most important elements in successful recovery after cruciate ligament surgery is adhering to an exercise and rehabilitation program for 4 to 6 months. Such a program may involve the use of special exercise equipment at a rehabilitation or sports center.

Massage Strategies

Use specific strategies for the knee (see page 561).

DISLOCATED KNEE

A **dislocated knee** is an extremely severe traumatic injury to the knee, and one of the few true orthopedic emergencies. Total dislocation of the knee, in which the whole knee is torn out of the socket, is caused by a severe blow. The lower leg moves away from the upper bone, and only the skin is holding the lower leg together. This can cut off the blood supply to the lower leg and necessitate amputation.

Massage Strategies

This is a medical emergency. Once this has been addressed, follow strategies for dislocation (see page 470).

DISLOCATED PATELLA

The back of the patella is shaped like a wedge and rides in a V-shaped groove in the front of the lower end of the femur between the two condyles. If the patella is hit at an angle, it can be knocked out of this groove. The patella almost always dislocates to the outside, as the outer lip of the groove is much shallower than the inner lip. Interestingly, the patella groove is much shallower in females than in males, so dislocation is a more common and recurrent problem in women.

A **dislocated patella** causes pain, and the knee will appear deformed because the patella will sit way out to the side. Usually it can be popped back into place by a physician without too much difficulty. It may even pop back in by itself on the way to the doctor's office or emergency room. Even if it pops back in, however, it must be x-rayed to make sure that a piece of bone has not been knocked off the undersurface. Occasionally, the patella is locked out of place so severely that surgery is needed.

Treatment requires immobilization of the patella in a splint for about 3 weeks to allow the tissues on either side of the bone to heal. These tissues hold the patella in place, and if they remain torn, the patella will be prone to recurring dislocation.

After a period of rest, the athlete must strengthen the quadriceps with rehabilitative exercises. These exercises will increase the tone of the muscles pulling on the tendon underneath the patella. This will hold the patella in the groove so that it won't be likely to pop out again.

Massage Strategies

Use specific strategies for knees shown on page 561 and for dislocations on p. 470.

BROKEN PATELLA

The patella may fracture from a head-on blow, causing pain and swelling. X-rays confirm the fracture.

A **broken patella** needs to be immobilized and may even need surgical repair, depending on the direction of the fracture line. If the fracture line is vertical, immobilization should be enough. If the fracture line is horizontal, then the two pieces will be pulled apart by the quadriceps and will need to be wired together until they unite.

Massage Strategies

Use presurgery and postsurgery strategies, if needed, and normalize firing patterns in the subacute healing phase.

LOOSE BODY IN THE KNEE

If an athlete has sudden episodes of knee pain and knee locking, a loose body may be floating inside the joint. The loose body may be a piece of cartilage that has torn off or a piece of bone that has chipped off the tibia, femur, or patella. The bone may have been previously injured. It gradually dies, and a piece can fall off the bone and float inside the knee.

The onset of these symptoms may not appear until months to years after a traumatic injury such as a blow to the knee. Just as suddenly as the pain appears, it disappears and full range of motion returns.

These on-again, off-again symptoms are due to a **loose body** in the knee getting caught between the upper and lower bones. When the loose body floats back up into the hollow space in the knee, out of the way, the pain is relieved.

The loose piece may feel like a pea that suddenly floats into the knee under the pressure of the person's weight and then suddenly disappears.

Arthroscopic surgery is necessary to remove the loose body.

Massage Strategies

Use presurgery and postsurgery strategies (see Chapter 19), and normalize firing patterns. Also, see knee strategies on page 561.

OSGOOD-SCHLATTER DISEASE

Seen only in adolescents, **Osgood-Schlatter disease** is not really a disease but a syndrome. It is an overuse syndrome related to the growth process.

The lower end of the patellar tendon attaches to a knob on the surface of the tibia, called the *tibial tuberosity*. As a child grows, this knob becomes larger to increase the surface to which the tendon attaches. The constant yanking on this tendon from running and jumping can cause some irritation in the knee. Every time a child with this syndrome straightens the leg, as when going up stairs or riding a bicycle, the pain becomes worse. Also, growth of the knob becomes stimulated by

the constant irritation, and the knob may protrude as a lump on the shinbone, which will be tender to the touch.

This is a self-limiting syndrome. It always disappears by late adolescence, when the knob stops growing. By then, the tendon is yanking on a solid piece of bone, and the pain goes away, although the protuberant knob will remain.

A few weeks of rest is required only if there is severe pain. Casting and other aggressive treatment is usually unnecessary.

Massage Strategies

Use general message for pain control. Do not aggressively massage the area.

ILIOTIBIAL BAND SYNDROME

Pain along the outer side of the knee is often due to the **iliotibial band syndrome**, particularly among runners. The pain usually begins 10 to 20 minutes into the run and gets progressively worse.

The cause of the pain is an overly tight IT band. The IT band starts at the rim of the pelvis, crosses the point of the hip (greater trochanter of the femur), comes down the thigh across the outer side of the knee, and attaches below the knee. This attachment includes the fibular head.

Sometimes the band overdevelops and tightens with exercise; it may rub hard enough to irritate the knee, causing pain. It may cause similar pain over the point of the hip.

Massage Strategies

Use massage to reduce motor tone in all muscles that influence the IT band (i.e., gluteus maximus, tensor fasciae latae, lateral hamstrings and quadriceps, and opposite side of latissimus dorsi). The IT band is connective tissue and responds to shear, bend, and torsion forces to increase pliability. Tension or compression forces (gliding or direct pressure) are not effective. The side-lying position is best for treating the IT band.

OSTEOARTHRITIS/ARTHROSIS

Osteoarthritis/arthrosis of the knee is wear-and-tear degeneration of the knee, otherwise known as *degenerative joint disease*. Spurs of bone form along the edges of the knee joint and wear down the cartilage. This can be aggravated by an injury to the knee. Bowlegged people may develop severe osteoarthritis of the knee because the bowing causes increased pressure of the inner part of the tibia against the medial femoral condyle. This wears out the inner cartilage and causes bone to grate on bone, leading to arthritis.

Bone spurs or pieces of worn-down cartilage can break off and become a loose body. This causes pain during activity and swelling of the joint. Anti-inflammatory medications can ease the pain. If an x-ray reveals a large amount of debris in the knee, arthroscopic surgery can clean out the joint and provide relief for a few years.

If the pain becomes so severe that it interferes with activity, the knee may have to be replaced with an artificial joint. Knee replacement is a common reason for people to be in physical rehabilitation programs.

Massage Strategies

Use the protocol for arthritis (page 468). If knee replacement is necessary, apply presurgery and postsurgery strategies (see Chapter 12). Pain control should also be the focus of massage. Also, see knee protocol on page 561.

PRE-PATELLAR BURSITIS

A large sac of fluid may form in the front of the patella (**pre-patellar bursitis**) as the result of a sudden blow or other trauma to the knee. This condition is common among roofers and carpet layers, who work on their knees; it was called "housemaid's knee," a reference to maids scrubbing floors on their knees.

Trauma to a bursal sac in front of the patella irritates the patella and causes fluid to form in the sac. Treatment is drainage of the bursal sac and then injection of cortisone into the sac if it continues to fill with fluid. If the condition persists, the sac is removed surgically.

Massage Strategies

Lymphatic drain methods may be helpful.

TORN CARTILAGE

A blow on the outer side of the knee causes the inner side to stretch. This can cause one of two things to happen. The MCL, which is attached to the cartilage, can tear the cartilage as it stretches, or, when the stretching force is removed, the inner side of the knee can close again with some force, driving the condyle back into the cartilage. The grinding action on the knee as it rotates can also damage cartilage. The same thing happens when the femoral condyles rotate on the tibia with body weight compressing it.

The pain from the **torn cartilage** may be on the inside or the outside of the knee, depending on which cartilage has torn. There may be a clicking sound inside the knee during movement as the bone rides over the torn part of the cartilage. A common symptom is the inability to make a sharp turn even when walking.

Most cartilage tears do not heal by themselves. This is possible ONLY if the tear is at the outer edge of the cartilage, or if it is small. Cartilage has a poor blood supply except at the outer rim, so about 90% of cartilage tears have no ability to heal, and the torn piece needs to be surgically removed.

Treatment includes participation in a rehabilitation program to restrengthen the muscles around the knee.

Massage Strategies

Focus on procedures for pain relief as well as presurgery and postsurgery strategies, if necessary. Also see knee protocol on this page.

BAKER'S CYST (POPLITEAL CYST)

A **baker's cyst,** or popliteal cyst, is a collection of fluid in the back of the knee joint. It is usually a symptom of another problem, or it may be an incidental finding with no significance.

Most often in adults a baker's cyst is found in conditions in which there is chronic swelling or fluid accumulation in the knee joint. These conditions include knee arthritis, meniscus injuries, and ligamentous injuries. Treatment of a baker's cyst that is the result of a problem within the knee consists of treating the underlying problem.

If conservative treatments fail to correct the cyst, an operation to remove the cyst can be performed.

Massage Strategies

If the cyst is removed surgically, presurgery and postsurgery strategies are appropriate. Do not massage on the cyst.

MASSAGE FOR KNEE INJURY AND PAIN

Knee injuries that involve strains and sprains are addressed with the strategies described for these type of injuries (see pages 458). Knee surgeries are mostly arthroscopic procedures, and presurgery and postsurgery massage strategies are appropriate in these cases. These are relatively straightforward applications for easily diagnosed knee conditions.

More complex is the knee aching experienced by many athletes and those in physical rehabilitation. The beginning stages of patellofemoral syndrome fall into this category. The general protocol described in Unit Two supports knee function. Those methods are expanded here in relationship to knee pain, injury, and function.

Muscle activation sequences (firing patterns) of muscles around the knee joint need to be optimal for pain free joint function. These firing patterns are often disrupted, and the problem usually begins with the core muscles, as described in relation to low-back pain and hamstring injury. There are two reasons why the knee is just as common a location for pain as the low back.

First, the knee is the middle joint in a closed kinetic chain that involves the hip, knee, and ankle. If the mobility or stability of the hip or ankle is compromised, the knee has to adapt to the changes in force distribution. So if the hip or the ankle is hypomobile, the knee becomes more mobile to continue to allow movement—as a result, stability is decreased and injury potential increases. This situation occurs during the injury process, as traumatic forces are transmitted through the hip, knee, and ankle complex; if hypomobility exists in the hip or ankle, the knee will be the weak link in the chain and incur the most force and therefore the most trauma.

Conversely, if the hip and or ankle is hypermobile, the stability of the structure and muscles of the knee increases, making the knee more vulnerable to injury because there is insufficient flexibility and pliability in the tissues to absorb traumatic forces.

Second, as previously mentioned, core instability affects knee function. Here is how the progressive degeneration of function spreads: the inner abdominal muscles responsible for core stability are weak and inhibited. As a result of the adaptive process, the next functional group of synergists become dominant—that is, the psoas and the rectus abdominis. If these muscles are tight and short, the gluteus maximus is inhibited and cannot function as a hip extensor, which is especially important in running. Also, the gluteus maximus functions to support knee stability by keeping an appropriate tautness on the IT band. When the gluteus maximus is inhibited, weak, and long, the abductors and deep lateral hip rotators become short. The orientation of the femur is changed, usually to external rotation, which will change the fit of the

patella and tibia at the knee. Rubbing of the bones within the knee capsule begins and creates problems with patella tracking. The hamstrings and vastus lateralis become dominant, and the vastus medialis is inhibited and weak.

Also, the erector spinae in the lumbar area become overactive to assist hip extension. Firing patterns are disrupted, with the hamstring and erector spinae firing first during hip extension, and the gastrocnemius firing first in knee flexion. The vastus lateralis fires first in extension and pulls the patella laterally. The vastus medialis is unable to balance the lateral pull, further increasing patellar tracking problems. Pain can occur behind the knee at the attachments of the gastrocnemius on the femur and the hamstring on the tibia. The IT band is too taut and the normal position of the fibula is altered, eventually affecting the ankle. The tibia now becomes twisted into external rotation, and internal rubbing within the knee capsule increases.

Because the gastrocnemius is functioning primarily at the knee, the soleus is responsible for ankle plantar flexion. Rubbing between the two muscles can cause the fascia to adhere, making them function as one muscle pulling in different directions. The Achilles tendon becomes short and painful and can lead to irritation of the plantar fascia. Both of these conditions reduce ankle mobility, which needs to have a minimum of 10 degrees of dorsiflexion (15 to 20 degrees is much better) to allow proper knee function. The ankle becomes hypomobile and the knee is further strained. The rectus femoris of the quadriceps group tries to balance the increasing lateral pull on the patella. This muscle also functions as a hip flexor. The friction against the underlying fascia over the vastus intermedialis results in the adherence of these two muscles as they stick to each other and shorten. The adductors and the sartorius attempt to support knee function but are ineffective, and the pes anserinus attachment of the sartorius, gracilis, and semitendinosus becomes irritated and inflamed. The sartorius can actually shift position, with the distal end moving anteriorly over the medial condyle on the tibia. Typically this occurs if the femur becomes externally rotated and the tibia is internally rotated. Pain occurs just below the knee on the medial side.

To complicate matters even more, attempting to stretch inhibited muscles while the synergists are dominant does not work, because the overactive muscles are generating reciprocal inhibition. This is where massage sequencing becomes important.

Comprehensive treatment must start at the beginning of the progression: stabilize the core and reset the firing patterns. If the condition is chronic, the connective tissue will be dense and adherence between adjacent muscle layers will be common. Massage needs to normalize the connective tissue, ensuring that all muscles are able to slide freely over each other. The short and tight muscles—usually the psoas, quadratus lumborum, rectus abdominis, hamstrings, gastrocnemius, vastus lateralis, abductors, and deep lateral hip rotators—need to be inhibited and lengthened. Then strengthening exercises for the transversus abdominis, abdominal obliques, gluteus maximus, and vastus medialis can begin. Firing patterns can be reset and reinforced, which may be required at each massage session in the series of treatments, until the neuromuscular relationship is reeducated. Once the soft tissue will allow movement, the trainer, physical therapist, physician, or chiropractor can begin to reorient the bones. The pelvis is usually rotated: the symphysis pubis is offset, the femur and tibia are excessively rotated, and the fibula is fixed in place. Massage can support this intervention using the methods described for joint play as well as indirect functional methods for the pelvis and other joints.

Factors other than core instability can contribute to knee problems, including any ankle sprain, with a high ankle sprain being more serious. Ankles that are hypomobile for any reason will increase the tendency for knee pain. This is because the fibula changes position, which changes force distribution through the knee. Also, compensation for ankle sprain will change firing patterns at the knee. Low-back pain can strain the knees, and, conversely, knee pain can strain the back.

Note that relationships of functional change flow in all directions—up, down, across, and diagonally—influencing adaptive changes remote from the original change.

Inappropriate strength programs that focus too much on the biceps and triceps will stimulate gait reflexes to reflexively shorten the hamstrings and quadriceps. Usually the biceps are overworked.

Make sure when applying massage that the elbow flexors and extensors are massaged in conjunction with the knee flexors and extensors.

Squats and lunges strain the knee when they are performed incorrectly or overdone.

Changing shoes changes how the foot is positioned, and the force translates to the knee if the ankle is hypomobile or hypermobile.

Specific Massage Applications for the Knee

Massage needs to address the soft tissues so that therapeutic exercise and joint mobilization are effective. Working with the knee is truly a full-body massage application. To support knee function and rehabilitation, follow these strategies as appropriate for acute, subacute, and remodeling stages of healing. Apply lymphatic drain methods because any swelling in the knee can inhibit muscle and joint function.

- Make sure that all muscle layers that cross joints of the lower extremity are sliding freely over the underlying tissue. Use kneading and compression plus movement to introduce bend, shear, and torsion forces to the muscle layers. Specifically address the IT band by first reducing motor tone in the muscles that attach into the band (i.e., the gluteus maximus, tensor fasciae latae, and others). Then knead across the IT band to increase pliability of the tissue.
- Assess and correct all muscle firing patterns. Overactive synergists respond to compression and muscle energy methods.
- Shaking is an underused massage method, and these muscle respond well to aggressive but pain-free shaking. This is best accomplished by placing the knee in a slightly flexed position, instructing the client to be passive. Then manually shake the hamstrings. Shake the gastrocnemius both manually and by moving the lower leg.
- Make sure that the ankle is mobile to at least 10 degrees of dorsiflexion. Help the foot joints to function freely by massaging all the fascia and muscles of the foot, using joint movement for each joint in the foot.
- Massage the attachments of the hamstrings and gastrocnemius at the back of the knee, being cautious of applying excessive pressure onto the popliteal space. If any internal or external rotation of the tibia exists, the popliteus muscle will be affected.
- Trigger points in the quadriceps can refer pain under the kneecap. Assess and treat only those that increase symptoms.

THE LEG

Practically all of the pains that occur on the inner side of the tibia are due to improper foot strike. Most are classified as overuse injuries. Excessive pronation can lead to three leg injuries: shin splints, tibial stress syndrome, and tibial stress fracture. Pronation is the inward roll of the foot as it hits the ground. Aside from congenital abnormalities such as a clubbed foot, two foot problems cause excessive pronation. A person with a **pronating foot** has an overly mobile foot and ankle and loose ligaments, and the foot rolls to the inside.

The other problem is Morton's foot, in which the second toe is longer than the big toe. This causes the foot to roll to the inside when the toes push off for the next step.

SHIN SPLINTS

"Shin splints" is a catchall term for any pain on the inner side of the shin. A true shin splint injury is quite rare. What people call shin splints are actually pains in the muscles near the shin bone. They can be caused by running or jumping on hard surfaces and by overuse.

The pain is felt on the inner side of the middle third of the shin bone, which is where the muscle responsible for raising the arch of the foot attaches. When the arch collapses with each foot strike, it pulls on the tendon that comes from this muscle.

In the pronating foot, the arch stays down because the foot is rolled to the inside. Consequently, the muscle starts to fire while there is still weight on the foot, and it is unable to bring the arch up. Because of these multiple firings during each foot strike and the pull against great weight, some of the fibers of the muscle are torn loose from the shin bone. This causes small areas of bleeding around the lining of the bone, and pain.

The key element of treatment is an arch support to prevent excessive pronation and pull on the tendon. This usually solves the problem almost immediately. Many athletes do well with a simple commercially available arch support. Those who have a more serious problem may need an orthotic device custom-made by a sports podiatrist.

Massage Strategies

Caution: Make sure that the condition is not compartment syndrome. Apply massage as described for muscle strains on page 458.

TIBIAL STRESS SYNDROME

Most runners with shin pain have **tibial stress syndrome**. Excessive pronation causes the shin bone to rotate inward with each step while the upper part of the leg remains almost fixed. This abnormal twist of the bone, coupled with repetitive impact trauma, puts stress on the shin bone and causes irritation and pain.

Treatment includes wearing an arch support or orthotic device, depending on the extent of foot disability. This will support the foot and stop the rotation of the tibia. As soon as the rotation stops, the soreness will begin to disappear, often in as little as 2 to 3 weeks.

Massage Strategies

Even though this syndrome isn't a muscle strain, massage for muscle strains (page 458) is effective.

PAIN ON THE OUTSIDE OF THE LEG

Another type of pain occurs on the outside of the leg and is due to stress on the fibula from pounding and shock transmission up the outside of the leg, rather than twisting.

When the foot rolls to the outside (supination) because the arch is too tight, pain can result. If the client's shoes are turned over to the outside, the client lands on the outside of the foot when running. A high-arched, rigid foot will not collapse on impact. Because the arch of a supinated foot does not collapse to sustain the shock of the foot strike, the shock is transmitted up the outside of the leg and can result in bone pain and a possible stress fracture of the fibula.

Treating this condition is difficult. The best treatment is to provide maximum padding for shock absorption at the outer side of the foot.

Fibula pain is less debilitating than tibial pain because the fibula is not a true weight-bearing bone. The pain should disappear in 2 to 3 weeks with proper padding under the foot.

Massage Strategies

Use strategies for fractures (see page 472) because the injury is to the bone.

COMPARTMENT SYNDROME

Compartment syndrome occurs when an overdeveloped muscle crowds the connective tissue sheath that surrounds it, causing pressure and pain. It can be acute or chronic.

The leg is unique in that the various muscles are contained in thick, fibrous tubes called *compartments*. The design of these compartments doesn't allow them to expand very much, so overdeveloped muscles will be somewhat compressed within the compartments.

Acute Compartment Syndrome

During exercise the leg muscles become engorged with blood, and the pressure on the veins doesn't allow the blood to leave the affected muscle. Blood continues to enter the muscle from the arteries, where the pressure is higher than that inside the compartment and builds up until blood from the arteries can no longer nourish the muscle. When oxygen cannot be transported by the arteries, the muscles can become damaged. Eventually, the muscle fibers die if the condition is not corrected. Compartment syndrome can also be caused from impact trauma or a muscle tear to the area.

Pressure inside the compartment causes pain in the anterior muscles of the leg. This area swells and becomes very sensitive to any pressure.

This is a surgical emergency. If the compartment is not opened up to relieve the pressure within, the affected muscles will die, with permanent loss of function.

Massage Strategies

Massage is contraindicated in these cases. However, as a preventive measure, massage can increase and maintain pliability in the muscle sheath.

Chronic Compartment Syndrome

This injury mainly occurs in runners. Symptoms consist of pain that gradually develops during a run, getting worse until it is impossible to continue. After a period of rest, the pain disappears only to return when the athlete tries to run again. The cause is usually training too much too quickly. An athlete who has laxity in the ankle ligaments, usually from multiple sprains, is prone to this condition.

Treatment includes rest until pain subsides and antiinflammatory medication.

Surgery is necessary only if pressure increases in the compartment.

Massage Strategies

Use connective tissue methods to manually stretch the muscle sheath. Carefully monitor for increase in symptoms; if this occurs, refer the client to a physician immediately.

LEG MUSCLE PULLS AND TEARS (STRAINS)

Leg muscle pulls and tears commonly occur in the major muscles of the calf, the gastrocnemius and soleus. Pulls and tears represent different degrees of the same injury, which occurs when muscles are suddenly overstretched beyond their limits. The degree of overstretching determines whether the muscle is pulled or actually torn.

Treatment depends on the severity of the injury and consists of rest for a few days and then a gentle, gradual stretching program.

Massage Strategies

Use the strategies for muscle strains (see page 458). Prevention—the best treatment—is reinforced by using massage to maintain the normal resting length of the muscle, as well as the pliability and elasticity of the connective tissue in the area. It is also necessary to make sure that firing patterns are normal and that the muscles are not adhered together. If using bending, shear, and torsion forces to separate the muscles, place the gastrocnemius in passive contraction—knee flexed and ankle plantar flexed—to facilitate movement over the soleus.

CALF CRAMPS

Calf cramps are dangerous because the sudden muscle pain can be so severe that an athlete may fall and risk other injury. A number of factors may cause cramps, including dehydration, electrolyte imbalance, poor physical conditioning, and improper diet. Calf cramps usually occur after periods of repeated heavy exercise.

Massage Strategies

When the calf muscle twitches uncontrollably, this is a sign that it may go into spasm.

- When the muscle does cramp, apply broad-based compression to the belly of the muscle.
- Then massage the muscle from the top down toward the feet until the pain subsides.
- Gently stretch the calf.

Refer the athlete to the trainer or physician for hydration and electrolytes.

ACHILLES TENDINITIS

The Achilles tendon is the large tendon at the back of the ankle. It connects the gastrocnemius and soleus muscle to the calcaneus bone. **Achilles tendinitis** (inflammation) can be acute or chronic.

The inflammation usually develops just above the point where the tendon attaches to the heel bone. Signs of Achilles tendinitis include pain when pushing off during walking or when rising on the toes, redness and swelling over the tendon, and a crackling or creaking sound heard during movement of the tendon.

Achilles tendinitis results from repeated stress on the tendon, which may be caused or aggravated by the following:

- Overuse
- Running on hills and hard surfaces
- Poor stretching habits
- Tight, short calf muscles
- Weak calf muscles
- Worn-out or ill fitting shoes
- Flat feet

In addition, Achilles tendinitis can develop as the result of participation in sports involving stop-and-start footwork, such as tennis, racquetball, football, and basketball.

If the feet overpronate, this can increase the strain on the Achilles tendon because the tendon is twisted as the foot rolls in.

If the warning signs of Achilles tendinitis are ignored, or if it is not allowed to heal properly, the injury can become chronic. Because the Achilles tendon has a poor blood supply, it heals slowly. Chronic Achilles tendinitis is a difficult condition to treat. The pain experienced during the acute phase of the injury usually disappears after warm-up but returns when training has stopped. The injury gets worse until eventually it becomes impossible to run.

Symptoms of acute Achilles tendinitis include:

- Pain in the tendon during exercise
- Swelling over the tendon
- Redness of the skin over the tendon

Symptoms of chronic Achilles tendinitis include those of acute tendinitis as well as:

- Pain and stiffness in the tendon, especially in the morning
- Pain in the tendon when walking, especially uphill or up stairs

A major predisposing factor is overtraining. As a general rule, athletes who increase their training stress by more than 10% weekly run a 50% risk of injury occurring after 4 weeks. Achilles tendinitis can occurs in any athlete–both professional and amateur–who may have increased speed workouts, hill running, jumping, or total training volume. The Achilles/calf muscle tendon group is responsi-ble to a large extent for the push-off that leads to the airborne or "leaping" phase of running.

Treatment begins with PRICE therapy. Next, reduce training by 50%. Then gradually reinstate training intensity by 10% per week as treatment continues. Continued icing helps reduce swelling and inflammatory change.

Short-term use of NSAIDs is helpful, usually for no longer than 14 days. After this time, most of the changes seen in these conditions have more to do with tissue breakdown than inflammation. Steroid injection is sometimes used but is not recommended. Some specialists believe this can increase the risk of a total rupture.

Specific rehabilitation exercises help restore the strength of supporting muscle groups. These exercises emphasize strengthening the muscles that support the foot, arch, and lower leg. In general, exercise needs to work on both concentric (contracting) and eccentric (lengthening) strength.

Stretching should be done cautiously while any tissues are inflamed and should be directed at motion deficits. Begin by performing two to three pain-free stretches lasting 30 seconds of affected muscle groups, then increase repetition slowly.

Massage Strategies

In the acute stage, do not use any massage methods that increase inflammation. Lymphatic drain procedures are appropriate in the painful area. Focus on the short structures, muscles, and/or connective tissue causing the inflammation. The calf muscles are almost always involved. Make sure that the gastrocnemius and soleus are not adhering to each other. The cause of the shortening of the calf muscles needs to be addressed as well.

Disrupted firing patterns such as described for the knee are usually involved and need to be normalized. Once the inflammation is reduced and the acute phase has passed, bend, shear, and torsion forces can be introduced during massage.

Light massage can usually be performed daily; however, for deeper techniques alternate days may be more appropriate, giving the tissues time to recover. See massage sequence for tendinitis on page 466.

ACHILLES BURSITIS

Inflammation can occur in the bursa between the heel bone and the Achilles tendon. This is called **Achilles bursitis** or *retrocalcaneal bursitis*. Initially, there is pain and irritation at the back of the heel. There may be visible redness and swelling in the area, and the back of the shoe may further irritate the condition. Achilles bursitis can lead to increased swelling, pain, and disability.

Treatment consists of a combination of self-care measures. Surgery is rarely needed. Cortisone injections may occasionally be beneficial, but repeated injections are not recommended because of the increased risk of rupture of the tendon.

Massage Strategies

Use the sequence for bursitis (see page 466).

ACHILLES TENDON RUPTURE

The athlete can overstretch the Achilles tendon, and tear (rupture) it. A rupture can be partial or complete. **Achilles tendon rupture** typically occurs just above the heel bone, but it can happen anywhere along the tendon.

With a complete rupture, typically there is a pop or snap, with immediate sharp pain in the back of the ankle and lower leg, making it impossible to walk properly. Complete rupture of an Achilles tendon is usually treated with surgery. Ideally, surgery should occur within 2 weeks of the injury. The procedure generally involves making an incision in the back of the leg and repairing the torn tendon.

Postsurgical rehabilitation includes a period of 6 to 12 weeks with the leg immobilized in a walking boot, cast, brace, or splint. To prevent the tendon from healing in a stretched position (which would making it useless), the foot initially may be pointed slightly downward (plantar flexed) in the boot or brace, and then gradually moved to a neutral position . . . For the first few weeks, the cast will likely extend above the knee, and then it will be reduced to below the knee.

Following removal of the immobilization device, range-of-motion and stretching exercises can begin. It is usually 6 months to a year before the athlete can return to activity.

Nonsurgical treatment of an Achilles tendon rupture typically involves wearing a cast or walking boot, which allows the ends of the torn tendon to reattach. Studies indicate that this method can be effective without the risk of complications, such as infection, that can occur with surgery. However, the incidence of recurring rupture is higher with the nonsurgical approach, and recovery can take longer. Surgical repair of a ruptured Achilles tendon is usually preferable, especially if the person wants to continue to take part in strenuous physical activities.

A partial rupture of the Achilles tendon can occur in athletes in all sports, including running, jumping, throwing, and racket sports. Following partial rupture, scar tissue forms, which is likely to lead to tendinitis. Often the athlete will not feel pain at the time, but will become aware of the rupture later when the tendon has cooled down . . . When the athlete resumes activity after a short period of rest, there may be a sharp pain that disappears after warm-up, only to return. There is often stiffness of the Achilles in the morning. A small swelling in the tendon may also be present.

Massage Strategies

Prevention is important. It is critical for normal gait that the ankle can dorsiflex at least 10 degrees; 20 degrees is optimal. A tight Achilles tendon may limit dorsiflexion and may predispose the athlete to ankle injury as well as strain in the knee, hip, and low back. Apply massage to stretch the Achilles tendon complex. Stretching should be performed first with the knee extended and then with it flexed 15 to 30 degrees. Use both longitudinal and cross-directional stretching.

If there is or has been a partial rupture, palpation may reveal a particular lump or bump in the tendon that is sensitive. Massage outcomes include reduced swelling, increased circulation, and prevention of adhesions. If pain and swelling increase, reduce massage frequency and intensity.

Achilles tendon massage will work best when applied in conjunction with massage of the leg muscles, especially the calf muscles.

Depending on the healing stage, apply massage as follows:

Acute stage: with fiber direction toward injury.

Subacute stage: with fiber direction away from the injury.

Remodeling: bend and shear force across the tendon.

Also, see sequence for muscle strains on page 458. Surgical repair of a tendon follows the pre- and post-surgery protocol in Chapter 19. The Achilles tendon will be thick and rigid after surgery, and massage needs to be performed slowly and gradually to increase tissue pliability. Do not overwork the area. It typically takes a year of rehabilitation, including massage, to restore function in the ankle.

TENNIS LEG

The popliteus tendon runs parallel to the Achilles tendon on the inside of the leg. The disability resulting from rupture of this tendon is called **tennis leg** because it is often seen in tennis players; the rupture occurs as the athlete takes the first, hard step toward the net. Popliteus tendon rupture is more common in older athletes.

Another cause of this condition is a blow or hit to the back of the calf, which may rupture the popliteus tendon. The injured person will be unable to stand on the toes and may have a gait similar to that seen with an Achilles tendon rupture. The base of the bulging muscle on the inner side of the calf will be quite tender, and black and blue areas may be seen.

Initial treatment consists of PRICE. A gentle stretching program can begin as soon as pain decreases, and should be continued until full flexibility is regained. Normally, the tendon will heal in 10 to 21 days.

This injury should be examined by a physician to differentiate it from an Achilles rupture.

Massage Strategies

Apply the general acute, subacute, and remodeling sequences for muscle strains (see page 458).

FRACTURES

Breaking the tibia or fibula is a traumatic injury that requires medical treatment. A fracture of the tibia is serious because this bone heals slowly, and sometimes poorly, due to the sparse blood supply in some areas of the bone.

A fracture of the tibia commonly seen in skiers is called a *boot-top fracture* because the leg breaks right at the top of the rigid ski boot. Before the advent of rigid boots, ankle fractures were common in skiers, but now the ankles are protected and fractures of the tibia are more common.

A fracture of the fibula is less serious than a fracture of the tibia because the fibula is not a true weight-bearing bone. Normally, an athlete can return to activity 4 to 5 weeks after a fibula fracture, with padding to protect the leg from further damage.

Massage Strategies

Use sequences for fractures (see page 472).

STRESS FRACTURES

If twisting of the tibia or fibula is severe and is repeated enough times, the bone will crack. This is known as a **stress fracture.**

The problem with identifying a stress fracture is that the crack is so small that it typically cannot be seen on an x-ray until it begins to heal itself a few weeks later. If the x-ray is negative but pain still exists, a bone scan is often necessary.

Suspect a stress fracture if the pain level resulting from the fracture suddenly increases, or if pain was noticeable only while running but now is noticeable when walking.

Treatment for a stress fracture of the tibia or fibula is reduced activity and rest. Severe pain may require the use of crutches. Typical healing time is 6 to 8 weeks.

Massage Strategies

See fractures on page 472.

TIBIALIS ANTERIOR TENDON SHEATH INFLAMMATION

The tibialis anterior muscle is the large muscle that runs down the outside of the shin. Its tendon can be felt at the front of the ankle. Inflammation can develop as a result of overuse, particularly when running on hard surfaces or in racket sports that require frequent direction of change.

Symptoms of **tibialis anterior tendon sheath inflammation** are pain during dorsiflexion and plantar flexion, and swelling and redness in the area over the tendon.

Treatment includes PRICE therapy.

Massage Strategies

Massage includes lymphatic drain methods, pain control, and strategies to manage compensation. Massage can help reduce the tension in the muscles of the lower leg, which in turn may reduce the strain on the tendon attachments to the bone, allowing the injury to heal and preventing it from returning once training resumes.

As always, it is important to assess the effects of massage both after treatment and on the following day. If there is an increase in pain or inflammation, reduce frequency and intensity.

THE ANKLE

In the ankle, three bones form a "mortise" joint. The dome of the ankle bone (the *talus*) sits in a squared-off socket formed by the tibia and fibula. The joint is held together by three moderately strong ligaments on the outside of the ankle and one very large, very strong ligament on the inside.

Because of the ankle's unique structure, the foot can move in many directions. The foot's up-and-down movement allows walking. First the foot swings "up" on its ankle hinge to permit the heel to strike the ground; then the foot rocks "down" so that the forefoot can push off the ground—thereby propelling the walker forward.

Other important ankle movements are rolling the foot to the inside and to the outside. This allows adjusting the foot to walking and running on uneven surfaces.

The ankle is susceptible to two main types of injury: sprains and fractures. It can be difficult to differentiate between the two injuries. A large, swollen ankle may only be sprained, whereas a healthier-looking ankle may be broken. Therefore, every ankle injury, except the most minimal sprains, should be x-rayed.

SPRAINS

If the foot rolls to the outside on an uneven surface, it may continue to roll over until the ligaments on the outside of the ankle are stretched or torn. The presence of small holes in playing fields leads to many sprains. Even on a flat surface such as a basketball court, a player can always step on someone else's foot and turn the ankle. Ankle sprains account for as much as one-fifth of the injuries. Although most sprains are minor and do not require surgery or extensive treatment, diagnosing the severity of the injury is difficult, and all ankle injuries should therefore be evaluated by a physician.

Signs and symptoms of the three degrees of ligament sprains are as follows:

First degree:
- Some stretching or perhaps tearing of the ligament.
- Little or no joint instability
- Mild pain
- Mild swelling (however, moderate swelling can occur)
- Some joint stiffness
- Mild muscle guarding
- *Quick check*—Able to stand on one foot (the one with the sprain) and be stable, although it hurts

Second degree:
- Some tearing of the ligament fibers
- Moderate instability of the joint
- Moderate to severe pain
- Swelling and stiffness
- Muscle guarding

- *Quick check*—able to stand on one foot (the one with the sprain), but it hurts and is unstable

Third degree:
- Total rupture of a ligament
- Gross instability of the joint
- Severe pain initially followed by no pain
- Severe swelling
- Significant muscle guarding
- *Quick check*—Cannot bear weight on the foot with the sprain

Outward Sprain. The most common ankle sprain is the result of a roll off the outer part of the foot that injures the ligaments on the outside of the ankle. There is swelling and pain in the outer area of the ankle, with black and blue marks around the injury. Within a few days, the foot and toes may also be discolored from blood from the broken vessels flowing downward due to gravity.

If pain occurs on the inside of the ankle as well, x-rays are necessary. When the foot rolls over, the central bone of the ankle can knock against the tibia on the inside of the ankle. This may bruise the bone or even break off a piece, which makes the injury a fracture.

Inward Sprain. An injury resulting from rolling off the inside of the foot is much less common than an outward sprain and usually results in a fracture rather than a sprain. The inside ligament is actually stronger than the inside bone, and rather than spraining, it may pull off a piece of bone where it attaches (*avulsion fracture*). This type of ankle sprain always requires an x-ray.

Forward Sprain (High Ankle). A third type of sprain results when the front of the foot rolls over the toes. This pulls the tendons in front of the ankle and tears the ankle capsule (the membrane that surrounds the ankle bones) and the sheath between the tibia and fibula. This is the most serious type of ankle sprain.

Calf muscles get tighter and weaker after an ankle sprain. Massage can normalize the imbalance. An outward sprain results in increased shortening in the medial tissues. An inward sprain results in shortening of the lateral calf. A forward sprain usually results in co-contraction of all muscles surrounding the ankle.

Inability to bear weight on the affected ankle should prompt further evaluation by a health professional to determine the extent of the injury. Referral is necessary if the client complains of:

- Numbness in the foot or ankle
- Increased swelling rather than a gradual decrease
- Reinjury of the ankle
- A sensation that the ankle "gives way" while walking or running

Early use of NSAIDs may actually cause increased bleeding into the area of injury, so use should be limited in the acute phase of healing. For recurring sprains, an orthotic device with a lateral flange or built-up area over the side of the heel can prevent the ankle from turning over. Persistent sprains may require surgical repair of the ankle ligaments.

People with tight ligaments, such as those with a supinating foot or Morton's foot (discussed later), may be prone to ankle sprains. In both cases, the supinating foot tends to land on the outside and predisposes the ankle to turn out over the foot.

Ankle sprains should be taken seriously. An aggressive rehabilitation program is necessary to speed recovery and reduce the chances of reinjury (Box 21-1).

Massage Strategies

Use sequences for sprains/strains (see page 458).

BROKEN ANKLE

An ankle can break if it is turned severely and with great force—for example, when a basketball player comes down from a rebound and lands on the side of another player's foot, turning the ankle with the force of his or her full weight. A football or soccer player can break an ankle if the cleats are dug into the ground and someone falls on or rolls into the ankle. In baseball, catching the cleats while sliding into a base is a common cause of a broken ankle.

Box 21-1   ANKLE EXERCISES

"Alphabet" Exercise: Draw each letter of the alphabet in the air using the big toe as the "pencil." Repeat the entire alphabet 5 times. Do this exercise 3 times per day.

Motion Exercise: Move by flexing and extending the ankle up and down, without pain, as far as it will go 10 to 15 times. Do this exercise 5 times per day.

Stability training: Stand on the unaffected leg first and maintain stability; then switch to the affected leg. To make this more challenging, close the eyes and repeat.

A broken ankle is difficult to diagnose and can be mistaken for a sprain. Common signs of a broken ankle include:

- A recurrent, diffuse ache in the ankle that increases with exercise or a continual ache
- Swelling after exercise, followed by pain-free periods
- Limited movement
- Bruising in the ankle

Massage Strategies

The ankle needs to be x-rayed and medical treatment applied, including embolization.

Use massage procedures for fractures (see page 472). Also, use sequences for sprains and strains (see page 458).

TIBIALIS POSTERIOR SYNDROME

The tibialis posterior muscle comes from behind the tibia and forms a tendon that passes behind the medial malleolus. Inflammation can occur around the medial malleolus and farther down under the foot where the tendon attaches. This condition is called **tibialis posterior syndrome.** Those who pronate are more likely to suffer from this injury. Treatment involves PRICE and possible use of orthotics.

Massage Strategies

Use lymphatic drain massage (see Unit Two) and sequences for sprains and strains (see page 458).

DISLOCATION OF THE FIBULARUS (PERONEAL) TENDONS

The fibularus tendons run behind the lateral malleolus. If the tissue that holds the tendons in place is torn by an ankle sprain, the tendons can slip forward over the malleolus. Repeated dislocations can result in inflammation. The injury is common in athletes with unstable ankles.

Symptoms of **dislocation of the fibularus tendons** include:

- Pain when the foot pronates
- Pain or tenderness behind the lateral malleolus
- Swelling and bruising

Treatment includes PRICE, followed by gentle stretching when the inflammation has decreased. Surgery may be required in severe cases to mend the tissue that holds the tendons in place.

Massage Strategies

Even though this is not a true strain or sprain, the strategies for strain and sprain are effective (see page 458).

THE FOOT

If their feet hurt, clients tend to be miserable. The foot absorbs the shock of the body's weight landing on it during walking, running, and jumping. The foot supports up to four times the body weight during running, and it bears at least 1,800 foot strikes for every mile. It also locks into a rigid position during toe push-off, acting as a lever for propulsion. The foot must roll from outside to inside as the body weight comes forward from the heel to the front of the foot.

A structural abnormality of the foot can cause stress all the way up the leg into the back. The lower extremity can be viewed as a set of building blocks– the foot, ankle, calf, leg, knee, thigh, hip, and lower back–placed one on top of the other. When one building block does not function as it should, the blocks above it also do not function properly because they have an insecure base. Nearly all overuse injuries of the lower extremities are due to an abnormality in the way the foot hits the ground.

In most people, bones, muscles, and tendons under the foot create an arch. Some people, however, are born with "fallen arches," or flat feet. Contrary to popular belief, flat feet are not a problem for athletes. Most experts believe that flat-footed people should not limit their activities and do not need special treatment. In fact, flat feet usually are more flexible, have greater range of motion, and are better able to absorb the shock of running and jumping than "normal" feet. However, athletes with high arches are more injury-prone. An unusually high-arched foot is more rigid and has limited range of motion during quick, agile movements.

One of the best ways to recognize foot problems is to look at the wear pattern in a pair of athletic shoes. A pronating foot wears out the inside of the heel and toe, and the shoe breaks over to the inside. If the shoe is placed flat on a table top, it will lean to the inside. A supinating foot wears out the outside of the shoe, from the heel all the way down to the toes. This shoe will lean to the outside. A Morton's foot wears out the shoe on the outside of the heel and midsole, and then straight across the sole to the inside of the big toe.

Orthotic devices containing carefully placed divots and bumps are designed to shift the weight in a way that forces more optimal movement. They are made from a variety of materials, from layered foam to leather-covered cork to hard plastic.

PRONATING FOOT

The **pronating foot** has loose ligaments and, because it doesn't have the proper support, rolls to the inside. The foot appears to be flat because the arch becomes compressed when the foot rolls over. However, when the weight is taken off the foot, the arch reappears. A person with true flat feet has no arch at all.

The inward roll of the foot causes the entire leg to rotate to the inside. The kneecaps point toward each other. Every structure in the person's leg and hip is pulled out of optimal alignment.

A pronating foot can be supported with an arch support under the inside of the foot. This keeps the foot in line when it strikes the ground and prevents the leg from rolling inward.

Massage Strategies

See Massage Strategies for the foot.

SUPINATING FOOT

The **supinating foot**, or cavus foot, rolls to the outside. The ligaments are tight, and the foot is rigid with a high arch, causing the person to walk on the far outer portion of the foot. Because the arch is too tight, it cannot collapse when the foot hits the ground. With no arch to absorb the shock of each step, the shock travels up the outside of the leg.

The supinating foot requires soft padding under the outside of the foot. This will cause the foot to roll back slightly toward the middle and will provide some padding to reduce the pounding on the legs. An orthotic device can take some of the weight off of the outer side of the foot.

Massage Strategies

See Massage Strategies for the foot.

MORTON'S FOOT

In **Morton's foot,** the second toe is longer than the big toe. The problem is that the bone behind the big toe (first metatarsal) is too short. This inherited trait occurs in about 25% of the population and causes problems in more people than the two previously discussed foot abnormalities combined.

Forward momentum during walking or running occurs by pushing off with the big toe ("toeing off"). Just before toeing off, all of the weight is on the head of the first metatarsal. In persons with

Morton's foot, the foot buckles to the inside, and the weight rolls along the inner side of the big toe. This is similar to what happens with the pronating foot, but a Morton's foot doesn't pronate until weight is placed on the toes.

People with Morton's foot first strike the ground with the far outer part of the foot. Walking on the inner side of the big toe often causes a large callus to form. Also, the big toe will also be pushed toward the second toe, and the pressure on the inside of the big toe may cause bunions.

Morton's foot is corrected with an orthotic device that has an arch support built up under the big toe joint.

Massage Strategies for the Foot

Massage the foot thoroughly. Make sure that the joints move freely and that the connective tissue structures are pliable, especially in a high arch. Trigger points can develop in the calf as a compensation pattern. Do NOT massage these trigger points until the foot position improves through exercise and orthotics. They are serving an appropriate compensation function.

METATARSALGIA

Metatarsalgia is pain in the front of the foot just behind the toes that can be due to the stress of placing weight on the toes during running. Usually the pain occurs in the second or third toe. The heads of the metatarsal bones in these toes may drop slightly, and the excessive weight placed on them when coming up on the toes causes pain.

A pad placed behind the heads of these toes will lift and take the weight off them, which usually relieves the pain.

Massage Strategies

Use procedures for contusion (see page 447).

METATARSAL STRESS FRACTURE

A **metatarsal stress fracture**, as the name implies, results from an excessive amount of stress on a metarsal bone. When excessive force is transmitted to the second, third, or fourth metatarsal bone, the bone can crack from overfatigue.

If mild pain is felt in the foot for days or even weeks during activities, and then a sudden, severe pain in the front part of the foot is felt, a stress fracture of the foot probably occurred.

In a metatarsal stress fracture, both the upper and the lower surfaces of the foot will be tender, with some swelling. An x-ray of the foot, and some-

times a bone scan, is needed to confirm the diagnosis.

Treatment includes rest for 4 to 6 weeks to allow the fracture to heal. Crutches are necessary only if severe pain occurs when walking. Casting is usually not necessary. Early use of an orthotic device will give relief while the fracture heals.

A stress fracture of the fifth metatarsal, behind the little toe, is a more serious injury. This results from an excessive load on the outside of the foot, such as occurs in the supinating foot.

These fractures heal poorly and require immediate medical attention. Simple rest is not the answer. Casts and crutches for anywhere from 6 weeks to several months may be required. Many of these fractures need to be treated surgically, with a screw used to hold the fragments together.

Treatment of metatarsal stress fractures includes placement of metatarsal pads in the shoes. These are placed behind the metatarsal bones so that during walking the body weight comes down on the pad of the foot, instead of on the bone, thus relieving mechanical stress. In some cases, walking boots with a rocker bottom or rounded soles are used.

Broken bones in the foot other than the toes require immediate medical attention and casting. Immobilization of the foot for 4 to 6 weeks is customary.

Massage Strategies

Use sequences for fractures (see page 472).

BROKEN TOE

A **broken toe** is usually buddy-taped to the toe next to it. Gauze is placed between the two toes before taping them together; otherwise, sweat will cause the skin to soften and flake.

Massage Strategies

Use sequences for fractures (see page 472).

BLACK TOENAILS

Athletes that run as part of their sport may have **black toenails** that may eventually fall off. The constant banging of the toenail against the toe box of the shoe causes bleeding under the toenail, which is why it looks black. The problem usually is caused by an undersized shoe.

People with Morton's foot have an additional problem. The toe boxes of running shoes are all designed with the assumption that the big toe is the largest toe. In the person with Morton's foot, the second toe is largest, so most athletic shoes do not fit properly. The condition is usually ignored, but making sure the shoes fit properly prevents this condition.

Massage Strategies

Massage is not applicable in these cases.

TURF TOE

Turf toe is a sprained joint at the base of the big toe. Turf toe can occur after very vigorous upward bending of the big toe. It got its name due to the fact that it occurs frequently in athletes that play and practice on artificial surfaces such as Astroturf. When running on natural grass with cleats on, the grass gives and some of the stress of toeing off is absorbed by the ground. The hard surface of artificial turf has no "give," and the entire stress of toeing off is transferred to the toe joint. The shoe grips hard on the surface and sticks, causing the body's weight to go forward, bending the toe upward.

Turf toe is also a common injury in martial arts.

When the toe is bent upward, this causes damage to the ligaments, which can become stretched. In addition, the surfaces of the bones at the joint can become damaged. An x-ray can determine whether a bone has been broken.

There is swelling and pain at the joint of the big toe and first metatarsal bone, as well as pain and tenderness when bending the toe or pulling (stretching) it upward.

Risk for this injury is increased when there is excessive range of motion in the ankle and when soft flexible shoes are worn. Playing on grass with shoes with short cleats decreases the risk

Turf toe is very painful and slow to heal. The athlete should rest until the pain is gone, but this seldom happens Recovery can take 3 to 4 weeks, depending on the severity of sprain. When it begins to heal, the trainer can tape the toe down so that it cannot extend upward.

If this injury does not heal properly then it may develop into *hallux limitus*, which is a decreased range of motion due to arthritis around the joint.

Massage Strategies

Massage is focused on full-body compensation patterns because of the change in how the client walks and runs, which strains all muscles involved. Often the low back or knees will ache. Address firing patterns at each massage session. Gentle, pain-free

traction seems to relieve the pressure and pain in the joint. Also use strategies for sprains and pain management (see page 458).

PLANTAR FASCIITIS

The plantar fascia is the connective tissue covering on the sole of the foot that holds up the arch. It runs the length of the foot, from just behind the toe bones to the heel bone. This shock-absorbing pad can become inflamed, a condition called **plantar fasciitis**, causing aching and sharp pain along the length of the arch.

The pain is due to overstretching or partial tearing of the plantar fascia. This injury usually happens to people with rigid, high arches. They feel the pain when putting weight on the foot or when pushing off for the next stride. As the arch starts to come down, it stretches the plantar fascia and pulls on its fibers. The torn fibers become inflamed and may shrink. The plantar fascia tears a little more with every step, resulting in intense pain.

Plantar fasciitis can affect anyone, but is more common in older athletes, overweight athletes, and those engaged in prolonged exercise. Distance runners, golfers, tennis players,, and basketball players are examples of athletes who frequently develop plantar fasciitis. Plantar fasciitis is particularly common among middle-aged people who have been sedentary and who suddenly increase their level of physical activity. Running and jogging lead to most of the injuries. Inappropriately fitting shoes or a weight gain of 10 to 20 pounds can also contribute to the condition. The condition is treated with ice and stretching. A cortisone injection may be used if necessary. Orthotics are often prescribed.

Massage Strategies

Inflammation is a symptom of this condition. Therefore, in the acute stage do not use any methods that increase inflammation, especially friction. Lymphatic drain application is appropriate in the painful area. Focus treatment on the short structures—muscles and/or connective tissue.

Disrupted firing patterns such as described for the knee are usually involved and need to be normalized. Once the inflammation is past the acute phase, bend, shear, and torsion forces can be introduced during massage to address the Achilles tendon and plantar fascia. Also make sure the gastrocnemius and soleus are not adhered to each other or short.

MORTON'S SYNDROME

Nerves that transmit messages to the brain from the toes pass between the metatarsal bones. If the arch is weak, the metatarsal bones can pinch a nerve, causing inflammation, or **Morton's syndrome**. This is most likely to happen between the third and fourth metatarsals, resulting in pain or a numb sensation on one side of a toe and the adjacent side of the next toe when the foot is squeezed. The pinched nerve causes pain or numbness on the sides of the toes nearest to the nerve

Treatment includes rest, orthotics, NSAIDs, and exercises to strengthen the arch of the foot.

Surgery may be required if other treatments fail.

Massage Strategies

Caution: do not massage over the painful nerve. Lymphatic drain methods may be helpful. Focus on management of compensation and causal patterns.

HEEL SPUR

A **heel spur** is a hook of bone that irritates the heel and is often caused by an irritated, overstretched plantar fascia.

The pain is located at the heel where the plantar fascia attaches into the heel bone. Constant pulling on the plantar fascia at this point can cause the heel bone to overgrow and form a spur, which is visible on x-ray.

Treatment includes an arch support, which can hold the plantar fascia and keep it from overstretching. Surgery is also an option in some cases.

Massage Strategies

See massage strategies for plantar fasciitis. Do NOT massage over the area of the spur.

HEEL STRESS SYNDROME

Heel stress syndrome occurs on both the inside and outside of the heel bone, but more severely on the inside. This syndrome is due to excessive pronation of the foot. The heel rolls to the inside, and the force of the weight is delivered at an angle rather than straight down. It feels like the heel is bruised.

Treatment includes the use of an orthotic device.

Massage Strategies

Focus on compensation patterns arising from changes in gait. Do NOT apply heavy pressure in the painful area. Treat as a contusion (see page 447).

TOE TENDINITIS

Tenderness and swelling along the top of the foot only are usually due to **toe tendinitis**, an inflammation of the tendons that raise the toes. Pain is intensified if the toes are held down and then pulled back up against resistance.

Shoes laced too tightly or poor padding under the tongues of the shoes can cause toe tendinitis.

Treatment consists of icing the tendons intermittently until the pain and swelling subside. Like many conditions of the foot, this condition relates to ill-fitting shoes (Box 21-2).

Massage Strategies

Massage as for tendinitis (see p. 466).

TARSAL TUNNEL SYNDROME AND ENTRAPMENT OF THE MEDIAL CALCANEAL NERVE

The tarsals are the long bones of the foot. The tunnel holding the medial and lateral plantar nerves is located just below the medial malleolus.

An overpronated foot rolls during walking or running, putting pressure on these nerves, which can become irritated and inflamed. When there is excessive pronation or pressure from shoes, the medial nerve can become trapped. Pain radiates from the inside of the heel out toward the center of the heel. This complex of the symptoms of irritation, inflammation, and pain caused by the entrapped nerve is called **tarsal tunnel syndrome.**

Symptoms include:
- Pain radiating into the arch of the foot, the heel and sometimes the toes
- "Pins and needles" or numbness in the sole of the foot
- Pain when running or standing for long periods of time

Tapping the nerve just behind the medial malleolus may reproduce the pain.

In the acute stage, treatment includes PRICE. If overpronation is present, an orthotic device should be worn.

Massage Strategies

Use sequences for nerve entrapment (see page 477).

PES CAVUS (CLAW FOOT)

Pes cavus (claw foot) is a genetic defect in the foot causing an excessively high arch and supination.

Box 21-2   CHOOSING AN ATHLETIC SHOE

Wearing proper athletic shoes can reduce the risk of all the injuries that stem from a poor foot strike and lead to pain all the way up the leg to the back. Following is a list of necessary features for sports-specific shoes:

Running Shoes

Look primarily for good cushioning and good stability. The soles should curve up in the front and back, with a slightly elevated heel; heel counters should be firm, and the edges should be sharp for stability. The shoes should be lightweight with soft, breathable, flexible uppers. They should have good midsole cushioning and soles that are grooved or studded. If the foot tends to pronate, choose a shoe with a straight last and extra firmness along the inner edge for more stability. If the foot tends to supinate, a shoe should be chosen with a curve that forces the foot inward and should have a soft midsole and heel counter.

Walking Shoes

Walking shoes support the heel-to-toe gait of walking. They should have adequate flexibility in the forefoot and adequate room between the toes and the top of the shoe. The shoes should be lightweight and have strong heel counters, good midsole cushioning, slightly elevated heels, and flexible soles that curve up at the heel and toe. The upper should be made of breathable materials with a hard, reinforced area to protect the toe.

Tennis Shoes

Tennis shoes are designed for good lateral support and good shock absorption. They should be heavy and strong with flat soles and a hard, squared-off edge. Also look for a reinforced front, a cushioned midsole, a firm heel counter, and a sole with circles to facilitate turning.

Racquetball Shoes

Look for lightweight uppers, good midsole cushioning, and tacky, round-edged soles that are thinner and more flexible than those of tennis shoes.

Volleyball Shoes

Volleyball shoes are lightweight and flexible with reinforced toes, well-cushioned midsoles, and soles made of ridged gum or rubber with rounded edges for good lateral support.

Aerobics Shoes

Aerobics shoes are a lightweight combination of tennis and running shoes. They should have good shock absorption; stabilizing straps may be good for the side-to-side action of low-impact aerobics. Good aerobics shoes will have slightly elevated heels; firm heel counters for stability; lots of midsole cushioning; and wrapped, soft rubber soles for lateral support.

Basketball Shoes

Basketball shoes are designed to be heavier than tennis shoes, with good shock absorption, ankle support, traction, and stability. This means good lateral support, hard rubber cup-ridged soles, and sturdy midsoles.

Football Shoes

Football shoes have thick, rigid, leather uppers with sturdy heel counters and spiked rubber soles.

Baseball shoes

These shoes have uppers made of leather or nylon and leather, soles with sharp edges for good traction, a long tongue flap that folds back over the laces to keep dirt out, and soles with cleats of molded plastic or hard rubber.

Cycling Shoes

Cycling shoes have stiff soles for efficient pedaling. Racing shoes should have a very stiff sole, and touring shoes should have a little more flexibility. The snug-fitting, stiff uppers should be made of leather or leather and nylon with no cushioning. Shoes for mountain biking may use more durable materials. Many cycling shoes have Velcro snaps for a snug fit. The shoe should also fit snugly into the toehold on the pedal, and the soles should have grooves to help grip the pedals.

Weight-Training Shoes

Weight-training shoes require a wide base for stability and a firm midsole for support. Stabilizing straps can lock in the heel to provide a firm footing.

Cross-Trainer Shoes

Cross-trainer shoes shoes are designed to combine flexibility, stability, and cushioning in one pair of shoes. Choose shoes with reinforced toes and with restraining straps for good lateral support.

Because of my level of experience, I am often involved with injury rehabilitation of athletes. I have stared at so many pictures and models of knees that the images appear during my dreams. My biggest nightmares are rib injuries and turf toe. Both hurt so much and there is so little that can be done. I am thrilled when working with an athlete who has a bone break because bone heals really well. If an athlete comes to me with a ligament injury, I cringe.

I have used lymph drain more than any other method. Once the client and I both fell asleep during the lymph drain process! The client was lying on the floor and I was kneeling beside him draining away. He fell asleep and apparently so did I. He woke me up and my hands were still on his ankle.

It may seem inappropriate to tell funny stores about injuries, but laughter is healing. I recall working very intensely (24 hours a day for 16 days) with an athlete recovering from arthroscopic knee surgery to remove a loose body. Time was critical, so out came the vitamins, essential oils, and arnica, the rescue remedy, the magnets, the ice, and the healing energies and intentions. The athlete and I spent so much time together that we did not even talk anymore. He slept, watched TV, or talked on the phone. I lymph-drained until I was drained. Massage was applied morning, noon, and night, encouraging firing patterns and range of motion. Every time the athlete saw me coming he opened his mouth to take something and lie down wherever he was for whatever massage he was going to get. He always smelled like a flower or piece of fruit because of the essential oils. Magnets were stitched into the elastic compression sleeve worn around the knee. He made the time deadline and never missed a practice or a game.

The outcome was very good but the process was often hysterical and ridiculous—maybe not then but especially now when I look back. I have no clue what worked and what didn't. I also know that there was more involved than what I did. Body, mind, and spirit combine for the miracle of healing.

Claw feet are relatively inflexible. The high arch is associated with very tight calf muscles at the back of the lower leg.

There may be pain in the feet during running and painful, and bent toes that cannot be straightened. Treatment is difficult and typically involves orthotics and in severe cases, surgery.

Massage Strategies

Focus on management of compensation patterns in the calf and maintain pliability and mobility of foot structures.

BUNION/HALLUX VALGUS

A **bunion** is a painful prominence on the side of the foot where the big toe begins. This condition is marked by soft tissue swelling and enlargement of the affected joint (at the first metatarsal head of the big toe). Both biomechanical factors and genetic anatomic defects may contribute to this abnormality.

Poorly fitting shoes will exert friction and pressure on a joint that already may be somewhat abnormal in function or size. The resulting swelling and tenderness will get even worse from wearing a shoe that is not wide or deep enough to accommodate the bunion.

Often the big toe is bent in toward the other toes—this deformity is called *hallux valgus*—or even can lie across them.

Excessive pronation and Morton's toe can lead to the formation of bunions.

Massage Strategies

General massage of the foot may be helpful. Do not irritate the bunion.

There are many different ways an injury can occur other than as a direct result of an athletic activity. People often get hurt just fooling around, during general daily activities, or when participating in a sport other than their primary activity. I remember a football player who strained his back while bowling and a basketball player who sprained her ankle stepping on her child's toy.

The only way to be truly effective using massage during injury rehabilitation is to be able to use your problem-solving skills. The workbook section in this chapter asks you to manipulate the information in multiple ways to help you proceed with the information in different contexts. You may get tired of flipping through the chapter pages while completing the workbook questions—but, oh well—repetition is part of excellence. It is true that repetition can be tedious, but so is lymphatic drain if you are doing it right.

Nevertheless, if a basketball player sprains an ankle by stepping on another player's foot or one of her child's toys, I still end up using massage strategies for sprains.

SUMMARY

This chapter describes the most commonly occurring sports injuries encountered by the massage professional. Most of these injuries should be treated and monitored by the physician or athletic trainer, and the role of the massage therapist is usually supportive.

In all injury situations, rest and appropriate rehabilitation are important for proper healing. Massage supports both. It is hoped that this chapter will be used often as a reference. If you have a client with any of these injuries, use this textbook to begin your research and then access other resources to expand your knowledge. In general, it is best to undertreat, not overtreat injury. The sooner massage can begin after injury, the better the outcome. Old injuries that are symptomatic need to be taken into a controlled acute phase with precise frictioning, and then addressed as an acute injury. This process is repeated over and over, and this takes patience and persistence. Preventing injuries is always better than having to treat the injury. When in doubt about what to do, apply lymph drainage methods and use sequences that entrain healing energies.

1 List at least five major benefits of massage that support healing mechanisms.

_____

_____

_____

_____

2 List 10 injuries that are treated with strategies for wounds.

_____

_____

_____

3 List 10 injuries that are treated with strategies for tendinitis.

_____

_____

_____

_____

4 List 10 injuries that use lymphatic drain as the primary treatment method.

_____

_____

_____

_____

5 List 10 injuries that are medical emergencies.

_____

_____

_____

_____

6 List 10 injuries most likely to occur from trauma.

_____

_____

_____

_____

7 List 10 injuries most likely to occur from repetitive strain.

_____

_____

_____

_____

8 List 10 injuries where core stability is a factor.

_____

_____

_____

_____.

9 List at least five errors made during massage treatment of injuries.

_____

_____

_____

_____

10 Based on the typical strain and injury potential of a specific physical activity, identify five injuries you feel would be common in the following sports or exercise programs.

Aerobic dancing

_____

Baseball

_____

Gymnastics

_____

Golf

_____

Tennis

_____

Football

_____

Soccer

_____

Running a marathon

_____

Long jump in track and field

_____

Weightlifting

_____

Volleyball

_____

Rowing

_____

Hockey

_____

Biking

_____

Race walking

_____

Skateboarding

_____

Surfing

_____

Rollerskating

_____

11 Identify your favorite sport or exercise activity and list five common injuries that may occur while performing it.

_____

_____

_____

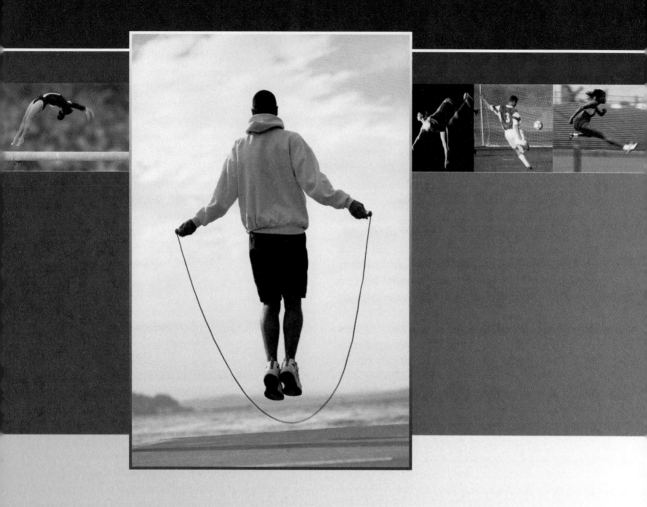

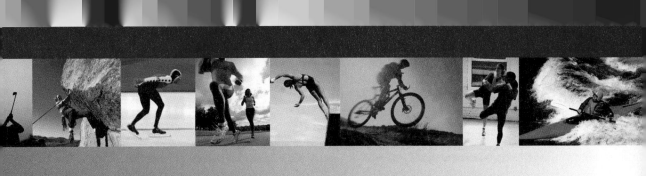

UNIT FOUR

CASE STUDIES

STORIES
from the field
CHARLIE BATCH

All persons—athletes included—have a story. Each individual's story shapes his or her life. Because when working with so-called celebrities, one commonly focuses on what they do instead of who they are, I have included a few stories of individuals, who are also athletes, to put into perspective the importance of the professional relationship the massage therapist achieves and maintains with this type of client. We do not provide massage to a football player or basketball player or golfer. We support individuals in their own personal quest for achievement. The stories I have chosen to tell are about those with whom I have spent the most time and therefore know the best. The stories are from my point of view and with their permission.

I first met Charlie at the onset of the educational programs with the Detroit Lions that began in 1998/99. He had been drafted that previous year, and through various circumstances, he had been the starting quarterback as a rookie. I soon learned that rookies are just kids, and being the quarterback on an NFL team put this kid in the spotlight. During his rookie year, he had performed extremely well. He had the opportunity to play with Hall of Fame running back Barry Sanders and is the first to acknowledge that a part of his rookie success was due to having Barry on the team. I met Charlie the next year when the team was in transition because this was the year that Barry Sanders retired. Especially with team sports, a change like this is especially difficult for a young player.

The first time I worked with Charlie, he had a kink in his neck. I had no idea who he was, and I was swamped with a bunch of other players with aches and pains. I do remember thinking how young he looked as I applied compression to the scalenes. This was the beginning of a long, involved professional relationship that has spanned many years.

Various circumstances over the years resulted in Charlie playing with a series of painful injuries, and massage was an ongoing part of how he continued to play. At the same time, the team was undergoing many organizational changes. Stress levels were high for

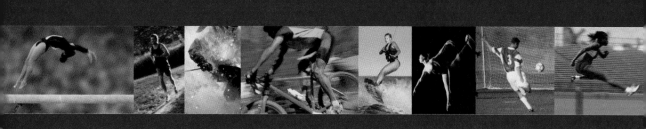

everyone, which added to the typical strain of the ongoing football seasons. The cumulated injuries had affected his ability to perform at his peak. In 2002 he undertook a major commitment to rehabilitation and spent months at the IMG training facility in Bradenton, Florida. I have experienced only a few persons in my long massage career who worked so hard to rebuild their bodies. It was during this time that I became involved with this group of sport medicine professionals, and the educational program for advanced sports massage was developed with my school.

In 2002 Charlie left the Detroit Lions and joined the Pittsburgh Steelers. He was in the best physical condition I had ever seen him, and he had matured from a kid to a man. For a major part of his career in Detroit, he had been the starting quarterback. In Pittsburgh his initial role on the team was third quarterback. He had to adjust professionally and personally to the status change, knowing that he was in the best playing shape of his life but likely would not see playing time and in fact was last in line. He made the adjustment from top dog to background support with grace and maturity.

An old knee injury, likely from when he was in high school or college, resulted in a loose body in his knee, and arthroscopic surgery was performed less than 3 weeks before the beginning of training camp with his new team. Excellent medical care and 24-hour-a-day massage care resulted in him reporting to camp and never missing a practice. That was a long and intense 2 weeks. I performed lymph drainage on his knee and managed compensation hour after hour. He participated and at times endured (with only a bit of grumping) scar tissue management, ice application, and range-of-

motion methods. Many funny stories resulted from that intense 2-week period because circumstances were just not typical. We got tired of each other but persisted anyway.

Massage was provided on the massage table but also on the floor, on the sofa, at the computer, and so on. The effort put forth was incredible.

I wonder what motivates or drives these athletes, so in brief here is the rest of his story.

Charlie grew up with a committed single mom. He and his mother are very close, and she supported him in his career from the time he was little. Needless to say, those days were hard and do not need further explanation here. Charlie excelled in sports and was awarded a scholarship to Eastern Michigan University. He survived a life-threatening illness from toxic chemical exposure at a summer job and managed to returned to football, breaking almost every quarterback record at the school. Even more devastating was the tragedy to hit his family next.

In 1996, when Charlie's sister, whom he adored, was walking along his hometown sidewalk with a friend, a gunshot intended for her companion struck her in the head and killed her. She was 17 years old. The shooter never has been brought to justice.

Charlie had left the neighborhood he grew up in for college before the neighborhood was torn apart by guns, drugs, and a feeling of hopelessness. Grief for his sister motivated him to wonder how he could make things better.

When his sister was killed, Charlie told his mother that he was leaving college to come home and provide for the family, but she would not permit it, reminding him that his sister was so proud that he had made it to college and never

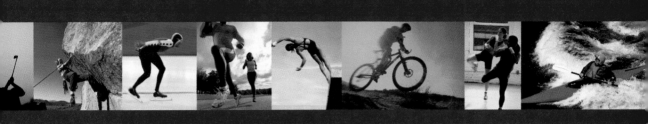

thought he was a quitter. So he found another way not only to support his family but also the community that he loves.

Charlie started the Best of the Batch Foundation that targets low-income families and youth in the Homestead area where idle hands often can get in trouble.

The foundation took early roots in Detroit when Charlie played for the Lions, but he started to focus on home when he joined the Steelers in 2002.

The foundation has started after-school programs that promote literacy by conducting registration for library cards. But that is only a small part of it. The foundation also provides scholarships, restores playgrounds, takes kids to the movies, and conducts a popular summer basketball league for boys and girls between the ages of 7 and 18. The league is run through an arm of the foundation called Project C.H.U.C.K. (Constantly Helping Uplift Community Kids).

I know Charlie shows up at the playground almost every night to talk to the kids or just shoot baskets with them. He also mentors students in one-on-one sessions at Steel Valley High School, reads to them at the library, and simply hangs out with them at the park. I have seen him go from kid to kid asking for a report on grades and conduct. He is tough. If they do not follow the rules, they have to answer to him, but because he is there, the kids know he cares.

I was there when he took 50 elementary students to the circus and again when he took 50 more students to the movies. The kids who went had made the grades and attendance requirements at school.

Even though Charlie just turned 30 years old, as of this writing he has played football for 21 years. By nature he is quiet and not one to talk much, including about himself, but he did say during an interview, "If you can save one person, that changes somebody's life. If you can make an impact on somebody's life forever, that's something I want to do."

As of this writing, Charlie wants to play football a few more years and is beginning to plan for the next stage of his life—not being a football player. He has role models to whom he looks for guidance, just as he is a role model to the kids with whom he interacts. ∎

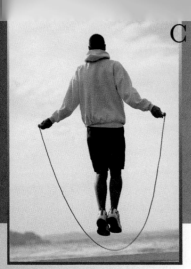

22

CASE STUDIES

This unit presents a unique perspective for a textbook. The unit is written more like a series of stories that chronicle the clinical practice of massage therapists specializing in sport and fitness massage. The content is technically correct and is presented in an interpersonal context of experienced massage therapists who are continually learning. The client profiles are often composite characters drawn from actual experience, designed to represent accurately the real-world application of information presented in this text. The goal is to involve the reader in a clinical reasoning outcome-based massage approach that is a realistic representation of the sport and rehabilitation environment and the persons involved. This is the best way for me, the author, to shift from teacher to mentor.

Each case in this unit is a composite of many different clients, but all the situations are ones with which I have been involved personally. As I reflect on all the sport stories I have read or watched, the underlying story is about the personal sacrifices and triumphs and the persons behind the scenes—the doctors, trainers, coaches, family, and massage therapist and others who contributed to the outcome, be it regaining fitness, ability to overcome injury, winning, and losing. Shakespeare coined the metaphor of the "play within the play," and these vignettes can be thought of as the play within the competition. I purposely have used a variety of formats for these case studies so that the reader can become familiar with different narrative and documentation styles.

First, I will describe each of the clients, and then the text will follow a period of time using a charting format of the therapeutic massage session for each client. Individual methods such a lymphatic drainage or joint play will not be described. Instead, the reader needs to refer to those areas in the text or other textbooks that are recommended to support this text. Because there is no way to develop precise protocols, a clinical reasoning model is used.

CASE ONE

MARGE—CARDIAC REHABILITATION

Marge is an 84-year-old woman with age-related cardiac insufficiency. The coronary arteries are somewhat blocked, but surgery is not the best option and the condition is being controlled with medication. Previously she underwent procedures to unblock arteries in her left leg and participated in a cardiac rehabilitation program.

Marge was a high school teacher for many years. She has been moderately active and basically healthy over her life span. She smoked for many years but quit in her 40s. When she was in her 60s, she fell and severely sprained her right wrist and left ankle and bruised her back. She did not receive rehabilitation after the fall and only had medical care for the acute phase of healing.

She cared for her husband during a long-term illness until he passed away. When Marge was in her mid-70s she found herself a widow, fatigued, and deconditioned. In addition, she had developed a kyphosis to which she is genetically predisposed and that had worsened during her years of caring for her husband. Being an intelligent and determined woman, she slowly began to reconstruct her life. She began by seeing an osteopathic physician for the kyphosis. The doctor recommended massage as part of the care. Consultation between the massage therapist and the doctor resulted in the following assessment:

- Age-related loss in muscle mass; osteoporosis: alendronate (Fosamax) was prescribed.
- High blood pressure: A diuretic and beta-blockers were prescribed.
- Circulation impairment in lower extremities, more so on the left side to be monitored with surgery as an option
- Therapeutic exercise and referral to a physical therapist
- Compression of internal organs from the kyphosis, reduced respiratory capacity managed with osteopathic manipulation
- Persistent upper thorax pain and brachial plexus impingement: Condition was treated with massage therapy.

In addition, the doctor indicated that Marge was prone to falls because of the changes in her head position from the kyphosis (forward head) and ongoing cardiovascular symptoms. Strength and balance training was necessary to slow the progression and was provided by the physical therapist.

Massage assessment identified upper and lower crossed syndrome, which is difficult to manage because of the structural change in her spine. The pattern of short and tight muscles coupled with weak inhibited muscles that are necessary for stability during walking did not help the balance problems or support rehabilitation to strengthen the core, gluteal, and quadriceps area. Without a confident gait, the cardiovascular rehabilitation that relied on walking was compromised. Accommodation in physical therapy was to use a treadmill with side rails so Marge could maintain her balance. However, with the arms fixed during exercise, firing patterns and gait reflex were consistently out of balance.

Initially Marge used a cane to provide additional stability, but over time she regained strength so that she used the cane only if she had to walk long distances or if the weather was raining or snowy. Life went on over the next 10 years. Marge increased her strength, was diligent with her exercise program, and purchased a treadmill for her home. She resumed social activities and volunteered for hospice and enjoyed life. The osteopathic physician moved, and Marge began seeing a chiropractor. She continued with weekly massage sessions to manage soft tissue compensation from the kyphosis. The kyphosis gradually worsened, but continued activity allowed Marge to live a full, independent, and productive life.

The current situation is as follows:

Marge is now 84 years old.

The past winter was severe, and she was not able to attend her cardiac rehabilitation and strength training program. She began to be more sedentary. She did not drive in the bad weather, so she was more house bound than normal and did not make all of her massage and chiropractic appointments. She became dizzy one day and fell and was taken to the hospital. The dosage of her cardiac medication was changed, and she went to a nursing facility for observation and therapy to regain her balance and strength. She is being taught how to use a walker.

Physical therapy involves progressive strength training for the lower extremities and modified cardiovascular training using a bike. She is noticeably frail. Some nerve entrapment pain occurs in her brachial plexus, and she is taking pain medication.

Marge realizes that she will not be able to return to full independent living and is making arrangements to move into an assisted-living facility. The facility offers various services including physical therapy. During the 10-year relationship with her massage therapist, the ongoing consistent outcome of treatment has been managing progressive changes in posture, including persistent upper and lower crossed syndrome with breathing difficulties from structural changes in the thorax. Goals also have included continued circulation support, primarily for the lower extremities, and pain management for recurring nerve entrapment pain. A close professional relationship has formed between the two. The massage therapist has agreed to begin seeing Marge at her residence once she is released from the short-term care in the nursing facility.

The current goals for the massage are to support the physical therapy that is targeted to increasing strength in the legs, learning to use the walker, and improving overall strength and balance.

Marge indicated that her legs are achy from the new exercises and her forearms are tight, which she suspects is from the walker. Her shoulders are elevated from pushing the walker. She is a bit groggy from the pain medication and often out of breath. She fears that she will fall again.

Previously, Marge received a 1-hour massage once a week. Accommodations were made in positioning because she could not comfortably lie on her back or stomach, so the side-lying and seated positions were used primarily. A general massage approach to increase circulation, support pain management, and reduce tension in short muscle provided the bulk of the massage. Connective tissue binding in the chest was not addressed specifically because there was no realistic expectation of change and her adaptive capacity was minimal. Instead, a more general massage was used to soften the tissue temporarily. The nerve impingement area in the shoulders received general massage to activate hyperstimulation analgesia. This was accomplished with repetitive stroking of the skin and kneading and compression with a capsicum-based ointment.

The lower body still had some adaptive capacity, so careful use of muscle energy methods and active movement targeted the weak gluteus maximus, quadriceps, and short hamstrings. General massage for pain control and circulation will continue, but the forearms will need additional attention until Marge adapts to the walker. Marge especially enjoyed having her lower legs and feet massaged. The altered treatment plan increased massage frequency to 2 times per week for 45 minutes at her residence.

Assessment and treatment of firing patterns and her gait reflexes will depend on her ability to participate. More passive application to encourage muscle balance may replace the active participation if Marge is especially tired. Marge has a combination of anxiety over the move into the new apartment and depression over the decline in her condition, and massage will target neurotransmitter function to help stabilize mood if possible.

The massage therapist needs to know the following for the clinical reasoning process:
• What is cardiac insufficiency?
• What medication is Marge taking, and what are the possible interactions with massage?
• What exercises are involved in the cardiac rehabilitation program?
• What strength and balance exercises is Marge doing?
• What are the special concerns because of the osteoporosis and high blood pressure?
• What is the correct method for using a walker or cane?
• What is the medical team's prognosis and recommendation for massage?

These questions are answered in multiple ways. The medication and the cardiac condition can be researched in reference books and on the Internet. The nurse in charge of Marge's case can answer questions.

Marge can teach the massage therapist how to do her exercise and use the walker and cane. The massage therapist can attend a physical therapy session with Marge and observe and ask questions.

Marge can provide information on the prognosis and recommendations from her physician or give permission to speak with the doctor. The massage therapist needs to be concise with the question and should prepare questions in advance before speaking to the doctor.

Session notes since being released from short-term care are as follows:

Session One

S—Client reports that she is tired and her arms and legs ache. She does not want to do her exercises. She knows she is depressed. The doctor is concerned about medication side effects, especially the pain medication, and would like the massage to target pain management.

O—Client displays difficulty moving from the chair to standing position, and her balance is compromised. She is gripping instead of holding the walker. Her feet and ankles are moderately swollen with venous congestion evident by prominent veins. She was able to lie on the massage table if it was lowered. General massage targets parasympathetic dominance with support for neurochemical mood elevators, pain control, lymphatic drain, and venous return. Active assisted range of motion is used on lower extremities, and slightly deeper compression is used on forearms, while the wrist is actively moved in circles.

A—Client's mood lifted as the massage progressed, circulation increased with assisted movement, swelling substantially decreased, and the forearm muscles relaxed.

P—Alter massage frequency to 2 times per week for 45 minutes.

Session Two

S—Client seems disoriented. Pain medication seems to be the likely cause. She is not eating well and continues to have swelling in lower extremities. Visiting nurse will be there this afternoon.

O—Client seems weaker and needs assistance getting up from the chair. Mild edema is evident in lower extremities with venous congestion. General massage should follow same pattern as last session.

A—Client does not respond as well to the massage; however, she is steadier with the walker after the massage. She really enjoys having her feet massaged and asks for more time in that area.

P—Continue with current plan.

Session Three

S—Marge is more energetic and says she is eating better and feels stronger. She reports that she has started participating in Meals on Wheels and has been eating smaller, more frequent meals. She missed the doctor's appointment, but talked with her physician on the phone. She was told to not take the pain medication. Her right shoulder is bothering her.

O—Marge is walking more confidently with the walker but continues to grip the handles. Getting up from the chair is still labored. She is less swollen and congested in the ankles. General massage targets active resisted movement for lower limbs and positional release near scalenes on tender point that increased shoulder symptoms. Also treated are bilateral tender points in pectoralis minor and lymphatic drain on lower extremities. Increased time is spent on the feet.

A—Marge is more interactive with the massage and stronger during active assisted range of motion. Pain reduced significantly in her shoulder.

P—Continue massage as previously determined.

Session Four

S—Client requests massage 3 times per week. She says she feels better and sleeps better after the massage. She indicates that finances are not a problem, and the doctor approves. She is still experiencing pain in her right shoulder, but her forearms do not feel as tight to her. Visiting nurse has been coming every other day. She continues to get meals from Meals on Wheels.

O—Marge appears more confident with the walker, and when she demonstrates the pedaling device she used from her chair, movement looks more symmetrical. She is able to resist light pressure applied to assess shoulder flexors and hip flexor strength. Massage continues to address circulation, lymphatic drainage, and pain management. In addition, active resisted range of motion is added for legs and arms.

A—Only one sequence of active resisted range of motion is used to prevent fatigue and muscle soreness. Marge enjoys the massage interaction and is cooperative.

P—Increase massage sessions to 3 times per week.

Session Five

S—Marge reports that she experienced no ill effects from the active resisted methods. She is eating and sleeping well. She has been able to reduce pain medication so she only takes it before going to bed. Using public transportation, she has begun to go to cardiac rehabilitation at the hospital. She has resumed the treadmill and bike workout, but at a reduced duration. She is pleased with her progress.

O—Assessment indicates Marge is adjusting to the walker. She is beginning to use her legs more and is using her arms only for balance. As a result, pain in her arms is reduced. Edema in her legs is reduced. Massage is nonspecific and full body.

A—Because progress has been good and the exercise is showing progressive increases in strength, a general nonspecific massage achieved the goal of physical stimulation, relaxation, and support for circulation without straining adaptive mechanisms.

P—Continue with nonspecific massage.

Session Six

S—Marge reports that she is doing fine.

O—Assessment does not indicate any significant changes in progress. General nonspecific full-body massage is used.

A—Client reports feeling well and enjoys the massage.

P—Continue nonspecific approach and reduce frequency to 2 times per week.

Session Seven

S—Marge reports that her checkup with the doctor went well and there were no changes in medication. They did discuss the benefits of Marge moving to an assisted-living senior complex.

O—Marge discussed the pros and cons of the move during the massage. The massage application remains general full body.

A—Marge enjoys the massage and comes to the decision to make the move to assisted living.

P—Continue maintenance care.

Session Eight

S—Marge indicates that she did not sleep as well but attributes it to decision making over the move. She continues with home and cardiac rehabilitation exercise. She asks for attention to her feet.

O—Marge appears more fatigued and a bit anxious. She again discusses the move to assisted living in terms of process. She displays a bit of upper chest breathing. Massage remains general full body with attention to shoulders and neck to decrease upper chest breathing tendency. There are tender points in the mid and upper trapezius. Extra attention is given to the feet. Marge begins to cry softly during the massage. The massage continues, and there is no discussion about the emotional display.

P—Continue with general massage with reevaluation of breathing.

Session Nine

S—Client reports she has been cleaning out closets and her back hurts. She missed going to cardiac rehabilitation because she was sorting through "stuff."

O—No apparent decrease or increase in arm and leg strength is apparent, but therapist does notice that Marge uses the walker mostly for balance. Tender points exist in lower lumbar multifidi and quadratus lumborum. General massage is performed with positional release to tender points. Breathing is mildly dominant in the upper chest. Tender points exist in the upper trapezius and pectoralis minor. Inhibitory pressure is used in both areas. Inform Marge that these areas may be tender to the touch for a couple days.

A—Marge reports that her back feels better and that the tender areas in her trapezius or pectoralis minors are really sore, but she can move her shoulders better.

P—Continue with general massage; reevaluate breathing and low back.

Session Ten

S—Client reports that she feels okay but a bit overwhelmed. She again missed the cardiac rehabilitation appointment. She has been informed that an efficiency apartment is available at the assisted-living facility she likes. The actual move will begin in 2 weeks.

O—Marge appears stable physically but is understandably a bit anxious. Massage is targeted to support parasympathetic dominance. Marge discusses life changes a lot during the massage.

A—Marge feels more relaxed and in control of her situation. She decides to donate what household items she would not need to her church for the new recreation center and also solidifies plans for obtaining assistance for the actual move. As the massage therapist is leaving, Marge is already on the phone finalizing the plan.

P—Continue with general massage.

The Rest of the Story

Marge successfully made the move. Her condition stabilized but did not improve significantly. She eventually reduced massage frequency to once per week. She continues to be active in the assisted-living complex activities and participates in the various exercise programs. Her newest endeavor is weight training. Age-related changes are evident, but she continues to take them in stride.

CASE TWO

TOM—GOLFER

Tom is a professional golfer. He is 31 years old, in good health, and usually is actively involved in effective strength and conditioning programs. He will slack off periodically and then overtrain to compensate. His core strength is excellent, and firing and gait patterns are usually normal. Tom occasionally gets fatigue-induced gait and firing pattern changes if he has to play on an extremely hilly course, has to play back-to-back rounds, or has overtrained at the gym. When this occurs, he complains of heavy legs, tight calves, and achy feet. He has had plantar fasciitis in both feet successfully treated with cortisone injection and orthotics. He is an intense, emotional competitor and has a tendency for breathing dysfunction. He recently fell while skiing and broke his left fibula near the ankle. The fracture did not require surgery.

Like most golfers, Tom has a pelvic rotation and shoulder girdle rotation that is sport related and asymptomatic. His forearm muscles co-contract on the golf club and become short and tight. He is prone to an occasional migraine headache and has seasonal sinus headaches and periods of tension headaches.

Tom travels a lot during the tour season, sleeping in different beds. This interferes with restorative sleep. Most of his complaints are related to being stiff, restless, and unable to relax. He relies on massage for tissue pliability and normal muscle resting length because he is not consistently compliant with a flexibility program even though he is consistent with aerobic and strength training. Tom sees a chiropractor regularly. He prefers massage 2 times a week when in town with outcome goals concentrating on the restorative properties of the general protocol. Each session he identifies a different focus area. Sometimes the focus is his left shoulder or mild low back pain. Often his hamstrings, calves, and feet are the focus.

Tom is ritualistic, as are many elite athletes, and wants everything as sequential and familiar as possible when he gets ready to play. He is also accommodating and understands his demands on the massage therapist. He only travels with the massage therapist if he is especially tired or has some nagging, achy areas that are interfering with his golf performance. Otherwise, when on the road, he will get a massage from a massage practitioner in the area, based on other local golfers' recommendations. He has been hurt once by a massage that was aggressive and too deep, and he was sore the day of that tournament. Most of the time, if the massage is ineffective, he complains that the massage does not really make him feel looser. When Tom is at home, his massage therapist goes to his residence for the massage sessions. He usually watches the golf channel on ESPN on television during the massage. Occasionally he will fall asleep.

Questions that need to be answered are the following:

1. What biomechanics are involved in golf?
2. What are the various tournament locations and schedules?
3. When is Tom home and on the road?
4. What other endorsements and publicity obligations does Tom have?
5. Are there any cautions for working with the broken leg?
6. What does Tom's strength and conditioning program include?
7. Are there any recommendations from the chiropractor?

Current Assessment and History

Client is 3 weeks postinjury and is still in a cast. Surgery was not required. He complains of tension headache, low back pain, and is restless. He is not sleeping well. Client is home recovering. He is not taking any pain medication. Healing progress for the fibula is on schedule. Tom is obviously overbreathing and out of sorts. He seems to be experiencing increased sympathetic dominance in

response to reduced activity. He also is frustrated about missing tournaments, because he is losing opportunities for professional advancement and finances. Overall, he is miserable.

The following revised treatment plan and series of massage sessions will support the final healing of the fracture and beginning stages of rehabilitation before a return to competition.

Subjective Assessment. Client reports that he is not sleeping well and knows he is breathing with his upper chest and is irritable. He has a recurring headache that he thinks is a combination of sinus pressure and muscle tension. His shoulders, axilla area, and low back ache from using crutches, the walking cast, and lying around. The doctor is satisfied with the healing progress and expects the cast to come off next week. The physical therapy will begin immediately and last 8 to 12 weeks.

Objective Assessment. The objective assessment found the following:

- Upper chest and shoulder movement occurs during relaxed breathing.
- Client is restless and fidgeting. Left hip is elevated and anteriorly rotated.
- Gait is abnormal. Trunk, hip, knee, and shoulder firing patterns are synergistically dominant.
- Psoas and scalenes are short bilaterally; quadratus lumborum is short on the left.

Analysis of Assessment and History to Develop Treatment Goals

This client previously has responded to massage as described in the general protocol in this text. Assessment information is influenced by the fibula fracture and compensation and does not necessarily indicate his postrehabilitation status.

Until the cast is off and rehabilitation begins, it is ineffective to specifically address the gait dysfunction. Two weeks into rehabilitation likely would be an appropriate time to assess gait and firing patterns and to begin to provide specific intervention. Firing patterns that would influence shoulder function and breathing would be addressed, even if the results were temporary.

The main immediate goals are to address the breathing pattern and reduce the aching from adapting to the cast and reduced activity. Benefit in these areas should support better sleep, reduced irritability, and support productive healing.

Short-Term Goals. Manage discomfort from compensation caused by fracture as reported each session by client. Normalize breathing and support restorative sleep.

Long-Term Goals. Support rehabilitation and return to competition. Reverse fibrotic changes in left lower leg. Normalize all firing patterns and gait reflexes.

Manage preexisting golf-related compensation for areas of tissue shortening, low back pain, plantar fascia pliability, and tendency toward headache.

Manage and support final healing phase of fracture for 6 to 8 months.

Massage Frequency and Duration

Start with 3 times per week for 1½ hours in the client's home. Reduce frequency to 2 times per week when sleep improves and rehabilitation progresses.

The general protocol is the foundation of the massage with the addition of the strategies for breathing dysfunction, restorative sleep, bone fractures, headaches, and low back pain. Each session also will address specific goals the client identifies concerning his condition that day.

Session One

S–Client reports irritability, restlessness, headache (sinus and tension); low back, neck, and shoulder stiffness; and aching. He also indicates constipation and intestinal gas. He is doing some upper body activity with light weights but indicates that he does not know how to perform an intense cardiovascular workout with his leg casted. The doctor is not concerned with the cardiovascular deconditioning because it is minor and rehabilitation will begin soon.

O–Client is breathing with the upper chest. Neck and chest palpate as tense and restricted. Scalenes, anterior serratus, and quadratus lumborum are short. Left hip is elevated and anteriorly rotated. Edema is present in the left leg above the cast. Fullness in large intestine is palpable. Firing patterns and gait reflexes were not assessed.

Massage consists of general protocol with regional contraindication for the area of the fracture. The entire breathing protocol is integrated into the general massage session. The left leg receives lymphatic drainage. The foot not covered by the cast is addressed with rhythmic compression and active and passive range of motion.

Reflexively, the right forearm and wrist are massaged specifically to influence the area of the fracture.

Scalene, sternocleidomastoid, psoas, and quadratus lumborum releases are performed bilaterally.

The vascular and tension headache sequence is performed.

Energy work over the cast, combined with rhythmic passive range of motion of the left knee, targets the area of the fracture.

Abdominal massage addresses constipation.

A–Client reports that his headache is almost gone. He feels less stiff and achy. His left foot is itchy. (Note: Massage likely increased circulation).

Observation and palpation indicates 75% improvement in breathing function; edema is reduced in left leg by 50%. Client is sitting still and talking slowly. He is laughing and joking. The massage duration was 2½ hours. This is typically too long, but client seemed to respond well.

P–Continue with general massage focus and breathing function strategies. Reassess for edema. Check with client about sleep function and if there were any negative effects from the long massage.

Session Two

S–Client reports that he will get the cast off next week. He also indicates that after the last massage he slept better for two nights but was restless again last night. He has not had a headache and is not constipated, but his low back is aching. He was tired after the last massage, but in a pleasant way.

O–Upper chest breathing is evident through observation and palpation of shoulders. Firing patterns for the shoulder are displaying synergistic dominance. Edema is evident again in the left leg. Connective tissue bind is palpated in lumbar and pectoral fascia.

General massage protocol performed with sufficient pressure applied to support increased serotonin release. Lymphatic drainage on the left leg. Scalene, sternocleidomastoid, psoas, and quadratus lumborum releases are performed to address low back aching. Direct connective tissue methods, bend, tension, and torsion are used to increase pliability in fascia. Energy-based modality is used over cast between left lower leg and ankle and between right forearm and wrist. All breathing strategies are incorporated.

A–Breathing assesses as normal with inhale to exhale ratio of 1 : 3. Edema is reduced in left leg by 50%. Connective tissue pliability has improved. Client reports feeling good and less stiff. He is sleepy and plans to take a nap.

P—Continue with general protocol. Client will have cast off by next session. He will discuss specific recommendations for massage with the doctor.

Session Three

S—Client had cast removed this morning. He begins rehabilitation in 2 days. The doctor instructed him to move his ankle in pain-free circles. The doctor also requests that massage avoid the area and not perform lymphatic drainage there until after physical therapist evaluates, and then to follow the physical therapist's directions.

O—Moderate lower left leg muscle atrophy is observable. Client is using one crutch as needed. He appears apprehensive about weight bearing on his left leg even though he has been in a walking cast for 3 weeks.

Left hip remains elevated and anteriorly rotated but not as pronounced. Breathing is generally good for this client. He is sleeping better and is less restless.

General massage protocol: Avoid the left leg; no specific focus, and target general support of parasympathetic dominance.

A—Client is preoccupied with what is expected at rehabilitation, how long before he can begin to play golf, and his leg muscle atrophy. He talked a lot during the massage and did not seem to relax, even though he reports feeling looser.

P—Have client get specific massage instructions from the physical therapist and a copy of the rehabilitation plan, including types of exercises and modalities.

Session Four

S—Client reports that he has begun physical therapy, including cardiovascular work with the stationary bike. The physical therapist indicates only lymphatic drainage and circulation-focused massage should be done below the left knee. No other recommendations are given. Client forgot to get rehabilitation plan but indicates they did passive and active range of motion and he was given homework of drawing the alphabet with his toes.

O—Ankle mobility on the left is decreased. Edema is observable. Breathing function is normal for this client. Thigh muscles are bilaterally tense: they are co-contracting. Sacroiliac joint movement on the left is restricted, and the lumbar fascia and pectoral fascia are binding.

General massage is done with a focus on breathing and increased connective tissue pliability; do not address thigh muscle tension specifically, which seems to be guarding response. Will monitor. Incorporate passive mobilization for sacroiliac joint.

Full sequence of lymphatic drainage and venous and arterial circulation is performed, but did not passively move left ankle. Ask client to move ankle during lymphatic drainage.

Specifically address right forearm and wrist to affect left leg and ankle reflexively.

A—Client wants me to work more on left leg, but we discuss importance of following physical therapist's instructions. Fluid movement improved in left leg. Sacroiliac joint restriction improved 50%. Will continue to monitor. Suggest client point out SI joint restriction to physical therapist. Client reports that his legs still feel tight. Explain that this may be appropriate compensation and it would be assessed again next massage.

P—Continue general massage. Reassess sacroiliac joint. Reduce massage to 2 times per week.

Session Five

S—Client is sore from rehabilitation, especially cardiovascular workout and weight training. Client is beginning proprioceptive training. Physical therapist okays massage in fractured area as long as it does not result in pain or inflammation, with caution given against heavy pressure over fractured area. Client has a tension headache but is sleeping well. He reports that he is anxious to get back to golf. Because the fracture occurred during a nonrelated activity (skiing), the doctor feels that he should be able to begin golf-related activity as long as there is no pain during or after activity in the area of the fracture. Physical therapist manipulated sacroiliac joint.

O—Range of motion in left ankle is 90% normal. Atrophy there is beginning to reverse. Tension in both thighs is reduced. Breathing is mildly disrupted. Left calf tissue pliability is reduced. Gait reflexes assessment indicates that opposite side function is normal, but unilateral assessment indicates that arm and leg flexors do not inhibit in response to activation of corresponding flexion pattern. Also adductors do not inhibit when abduction is activated. Trunk firing is normal, but hip extension, hip abduction, and knee flexion are synergistically dominant. Knee extension and sacroiliac joint movement are normal.

General massage protocol used: Address all firing patterns and gait reflexes. Begin kneading (torsion force) of left calf to increase tissue pliability. Include breathing protocol and tension headache strategies. Apply lymphatic drainage to all areas of delayed-onset muscle soreness.

A–Client feels more stable on his feet, especially on the left. Left calf is itchy and prickly (histamine response).

P–Continue general massage. Reassess firing patterns and gait reflexes. Monitor sacroiliac joint function and breathing. Begin to introduce golf-specific focus as client begins to practice.

Session Six

S–Client is doing well in rehabilitation. Physical therapist again adjusted left sacroiliac joint. Client went to driving range and hit a bucket of balls yesterday. Body and neck are tight, forearms are stiff, and low back is achy. Client indicates that it feels good to ache like he has played golf. No pain occurs in left ankle.

O–Client has a left anteriorly rotated pelvis consistent with golf activity. Firing patterns and gait reflexes returned to same dysfunction as last massage. Eye/neck reflexes do not inhibit as they should in flexion/extension pattern. Wrist flexors and extensors are short; psoas and quadratus lumborum pressure reproduces achy low back symptoms.

General massage is performed, including correcting firing patterns, gait reflexes, and eye/neck reflexes. Muscle energy (contract relax, antagonist contract) used on forearms, and compression used with active movement of forearms.

Scalenes, quadratus lumborum, and sternocleidomastoid/psoas were released. Kneading (torsion force) applied to calves bilaterally. Addressed breathing.

Used indirect function technique to reduce anterior pelvic rotation.

A–Client reports that he feels great. He is cautioned to not overdo it.

P–Reassess all gait and firing patterns; perform general massage.

Session Seven

S–Client overdoes it. He is sore and there is mild edema in left ankle. Physical therapy is reduced to every 3 days. Physical therapist discussed the importance of moderation during activity. Client is achy, stiff, and sore. He is irritable, but breathing is normal for this client.

O–Client appears frustrated and stiff all over. His adaptive capacity does not appear sufficient for beneficial response to focused massage. General massage protocol is used instead, with focus on relaxation and lymphatic drainage.

A–Client fell asleep during massage. I left him sleeping on the massage table and told his wife to make sure he stays hydrated.

P–Monitor for adaptive strain and then determine massage focus.

Session Eight

S–Client is 10 weeks postinjury and is doing well. Doctor and physical therapist are pleased with his progress despite the setback from overexerting last week. No more cautions are in effect for the fracture area. Client has a sinus headache.

O–Client's firing patterns continue to show synergistic dominance but correct easily. Gait reflexes are normal. Eye reflexes do not inhibit in flexion when eyes are rolled back. Client displays familiar golf pattern: low back pain, pelvic rotation, and high shoulder on the left, with inhibited scapula retraction with attachment tender points, short pectoralis minor and anterior serratus. Client also displays co-contraction of wrist flexion and extension, short calves, inhibited gluteus maximus, dominant hamstrings during hip extension, and binding plantar fascia.

General massage protocol targets each area as needed.

A–Client says he is beginning to feel like himself. He plans to play a round of golf before the next massage. Client is beginning to resume adaptive patterns consistent to his golf style and compensation in response to the fibula fracture is only mildly evident.

P–Return to general maintenance massage with monitoring of tissue pliability in left calf and ankle range of motion.

Session Nine

S–Client reports that he played golf and was rusty, but no lingering effects are apparent from the time off. He is frustrated, did not sleep well, and was restless in his sleep. He is going to play 18 holes in a charity golf tournament in 2 weeks and hopes he does not embarrass himself.

O–Firing patterns are normal except for the knee flexors. Common pattern of muscle imbalances related to golf persists, as described in previous session. Upper chest breathing is evident.

General maintenance massage will be done with connective tissue focus to calves, addressing knee flexion firing patterns.

A–Client is restless and talkative during the massage. He does not relax, but this is not uncommon for him. Firing pattern for knee flexion is corrected easily. Breathing improves.

P–Client requests three massage sessions this week because he needs to get ready for the tournament.

Session Ten

S–Client reports golf game is improving. He is fatigued.

O–Firing patterns are normal except for the knee flexors. Common pattern of muscle imbalances related to golf is found. Upper chest breathing is evident.

General maintenance massage was performed with connective tissue focus on the calves, addressing knee flexion firing patterns.

A–Client falls asleep and is left on table. Wife will monitor.

P–Continue with pre-event preparation massage focus. Continue general massage application and methods to reduce anxiety.

The Rest of the Story

This client occasionally will experience aching in his left ankle if he is on his feet a lot, especially if the golf course is hilly. He continues to play in the PGA, has yet to win a major tournament, but is doing generally well. He still gets headaches, over-breathes, gets constipated, has forearm tension, low back ache, and golf-related musculoskeletal imbalances. He is a typical professional golfer. He maintains a solid conditioning program and still does not stretch like he should. He has a new baby; therefore, he now has an excuse for not sleeping. This client will want massage regularly his entire career and beyond.

CASE THREE

DARREL—BASEBALL

Darrell is a 23-year-old minor league baseball pitcher. He played Little League, high school, and college baseball. He is intent on moving up to the majors. The only major physical problem is recurring bursitis in his right shoulder. This is problematic because it is in his pitching arm. The trainer has used ice and various other treatments, and the pain is reduced, although the pain returns if he plays consecutive games. Darrell had one cortisone injection 12 months ago that was helpful, but additional injections are not advised. He is taking valdecoxib (Bextra). Darrel also has modified his pitching style somewhat so that his shoulder is not bothering him as much. Lately, he has noticed an increased tension in his forearm. Massage has not been used specifically to address the underlying factors causing the bursitis. The goals for massage intervention will be targeted on reducing the irritation causing the bursitis and general athletic performance support. Darrell received therapeutic massage occasionally when on vacation. Darrell will come to the office for the massage sessions.

Questions that need to be answered are the following:

1. What is causing the bursitis?
2. Why are there increased feelings of tension in Darrell's forearm?
3. What is the proper form for pitchers to prevent injury?
4. What effects is valdecoxib (Bextra) having?
5. What is Darrell's training and playing schedule?
6. What has the trainer been doing, and why have the results been mixed?

History and Assessment

History: No major childhood illnesses. No current illness. Family history of cardiovascular disease.

Injuries: Car accident when 12 years old with a broken left wrist that successfully healed. Various contusions from playing baseball since 8 years old. Right ankle deltoid ligament second-degree sprain at 14 years old. Ankle healed but aches occasionally.

Current: No injury. Bursitis in right shoulder. Being treated with ice and antiinflammatory drugs. Restless sleep. Excessive caffeine consumption.

Medications/Supplements

Valdecoxib (Bextra)

Megadose multivitamin, protein sports shake, and extra antioxidants.

Physical Assessment

Posture: Mild rotation of shoulder girdle to the right, pelvic girdle to the left, which is common training and performance adaptation for right-handed pitcher. Externally rotated right leg and mild forward head position.

Gait assessment: Arm swing is limited on the left. Left hip flexors do not inhibit when assessed against right shoulder extensors.

Range of motion: Right arm internal rotation limited by 20%. Flexion and abduction are normal but painful at end range. Right ankle is hypermobile. Sacroiliac joint is restricted on the left, with medial hip rotation limited with hard end feel.

Muscle testing: Right arm abductors are painful to resistance testing but do not test weak. Hip flexors are weak at maximal pressure bilaterally.

Firing patterns: Hamstring dominance is bilateral, and calf is dominant for knee flexion on the right. Trunk firing is rectus abdominis dominant. Shoulder firing on the right is upper trapezius dominant. Hip abductors on the left show quadratus lumborum dominance.

Palpation: Right shoulder is warm with reddening and increased sweating during drag palpation. Left and right forearms are taut and binding with increased tension in flexion groups. Pain, point tenderness, and heat are displayed at medial epicondyle on the right. Pain and point tenderness exist on the medial head of the right gastrocnemius. Calf muscles are adhered on the right. Upper chest breathing pattern exists. Fascial bind starts from occiput down spine to lumbodorsal fascia to right hip and iliotibial band. Mild edema is felt at bursae in right shoulder.

Analysis of History and Assessment

Darrel is highly focused on moving to the major leagues. He loves baseball and seems to overpractice. He has excessive caffeine intake, primarily coffee and soda, which may be contributing to the restless sleep and to the upper chest breathing. Darrell exhibits sympathetic dominance by being fidgety and talking loudly, with a description of a typical day as follows: up early, treatment by the

trainer for the bursitis and the strength and conditioning. Often there is team practice and then more treatment by the trainer. Preseason begins in 4 weeks, with season consisting of around 120 games. Darrel wants to be ready for the season to show off his skills and to be called up to the majors by midseason if luck goes his way. He is healing but is beginning to show signs of reduced recovery.

Darrell's overtraining coupled with the playing schedule is a concern: whether he is recovering well enough not to become injury prone and excessively fatigued, which will affect performance. He does not have major adaptation issues at this time, and the various changes in posture, range of motion, and tissue texture seem appropriate with the sport activity. The exception to this is the point tenderness at the medial epicondyle on his throwing arm and the sacroiliac joint restriction. The sacroiliac joint restriction may indicate excessive rotation at the pelvis. The firing patterns in general indicate a tendency to synergistic dominance, and the trunk firing pattern indicates a weak core muscle function. The upper chest breathing pattern is a concern and could be contributing to the shoulder problems and the recovery issue. Stress and emotional issues are a likely cause. Massage can address the general sympathetic dominance, the firing patterns, and connective tissue bind. Massage cannot address the bursitis specifically but can reduce rubbing, which is causing the problem.

Massage would need to be combined with appropriate therapeutic exercise and flexibility program to be most effective.

Darrel is highly motivated, and the trainer is supporting massage if a treatment plan is provided for approval, because the massage therapist is not employed directly by the team.

Treatment Plan

Short-term goals: Reduce sympathetic arousal. Normalize firing patterns.

Long-term goals: Support recovery. Normalize connective tissue bind. Maintain normal firing patterns. Increase range of motion of the shoulders by 50%. Reduce pain in shoulder by 50%. Support therapeutic exercise and flexibility.

Methods used: Therapeutic massage, muscle energy methods, trigger point methods, connective tissue approaches, and lymphatic drainage

Frequency and duration: 2 times per week, 1½ hours for 6 weeks, then once per week as available during season.

Progress measurement: Firing patterns, gait assessment, range of motion, pain scale, breathing assessment, and feedback from client's trainer.

Session One

S–Client reports no change in bursitis pain since assessment. Forearms remain tight. Sleep patterns are the same as previously. Trainer does not want direct work on bursitis area. Client was hit with baseball on right hip.

O–No changes in assessment since intake session. Client has bruise on right hip. General massage protocol, including specific breathing pattern sequence. Normalize firing patterns. Perform lymphatic drainage over bruise.

A–Breathing pattern is improved as indicated by reduced movement of auxiliary breathing muscles during inhale. Range of motion of right arm has not changed. Bruised area on right hip is less swollen and painful. Firing pattern for right shoulder is normal, but other patterns did not change.

P–Continue with full-body general massage. Reassess breathing and continue to address firing patterns. Add gait reflexes to assessment and treatment.

Session Two

S–Client reports improved sleep for one night. Bruise feels better, and calves are tender to the touch 1 day after massage, but feel loose. No change in bursitis. Forearms feel relaxed for 1 day.

O–Upper chest breathing is improved slightly. Firing patterns remain synergistically dominant. Gait assessment continues to show right shoulder extension not signaling inhibition to left hip flexors. General full-body protocol performed. Specific attention given to calf/forearm patterns with connective tissue focus. Shear of right gastrocnemius off soleus done. Addressed firing patterns and gait patterns.

A–Forearms and calves are more pliable but may be sore to the touch for 24 to 48 hours. Trigger point activity is still present in gastrocnemius. Gait patterns are normalized. Shoulder, hip abduction, and left calf firing patterns are improved. Other patterns would not reset. Client appears to be sleepy and reports that he is sleepy.

P–Continue with general massage, targeting firing patterns, connective tissue pliability, and breathing dysfunction.

Session Three

S–Client reports that calves were sore to the touch and during movement. Left forearm is better. Low back is aching around the left lumbar area. Sleep is improving. Trainer is concerned about calves being sore during movement. Asks that massage intensity be reduced.

O–Upper chest breathing is improved, and auxiliary muscles are not active during relaxed breathing. Firing pattern for shoulder normal, but hip abduction and extension remain in synergistic dominance. Quadratus lumborum active on the left; point tenderness present at left sacroiliac joint. Calves pliable but mildly swollen. Right gastrocnemius beginning to move independently of soleus. Trigger point in gastrocnemius less tender. Forward head improved slightly. Right shoulder less tender to the touch, but right forearm muscle is tense with point tenderness at medial epicondyle. General massage protocol: Quadratus lumborum and psoas release done bilaterally, and scalenes and sternocleidomastoid addressed. Inhibitory pressure used on trigger point in multifidus near left sacroiliac joint, and lymphatic drainage performed over shoulder and calves. All firing patterns and quadratus lumborum and psoas addressed. Also rectus abdominis is inhibited, and then trunk firing patterns reinforced.

A–Psoas, quadratus lumborum, and rectus abdominis inhibition seems to allow firing patterns to respond to treatment. All but the right calf is normalized. Reassessed gait patterns, and they were normal. Forward head position is improved. Right forearm remains tight and painful. Range of motion of right shoulder increased by 10% before becoming painful. Left sacroiliac joint remains painful to touch, but lumbar aching is improved.

P–Next session: Address short muscles in right shoulder. Continue with general massage and firing patterns. Resume connective tissue work. Suggest that client begin scapular retraction exercises and core training. Referred client to trainer for strength exercise program. Also asked client to have trainer evaluate right forearm and elbow tendonitis.

Session Four

S–Client reports that team chiropractor adjusted low back and sacroiliac joint and that they feel better. Trainer increased rotator cuff strengthening exercises and added scapula protraction sequence. Client indicated mild delayed-onset muscle soreness in the area. Calves are no longer sore. Sleep was restless, but client thinks it was from upper body aching caused by the increased exercise. Trainer did not increase core strengthening but intends to add exercises next week. Trainer thinks client is throwing too many pitches during practice and this is making his arm sore. He has been icing shoulder when it is sore.

O—Forward head position has returned to original assessment position. Shoulder remains rotated right, but pelvis has improved slightly since the chiropractic treatment. All firing patterns again are synergistically dominant. Gait pattern normal. Right forearm and medial epicondyle remain tight and sore to the touch. Bilateral muscle testing of wrist flexors and extensors indicates right side is overly strong, both being hyperresponsive to resistance pressure and painful at medial elbow. General massage with scalene/quadratus lumborum and psoas/sternocleidomastoid releases bilaterally. Deep lateral hip rotators and shoulder external rotators released (inhibited) and gently lengthened bilaterally. Pectoralis minor inhibited and lengthened bilaterally. Addressed all firing patterns. Connective tissue work done on lumbodorsal and anterior thorax fascia. Lymphatic drainage performed on areas of delayed-onset muscle soreness.

A —Right shoulder strength and pain are improved according to shoulder abduction assessment. Firing patterns have normalized. Forward head posture is reduced by 90%. Shoulder rotation and pelvic rotation have improved, with shoulder rotation 10% from normal and pelvis asymmetry only slightly dysfunctional, but inflare on the right is identified in postmassage assessment. Wrist flexion on the right painful at normal resistance, but no longer hypersensitive. Point tenderness at medial epicondyle remains. Hip flexor strength is improved.

P—Continue with full-body massage with specific focus for normalizing and stabilizing firing patterns and connective tissue bind. Concern is expressed about forearm pain, and client is referred to trainer for reevaluation.

Session Five

S—Client reports upper pectoralis area and abdomen are sore to the touch but not to move-

ment. Right shoulder does not hurt to sleep on it. Sleep is again better and not as restless. Delayed-onset muscle soreness is better. Client reports that he is a little stiff around his shoulder until he warms up. Client continues to receive chiropractic adjustment for lumbar and sacroiliac joints.

O—Firing patterns for hip abduction and shoulder are normal. Hip extension and trunk firing patterns remain synergistically dominant. Hip flexors and shoulder abductors are strong and nonpainful at normal resistance. Right shoulder cannot sustain pressure as long as left. Gastrocnemius adherence and trigger point activity are decreased by 75%. Shoulder rotation has regressed to previous position, but pelvis remains stable. Performed general massage with inhibiting pressure to release scalenes, psoas, sternocleidomastoid, rectus abdominis, infraspinatus, teres minor, triceps, pectoralis minor, and deep lateral hip rotators. Performed passive range of motion of acromioclavicular and sternoclavicular joints bilaterally. Also inhibited hamstrings and biceps while resetting firing patterns. Used positional release on the tender points in the right forearm. Also used positional release on anterior serratus to improve ability to retract scapula. Specifically addressed fascial pliability in anterior and posterior thorax into iliotibial bands bilaterally primarily with kneading (bend and torsion force). Addressed shoulder and elbow through reflexology points on the foot and hand. Applied compression along meridians in arms and legs. Used indirect functional technique on shoulder rotation and right pelvic inflare.

A—Positional release effective for anterior serratus and forearm tender points except at right elbow medial epicondyle. Firing patterns are all normalized. Shoulder rotation improved again to within 10% of normal. Inflare improved slightly. Connective tissue bind decreased in thorax but remains in lumbodorsal fascia.

P—Continue with current plan. Again refer client to trainer for right elbow pain. Also encourage chiropractic appointments, core strength training, and rotator cuff and scapular retraction strength exercises.

Session Six

S—Client reports that he was restless for the last two nights and did not sleep well. He also feels like he is getting a cold. Preseason begins next week.

Trainer continues to ice right shoulder and arm and is stretching shoulder, elbow, and wrist muscles. Core training began 2 days ago, and client is sore. He reports that he is in a bad mood.

O–Client again displaying an upper chest breathing pattern. Rib cage less mobile than typical for this client. Firing patterns are stable, but gait reflexes are not holding strong in the shoulder flexion/hip flexion diagonal pattern. Client not as cooperative as usual. General massage given to address lymphatic drainage, pain management, mood elevation, and parasympathetic dominance pattern, but no specific work targeted due to cold.

A–Client falls asleep during massage and is groggy when he wakes up. Gave him some hot tea to drink. Also gave him eucalyptus and lavender essential oil to take home to inhale and rub on his chest. Did not perform postassessment.

P–Reevaluate: This was last session of 2 times per week schedule. Need to adjust treatment plan for once per week and to accommodate beginning of season.

Session Seven

S–Client has a cold, but it is not in his chest, just in his head. He indicates that he has a minor sore throat and sinus headache but feels better than last session. He would like more of the essential oil to take home. His shoulder is better as long as he continues to ice it. The trainer told him that he was pleased with the progress. The right forearm remains sore and tight. He is stiff and slightly sore from the core and rotator cuff and scapular retraction strengthening exercises, but it is better than it was. Client says he is not sleeping well. He believes it is a combination of the cold and muscle aching and that he is anxious and excited about the season starting. He is frustrated that he does not feel like practicing hard because of the head cold and headache.

O–Assessment indicates posture is forward head and shoulder/pelvis rotation stable. Firing patterns are slightly synergistically dominant. Client appears sluggish. Session includes full-body massage with lymphatic drainage focus and headache sequence for sinuses, release psoas and sternocleidomastoid, and address diaphragm. Performed inhibition by compression on hamstring and biceps; deep lateral hip rotators and lateral shoulder rotators; and deep compression on serratus postior inferior bilaterally (tender from sniffing). Mobilized facet joints with rhyth-

mic compression and decompression of ribs. Massaged sinus, neck, and head reflex points on feet. Applied rhythmic compression to L1 and L4 acupressure points in hand. Continued to focus on parasympathetic dominance and restorative sleep.

A–Client reports headache is better. Firing patterns have improved. Client wants to take a nap.

Did not do revision of treatment plan this session. Client is fatigued and wants to relax during massage.

P–Do reassessment and treatment plan revision next session.

Session Eight

S–Client reports that cold is better, but he still has a headache. He is going to be pitching in 2 days and asks for increased focus on his right arm. It has been sore but now is better.

O–Reassessment:

Forward head position is nearly normal.

Shoulder girdle right rotation is mild, and pelvic girdle left rotation is slight. Right leg external rotation has reduced to slight.

Arm swing still reduced on the left, but gait patterns are normal.

Internal shoulder rotation is limited by only 10%, which is acceptable. No pain occurs at end range of shoulder movement, but pain remains upon slight overpressure in the right shoulder.

Muscle strength testing is normal. Firing patterns continue to assess synergistically dominant but will correct easily, especially when obliques and transverse abdominis fire. Core training should continue to improve this situation.

Right shoulder at the area of bursitis is less point tender but continues to redden during drag palpation and remains slightly swollen.

Right forearm seems worse during persistent wrist flexion/extension, and there is point tenderness at medial epicondyle.

Gastrocnemius trigger points have resolved, but mild fascial adherence remains in fascial planes. Fascial planes are more pliable but still bind. Upper chest breathing pattern is intermittent.

Overall Impression

The client has improved slightly to moderately in all target areas. The posture has improved, and antagonist/agonist patterns have balanced around the shoulder. The irritation on the bursae is reduced, and the inflammation is improving and responding to the ice and antiinflammatory medication. The reduction of shortening in the flexion and rotational patterns is allowing the therapeutic exercise to be increasingly effective. The client has been fairly compliant but does display some symptoms of overtraining. Because the massage application thus far has been moderately successful for the original treatment plan goals, it would be prudent to continue and add specific treatment to the pitching arm to attempt to reduce muscle tension and pain. A concern is that the arm is this dysfunctional and the season is just starting. The shoulder is improving, but the symptoms at the elbow are not improving. Although symptoms are not yet getting worse, the strain of competitive play may override current adaptive capacity. It would be best to speak with the trainer to coordinate a treatment plan to support performance during the oncoming session.

Results of conference with trainer: Client does have some form issues with his pitching style that increased when he accommodated to the bursitis pain. The coaches are working now to adjust the pitching form. The bursitis is improving, and Darrel is encouraged Note: Not included in the chart was the discussion with the minor league coach that indicates Darrel will be called up within the next month. This information influenced the treatment plan in that the time frame is more urgent.

The trainer suggests that the massage continue as before and also to keep the flexor muscles in the right forearm loose. We agreed that friction at the medial epicondyle was not appropriate at this time.

Session Nine

S—Client reports that he is feeling good. His shoulder only hurts a little after practice, and ice takes care of it. His forearms are tight, but he can deal with that. He continues to see the chiropractor once a week. He will be pitching in 2 days. He is sleeping well.

O—Assessment indicates that firing patterns are stable. Hip extension is a bit hamstring dominant, and rectus abdominis wants to fire during initial trunk flexion but inhibits easily and firing patterns normalize. Right elbow extension painful during the last 20 degrees of extension, and forearm remains tense and binding. Point pain at epicondyle improved slightly.

General massage protocol given with reflex application at left hamstring to reduce pain in right elbow extension. Also biceps and triceps are inhibited. Worked on reflexology points in the foot for the shoulder and elbow.

A—All firing patterns and gait reflexes normal, with breathing slightly from upper chest. Client excited about season starting. Client reports that forearms feel looser and elbow is less painful. He does report that full elbow extension feels stiff at end range.

P—Continue with current massage plan.

Session Ten

S—Client reports that he pitched well. Shoulder was only slightly sore the next day. His low back hurts deep, especially when he sits for awhile and then stands up. His legs feel heavy but not sore. His elbow hurts when extended, but he can deal with it. He will miss the appointment next week because of road trip.

O—Trunk flexion and hip extension firing patterns synergistically dominant, and gluteus maximus inhibited. Slight increase in shoulder/pelvic rotation pattern evident. Right forearm and shoulder slightly swollen.

General massage protocol performed with restorative/recovery focus: apply indirect functional technique for shoulder and pelvic rotation; inhibit rectus abdominis, psoas, hamstring, and sternocleidomastoid; reset firing patterns; performed lymphatic drainage on right arm; provided positional release for tender point in forearm; and perform cross-directional tissue stretching of forearms and calves.

A—Firing patterns normalized, and low back pain resolved. Client slept for half of massage. Muscle stiffness in right arm better, but guarding and flinching remain at medial epicondyle tender points.

P—Next massage is in 10 to 14 days. Client will call. Continue with massage as in previous session. Gave client eucalyptus and peppermint essential oil combination for his arm. Also taught him how to use a roller to massage out his forearm and how to do positional release.

Note: Client called and is despondent. He pitched four games and blew out his elbow. He is on his way for surgery and will get ahold of me later.

The Rest of the Story

Darrel became dehydrated from excessive sweating. Potassium/sodium imbalance must have occurred, and his muscles cramped. The muscle pulled away from the medial epicondyle, and he tore his medial collateral ligament. The injury will be corrected with what is called Tommy Johns surgery. The muscles are reattached, and the palmaris longus tendon is used to reconstruct the medial collateral ligament. There will be a year of rehabilitation before the arm is healed completely.

The treatment plan will need to be revised to include postsurgical healing–acute/subacute/and remodeling stages–along with the rehabilitation process. In addition, Darrel is depressed and angry but is determined to play again.

Massage will begin again about 1 week after surgery and continue 1 to 2 times per week throughout the rehabilitation process. The massage approach will be similar to the previous 10 sessions, and as soon as the doctor and trainer approve, scar tissue management will be incorporated.

The emotional state of the client is important to support healing. Energy-based modalities seem to support tissue regeneration and emotional well-being. The intentional and focused touch during massage needs to support well-being as well. Tissue regeneration and mood-elevating essential oils, homeopathy (particularly arnica), and magnets to support the healing process may be used. It would be wise for Darrel to see a sport psychologist during the rehabilitation.

Finances are going to be a concern. Minor league players do not make a lot of money. The team will cover the surgery and rehabilitation cost and pay Darrel's contract, but the massage and psychologist are not paid, and Darrel will have to find resources to cover these costs. Working with an athlete through an extended rehabilitation process is tasking and requires commitment. Boundary issues need to be monitored and once the healing has taken place, the injury mentality of the client and massage therapist must return to supporting performance. Many athletes will not return to preinjury performance and will have to come to grips with a career-ending event. Many traumatic injuries become chronic and require ongoing care.

For the reader: Although this is a hypothetical case, it is based on clients with whom I have worked. The person I modeled this case after did recover and played again in the minors. He was called up to the majors briefly, but did not perform well. He was traded and played awhile in the minors and then moved on with his life. Currently, he coaches high school baseball.

CASE FOUR

TANIA—SOCCER

Tania is a healthy 32-year-old woman and recreational soccer enthusiast. Her two children play in local youth soccer programs, and she plays year-round in an indoor and outdoor league. She plays on a competitive women's recreational travel league and a coed home league. She also coaches soccer and participates in youth soccer camp. Tania played high school and college soccer. When she was in high school and college, soccer was just beginning to become popular in the United States. She has avidly followed the progress of amateur and professional soccer.

Tania is financially secure from an inheritance that she invested wisely. She is an accountant working part time. She uses the physical and competitive nature of soccer as a social interaction and for physical fitness and stress management. Tania has received massage for many years and wishes to continue weekly massage on a long-term basis as part of her wellness lifestyle. She is a sequential and logical person and expects results from massage that she can identify in a tangible manner. Tania is well-educated about her sport. The anatomy, physiology, and approach of the massage must be presented to her in an analytic and scientific way. She has changed massage therapists often because they were not able to meet her expectations for pressure, focused outcomes, and symptom management for her active life. This is the third month (12 to 14 massage sessions) mark with her current massage therapist, and she is pleased with the results of the massage sessions so far. The treatment plan usually has followed the general protocol of this text with weekly focal areas indicated by Tania. Lately, she has had some pain around her pelvic bone. The pain is more of a nuisance than constant pain. She has had osteitis pubis (pubalgia) before. She is a demanding but loyal client who has a weekly standing appointment at the office.

Questions that need to be answered are the following:
1. What are the physical demands of soccer?
2. What is osteitis pubis (pubalgia)?
3. What are the concrete explanations of massage benefits?

Overview of Client's Current Condition

Client has had various traumatic injuries since childhood. Both ankles have been sprained, but never a grade three injury. She had osteitis pubis in college that was slow to respond to treatment because she would not rest long enough. It eventually cleared up. She had similar symptoms during the last month of her two pregnancies and for about a month afterward.

Her pelvis is rotated anteriorly on the right and rotated posteriorly on the left, with tendency for shearing at the symphysis pubis. Sacroiliac joints occasionally fixate, but chiropractic adjustment is effective treatment. Gait reflexes, firing patterns, and range of motion are generally normal. They become disrupted if she has become fatigued, and then she complains of heavy legs or an aching back. She consistently shows erector spinae dominance during right hip extension. Strength assessment is normal except for gluteus maximus on the right. She has adapted to overexercise by maintaining a consistent core stability and flexibility program.

She takes various nutritional supplements intelligently and in moderation. She is not vulnerable to sport fads and gimmicks. She does not take medication regularly; however, she occasionally will use ibuprofen (Motrin) or naproxen (Aleve) for headache or muscle aching.

Breathing function is good if she can play soccer consistently, but she will have upper chest breathing if forced to be relatively inactive. This rarely occurs, but when it does, she is irritable and usually gets a headache.

An area of point tenderness currently exists near the rectus abdominis inferior attachment on the right. It seems to have gotten more irritated after she attended a series of business meetings and wore shoes with a 2-inch heel. No regional or general contraindications are present.

Treatment Plan

Short-term goals: Address lower abdominal groin-type pain.

Long-term goals: Enhance sport performance and recovery. Reverse and stabilize pelvic rotation adaptation, and reduce firing pattern dysfunction.

Methods: General massage protocol with heavy broad-based pressure for serotonin and endorphin effect; indirect functional technique for pelvis; firing pattern correction.

Frequency and duration: Weekly standing appointment for $1\frac{1}{2}$ hours.

Progress measures: Client-reported pain scale and satisfaction.

Session One

S—Client reports that she has been functioning well. Sleep, breathing, and soccer performance are satisfactory. She is bothered by the tenderness in her symphysis area. She has been using ice but not taking any antiinflammatory medication. She requests her typical full-body session with attention to the sacroiliac joints and muscles attaching to the symphysis pubis.

O—Client displays typical pattern of pelvic anterior rotation on the right, posterior rotation on the left, slightly longer right leg, symphysis pubis shearing, and point tenderness. Left lumbar muscles are dominant for hip extension on the right, and gluteus maximus is weak. In addition, there are kinetic chain-related tender points in the left pectoralis major, pectoralis minor, and coracobrachialis. The muscles on the left posterior shoulder are long but asymptomatic. Full application of the general massage protocol included the following: inhibiting pressure on rectus abdominis attachments at ribs and pubis; bilateral psoas release, with bilateral stretching of sternocleidomastoid; and inhibition of left lower lumbar with broad-based compression in shortest area, combined with left hip extension (with knee flexed) active movement.

Used positional release on tender points in left anterior shoulder area and indirect functional technique and sacroiliac joint mobilization to address pelvis.

A—Client reports that massage was effective. Point tenderness remains at symphysis pubis, but movement is not painful. Client indicates that she thinks she will see the chiropractor. Firing patterns normalized, but pelvis resistant to mobilization. Indication of mild inflammation (heat and slight bogginess) present at muscle attachments at the right symphysis pubis. Only rectus abdominis actively tender to palpation, but right adductors took longer to lengthen than the left adductors.

P—Client to see chiropractor, and massage is set for next week.

Session Two

S—Client reports right sacroiliac joint was resistant to chiropractic adjustment and took three visits before it normalized. Leg length also normalized. She does not feel the pain at the symphysis pubis unless she exercises or plays soccer while fatigued. She indicates that her adductors feel tight. Client is 2 days into menstrual cycle.

O—Adductors assessed are mildly short on the left and moderately short on the right. Consistent pattern as described in previous session exists. Client has some generalized edema as typical during the menstrual cycle. Left shoulder tender points are present but not as prominent.

General protocol with lymphatic drainage included the following: correct firing patterns, mobilize pelvis, apply muscle energy (pulsed) to adductors with compression and lengthening, inhibit pressure on rectus abdominis attachments and adductor attachments on the right, and apply compression on left anterior shoulder muscles with connective tissue stretching (active release).

A—Client reports she is tired but feels okay. Massage application effectively addressed assessment findings.

P—Suggest chiropractic adjustment this week, and expect to use same massage protocol pattern next week.

Session Three

S—Client had one chiropractic adjustment. Chiropractor is concerned about pelvic instability and symphysis pubis shearing. He prescribed some sacroiliac joint–stabilizing exercises. The right sacroiliac joint is most unstable. Chiropractor suspects high heels destabilized the pelvic adaptive mechanism. Because the sacroiliac joint is stabilized in a force couple between the left latissimus dorsi and the right gluteus maximus and because both of these muscles assessed weak, strengthening should help restabilize pelvis.

O—Confirmed chiropractor assessment. Left latissimus inhibited by upper trapezius and pectoralis major and pectoralis minor and coracobrachialis on the left. Gluteus maximus on right inhibited by short rectus abdominis and psoas. More focused assessment in relationship to high heels indicates short gastrocnemius/soleus with some binding and reflexive shortening in the forearms. General massage protocol with: Firing patterns, belly trigger point inhibition to short muscles, connective tissue stretching, psoas release, sternocleidomastoid release, and stretching of superficial fascia of left lumbar area.

Activate right gluteus maximus and left latissimus together, using pulsed muscle techniques, and lengthen and stretch psoas and latissimus bilaterally.

Did not do indirect functional technique or sacroiliac joint mobilization because client is under active chiropractor care.

A—Client reports that she feels off balance but believes it to be adaptive and will report back next session how long the sensation lasted. She is not playing soccer today, so she does not have to be at high performance. Firing pattern for right hip extension response improved.

P—Massage next week. Pay closer attention to right sacroiliac joint force couple.

Session Four (3 Days Later)

Client calls and requests a second appointment. Chiropractor noticed improvement and asks for the previous massage to be replicated.

S—Client reports that she agrees with chiropractor and wants same massage sequence as 3 days ago.

O—Repeat session as requested.

A—Client reports that she feels like she typically does after a massage. She responded well to the session.

P—Massage as previously scheduled.

Session Five

S—Client reports some aching in the sacroiliac joint area bilaterally but reduced point tenderness at symphysis pubis. Chiropractor is pleased with progress and requests similar massage sequence. Client has a mild tension headache.

O—Connective tissue bind in scalp appears related to occipitofrontalis shortening. Temporalis and masseter trigger points are found bilaterally. Repeat same massage sequence format as last two sessions plus tension headache sequence.

A—Headache improved but is not gone: 75% reduction in pain. Right sacroiliac joint force couple much improved. Point tenderness at rectus abdominis remains.

P—Next scheduled massage.

Session Six

S—Client sprained left ankle 2 days ago during soccer game: grade one sprain with outward rotation. Otherwise, nothing new to report. Client continues to see chiropractor 2 times per week but says appointments will begin to be reduced over next 4 weeks.

O—Mild edema, point tenderness, and muscle guarding are present in left ankle. Right hip extension firing pattern normal. Point tenderness at rectus abdominis attachments bilaterally slightly increased. Massage protocol used same as last three sessions, plus acute treatment for ankle sprain and addressing of kinetic chain pattern in relationship to left ankle (right lateral thigh, left lateral hip, right lateral lumbar, left lateral thorax, right lateral clavicle, left lateral head).

A–Client fell asleep. This is a rare occurrence. No noticeable change in ankle pain.

P–Session next week. Discuss proprioceptive training for ankle stability.

Session Seven

S–Client reports she played on the sprained ankle and experienced only mild discomfort. She has been keeping it wrapped and consistently icing it. She indicates that her left medial calf is tight and left hip is stiff. She also has a mild upper respiratory infection and sore throat. When questioned about change in daily demands, she replied that the team she coaches is going to qualify for the playoffs, so there has been an increase in practices. When asked about her personal performance during games, she indicates she is a bit flat.

O–Left ankle bruised and mildly swollen. Kinetic chain compensation patterns include reflex shortening in the left gluteal area, right psoas, left latissimus, and right cervical area. Guarding remains in the left calf. Firing patterns are synergistically dominant. Client appears sluggish and displays overtraining symptoms. She is breathing with the upper chest. Massage followed general protocol with subacute treatment of left ankle, corrective firing patterns work, and breathing dysfunction strategies. Educated client about overtraining symptoms and proprioceptive exercises for her ankles (one foot standing sequence).

A–Client responded well to massage and realizes she is fatigued. This frustrates her. She indicates she will analyze her current workload, soccer playing, coaching schedule, and personal demands to see where she can reduce demand.

P–Massage next week.

Session Eight

S–Client is irritable, is cold and can't seem to get warm, has a headache. In response to question about lifestyle demands, she is abrupt and says she is working on it.

O–Upper chest breathing is evident. Sympathetic autonomic nervous system is dominant. Left ankle is healing but a bit slowly. Full-body massage given with serotonin/endorphin focus: nonspecific broad-based deep compression, breathing dysfunction strategies, and subacute treatment of left ankle sprain.

A–Client's conversation indicates she is overloaded, has done this before, does not know why, and is concerned because she is impatient with the kids she coaches. As massage progresses and client relaxes a bit, she becomes introspective and quiet. She asks if I know of a good psychologist who understands athletes. I also suggested a complete physical to rule out an underlying medical condition.

P–Make referral to three psychologists. Massage next week.

Note: Client called and cancelled standing appointment, indicating she was having some medical tests performed.

Session Nine

S–Client reports that she has a mild thyroid deficiency, and she has begun taking thyroid replacements. She is still cold and can't get warm. She also is seeing one of the psychologists for a short-term behavior modification program. She has not made any significant lifestyle changes but is considering not continuing with the traveling team and concentrating on the home league. She requests the same kind of massage as last session because after the last massage, she felt more focused and less scattered for a few days.

O–Client less irritable and more relaxed. She appears fatigued. Breathing is slightly dysfunctional, and ankle is healing. Repeat last session and move to remodeling phase for ankle sprain.

A–Client dozes on and off during the massage. Breathing is slowed. Ankle seems somewhat hypermobile.

P–Encourage proprioceptive training for ankles bilaterally. Massage next week.

Session Ten

S–Client reports she is feeling better. The thyroid medication is helping. Left ankle is still a bit sore, but client is sore nowhere else. She says she is sleeping better but is a bit emotional at times, which is unlike her. She has no specific request for massage. She did not mention being cold.

O–No obvious postural deviations. Left calf continues to guard a bit. Knee flexion firing pattern on the left is synergistic dominant.

Full-body massage protocol with heavy pressure parasympathetic focus, remodeling stage treatment of ankle sprain. Encourage proprioceptive training for ankles.

A—Client relatively calm. Ankle healing progress is more normal. Breathing normal.

P—Massage next week.

The Rest of the Story

This client did have to deal with some psychological issues around her intense focus on soccer. Although she continues to be a soccer lover, she did stop traveling with the recreational league and concentrated more on playing locally. She will occasionally overtrain but recognizes it and is somewhat more moderate in her activities. She undergoes a weekly maintenance- and performance-based massage because she appreciates the relaxation quality benefits and the performance benefits. The ankle hypermobility continues to be a problem, and the compensation patterns need to be managed each session. The team she coached did make it to the playoffs but did not win the championship.

She still coaches, and her kids enjoy playing soccer. She is observant of them becoming burned out and monitors their life to make sure there is an element of balance similar to that which she is learning herself.

CASE FIVE

JOE—FOOTBALL

Joe is a professional football starting middle linebacker

Note: Football is the primary sport in which I work. Physical and mental demands of this position are huge. I have worked with many linebackers, and among them I have seen the most injuries. The player, Joe, who is described in this case study, is a representative of a multitude of football players with whom I have worked. The composite player history is realistic even though it sounds exaggerated.

Joe is 28 years old and is in his sixth year of professional football. He has been with two NFL teams. He also played high school and college football. His history includes the following major sport injuries:

- Right anterior cruciate ligament tear, and surgical repair successful except for lingering aching behind the knee
- Grade three right shoulder separation that was not repaired surgically and remains somewhat lax, but rehabilitation exercises provide sufficient stability. The shoulder aches on occasion.
- Two severe episodes of turf toe
- High ankle sprain on the left

- Slight bulging disk at L4 that has an acute episode about once a year
- Loose body removed from the left knee
- Hyperextended left elbow with a stress fracture in the olecranon process. This injury healed successfully, but it reduced range of motion in the elbow that does not affect professional playing and bothers him just because it is different from the right elbow.

Currently, Joe has some traumatic arthritis developing in his left ankle. Because his permanent home is in a location different from the location of the team for which he plays, he only receives massage during the season. He gets a massage at least once a week and as the season progresses, the frequency increases up to every other day when possible. In this case, Joe is beginning training camp and the seasonal massage program.

Goals for the massage: Support recovery, manage chronic pain, and enhance performance. Massage on Tuesdays is at Joe's residence at 9 PM after the children have gone to bed (if all goes well). He has a 4-year-old daughter and a 2-year-old son, and his wife is expecting their third child in 6 months. They also have two dogs that are always in the massage area. The family stays with him during the football season in a small condo near the stadium. This is the third year working with Joe. Joe usually falls asleep during massage.

Questions that need to be answered are the following:

- What are the demands of Joe's football position?
- What are the stress demands of the family in relationship to the work stress, including celebrity status?
- What are the treatments used by the athletic trainer to manage the cumulative football traumas?
- What are the limits of performance and the cautions for massage from the bulging disk?
- What are the specific demands of training camp?

Current Analysis of Condition

The client has participated in the off-season conditioning program and two preseason minicamps. He has returned to begin training camp, and the family will follow in about 2 weeks. He has received a series of three massage sessions in preparation for training camp. Because of the camp schedule, he will be able to receive massage only periodically. When the season begins, the regular schedule will begin.

History Update from Last Year

No new events are in Joe's life other than expecting the new baby. He has been participating in a yoga stretching program on his own, and the strength and conditioning coach has increased the focus of functional core training.

Despite the cumulative injuries, Joe indicates that he feels better beginning this season than he did last season. He tried to get massage when he was home but was disappointed in the pressure levels. He felt beat up, poked, dug on, over-stretched, and over–trigger pointed, or the massage was too superficial. He has found the yoga program has helped with stamina and flexibility.

He has begun to take glucosamine and creatine.

Physical Assessment

Knee extension firing pattern is bilateral vastus lateralis dominant. Knee flexion on the right is gastrocnemius dominant. Hip extension is hamstring dominant but improved from last year. Guarding is present in erector spinae and multifidus around bulging disk, with sacroiliac joint bind on the left and slight anterior pelvic rotation bilaterally. Left elbow reduced range of motion remains constant with hard end-feel. Left ankle dorsiflexion is only 10%, and rotation has crepitus.

Joe has gained about 10 pounds. His tissues are a bit boggy (creatine water gain). Gait reflex assessment indicates that shoulder extensors do not inhibit hip flexors, and the shoulder and arm abduction does not inhibit hip/leg adduction. However, hip adduction responds correctly to head and eye moved into flexion (strong) and extension (inhibited).

Increased tissue density exists with some fibrosis identified in lumbar fascia, upper trapezius bilaterally, biceps, triceps, and forearms bilaterally. Joint capsule area of both knees is binding.

Breathing is normal for this client, with mild upper chest breathing tendencies.

Client is sleeping well for the most part. The kids get in bed with him in the middle of the night occasionally, and this disturbs his sleep.

Session One

S–Client leaves for training camp tomorrow and asks for a full-body session addressing everything. He also would like to take a nap and asks for the massage to be done on the mat where he is more comfortable. He requests extra time on ankles, feet, hamstrings, and gluteus.

O–Assessment is as previously described. Provided full-body protocol with generalized lymphatic drainage. Use pattern for sleeping client 2½-hour massage (client uses restroom once and goes right back to sleep).

A–Client reports that he feels great and ready to go. Discuss effects of creatine with him, and ask him to discuss with trainer. Remind him to take his arnica.

P–Will see him on his next day off. He will call.

Session Two (8 Days Later)

S–Client is sore everywhere: legs are heavy and skin feels fat; low back and left ankle are stiff; and hamstrings are tight bilaterally. Client requests mat, a nap, and work on feet and head.

O–No specific assessment done because client is fatigued. Palpation indicated edema in tissue, with delayed-onset muscle soreness. Therapist assumes all firing patterns and gait reflexes are off. Massage incorporates general support for normal function using general protocol, lymphatic drainage, and sleeping client strategies.

A–Client feels less stiff and achy and wants to go to bed.

P–Wait for call.

Session Three (10 Days Later)

S–Client is tired and irritable, tending to display electrolyte and dehydration cramps. He had a mild heat exhaustion episode 3 days ago. He just wants a good massage and does not want to talk or participate. He wants to go to sleep and wants massage on mat but does not want to lie on his side. Because his low back is achy, he wants bolstering under the abdomen. He does not want a sheet drape because he is hot, so the plan is to cover him up when he gets cold and let him sleep after massage.

O–General protocol focused on parasympathetic dominance; support serotonin, endorphin, and oxytocin release; pampering; and sleep, following suggestions for sleeping client. Incorporate energetic modalities and essential oil (lavender).

A–Client falls asleep almost immediately and is asleep when I leave.

P–Wait for call.

Session Four (10 Days Later, Day after First Preseason Game. Client Played First Half.)

S–Client has a thigh bruise and low back pain. He is happy with performance, and family arrived for the game. He wants good, all-over massage and only has 1½ hours.

O–General massage protocol to include psoas, quadratus lumborum, and sternocleidomastoid releases; correction of hip extension firing patterns; use of sacroiliac joint mobilization pattern; broad-based compression on legs and arms (knees and feet used to provide compression) with movement by the client; and lymphatic drainage performed on bruise. Massage performed on mat.

A–Client is in much better mood and is less fatigued. He responds well to massage.

P–Will call.

Session Five (12 Days Later. Camp Breaks Next Week.)

S–No new conditions. Client is fatigued and wants the all-over treatment on mat. Doctor put him on rofecoxib (Vioxx). Asks to be left asleep on the mat after massage.

O–Mild fibrotic development is occurring in thigh bruise area. Use kneading to increase pliability. Identified mild upper chest breathing patterns. Corrected lower body firing patterns: hip abduction/extension, knee flexion/extension, and shoulder. Did not assess gait reflexes. Palpate heat and mild edema in both knees, left elbow, and ankle. Client fell asleep.

A–For fibrotic tissue, increased pliability by 75% before becoming too hot to continue work. Edema improved by 50% around affected joints. Breathing is more normal.

P–Begin weekly sessions.

Session Six (Game One)

S–Client reports he is satisfied with performance. His back is stiff, and his feet and ankles hurt. He wants general massage with attention to low back and feet. He jammed third finger on left. He asks for some essential oil: eucalyptus and lavender. Client found his arnica after losing it for 2 weeks. Massage is done on the mat. Okay for family to watch a movie with him during the massage.

O–Hip extension firing pattern and trunk flexion are synergistically dominant. Psoas short, and there are trigger points in lumbar multifidus and gluteus medius bilaterally. Anterior pelvic rotation increased on right. General massage: Released psoas and stretch sternocleidomastoid. Increased pliability in lumbar fascia 50%. Used indirect functional technique and joint play on jammed finger. Perform indirect functional tech-

nique to correct pelvic rotation with symphysis pubis reset. Some adhesion exists between gastrocnemius and soleus in the left, so use shearing and torsion to release bind. Used kneading and stretching for plantar fascia, which is short and binding. Addressed tenderness around large toes with joint play.

A–Client feels fine. Range of motion increased in left ankle by 5%, but did not treat trigger points, which seem to be resourceful adaptation for sacroiliac joint function. Will monitor.

P–Requested client to have trainer assess sacroiliac joint function. Massage next week.

Session Seven (Game Two)

S–Client reports sacroiliac joint is fine and that he went to trainer, who sent him to team chiropractor for adjustment. He banged the shoulder that had the previous injury. The shoulder is sore and stiff, and he cannot raise his arm easily.

O–Acromioclavicular joint on the right is binding. When addressed with indirect functional technique, client reported a pop at sternoclavicular joint, and afterward area can move better. Trigger points remain in gluteus medius and lumbar multifidi: treated with inhibition pressure and local tissue stretching. General massage protocol given, and client fell asleep.

A–Left client sleeping on mat. Clavicle seems to be displaced, but return it to normal joint play with indirect technique. Will need to monitor response to trigger points because sleeping client gave no feedback.

P–Next week, assess for trigger points.

Session Eight (Game Three)

S–Nothing new: Client requests, "Patch me up so I can play again and again and again." Low back is improved.

O–Trigger point activity remains, but not as point tender. Lower body appears to move in labored manner when observing gait. Client is off balance during one-leg standing, more on the left: left hip adductors are short. Adduction firing pattern is not inhibiting when appropriate. Client has bruise on left hip. General massage: Performed lymphatic drainage over bruise. Corrected adduction firing pattern and use contract/release stretch on adductors.

A–Client is steadier on feet during one-leg standing.

P–Massage next week.

Session Nine

S–Client has a concussion from game last Sunday. He has a headache and sore and stiff neck and is fatigued. He will be evaluated pregame to see whether he can play. The doctor is holding him out of practices. Client requests a calming massage, something for the headache. He asks for essential oils, so used peppermint and lavender and provided rescue remedy. He reports that he has been taking arnica.

O–Client is holding head rigid, and upper body is stiff during walking. His eyes seem to track well, but his movements are slow and deliberate. Ability to balance on one foot is diminished, and he can maintain it only for 3 to 5 seconds.

General massage: focused on parasympathetic dominance; avoided oscillation and instead used tension headache strategies but with reduced pressure and duration; incorporated energy-based modalities.

A–Client indicates headache a bit better, but neck remains stiff. His balance seems better.
P–Massage next week.

Session Ten (Client Calls for a Massage Early on Thursday.)

S–The only concussion symptom that remains is a headache, and the doctor thinks it may be from muscle tension in client's neck and requests that client get a massage before evaluation on Friday. Target is upper body stiffness, but with caution about abrupt movements of the neck and head.

O–Client is a bit irritable and more sensitive. (He yells at his children, which he seldom does). Upper body remains rigid, and movement is cautious. General massage incorporated positional release for upper body stiffness as requested. Used tension headache strategies and had client apply gentle pressure to eyeballs (with his eyes closed) while rolling eyes in slow clockwise and counterclockwise circles to balance eye muscles. Assessment identified upper chest breathing pattern. Use breathing dysfunction strategies.

A–Client is able to stand on one foot for 25 seconds on left and 40 seconds on right. Reassess for abduction firing pattern on left. Quadratus lumborum is dominant. Trigger point located in tensor fasciae latae. Quadratus lumborum released with gentle stretching of scalenes by inhibiting pressure and direct tissue stretch on scalene trigger points. Reassessed and right leg increases for one-foot standing to 45 seconds.

P–Adjust massage next session based on whether client plays or continues to have postconcussion symptoms.

The Rest of the Story

This client was held out of the game to prevent the possibility of a repeat injury. He had never had a concussion before, but the physician was cautious. His symptoms dissipated over the next 2 weeks, and he played as the starter for the season. He continues to play in the NFL.

CASE SIX

LAURA—WEIGHT LOSS

Laura is a 27-year-old woman. She is currently a university student majoring in biology and education. She experiences pain and aching in her hips and low back.

As an adolescent she was involved in jazz and tap dancing and cheerleading.

She had a severe ankle sprain (left) during this time. The ankle healed, but it remains unstable.

At the age of 18 she entered the Army. Before enlistment she lost 20 pounds and during basic training lost another 20 pounds. She was required to complete a physical training program that included strength training and running. Physical fitness had to be maintained during her military commitment.

After 5 years in the Army she developed a medical condition related to her job responsibilities as a mechanic and received a medical retirement. Without the superimposed requirements and discipline of the Army, she has lost a significant amount of conditioning and has gained weight.

The demands of her schooling added to the deconditioning because she sits a lot in class and is extremely busy with various school responsibilities.

She currently is attempting to regain a degree of physical fitness appropriate to nonmilitary life and to stabilize her weight.

The nature of the medical condition is an inflammatory skin and joint issue. She has taken a substantial amount of cortisone-based medicine, topical and internal. She is concerned about developing arthritis. She currently has reduced the amount of cortisone use and is taking an immune-suppressant medication that is at this point controlling the condition. She is just getting over a bout of bronchitis where she coughed a lot and hard. She has been complaining of midback and thorax muscle pain.

Overall assessment indicates that she has inherent joint laxity with multiple areas of instability, primarily in the lower body to include lumbar vertebras, sacroiliac joints, hips, knees, and ankles but also elbow and to a lesser extent, shoulder. She "cracks" these joints frequently.

The worst areas are her knees, which hyperextend during standing, and her left ankle.

She has a bilaterally anteriorly rotated pelvis, short quadriceps and psoas, and long and weak hamstrings. Calves are short and tight.

Her trunk, hip, and knee firing patterns are synergistically dominant. All gait reflex patterns do not inhibit when appropriate.

Postural assessment identified a forward head position, slightly protruding abdomen, increased lumbar curve, and evidence of upper and lower crossed syndrome.

She is unstable during one foot standing, more so on the left.

The main issue seems to be the core instability, anteriorly rotated pelvis and the hyperextended knees. The other assessment findings seem to be compensation.

Client is on a fixed income, and finances are a big issue.

Treatment Plan

Short-term goals: Eliminate thorax aching and pain associated with coughing.
Long-term goals: Normalize firing patterns and gait reflexes; shift anterior pelvic rotation to be more normal; lengthen and stretch short, tight structures; and support strengthening exercises for core and hamstrings and ankle stability.

Methods Used

General massage: Neuromuscular and connective tissue approaches
Frequency and duration: 1 time per week, 1½ hours each session, 10 sessions, and then reassessment
Progress measurements: Self-reporting of pain scale; firing pattern and gait assessment; and postural assessment
Questions that need to be answered are the following:
1. Where is Laura going to obtain guidance for strength training?

2. What is the influence of the inflammatory condition, and how does that affect the massage approach?
3. What are the implications of the cortisone use and current use of immune-suppressing treatments?
4. What is the motivation, time commitment demand, and influence of financial limitations on the course of treatment and potential outcomes?
5. What approach is Laura using for weight management, and what are the exercise requirements for this program?

First Session after Intake Assessment

S—Client describes pain in lower posterior thorax more on the right. Her primary goal is to reduce this pain.
O—Client's hand placement indicates posterior serratus inferior. She continues to have a deep, hacking cough. Upper chest activity is observable during normal relaxed breathing. Firing patterns and gait reflexes remain dysfunctional. Postural assessment has not worsened or improved. Palpation during massage identified areas of superficial connective tissue bind in lumbar and upper chest. Lymph nodes in her neck on the left are palpable. The quadriceps muscles and gastrocnemius/soleus are adhered. Provided general full-body massage with breathing pattern dysfunction strategies. Perform trigger point inhibition and manual direct stretching of posterior serratus inferior. Addressed gait reflexes to support appropriate inhibition response. Targeted contralateral shoulder extensors to inhibit hip flexors. Used bind and shear forces to begin process of reducing adherence of rectus femoris to vastus intermedialis and gastrocnemius to soleus. Did not address firing patterns this session. Taught simple core draw-in maneuver. Client knew this from military training.
A—Client reports significant (75%) improvement in lower posterior thorax pain and easier breathing. She continues to cough, so likelihood of recurrence is strong. Was able to achieve inhibition of hip flexors when paired with contralateral shoulder flexors, but it took extensive overpressure on the hip flexors, and client had to be reminded repeatedly not to hold her breath.
P—Client will target lower abdominals with draw-in exercises and stretch quadriceps using prior military experience. Massage next week at scheduled time.

Session Two

S—Client reports that back is aching again but not as badly. She would roll on a tennis ball in the trigger point area in the posterior serratus inferior. She did practice core activity of draw-in and stretched quadriceps 4 out of 7 days. She also reports she has joined a weight management program that is based on a well-rounded nutritional plan, portion control, weekly weigh-in, and peer support. The program includes a moderate general exercise program of walking 10,000 steps per day. Laura has purchased a pedometer and typically walks about 7000 to 8000 steps daily.

She would like to continue to focus on the back pain and breathing this session and feels that the work with the gait reflexes was valuable. Her calves are sore to the touch but not when she moves.

O—Client's posture remains the same; she continues to breathe with the upper chest and cough but appears improved. Serratus posterior inferior continues to have trigger point activity. Gait reflex assessment indicates that patterns do not inhibit when indicated. Did not assess firing patterns. Superficial fascia in upper anterior chest and lumbar remains short and binding. Quadriceps still are adhered. Calves are adhered and a bit boggy. Repeat general massage treatment as previous session and included lymphatic drainage on calves and skin rolling connective tissue application on lumbar area. Used ease/bind method in upper chest.

A—Lumbar area had excessive reddening (histamine/vasodilator) response after skin rolling. Client experienced itching and picking in the area. Hip flexors inhibited, but it took similar effort as in last session. Client reports that she feels more relaxed. She can get a deep breath and twist without her back grabbing. She indicated that her legs feel wobbly.

P—Continue with core strengthening: draw-in only and quadriceps stretching.

Session Three

S—Client reports that she lost 3 pounds, maintained daily 10,000 steps or more, and is not aching as much. Her backache is mild, and she can reduce it with the tennis ball. She indicates that her calves hurt to the touch and when moving, and her knees ache at night.

O—Breathing is more normal; calves are displaying edema and tautness. Assessed trunk and hip extension firing pattern, which remains synergistically dominant. Gait reflexes remain dysfunctional. General massage involved the following: continue to address contralateral hip/shoulder gait pattern; apply connective tissue shearing of rectus femoris to reduce adherence; perform lymphatic drainage and moderate shearing of gastrocnemius off soleus; perform psoas release and inhibit rectus abdominis to support appropriate trunk flexion; and stimulate gluteus maximus with pulsed muscle energy to activate firing. Did not address knees specifically.

A—Gait reflexes: Stimulate shoulder extensors to inhibit contralateral hip flexors, which corrected easily; added hip flexors to inhibit contralateral shoulder extensors, and this application took even more effort than previous application to get hip flexors to inhibit. Client discussed difficulty she had with push-ups as part of military physical training and wonders if this might be one of the causal factors. Trunk flexion is firing fairly normal: palpation indicates that lower abdominals are firing. Gluteus maximus did fire with pulsed muscle energy but did not hold against counterpressure.

Client continues to experience reddening with superficial connective tissue application. Calves are sore and swollen but more pliable.

P—Continue with weekly massage. Client will add intensity to lower abdominal strengthening by using protocol she learned in military and be specifically diligent about draw-in during exercise. She also will add strengthening exercise for gluteus maximus and continue to stretch hip flexors.

Session Four

S—Client reports she lost 1 pound and maintained 10,000 steps for 6 or 7 days. She did strengthening and stretching exercises 5 out of 7 days. Her knees and calves ache.

O—Trunk flexion is firing well, but she cannot sustain for more than 15 seconds. Gait reflexes are abnormal, with no inhibition: hip extension and lumbar muscles are dominant, and knee flexion indicated gastrocnemius dominant. Calves are taut but have some movement between gastrocnemius and soleus. Pelvis tilted anteriorly bilaterally, but more on the right. General massage targets inhibition pattern for contralateral gait reflexes and hip extension firing pattern. Used broad-based compression on lumbar muscles to inhibit while client activated gluteus maximus by first flexing the knee and then lifting her foot toward ceiling (client in prone position). Also applied percussion to gluteus maximus to increase stimulation. Applied inhibitory pressure to attachments of gastrocnemius. Continue to shear gastrocnemius to separate from soleus and promote lymph drainage.

A—Client reports feeling off balance when standing. Both hip flexors and shoulder extensors are inhibited as appropriate with less pressure than previous sessions. Client indicates that knees do not ache as much.

P—Continue with last session plan and add calf stretch.

Session Five

S—Client reports that low back, knees, and left ankle hurt at night. She wonders if massage is helping. She lost 1 pound and maintained 10,000 steps 6 out of 7 days but only did stretching and strengthening 4 out of 7 days.

O—Client's posture is beginning to shift, with anterior pelvic tilt showing minor improvement. Calves are less taut and more pliable; lumbar fascia is more pliable; trunk muscles are firing well but still cannot sustain against counterpressure; hip extension remains synergistically dominant with opposite lumbar muscle group activation, gluteus maximus is not firing until at 20 degrees of extension. General massage involved the following: connective tissue methods to lumbar fascia; indirect functional technique to pelvis; addressed firing patterns same way as last session; and added massage application specifically to inhibit vastus lateralis and increase iliotibial band pliability.

A—Client complains of burning in iliotibial band during massage application. Client finds broad-based compression intense and painful when focused on vastus lateralis but indicates that it felt right. Client pushes hard and enjoys the indirect functional method. She can feel the difference in pelvis alignment. The symphysis pubis made a loud pop when she activated adductors bilaterally against resistance. She feels wobbly when standing on her legs. Firing patterns are improving. Moderate movement of the pelvis occurs posteriorly, a bit more on the left. Gait reflexes normalize easily.

P—Next session begins to address unilateral gait reflexes and adduction/abduction patterns. Client will do the same self-help patterns as last week.

Session Six

S—Client reports pain in sacroiliac joint area and upper gluteal area. She was more diligent with exercises and did not discuss weight management. She indicates that her knees ache, but differently, and cannot seem to explain how. Says she did well with exercise but does not provide details.

O—Assessed joint play of head of fibula and tibia rotation. Fibula movement is restricted on left and both tibias bind during internal rotation. Contralateral gait reflexes are adequate but slow to respond. Unilateral and adduction gait reflex patterns do not inhibit as they should. Connective tissue in general is more pliable. Gastrocnemius continues to be dominant during knee flexion. Hamstring assessed short but weak. Gluteus maximus firing normal. Trunk firing normal but still cannot sustain against counterpressure. Psoas and quadratus lumborum short bilaterally. Pelvis reverted to previous anterior rotation position. General massage involved the following: psoas, quadratus lumborum, scalene, and sternocleidomastoid releases; reinforcement of contralateral gait reflexes, correction of unilateral and adductor/abductor patterns; reinforcement of trunk and hip firing; continued inhibition of lumbar paraspinals, with inhibiting pressure on multifidus trigger point bilaterally with sacroiliac joint mobilization sequence; and indirect functional technique for pelvis, fibula, and tibia.

A—Client is fatigued after massage. She feels top heavy and as if she is standing on her heels. Contralateral gait reflexes are normalizing with little effort. Unilateral pattern did normalize; however, client again experienced pop when symphysis pubis is addressed. Hamstrings and midscapular region cramped. Applied cramp release methods. Pelvis, fibula, and tibia responded well to joint play/indirect functional techniques.

P—Continue as previously and add gluteus and hamstring strengthening. Client will use a military exercise pattern.

Session Seven

S—Client reports that knees are less achy, but hamstrings are really sore and describes delayed-onset muscle soreness. She asks if she can just have a good massage with no effort on her part. She lost 3 pounds and says she deserves a treat.

O–No specific assessment. Follow general protocol and strategies for sleeping client.

A–Client reports that massage was great. Appears client needs some integration time for neurologic and structural changes.

P–Appointment as scheduled next week. Evaluate at that time as to focus.

Session Eight

S–Client says she is feeling better and would like to repeat last week's session. She has a moderate headache radiating from base of skull to her forehead. She is on second day of menstrual cycle and is a bit crampy. She would like a psoas release because she says it helps the cramping.

O–Scalp movement is restricted: tender points in frontalis and occipital area. Palpate mild to moderate edema bodywide, more in lower extremities. Provided general massage with sleeping client strategies. Performed psoas release at beginning of massage. Included bodywide lymphatic drainage and strategies for tension headache.

A–Client is tired and goes home to take a nap. She feels better. Did not provide any more details. From what would be assessed with passive approach, client's condition appears to remain stable, and she is likely integrating changes.

P–Obtain update on exercise program. Reevaluate if client is ready for therapeutic change application or if massage should remain on management level.

Session Nine

S–Client reports she is feeling better, has maintained exercises, and is noticing that her legs feel stronger. She has not lost weight but has not gained either. She would like all firing patterns and gait reflexes reassessed and addressed.

O–One-foot standing is improved from initial assessment. Laura can stand with eyes open 20 seconds on right leg and 15 seconds on left. She has obvious ankle instability on the left. Trunk flexion, hip extension, and shoulder flexion firing are normal. Hip abduction and knee flexion remain synergistically dominant. Gait reflexes: Contralateral, unilateral, and adduc-

tion/abduction are improving. They either respond slowly, or Laura holds her breath and has to be reminded to not use other muscle groups. Added eye/neck reflexes assessment, which is normal for flexion, but would not inhibit in extension or rotating left or right. During assessment, she recalls being hit in the face during a weapon drill and that she cracked a tooth. Palpation indicates restricted tissue texture in general. Increased pliability exists in sacroiliac joint area, and sacroiliac joint movement improved when force couple of same side gluteus maximus, opposite side latissimus dorsi is activated. May need to back off of connective tissue lengthening in sacroiliac joint area to prevent destabilization. Pelvis remains anteriorly rotated, but 50% improvement is noted. General massage protocol involved the following: eye/neck reflexes and all firing patterns, reinforced gait reflexes; released quadratus lumborum/scalenes; inhibiting pressure applied to proximal attachment of gastrocnemius; and promote joint play at left fibular head.

A–Client appears a bit emotional after massage. She speaks again of being hit in the face during military training. State-dependent memory is evident during the portion of the massage that includes the eye and neck application. Did not pursue issue. Client is fine and does not appear distressed when leaving office after sitting and drinking some water. Reflex mechanisms in general are functioning better. Strengthening for lower abdominals has been successful, and gluteus maximus and hamstring strength is improving. The knees continue to hyperextend: considering referral for more extensive evaluation of this condition.

P–Client will continue self-help activities as previous session. Massage next week as scheduled.

Session Ten

S–Client reports that she feels good and thinks things are beginning to work. She is sleeping better in general, although she did dream about basic training after the last massage. She knows that her hyperextended knees are a difficult issue and can tell that this is why her pelvis tips forward. Would like similar massage as last session including eye reflexes.

O–Repeat previous week's massage approach.

A–Client reports feeling good. She checks herself for one-foot standing stability and indicates that she feels better. It appears that massage has reached a condition management situation and can maintain and support the exercise, but until the knee/ankle issue is addressed, compensation will likely continue to develop.

P—Suggest client see an orthopedic specialist. She indicates that that will be time-consuming using the military health service, but she agrees. Continue with weekly session to support and maintain current status.

The Rest of the Story

This client did receive some physical therapy that improved the knee and ankle condition, but it continues to be an ongoing management situation. Most of the time, she is diligent with the core exercises strengthening program but has periodic lapses. There was no additional response or discussion concerning the injury to her face. She has maintained her moderate weight loss for the most part but as is common, has periods when she is less diligent. The inflammatory skin and joint condition is stable, but she continues to take the immune-suppressant medication.

She is prone to upper respiratory infection with coughing, and during these periods, the posterior serratus inferior and quadratus lumborum become short and painful. The situation responds well to massage.

CASE SEVEN

EMMA—FIGURE SKATER

Emma's mother has been a client for years to manage chronic back pain and headaches. Emma's mother now wants to include regular massage for Emma, her daughter, as part of Emma's figure skating training program. Emma has had various falls and a grade one ankle sprain, but nothing serious. She is stiff and aching in the mornings. Emma is 13 years old.

Assessment

Observation. Emma is a small, compact adolescent. She is beginning to mature but has not yet had her first menstrual period. Some emotional tension between mother and daughter is observable.

Interview and Goals. During the interview, there were minor disagreements between mother and daughter. These centered around scheduling and accuracy

of information. Mother and daughter agree that massage would be beneficial. The most current complaint is that Emma is stiff and achy in the mornings. She finds it difficult to get up and hard to concentrate in school for the first couple of hours.

Emma's training schedule is intense, and when asked about the possibility of overtraining, both denied this as a possibility.

The goals for the massage are to reduce the stiffness and aching in the morning and support recovery from training and competition.

Physical Assessment

Posture is typical for this type of athlete. Emma has moderate lordosis and mild anterior hip rotation bilaterally.

Gait is normal except for a slight tendency to bear weight on the balls of the feet instead of the heel during heel strike phase.

Passive joint movement indicates general tendency to joint laxity. The muscle tone provides the most joint stability.

Palpation assessment identifies taut skin and reduced soft tissue pliability. Whether this is primarily fluid retention or changes in ground substance density or both is unclear. Muscles palpate the same way. Tendons and fascial sheaths are taut but pliable. Identifying individual muscle layers or moving surface structures over underlying tissue is difficult.

Ligaments and joint capsules are lax. Joints are hypermobile. The pelvis has a bilateral anterior tilt. Breathing appears normal.

Muscle strength assesses strong bodywide. However, firing patterns and gait reflexes are disrupted. Hamstrings are dominant for hip extension; gluteus medius is dominant for hip abduction. Lower abdominal muscles are slow to fire. Gait reflexes are normal during contralateral patterns but do not inhibit appropriately in unilateral patterns. At this point, whether this is a training adaptation response is unclear.

The symptoms of being achy and stiff are mostly related to the possible fluid retention and ground substance density.

Questions that need to be answered are the following:

1. What is the cause of the fluid shift?
2. Is the client displaying overtraining syndrome?
3. Are the changes in reflex patterns appropriate adaptation to training?

4. How is inherent joint laxity required for this sport countered by muscle tone and tension?

Quantitative Goals

Reduce tissue tautness from increased fluid retention and decrease ground substance density about 50%, or until stiffness and aching in the morning is minor.

Quantifiable Goals

Support training protocol and recovery so that client is able to sustain current training and competition intensity. This goal depends on the possibility of overtraining syndrome. Should training intensity need to be reduced, massage will support recuperation.

Treatment Plan

Client will receive 1-hour massage 3 times per week for 2 weeks to normalize fluid balance and shift connective tissue density.

Client will be reassessed for benefit. If benefit is observed, massage frequency will be reduced to 2 times per week for 2 more weeks and then reevaluated again. If benefit is sustained, then massage would occur 1 time per week with additional sessions as needed.

Massage will follow general massage protocol with lymphatic drainage and connective tissue methods. Rotation of the pelvis and gait and firing patterns will not be addressed specifically but will be monitored and any changes noted and compared with any noted increase or decrease in performance.

Because the client is a minor, a parent will be present during the massage session. Because the reason for the fluid retention is unclear, the client is requested to receive a checkup from the physician before massage begins.

Report from the doctor indicates hormonal changes consistent with onset of menstruation. The doctor also is concerned about client's body fat ratio, which is low, and signs of fatigue. The doctor suggests a 5-pound weight gain, increase in essential fatty acids (i.e., fish, eggs, and olive oil), and more sleep. The doctor approves of massage as presented in the treatment plan.

Session One

S—Client reports that she is stiff and achy in the morning as usual. She is not sleeping well and does not think she needs to put on weight or reduce training intensity. In fact, she has been trying to lose several more pounds.

O—Assessment finding from previous intake remains consistent with assessment this session, with added indication of upper chest breathing. Mother and daughter squabble a bit, and then the mother ignores daughter and reads a magazine. Massage was full-body approach with focus on lymphatic drainage with minimal use of connective tissue methods. The intention is to address fluid first and then address remaining stiffness with connective tissue strategies. The strategies for breathing pattern disorder are used during the massage.

A—Client relaxes toward the last 15 minutes of the massage as indicated by breathing shift to more relaxed breathing function. The calves are much softer to the touch, and the client identifies increased ankle flexibility.

P—Massage in 2 days; repeat sequence.

Session Two

S—Client reports that ankle flexibility lasted about 1 day and then she woke up feeling stiff again. She did sleep better. Mother reports that Emma is not eating like the doctor recommended.

O—Fluid retention has returned, as has upper chest breathing tendency. Client is irritable. Repeated lymphatic drainage in context of general massage and include strategies for breathing. Asked client where she feels most stiff: she indicates calves, hamstrings, and neck. Introduced connective tissue kneading into these areas.

A—Client reports that she liked the kneading and she feels much looser. She is less irritable. Tissue texture is less taut and dense. Breathing is normalized.

P—Alter massage application to include fluid and connective tissue methods. Massage every 2 days.

Session Three

S—Client reports that she felt less achy and stiff the morning after the massage, but it came back the next day. She says she feels fat and stiff. She also indicates that she does not like eating the fattening food. Her father is with her during the massage.

O—Client has some edema in lower legs and hands. Her abdomen is a bit distended. She has developed a mild acne breakout on her shoulders, which disturbs her. When questioned, she thinks it is caused from eating the extra fat.

A–Client reports feeling better and indicates that her breasts were sore when she lay on her stomach. She says she still feels fat.

P–Massage in 3 days.

Session Four

S–Client participated in a regional competition and performed well. She continues to complain about feeling fat. Mother and daughter argue a bit about the diet. Client also indicates that her left glutes feel tight.

O–Left gluteus medius is short and tight. Left adductors are also short and tight. Tender point is found in belly of gluteus medius. Breathing is normal. Emma has slight edema in extremities. Lower abdomen is slightly distended. Client feels as if she has lost weight. General massage involved the following method: lymphatic drainage and connective tissue; kneading body-wide; positional release of tender point at left gluteus medius; and contract-relax-antagonist-contract and lengthen adductors bilateral. Increase massage focus on reflex areas of right deltoid and bilateral pectoralis major and latissimus dorsi.

A–Client reports that she feels better, like she always does, and her glutes feel better. She can stand on that leg and maintain balance without pain.

P–Suggest that massage sessions be reduced to 2 times per week because tissue density is normalizing. Mother and Emma agree. Monitor the client's weight, and refer back to physician if continue to notice changes.

Session Five

S–Client reports she had mild stomach flu. Mother thinks it was a 24-hour food poisoning. She threw up and had diarrhea for 24 hours and then did not eat much the next day. Emma indicates that she feels better than she has in weeks. She is less stiff in the morning and does not feel fat.

O–Client's tissues palpate as dense but not taut. There are mild indications of dehydration, but this seems reasonable considering the intestinal episode. Client and mother report she is drinking enough water. Client appears and feels thinner. General massage with connective tissue focus.

A–Client reports that she feels great and really likes the massage where her tissues are twisted. It makes her feel like she has been stretched all over. Client is encouraged to stay hydrated to support the connective tissue pliability.

P–Session in 4 days. Emma's weight loss is a concern.

Session Six

S–Client reports that she feels great and wants the same massage. She also indicates that her training has been going well. She is preparing for a big competition in 6 weeks. Mother is encouraged but somewhat concerned about Emma's erratic eating.

O–Client appears and feels thinner. The tissue palpates as pliable with localized areas of bind and density. General massage is given with connective tissue focus, especially in local areas of density. Used indirect functional technique on binding tissue (ease and bind).

A–Client reports feeling flexible and calm. She indicates that she enjoys the massage and wants to keep coming. She just knows it helps her. She wants to continue 2 times per week until the competition in the regional finals next week. Discuss with mother the concerns about weight loss. Mother indicates that Emma resists eating the foods recommended by the doctor. Provide a pamphlet on disordered eating in female athletes. When asked if Emma has experienced her first period, the mother replies no, although she really thought it was going to happen several weeks ago. Explained to mother that it is common for there to be a few months where all the premenstrual symptoms are present but the actual period does not occur. She agrees that many of the symptoms seem to be premenstrual related.

P–Session in 3 days. Continue massage as applied in a condition management/recovery process.

Session Seven

S–Mother reports she caught Emma throwing up. Emma says that something she ate made her stomach hurt and she felt better after she threw up. This is a major development indicating the tendency toward disordered eating. Made it clear that Emma must see the doctor before the next visit and suggested that the mother speak with Emma's various coaches and dance teacher.

O–Emma is sullen and appears thin. Her tissue pliability is good, and there is no obvious indication of fluid imbalances. Spot check of muscle strength does not indicate weakness. There are some hangnails on finger and toes and abrasions that had occurred just before the last session that are healing slowly. Client is upset with her mother and the massage therapist. She just lies there during the massage and is uncooperative. Gave general massage with kneading as client enjoys. Did not attempt to encourage client in conversation.

A—Client would not respond to postassessment questions.

P—Massage in 4 days only if Emma has seen the doctor.

Session Eight

S—Mother reports that Emma has lost 7 pounds since her last visit to the doctor. Her body fat has dropped below the recommended ratio for females. The doctor is concerned about normal sexual development and bone density. Emma is reporting to the doctor weekly. If she continues to lose weight, she will be referred to a psychologist that specializes in disordered eating for the athlete. At this point there are no limitations on activity. Continued massage is recommended.

O—Client is sullen and a bit defiant. She will not respond to assessment questions and indicates that she is tired, has a headache, and wants to go to sleep. General massage to reduce connective tissue density and focused on mood regulation and relaxation is provided. Included tension headache strategies in the massage.

A—Client reports that her headache feels better, and then she starts to cry. She tells us that one of the girls in her gymnastics class has been teasing here about her "big boobs and butt." She felt so much better after the "flu" a couple of weeks ago, that the next time she felt fat she made herself throw up. One of the girls she trains with told her how to do it. Because she felt better afterward, she did it a few more times until her mother caught her. She has been performing well and is afraid that if her body continues to change, she will not be able to make her jumps. She is sorry she has been mean.

P—Suggest massage continue on a weekly basis and that Emma and her parents have a good talk with the doctor and coaches. Emma likely would benefit from education on body changes during adolescence. Also recommend at least some short-term intervention with a sport psychologist who also understands eating disorders.

Session Nine

S—Client reports she has maintained her weight and would like the usual massage (connective tissue pliability focus). She has a bruise on her right forearm from a fall but otherwise feels pretty good. She saw the psychologist once, likes her, and reports that she is a skater too.

O—Contusion on forearm is large and discolored. Breathing normal. Tissue density has somewhat increased, with mild fluid retention in extremities. General massage performed with connective tissue focus: lymphatic drainage targeted to extremities and contusion.

A—Client reports that she feels good but a little fat. Explain that fluid retention does make the skin feel taut or "fat." This is not really fat, but water. Young women have fluid fluctuation because of hormone shifts. It is natural.

P—Massage again in 4 days.

Session Ten

S—Client reports she gained ½ pound, but she thinks it is muscle and that is good. She indicates that her breasts are bigger and tender. Her bruise is better, but she jammed her right big toe in dance class. Her father came with her to the session.

O—Client's posture and muscle firing and gait pattern remain consistent. Likely cause is a training effect adaptation. Bruise is improving and is soft. Right toe has reduced joint play. Used general massage with connective tissue focus and indirect functional technique/joint play on right large toe. Performed lymph drainage in the anterior chest area. Explained that tender breasts are part of the hormone changes she is experiencing.

A—Client reports a clicking sound in her toe when she moves it around and that it feels better. Her breasts are still tender.

P—Massage after 3 days.

The Rest of the Story

Obviously, this case describes a potential eating disorder development and the role of the massage therapist in such a situation. Emma did experience her first menstrual cycle about 3 months after the last recorded session and experienced an accelerated growth phase. Emma currently is going to college and is skating in various entertainment productions. She did not achieve her goal of going to the Olympics.

CASE EIGHT

JAMAL—BASKETBALL PLAYER

The client is a 20-year-old rookie basketball player. He is a point guard. It is the second week of training camp. He reports to the trainer that he aches all over and has some cramping in his hamstrings and calves. The leg cramping goes away with increased hydration and ingestion of electrolytes. He has been referred to the team massage therapist for management of delayed-onset muscle soreness. The trainer for this team is especially good and very well respected. He also expects all treatment to be preapproved and his treatment requests to be followed exactly.

Assessment

Observation. The client is emotionally pumped up but seems fatigued. His movements are generally a bit stiff. He keeps trying to stretch out while talking. He displays upper chest breathing and is talking fast, and the exhale is shorter than the inhale.

Interview and Goals. When asked how well he is sleeping, Jamal reports that he is tossing and turning and cannot get comfortable. His history indicates high ankle sprain on the right during his freshman year of college when he stepped on a fellow player's foot and then rolled forward. He also had a grade two groin pull on the right the last year he played college ball, but the injury was not basketball related. He did it demonstrating martial arts kicks when he was not warmed up (he was goofing around and showing off a little). Both injuries healed well, but the groin continues to get stiff. He has to keep the area stretched out or he feels the pulling. He has been playing basketball since he was a little kid. He played well in high school and received scholarships to college and was drafted by the NBA. Nothing unusual is disclosed in the history form, except a recent tendency to constipation. On a pain scale of 1 to 10, he says he feels like a 12.

His goals for massage are to reduce the aching and stiff feeling and to enhance his athletic performance. The trainer's goal is management of delayed-onset muscle soreness. Contacted trainer requesting to include approaches for constipation, which was approved.

Physical Assessment

Posture: Appropriate for basketball positional demands
Gait: Slightly reduced stride on the right

Range of motion: Abduction of leg on the right is reduced by 10% compared with left leg and has a binding end-feel. Elbow and knee flexion bilaterally are reduced slightly because of soft tissue approximation (muscle tissue bumping into itself). Note: Most basketball players are muscular and toned but structurally long and lean. Point guards, however, may be more muscular and compact because of positional demands.

Palpation

Near touch: Client is generally giving off heat.
Skin surface: Generally damp with axilla, feet, and hand sweating
Skin: Generally taut
Skin and superficial connective tissue: Binding at clavicles, which may interfere with lymph flow. Tissue in general feels dense but boggy.
Superficial connective tissue: Dense
Vessels and lymph nodes: Difficult to palpate because they seem buried in tissue
Muscles: Muscle tone is appropriate to training effect. General tone is increased from when client was first seen a month ago, indicating a response to training effects during training camp. Gluteus maximus is short and tight bilaterally.
Tendons: General tenderness at musculotendinous junction in phasic (movement) muscles of arms and legs. Mild binding of Achilles tendon on the right.
Fascial sheaths: Mild binding during superior and inferior movement in sheath that runs from cranial base to sacrum and continues down iliotibial band into calves. Bind also noted in abdominal and pectoralis fasciae.
Ligaments: Normal
Joints: Aching increased with traction, indicating soft tissue as primary causal factor. Joints of the feet are especially sore. Right tibia is slightly externally rotated, which is consistent with history of high ankle sprain. Knee is asymptomatic.
Bones: Normal
Abdominal viscera: Abdominal muscle development makes palpation difficult; appears normal, with some fullness over descending colon.
Body rhythms: Fast upper chest breathing pattern

Muscle Testing

Strength: All muscles test strong, but excessive synergistic recruitment is evident.
Neurologic balance: Generalized hypersensitivity is evidenced by fast, jerky contraction pattern and inability to contract muscles slowly.

Gait: Normal, but inhibition pattern for arms is slow to engage (it takes a few seconds for muscles to let go).

Interpretation and Treatment Plan Development

Clinical Reasoning. The profile for this client is common for most training camp or early season situations. It does not seem to matter what the sport or level is–high school to professional. Basketball, track and field, football, soccer, baseball, rowing, rugby, lacrosse, horseback riding: the sport does not matter. What is important to note is that training camp, or the initial few weeks of any intense training and conditioning program, is not the time to introduce massage for therapeutic change. The adaptive capacity of the body is maxed out. The goal is to manage symptoms and help the athlete sleep.

As described previously in this text, delayed-onset muscle soreness is a complicated response to increased physical and muscular activity demands. Soreness can be local or generalized, depending on the activity. Remember, although the term *delayed-onset muscle soreness* would indicate a muscle problem, the situation more likely involves the circulatory, lymphatic, and autonomic nervous systems and breathing functions. Simple delayed-onset muscle soreness in local areas may result when a muscle moves repetitively in eccentric contractions like rowers or sustained isometric contraction like motocross. Inflammation occurs and possibly some microtearing of muscle fibers. Inflammatory mediators (primarily histamine) are released during physical activity, there is increased capillary permeability, and interstitial fluid accumulates, causing simple edema. The increased fluid pressure in the tissue stimulates pain receptors, making the person feel stiff and achy.

Metabolic by-product (not lactic acid) buildup from exercise irritates nerve endings as well. Increased muscle tone can result in pressure on lymphatic vessels, interfering with the normal lymphatic flow and further stressing the lymphatic system. In addition, increased sympathetic arousal, which is part of athletic function, especially in contact sports, increases arterial pressure and blood flow.

If the normal expansion in the capillary bed of the muscle is restricted because of increased motor tone and muscle tone and connective tissue thickening, more plasma flows out of the capillaries but cannot return, requiring the lymphatic system to

handle the increased interstitial fluid volume. When the body is in a sympathetic state, the ground substance of the connective tissue thickens to provide more resistance to impact. This process should reverse itself when arousal diminishes and parasympathetic dominance takes over, but often with athletes the arousal levels do not reverse and the connective tissue remains thicker, placing pressure on pain receptors and contributing to stiffness. The combination of fluid pressure and connective tissue thickening makes the tissue feel taut and dense. More complex patterns result with sustained sympathetic arousal. Upper chest breathing patterns and a tendency for breathing pattern disorders are common and perpetuate the underlying sympathetic arousal.

Management of this condition requires the reduction of any muscle tension (both muscle and motor tone increase) interfering with circulation and lymphatic flow, mechanical drainage of interstitial fluid and support for arterial and venous circulation, reduction of the sympathetic arousal pattern, and an increase in ground substance pliability. The massage must be accomplished without adding any inflammation to the tissues or straining adaptive capacity. Friction or use of any other methods that would cause tissue damage is contraindicated.

The delayed-onset muscle soreness in planned training programs is to be expected. Each sport, in this case basketball, places specific demands on certain movement patterns. That massage applications support the training effect and not interfere with it is essential. Although symmetry in form is ideal, specific sport demand causes hypertrophy in certain muscle groups, and bodywide compensation occurs during a normal training regimen. This has to be considered during assessment and application of massage.

This particular client/player is displaying symptoms of combined delayed-onset muscle soreness and sustained sympathetic arousal. His breathing is appropriate to training activity but is not reversing during down time; therefore his sleep is disturbed and he is constipated. Tissues are fluid filled, with thickened ground substance making the tissue feel dense. Connective tissue binding in the back and the groin also is occurring, especially on the right and in the chest in the area of the right and left lymphatic ducts. Reduced abdominal movement because of the upper chest breathing and the overdeveloped abdominal muscles (primarily rectus abdominis) does not support movement of the lymph in the abdominal cavity. The muscle strength, with synergistic recruitment and slow response to inhibition patterns, can be attributed to overtraining and sympathetic arousal, which is especially common in rookie athletes who are trying hard to be really good performers.

The client likely is excited about being in professional basketball and is trying to prove himself in camp, which contributes to the sympathetic arousal. (Reader note: Be aware of the psychological implications of performance anxiety here and how so many of these syptoms are physical manifestations of it.)

In combination with the athletic trainer's support and proper hydration, massage can be focused to achieve the following:
1. Reduce the sympathetic arousal.
2. Soften the connective tissue ground substance.
3. Increase lymphatic flow.

The massage likely will help but needs to be done in the evening before the client goes to bed. This will make scheduling difficult.

The player must stay hydrated, and increased urine production may awaken him at night, interfering with sleep. If the massage intervention is too intense, he may be sluggish the next day, and his performance will be compromised.

With general nonspecific massage, sleep should improve, which would reduce the recovery time. Reflexes should be more appropriate, and coordination and timing should improve, which supports performance. With reduced sympathetic arousal, constipation should reduce.

Training personnel referred the client; therefore they are supportive. The player has had massage before and liked it but is worried about anything that could affect his performance. The massage therapist feels that it is important to deal with the situation but does not enjoy beginning massage at 9:30 PM. The player is likely to respond to the nurturing and to notice a reduction in anxiety.

Treatment Plan
Quantitative Goals
1. Reduce pain sensation to a tolerable 5 (on a scale of 1 to 10).
2. Ease feelings of stiffness by 50%.
3. Normalize breathing.
4. Normalize elimination.

Qualitative Goals. The player will be able to perform at or near optimum levels and will be able to par-

ticipate in all training activities without excessive soreness.

Treatment Regimen
Daily massage will be given for 5 days just before bed for 45 minutes. The frequency then will be reduced to 2 times per week. Lymphatic drainage and circulation enhancement massage with rhythmic, broad-based compression deep enough to spread muscle fibers in all muscle layers and to increase serotonin and endogenous opiate (endorphin) availability will be provided. Application of all methods should not create any inflammation or alter the training effect. The focus will be on reduction of sympathetic arousal and normalization of muscle and motor tone, reflex patterns, and fluid dynamics in the body. Limited use of myofascial release in the binding tissue of the back, groin, and chest, along with controlled used of kneading, primarily to squeeze out the capillary beds and soften the ground substance, is appropriate. Abdominal massage to encourage peristalsis, with a specific focus on the large intestines to move fecal matter, is indicated. Breathing, muscle tone, fluid retention, firing pattern, reflexes, and sleep patterns will be monitored as indicators that the player is responding to massage.

Questions that need to be answered are the following:
1. What are the demands of basketball training camp?
2. What is the trainer's understanding of, and expectation for, therapeutic massage?
3. What are the performance demands of a point guard?

Session One
S—Client reports he is sore and tired. Trainer wants massage to target fluid retention and sleep.
O—Client's tissue palpates as taut. Skin is warm around knees and ankles. He continues to breathe with the upper chest. Full-body lymphatic drainage is the general approach, with attention to breathing pattern strategies.
A—Client has to get up twice to use restroom. He falls asleep on the massage table and then immediately goes to bed. Tissues palpate less taut after massage.
P—Repeat massage tomorrow.

Session Two
S—Client reports that he was a little less stiff in the morning but still feels like a truck hit him. His

low back hurts. Called trainer for permission to address low back pain. Trainer's instructions are to work only surface tissues for symptom management and use a counterirritant ointment.

O—No change in assessment findings. Low back pain is common in training camp. Repeated lymphatic drainage and breathing strategies and applied broad-based compression to lumbar and sacroiliac joint area.

A—Tissue tautness again is reduced. Client reports being less stiff and that low back feels better.

P—Repeat massage tomorrow.

Session Three

S—Client reports increased constipation and headache. Breathing is improved, and he is sleeping better. He is feeling less stiff and achy.

O—Client's abdomen palpates as constipated. Trainer has given him a laxative. Modify massage to the general protocol with limited focus on connective tissue. Concentrate on ease and bind and general kneading. Add abdominal massage for constipation and vascular headache strategies.

A—Client goes immediately to the restroom after massage and stays there awhile. Indicates he would see me tomorrow

P—Massage tomorrow: Reassess firing patterns.

Session Four

S—Client has a large abrasion with bruising on left knee. He reports that he is feeling better and his practices have been good. He is definitely not constipated.

O—Reassessment of firing patterns indicates synergistic dominance for hip extension and shoulder flexion. Tissue texture is more pliable. Knees are warm to the touch. Breathing is slightly from upper chest. He talks a lot during the massage. General massage protocol is nonspecific and avoids left knee.

A—Client is excited about his performance. There is a preseason game in 2 days, and he wants to do really well. Choose not to address the firing patterns directly because he is doing well in practice. Will continue to monitor.

P—Last sequential massage occurs tomorrow, and then reduce sessions to twice a week. This will be his last massage before the preseason game. Will switch to pre-event format.

Session Five

S—Client indicates that he feels good. He asks for a massage like the one yesterday.

O—Only minimal assessment is performed. Use pre-event strategies. (Note: This is not the time to identify deviation from the norm, which may make client nervous about ability to perform.) Used full-body general massage: no specific focus.

A—Client says he feels great.

P—Massage in 3 days, after event. Need to reassess how to massage in context of response to game activity.

Session Six

S—Client performed well in the game. He is sore in general but not stiff. He indicates that his chest feels tight. His nose is stuffed up.

O—Client appears a bit sluggish. These are definite sinus symptoms. The abrasion on his knee is healing a bit slowly, indicating strain in adaptive capacity. He has a contusion on his left shoulder. General massage has post-event focus, added attention to sinus congestion, and essential oil mixture of eucalyptus and peppermint for him to rub on his chest.

A—Client really likes the smell of the essential oil. (Note: Use of essential oils was preapproved by trainer.) He feels sleepy even though peppermint is a bit of a stimulant.

P—Massage in 3 days will again be a pre-event situation.

Session Seven

S—Client has a cold with a sore throat. He feels a bit feverish.

O—General relaxing massage

A—Client is a bit discouraged. Explain that a cold is common at this point of the season.

P—Massage in 4 days: postevent.

Session Eight

S—Spoke with trainer about status of player. He indicates that Jamal is coming along well in spite of the cold. There is some indication of overtraining syndrome, but that is common and should settle down once the actual season starts. He asks if two sessions a week were still necessary. Indicate that it may be best to not change the schedule on Jamal at this point. Two sessions per week are typical for this type of training intensity. He agrees. Client indicates that he is feeling better but still is stuffed up with a mild sore throat. Explain again that this is not uncommon with this type of training intensity.

He indicates that his neck feels tight and he has a spot in his back that is really tight and sore.

O—Assessed for shortening in posterior serratus inferior because client has been sniffing and coughing: general shortening is evident; the neck area is generally short. The abrasion and contusion are healing, so applied lymphatic drainage over contusion and subacute strategies for wounds on the abrasions. Provided general massage with broad-based compression on posterior serratus inferior, with added muscle energy methods by instructing the client to sniff and cough while the compression is applied to create postisometric relaxation. Then applied direct tissue stretching. Used muscle energy methods and eye position activation to reduce tension in neck muscles. Taught client how to roll on a tennis ball to relieve back symptoms.

A—Client reports that his back is much better and his head is not as stuffy. Asks for more essential oil mixture.

P—Massage in 3 days with pre-event focus.

Session Nine

S—Client is feeling better. He reports that he could not find his tennis ball and rolled around on his deodorant bottle instead. He said it worked but the area felt a little bruised. Explained that the tennis ball should be squished a little when used to apply compression, so the tissue does not feel bruised. The deodorant bottle was a good option but does not squish and so the compression is a bit heavy. Gave him another tennis ball. He says his ankles and feet ache.

O—The client's cold is improving, and he looks healthier. Some shortening in upper chest fascia and an active trigger point in the left gluteus medius are evident. Posterior serratus inferior is still short and a bit tender to the touch. Provided general nonspecific massage with myofascial release (ease/bind) on anterior chest, provided direct inhibitory pressure on gluteus medius trigger point (belly location) with reflex massage stimulus to right deltoid and extra attention on ankles and feet specifically targeting joint movement and range of motion.

A—Client is sleepy and not communicative. He gives little postassessment feedback. Gluteus medius trigger point released, but it seems like compensation. Palpated increased tone in hamstrings but did not specifically address this.

P—Massage in 4 days with post-event focus.

Session Ten

S—He just wants a massage.

O—No special assessment today: general protocol recovery massage.

A—Client falls asleep during the massage. Goes right to bed.

P—Shift to season schedule next session.

The Rest of the Story

This client continues to play in the NBA. He was traded two seasons later and has played for four other teams. He has stayed relatively injury free. He continues to get regular massage, asking for recommendations from fellow players at each team with which he signs. He is now pushing 32 years old and is beginning to feel the adaptive strain even though he has not had a major injury. He has been a reliable player, never a star, and has had to develop an inner peace over this situation. He would like to stay in the NBA 15 years, which would make him around 35 when he retires and moves on with his life.

CASE NINE

STEVEN—REPETITIVE STRAIN/OVERUSE INJURY: BURSITIS

The client is a 48-year-old man who has been diagnosed with bursitis of the left elbow. The bursa at the olecranon around the attachment of the triceps has become irritated and inflamed. The client fell and hit the elbow 6 months ago. The bursa was injured but healed with no apparent problems. The client recently began a weight-training program that includes biceps and triceps toning. He admits that he overtrained, doing upper body and lower body exercises every day, instead of following an alternate-day pattern. In addition, he used more weight than was necessary. He was given a cortisone injection at the inflamed site and is taking aspirin. He has been told to rest the area and maintain range of motion but not to lift weight with the arm. The client expresses concern about losing recently acquired muscle tone and bulking. He had become overweight and deconditioned in his early 40s after being fit in his 20s and 30s. He is determined to reclaim a fit body. He already is receiving massage weekly with the goal of managing stress and the muscle soreness caused by exercise. He intends to maintain the schedule indefinitely. Currently, he wants the outcome of massage to be focused specifically on reversing the bursitis.

Assessment

Observation. The client is a bit restless and impatient. Frustration is evident in his voice tone and word use over what seems to him to be a delay in his training program. He rubs the sore elbow often.

Interview and Goals. The client is taking a muscle-building supplement that contains various vitamins and amino acids. He slipped on the ice 6 months ago and severely bruised the left elbow. It was speculated that he may have ruptured the bursa at the olecranon. The bursitis is in the acute, possibly early subacute, stage. The history indicates a family tendency for cardiovascular problems, primarily arteriosclerosis. The death of a relative prompted the client to begin a diet and exercise program. His blood pressure is elevated slightly but is not being treated medically, and his doctor expects that it will fall into the normal range with weight reduction, stress management, and exercise.

Physical Assessment

Posture: Mild anterior rotation of left shoulder and moderate anterior rotation of left pelvis. Left elbow is carried in a flexed, loose-packed position.
Gait: Stride is short when client moves forward on right leg and counterbalances, with right arm moving into extension instead of left arm.
Range of motion: Flexion and extension of left elbow are limited to 100 degrees by pain. External rotation of left arm is limited to 70 degrees.

Palpation

Near touch: Bursa area in left arm is warm.
Skin surface: Damp and slightly red near bursal inflammation
Skin: Goose flesh with light skin stroking over bursal inflammation
Skin and superficial connective tissue: Skin binding at triceps attachment
Superficial connective tissue: Adhered at triceps attachment at elbow
Vessels and lymph nodes: Normal
Muscles: Short triceps and biceps on the left. Long, taut quadriceps and short, tight hamstring on the right. Muscle mass of biceps seems out of proportion to triceps. Internal rotators of left arm are short, with inhibition of external rotators.

Gluteus maximus on the left is inhibited and not firing appropriately during hypertension.
Tendons: Tender to moderate pressure at right hamstring attachment at the pelvis and at all attachments of left triceps
Fascial sheaths: Iliotibial band binding in all directions on right leg
Ligaments: No palpable problems
Joints: Compression of left elbow joint does not cause additional pain, but traction does; primary problem is likely to be the soft tissue.
Bones: Normal
Abdominal viscera: Normal
Body rhythms: Fast, with some indication of sympathetic arousal and upper chest breathing

Muscle Testing

Strength: Triceps on the left is inhibited and weak, and biceps is too strong; quadriceps is inhibited and weak, and hamstring is too strong on the right. Left gluteus maximus is weak. Trigger point activity is found in these same muscle groups, with the trigger point in the belly of the short, concentrically contracted muscles and at the attachments of the inhibited long eccentrically functioning muscles. This reflects the general pattern for trigger point location.
Neurologic balance: Client is unable to increase resistance gradually against pressure; he uses maximal force, and movement is abrupt and jerky. Abdominal muscles are not firing appropriately.
Gait: Gait patterns are normal, even though there is local inhibition and increased tone with individual strength testing of direct antagonist and antagonist patterns.

Interpretation and Treatment Plan Development: Clinical Reasoning

What Are the Facts? Bursitis is an inflammation of the synovial fluid-filled sacs located around joints, tendons, and ligaments. Bursitis develops with impact trauma, sustained compression (it is often found in the knees of carpet layers, carpenters, and others who do a lot of work on their knees), and repetitive strain. Repetitive movement causes friction and a tendency toward shortening of the muscle and connective tissue structures, which further increases the tendency for rubbing, causing inflammation. Bursitis also can occur if there is a change in the position of the bones of the joint and ligament alignment or an uneven pull of muscles on the joint structures.

This type of inflammation responds to applications of ice, nonsteroidal antiinflammatory drugs (e.g., aspirin), and if necessary, localized injection of a steroid. The medication, especially aspirin, thins blood. Massage pressure needs to be altered to prevent bruising during massage. Areas where the steroid was injected must be avoided, because the medication exerts its effect on the local tissues, and massage may disperse the steroid. Recently, transdermal patches of antiinflammatory and analgesic medication have been used successfully instead of injection, but the same cautions exist. The muscle and connective tissue elements around the inflamed bursa are usually short, and lengthening and stretching of this soft tissue are necessary. If the problem is localized and not the result of a more general posture shift, spot work may be helpful. However, as soon as the body begins to compensate for the condition, as this client has, full-body effects develop; therefore even localized bursitis is addressed best in the context of full-body massage.

This client displays connective tissue shortening around the olecranon, with agonist and antagonist for elbow flexion being short and tight on the affected side. A corresponding kinetic chain pattern does not display active symptoms in the opposite leg.

What Are the Possibilities, in Function and Dysfunction, and the Massage Intervention Options?
The previous injury may have caused some scar tissue and shortening of the triceps tendon. The rotational pattern of the shoulder and hip also increases the likelihood of the triceps rubbing at the attachment on the elbow. The short, tight muscles with trigger points in the muscle belly may be changing the joint angle and orientation of the connecting bones, increasing the likelihood of friction at the bursa. The repetitive strain of the weight lifting for the biceps and triceps is partly causal and likely is aggravating the scar tissue from the previous injury. The client admits to overtraining, and it is possible that he also is training the flexors more than the extensors of the affected elbow, setting up the muscle imbalance. Massage is indicated, and better results would be obtained if the sessions were scheduled for every other day during the therapeutic change process:

1. Friction and myofascial release are options in the areas of connective tissue adhesion.
2. Direct pressure combined with muscle energy methods is indicated for the trigger points in the concentrically short muscles.

3. Lengthening and stretching of the short muscles, with stimulation of the inhibited muscles, could be effective.

What Are the Logical Outcomes of Each Possible Intervention Option?
Massage to lengthen the shortened muscles and ease the connective tissue dysfunction would reduce the tendency for rubbing. If eccentrically strained long muscles are inhibited further and become longer, the situation can worsen if the tension/length relationship is disturbed further. Connective tissue binding is at the triceps, and further complications would need to be addressed in combination with muscle stimulation of the triceps and reduction of excessive shortening of the biceps.

Massage directly over the site of the steroid injection is contraindicated for at least 7 more days, which interferes with application of scar tissue release in the area. The client is taking aspirin and therefore may bruise with direct application of compression to trigger points. Alternate methods are needed to address the trigger point problem. The client needs to ice the area frequently.

Because this is a regular client, an increase in massage frequency is a time and cost burden. The massage therapist will have to find available scheduling to accommodate the more frequent appointments.

The additional appointments are acceptable to the client as long as results are readily apparent within a month. The client's expectations are a bit unrealistic. He resists ice application.

Decision Making and Treatment Plan Development
Quantitative Goals
1. Restore range of motion of left elbow and arm to normal.
2. Reverse any compensation caused by posture changes.

Qualitative Goals. The client should be able to resume work and moderate, appropriate exercise and weight training without causing irritation to the bursa or elbow.

Treatment Regimen
Therapeutic Change/Return to Condition Management.
Full-body massage appointments will be increased from once a week to 3 times per week for 1 month. The focus will be on generalized massage to address the

compensation patterns in the opposite leg and the rotational pattern of the shoulder and pelvis. Compression, gliding, and kneading will be applied to the short biceps and hamstrings with tense-and-relax and lengthening techniques.

Tapotement and pulsed muscle energy methods will be used after general gliding and kneading to stimulate inhibited muscles and to focus on reducing trigger point activity and lengthening short muscles. In 1 week, connective tissue work will begin on the elbow, with myofascial approaches and skin rolling used to soften the ground substance for the first four sessions of connective tissue application. No additional inflammation will be introduced.

After this application, if heat and other indicators of inflammation are reduced in the area, controlled use of friction (bending and shearing forces) of adhered tissue can begin. This process needs to be monitored carefully to ensure that the bursitis symptoms do not recur. Aspirin should be discontinued before the introduction of therapeutic inflammation, or the methods will not be as effective, because it is the inflammatory process that changes the connective tissue fiber structure. Depth of pressure will elicit a "good hurt" sensation, and all layers of the short and tight tissues need to be addressed, especially synergists and fixators in the deeper muscle layers.

Questions to Answer

1. What is the relationship of exercise to cardiovascular and respiratory wellness for this client?
2. What were underlying factors perpetuating the tendency to overbreathing?

Session One

S—Client indicates that the area is sore. He did not ice but did reduce workout.

O—Assessment findings are consistent with previous session. No improvement is noted. This will be the first session specifically targeting the bursitis in the left elbow. General massage included integrated muscle energy and indirect funcional technique for left shoulder and elbow. Assessment and treatment of hip extension firing patterns and connective tissue methods on binding fascia of the legs.

A—Range of motion for internal rotation of left shoulder improved slightly. Firing pattern did not respond. Connective tissue bind responds best to ease/bind application of torsion forces with kneading.

P—Strongly encourage client to ice the elbow. Need to reassess the trunk and hip extension firing patterns. Massage again in 2 days.

Session Two

S—Client reports that elbow has improved and asks if it is from the massage, cortisone, or aspirin. Respond that improvement was most likely from medical treatment because it is targeted toward managing symptoms. Massage is being targeted to reversing some of the causal factors. He did ice and has not lifted with the arm. He has increased his aerobic activity with a stair stepper. His legs are sore and heavy and feel fat.

O—Legs palpate as taut. Will treat as delayed-onset muscle soreness. Trunk and hip extension firing patterns are synergistically dominant. Rectus abdominis and left lumbar erector spinae are dominant muscles. Hip abduction is also synergistically dominant on left, with quadratus lumborum firing first. Quadratus lumborum displays latent trigger point activity. Subscapularis on the left and infraspinatus on the right are short with trigger point activity in the muscle belly. Subscapularis trigger point refers pain into the anterior shoulder, which the client recognizes as an ache, which he gets occasionally. General massage involved the following: integrated muscle energy and indirect functional technique to the left shoulder and elbow; inhibitory pressure on belly of subscapularis while client moved area in and out of internal rotation; inhibitory pressure on belly of right infraspinatus with active release; indirect functional technique for the right anterior pelvic rotation; psoas release and quadratus lumborum release bilaterally, with muscle energy application and lengthening to sternocleidomastoid and scalenes; resetting of trunk and hip firing patterns; inhibitory pressure used on biceps brachii with active release and increased tension force to lengthen. Hamstrings addressed with muscle energy (contract-relax-antagonist-contract), lengthening and stretching in addition to general massage. Lymphatic drainage applied to legs.

A—Fifty percent increase in range of motion of left shoulder and elbow. Firing pattern: Hip extension responds as did hip abduction for trunk flexion, which remains synergistically dominant. Client feels less achy in general.

P—Teach client core exercises of drawing in maneuver and encourage him not to do sit-ups for awhile until core stabilizes. Massage again in 2 days.

Session Three

S—Client reports that he is still sore in his legs and now in his lower abdomen. He did do the core exercises and incorporated the draw-in maneuver during his workout on the stepper. He is surprised how hard it is to do and how much effect there is. He wants to be taught more core exercises. Elbow is improving. Caution client that improvement likely from medication and injection. He needs to continue to follow the doctor's recommendations and not use the arm. Client also reports that he did ice the elbow at least once a day.

O—Palpation indicates that bursa is less inflamed, but direct massage remains contraindicated for a few more days. Tautness in legs is less but still evident. Will need to avoid connective tissue work on fascial bind this session. Range of motion restrictions returned to left arm, but anterior rotation of pelvis is improved. Gave full-body massage, targeting shoulder rotation and aching: repeat previous session.

A—Left shoulder and elbow regained range of motion similar to last session. Trunk firing pattern is improving. Hip extension is less lumbar (erector spinae) dominant and more hamstring dominant, but gluteus maximus does fire at 15 degrees of extension, which is acceptable. Client reports that he feels pretty good and is becoming encouraged with results. He also indicates that he is sleeping better.

P—Demonstrate how client can reinforce the range of motion for the left shoulder by stretching. Did not teach any stretching for the elbow. Will introduce direct elbow work next session. Teach him draw-in maneuver with alternate arm swing. Indicate that if he is really interested in core training, he should see whether the gym had a functional core-training program such as Pilates.

Session Four

S—Client only has 30 minutes for the massage. Asks if I can concentrate directly on the left arm.

O—It has been long enough since the cortisone injection so that it is reasonable to honor the client's request. Used integrated muscle energy and contract and relax to target the short biceps brachii and subscapularis. Also performed subscapularis release and used active release on the biceps. Began connective tissue approach to the

arm and forearm. Primarily used bend and torsion, in and out of bind, while client slowly moved elbow in the midrange. Did not address the bursa specifically.

A—Noted significant improvement in range of motion.

O—Massage again in 2 days.

Session Five

S—Client reports that his whole arm was sore, but a "good" sore. Asks for the same massage today along with the rest of the body. Improvement continues. He did ice the arm and is doing better since he got a wrap that he freezes and then can wear. His legs are not sore but his abdomen is. His gym does not offer a specific core-training program, but the personal trainer will give him private lessons.

O—Lower abdomen is sore to touch and movement but appropriate. Client can isolate lower abdominal muscles without contracting the rectus abdominis. The rectus abdominis palpates as binding and rigid. There is no indication of increased inflammation on the bursa. Range of motion decreased slightly from last session but is much improved in general. Trunk firing pattern is beginning to respond to exercise. Provided full-body massage with inhibitory pressure at attachments of rectus abdominis, with bending and torsion forces to reduce rigidity in the muscle. Upper rib attachments of rectus abdominis were surprisingly tender. Repeated specific massage to the left arm same as during last session and added increased connective tissue focus to triceps tendons at the elbow. Continued to avoid direct work on the bursa area. Lengthened and stretched the internal shoulder rotators, using pulsed muscle energy. Resumed connective tissue approaches for the binding fascia on the right leg. Addressed reflex patterns in the right leg to left arm.

A—Client reports that he is beginning to feel straighter. Reassessment of gait indicates normalization of arm swing to opposite leg swing. Range of motion of elbow is almost normal. Pelvis anterior rotation is significantly reduced and remains stable.

P—Assess gait patterns next session.

Session Six

S—Client reports that he has begun sessions with personal trainer. I asked that he demonstrate core exercises he is using. Methods appear valid, although there is a tendency for the rectus abdominis to fire prematurely with one move. I suggest that he avoid that exercise, and the trainer can call me for clarification if he wishes. Arm is feeling good. He has a doctor's appointment tomorrow. He is beginning to experience some burning in the stomach from the aspirin. Suggest he talk to the pharmacist about an enteric-coated aspirin that is a bit easier on the stomach. Also reinforce icing and indicate that he ask the doctor if he could reduce the aspirin dose more to support cardiovascular function if he was diligent with icing.

O–Client is displaying general all-over improvement. Gait assessment indicates that the activation of the right hip extensors does not inhibit the left shoulder flexors. This is corrected during the massage. Client wants to hold breath during the assessment and correction. He is disturbed by the normal inhibition patterns and says he is weak and needs more exercise. Educate client on functional movement and the importance of kinetic chain and gait function. Hip extension bilaterally hamstring dominant, but gluteus maximus does fire at about 15 degrees of extension. Suspect the stepper is overtraining the hamstrings and suggest alternate aerobic activity that uses a different muscle group pattern, such as swimming, on alternate days. Gave general massage with repeat of last session: increased shear force on triceps attachment, but avoided actual bursa area.

A–Client again reports that he feels straighter and lighter. He feels just a bit off balance, which is common when gait reflexes are addressed. Had him do some cross-body movement; that is, bringing left arm to right leg and reversing in a marching pattern, and he felt more balanced after about 25 repetitions.

P–Review doctor's report with client. Suggest that appointments be reduced to twice per week because improvement is good. Also suggest that next two sessions be more general to allow the body to integrate the changes. Will continue with connective tissue application to left arm.

Session Seven

S–Client reports that the doctor is pleased with results and has okayed return to exercise with the limitations of light weights, moderate repetition, and only in the midrange of movement. The doctor also encourages swimming and core program with trainer and requests that massage

address the scar tissue directly on only the left elbow for 2 weeks to see how it responds. Doctor reduced aspirin dose but will not eliminate it since part of the effect is cardiovascular, and doctor also recommended an enteric-coated product.

O–Followed the general massage plan with an integration focus following pattern in Unit Two of this text. In addition, skin rolling and specific scar tissue release applied to the binding tissue in the left elbow.

A–Postassessment indicated warmth and redness of the tissue around the olecranon, but not specifically on the bursa. Client felt a bit sleepy and dozes off during parts of the massage. Upper chest breathing is less evident.

P–Evaluate response to specific work on left elbow. Watch for bruising. Continue with integration phase for at least one more session.

Session Eight

S–Client reports that his session with the trainer has been a good educational process. He is learning about how to balance weight training and aerobic activity (cross-training). The personal trainer's background is military and formal athletic training, although he did not complete his degree. He has a moderate approach to fitness and weight loss. The trainer reports that he notices an improvement in the client's response to eccentric-based training after the massage. The client is cautioned to not "overdo." The goal is health and fitness, not performance. Client also reports that the elbow is sore to the touch, but not like the bursitis pain. He continues to ice twice a day and has changed aspirin products. His stomach is still burning a bit but is better.

O–Provided general massage with repeat of connective tissue methods on the binding tissue of the left arm. Increased shear force on the triceps tendon and stretched both biceps brachii and triceps for a sustained time, combined with intermittent use of muscle pulsing.

A–Client felt a give, but not quite a tear sensation, in his biceps brachii. Reassessment indicates more movement of the biceps over the brachialis and increased ability to extend the elbow. The triceps assessed as strong for the first time since sessions began. The anterior aspect of the elbow is slightly red. It seems as if some adhesions separated between the muscles. Tell client this may be sore for a couple of days and to flex and extend his elbow gently in the midrange on and off for the next 3 days. Also suggested that he not weight train until the next massage to prevent increased inflammation.

P—Need to assess the left arm for increased inflammation and acute conditions.

Note: Client called next day to report that his elbow in the front is really sore to the touch and has a slight bruise. Told him to keep moving the arm gently back and forth, keep icing, and if the condition gets worse, that he should see his doctor. Explained that it appears that some tissue tore loose during last session. Typically, this is a good response if it is treated as an acute process with PRICE (protection, rest, ice, compression, elevation) and is rehabilitated. The connective tissue tearing is not uncommon when there is a history of a past injury, but it needs to be monitored carefully.

Session Nine

S—Client reports that the bruise did not get worse but it was even more sore the day after he called. He did call the doctor but was told to keep icing and resting as long as he could move it though its normal range of motion. Client reports that his range of motion is great. He now can straighten out his elbow.

O—Area around the distal attachment of biceps brachii and brachialis on the left is slightly bruised and warm to the touch. There is slight swelling. Movement of the muscle layers is improved and client can extend elbow fully. Full-body massage, including: connective tissue methods on left triceps with acute care approaches for biceps attachment area at elbow; specifically addressed left hamstring, especially distal attachments for reflex response.

A—It appears that some adhesion has worked loose, and once the healing takes place, the outcome should be positive. Client is not concerned with the soreness and is thrilled with the increase in movement.

P—Continue icing the elbow and begin movement through full range but with no weight. Teach client how to roll the tissue of his arm to support pliability during healing. Shift to subacute treatment on elbow next session and continue with full-body maintenance.

Session Ten

S—Arm is only sore to the touch, and bruising is almost gone. Client had a cardiac update

appointment with the doctor, who looked at his arm and said that he could resume moderate weight training with full use in another couple of days. Client has lost 8 pounds, and blood pressure is almost normal. Bursitis is asymptomatic, but tendency for recurrence likely exists.

O—Client's posture and gait appear normal. No heat, sweating, or goose flesh is apparent over bursa area; however, red response and mild heat remain evident around biceps and brachialis attachment on the left. Began subacute massage application to this area: shifted to maintenance massage for the rest of the body, with ongoing attention to stabilizing range of motion, firing patterns, and gait reflexes.

A—Client reports he feels good: nothing unusual.

P—Reduce massage to once-per-week preinjury schedule with ongoing attention to the left elbow area indefinitely. Continue to monitor all firing patterns and range of motion as presented in general protocol of Unit Two. Support exercise program and continue to reinforce moderation.

The Rest of the Story

This client continues to have a tendency to overdo but backs off sooner and does not push through the pain. He does best when monitored by the personal trainer. He is fortunate to have found a skilled trainer. One must check credentials for personal trainers to make sure their education and approach are valid and appropriate. Unfortunately, this is not always the case. His blood pressure fluctuates but is typically okay. He gets a massage every week.

CASE TEN

MORGAN—JOINT SPRAIN WITH UNDERLYING HYPERMOBILITY AND LAX LIGAMENT SYNDROME

Morgan is a 16-year-old female cheerleader. She has been involved in dance and gymnastics since she was 5 years old. She fell during a routine and sprained her right ankle and knee. The deltoid ligament on the lateral aspect of her right ankle received a second-degree sprain when she landed on the outside of her foot. Her leg tangled in a fellow cheerleader's leg, resulting in a grade one sprain of the lateral collateral ligament of the right knee. She was on crutches for a few days until she could bear weight on her foot. Appropriate first aid was administered, and follow-up medical care included external stabilization and passive and active movement without weight bearing to promote healing with pliable scar tissue formation. Weight bearing has been allowed for the past 5 days. It has been 10 days since the accident. The client's mother cleared the massage with her doctor, who supports the intervention to manage some of the compensation from using crutches and to promote healing of the injured area. The client complains of neck, shoulder, and low back stiffness and pain. Antiinflammatory and pain medication was used for the first 3 days and then withdrawn because these medications can slow healing. The client is generally in good health but has a history of various sprains and strains. This particular ankle was sprained last year. She also sprained her left wrist when she was 10 years old.

Assessment

Observation. The client is limping slightly. Discoloration is evident around the ankle but not the knee. The ankle still appears swollen, but the knee looks normal. The client fidgets during the interview. Her mother is concerned but not overbearing, letting the client answer most questions and adding information where pertinent. The right ankle is wrapped with an elastic support.

Interview and Goals. The history notes multiple sprain injuries and a tendency for generalized hypermobility. The client hopes to participate in a cheerleading competition in 2 months. Her mother is more realistic, thinking it will be at least 3 months before the ankle is strong enough for competition. The client complains of being stiff all over. No unusually pertinent information is indicated on the history form.

The client's goals for the massage are to support healing of the injured ankle and knee, reduce the general stiffness, and reverse the compensation from limping and the crutches.

Physical Assessment

Posture: Client is not fully weight bearing on the injured leg. Her posture is very good except for a slight lordosis and hyperextension of her knees, which is common in gymnasts.

Gait: Limited by limping, pain, and sense of instability

Range of motion: Client is generally hypermobile, most likely because of training effects from dance training, gymnastics, and cheerleading.

Palpation

Near touch: Heat is detected at ankle and knee injury sites and in the shoulders.

Skin surface: Drag and dampness are present in areas of heat. Bruising surrounds area of ankle injury.

Skin: Smooth and pliable

Skin and superficial connective tissue: No areas of bind noted

Superficial connective tissue: Connective tissue is resilient. Localized swelling remains at lateral right ankle.

Vessels and lymph nodes: Normal

Muscles: Muscles feel elastic but generally shorter in the belly, especially the calves, hamstrings, and adductors. Trigger point activity is evident in the belly of the adductors, hamstrings, and quadriceps in the injured leg. Supraspinatus, upper trapezius, and pectoralis major and pectoralis minor are short bilaterally, with tenderness in the axillas where the crutches contact. Psoas is short bilaterally. Muscles of the right leg have increased tone, most likely because of normal guarding of the injured joints. Quadratus lumborum and the gluteal group on the left are tender to moderate pressure. A very tender area near the musculotendinous junction of the lateral head of the right gastrocnemius palpates like a grade one muscle tear.

Tendons: Tendons in the muscles of the right leg are tender to moderate pressure.

Fascial sheaths: Resilient but seem too long

Ligaments: Generally loose

Joints: End-feel is not identified until joints are in hyperextension. Increased joint play is noted in major mobility joints.

Bones: Normal

Abdominal viscera: Normal

Body rhythms: Normal

Muscle Testing

Strength and neurologic balance: Muscles test normal except for those guarding the injured knee and ankle, which is expected. These muscles are displaying increased tone and are not inhibited as expected. Left quadratus lumborum is firing before tensor fasciae latae and gluteus medius.

Gait: Disrupted by limping and crutches. Flexor patterns in the arms are facilitating together instead of following contralateral patterns. Flexors and extensors of the left leg do not inhibit when tested against the arms.

Interpretation and Treatment Plan Development

Clinical Reasoning. Ligament sprains and muscle strains are common injuries and are diagnosed as slight (first-degree), moderate (second-degree), or severe (third-degree). When a joint is sprained, it is common to have strain in the muscles that are extended during the injury. Protective spasms around the tear (tiny microtears to more severe tears) act to approximate (bring torn fibers together to support healing), protect, and guard the area. In general, all the muscles that surround the joint increase in tone to stabilize and reduce movement. This should dissipate as the injury heals but can become chronic, limiting range of motion of the area. It is important not to stretch muscles that are torn in the acute and early subacute phase of healing. Protective spasm (guarding) is intense and painful in first- and second-degree tears. If there is a total breach of a muscle or tendon, there may be little pain. First- and second-degree injuries are more painful and have a greater tendency for swelling than a third-degree injury.

Ligaments begin repair immediately, and the inflammatory response is an important part of this process. Some inflammatory mediators are vasodilators, which help blood reach ligaments. This is important because ligaments do not have a good blood supply. Muscle tears (strains) heal much easier because of the high vascular component of the tissue. It takes 3 to 6 months or longer for a grade two sprain to heal fully. Repeated injury contributes to ligament laxity and joint instability.

Sprains are common in persons with joint hypermobility. The hypermobility can occur in only one joint that has a recurring injury or can be more general, appearing in most joints of the body. Some disorders (e.g., Marfan syndrome) are characterized by lax connective tissue. Most ligament laxity is functional, such as an increased range of motion required in many sports or dance activities. Once the plastic range of a ligament has been increased, it does not return to the previous range, but remains long and lax. Joint play is increased, and instability results.

The client fits this profile. She will likely remain hypermobile, with increased compensating muscle tone to provide stability. This situation leads to general stiffness, especially if activity is reduced. Depending on the degree of laxity, the client may find that stretching does not reduce muscle tightness, because joint end-feel and longitudinal tensile force do not occur until the joint is hyperextended or reaches an anatomic barrier.

The client's gait changes seem to arise from the use of crutches. Because the injury is recent and the crutches are no longer used, gait dysfunction should reverse easily with massage and general activity.

The low back pain may stem from a dermatome distribution, referring back from the knee combined with posture changes from limping and the use of crutches. The tendency for low back pain may exist because the client's psoas muscles are short.

Interventions
1. Massage can support the healing process in the acute, subacute, and final healing stages by increasing circulation to the area, maintaining normal and appropriate muscle tone, and supporting mobile scar formation.
2. Referral for diagnosis of the suspected muscle strain is recommended.
3. Referral to a physical therapist or exercise physiologist for a sequential strengthening program for the vulnerable joints is indicated.

Massage intervention would need to be long-term to meet the client's goals, with an incremental treatment plan for the current acute and subacute healing stages.

Cost and time are factors, and the mother or father needs to be with the client during each massage because she is a minor.

The client has unrealistic healing expectations and likely will be frustrated with a 6-month intervention plan.

Decision Making and Treatment Plan Development
Quantitative Goals
1. Reduce generalized stiffness by 75%.
2. Reverse compensation from use of crutches.
3. Support circulation and mobile scar formation in injured areas.

Qualitative Goals. The client will be able to resume normal daily activities, but not sports activity, in 2 weeks and can resume limited cheerleading activities within 6 weeks, and full use of the area in 6 months.

Treatment Regimen
Condition Management/Therapeutic Change. Condition management consists of two phases. Therapeutic change is phase three.
- *Phase one: early subacute–current.* One-hour massage will be provided 3 times for the first week. Full-body massage will be used to support

circulation and reverse the muscle tension in the shoulders and chest caused by the use of crutches. Specific application of gliding will be used along the sprained ligament and associated strained tendons in the fiber direction of the muscle and toward the injury to help align the scar tissue. Lymphatic drainage in the swollen areas will support healing. Passive range of motion with rocking and gentle shaking to all adjacent joints will encourage mobility and healing in the injured areas.

Ongoing ice application will encourage circulation as a secondary effect of the cold. The injured areas would benefit from ice application for 20 minutes, 2 or 3 times a day.

Questions that need to be answered are the following:

1. What are the performance demands of dance, gymnastics, and cheerleading?
2. What are the current treatments for joint laxity?
3. Is age a factor in joint laxity?

Session One

One-hour massage following treatment plan for phase one

Session Two

One-hour massage following treatment plan for phase one

Session Three

One-hour massage following treatment plan for phase one

Reassessment. Client reports that she does not have the shoulder aching but her low back still aches. Generally she feels less stiff. Client can bear weight on the injured ankle with no pain, but experiences pain if she rotates the ankle. The knee remains tender to medium pressure but does not feel unstable when walking. The client's physician does not feel that there is a tear in the gastrocnemius.

- *Phase two: subacute phase to remodeling.* Ice applications will be valuable for 1 or 2 more weeks. Massage applications will be provided for full-body sessions, twice a week for 4 weeks. Very gentle gliding across the fiber configuration of the tissue will support mobile scar formation. The intensity of gliding and cross-fiber friction on the injured tissues gradually will increase as healing continues. Trigger points and general tone in the muscles that are guarding will be addressed with muscle energy methods, length-

ening, and broad-based compression. Kneading can restore the pliability of the connective tissue ground substance. The area of the gastrocnemius will be treated with caution because it remains tender even through the doctor did not think it was strained. No deep pressure will be used, but localized stroking across the grain of the muscle can support mobile scar formation. Because self-stretching is not effective without moving into hyperextension patterns, the client's muscle tissue can be stretched and lengthened manually during massage with compression and kneading that introduce bending and torsion forces into the soft tissue. The psoas muscles can be lengthened with muscle energy methods and psoas release. Core training is encouraged. Hypermobility is the main issue, and although massage can manage the symptom of muscle stiffness, the reason for the conditions is the body's attempt to provide stability. The client really needs a comprehensive therapetuic exercise program. Massage will proceed with caution to minimize discomfort but not reduce stability.

Session Four

Notes: Client reports no new conditions and is feeling better in general. Massage is given following phase two treatment plan.

Session Five

Notes: Client is just beginning menstrual cycle. Massage follows phase two treatment plan with more emphisis on lymphatic drainage and no psoas release.

Session Six

Notes: Client is just ending menstrual cycle. Resume phase two treatment plan, no psoas release, but use muscle energy and stretching to address the achy low back.

Session Seven

Nothing new to report. Continue with massage as outlined in treatment plan for phase two. Performed psoas release.

Session Eight

Notes: Client is doing well. Continue with treatment plan for phase two.

Session Nine

Notes: Last session for phase two. Will reasess next session and begin phase three.

Reassessment. Regarding posture, client is fully weight bearing on the injured leg but not participating in sport activity. Lordosis and hyperextension of her knees remain, but achy low back has improved. Gait is no longer limited by limping, pain, and sense of instability.

Client is generally hypermobile, which seems to be the underlying cause of injury potential. Massage is not the best modality for reversing this conditon; that is, massage is excellent for helping short and tight structures become longer. Massage is also excellent for helping taut, dense structures become more pliable, but massage is not particularly effective in addressing long, lax structures. Client needs some sort of therapeutic exercise program with massage as the secondary modality.

Trigger point activity continues to occur in the the belly of the adductors, hamstrings, and quadriceps in the injured leg. This recurrence is likely a stabilizing function. Psoas is short bilaterally. Point tenderness is absent or substantually reduced bodywide after massage, but within a week, the postural muscles are again short.

Connective tissue structures are resilient but seem too long with most ligaments being lax.

No change occurs in end-feel, which is not identified until joint is in hyperextension. Increased joint play continues to occur in major mobility joints. Firing patterns are normal. Gait reflex is normal.

- *Phase three: therapeutic change.* Six months of weekly full-body massage will be provided. Once healing of the injury is complete, the underlying hypermobility can be addressed. Systematic frictioning can be applied to lax ligaments to introduce therapeutic inflammation and encourage increased connective tissue fiber formation. This will be applied to the injured lateral collateral ligament and deltoid ligament, as well as the rest of the connective tissue stabilizing units of the ankle and knee. This needs to be done in small increments, and the area should not be excessively painful the next day. Pain to the touch with moderate pressure is appropriate, but there should not be pain with movement. This is a painful intervention and needs to be done frequently. Teaching a family member to perform the technique is appropriate. Antiinflammatory drugs should not be used, nor should ice be applied to the area, because the goal is creation of controlled inflammation to encourage collagen formation. Full-body

massage with direct tissue stretching should continue. At the end of the 6-month period, the frequency of massage intervention could be reduced to a maintenance schedule of every other week. The client will be encouraged to maintain a strengthening and stretching program and to reduce exaggerated joint movements to support restabilizing of the joints.

Session Ten
Begin phase three. Client is resistant to frictioning, and the compliance potential is not good. Resume general maintenance massage to support a therapeutic exercise program. Teach ankle stability activity, that is, standing on one foot and drawing the alphabet with toes.

The Rest of the Story
Clients with this condition are difficult to treat with therapeutic massage. Massage is great for lengthening short tissue but not good at shortening long tissue. Hypermobility results in stiffness only because the muscles are trying to stabilize the structure. Massage is difficult, because as soon as the muscle relaxes a bit, the client has increased instability. Massage is much better in a support role to manage the symptoms of the appropriate therapeutic exercise program. Using frictioning to create incremental inflammation is painful, tedious, and usually not tolerated well unless the area is small. This client struggled because the strengthening activities reduced her flexibility a bit, interfering with her performance. Because she was so performance driven, she did not maintain the strengthening program but did continue with weekly massage. She continued to sprain the same ankle over and over and eventually tore her anterior cruciate ligament.

CASE ELEVEN
SAM—OSTEOARTHRITIS
The client is a 67-year-old man with osteoarthritis in both knees. The left knee is more painful. In the future he may undergo joint replacement surgery, but for now he is exploring any methods that will allow him to remain active. Currently, he enjoys golf and racquetball. He does not want to use a golf cart because he enjoys the walking and knows he needs the exercise. He plays racquetball for an hour on Tuesdays and Saturdays, but really suffers with knee pain during in-between times. His condition

is worst at his early morning Sunday golf game. Initially, he is stiff, which interferes with his golf swing, but he warms up as time goes on.

He uses topical capsicum cream and takes aspirin for the arthritis and for a cardiac condition. Because of the heart issue, he needs to stay active and keep his weight down. He is currently 20 pounds over what his doctors would like him to weigh. The extra weight bothers his knees. He thinks that he has gained some of the weight because the knee pain has slowed him down. He has always been active and has a history of participating in high school and college sports. He ran track and played basketball. During this time, he had various minor to moderate injuries, including knee trauma. In his words, "I would just tough it out and play anyway." To compound the issue, he was in a car accident when he was 36 and broke his left ankle. He also spent 12 years in the U.S. Marine Corps as a sergeant. He has never had massage and has the support of his physicians. He is a sales manager, is financially stable, and has a flexible schedule. Admittedly, he is skeptical about massage. He says he is not one to be fussed over and just wants the job done.

Assessment

Observation. The client is tall, 6 feet, 4 inches. He has long legs, a short torso, broad shoulders, and a bit of a pot belly. His center of gravity is high, which would place strain on the knees. He carries himself like a Marine. He is loud and gruff but seems kind underneath the facade. He seems a bit nervous about massage therapy. His shoulders move when he breathes.

Interview and Goals. The client says he aches all over but that he has lived hard and should expect to be creaky. The joint pain is worse in the morning, gets better as he moves around, and then gets worse again. He has had various and numerous joint injuries and soft tissue trauma. Four years ago his blood pressure rose, and he had angioplasty to unclog two coronary arteries. He takes aspirin to keep his blood thin and to manage the arthritis. He indicates that he does not seem to bruise easily. He was taking blood pressure medication but did not like the sexual side effects and insisted he go off it. The doctor agreed as long as the client could keep his blood pressure down with diet and exercise. He has done a good job of this. Nothing else of concern is indicated on the history form. He used

to smoke but quit 10 years ago. He used to drink heavily, but now drinks only some red wine. His sleep is restless because his knees ache. Heat application helps.

The client's goal for the massage is management of his knee pain.

Physical Assessment

Posture: Overall, client has decent postural symmetry. Cervical curve is flat. Left foot is a bit flat. Ribs are held tight and rigid.
Gait: Client walks stiffly, with reduced knee flexion and extension.
Range of motion: Range of motion in most jointed areas is in the acceptable range for daily activities, but stiff and resisting for any exercise. The left ankle is moderately restricted in eversion and inversion.

Palpation

Near touch: Heat is noted at knees and between scapulas.
Skin surface: Rough
Skin: Evidence of many traumas; various scars in many body areas
Skin and superficial connective tissue: Binding almost everywhere, with edema at the knees
Superficial connective tissue: Reduced pliability bodywide–almost an armorlike feel, with edema at the knees
Vessels and lymph nodes: Seem normal, but ability to palpate is restricted by tissue density
Muscles: Well-developed but dense and inflexible. Trigger point activity is evident in quadriceps and gluteal muscles. Muscles that surround the knees have increased tone and isometric contraction in antagonist and agonist patterns. Apparently these muscles are attempting to guard the knee joints.
Tendons: Tender to moderate pressure around the knees and scapular attachment
Fascial sheaths: Thick and inflexible
Ligaments: Mild laxity at injured ankle and knees
Joints: Most are within the normal range of motion, but crepitus is common, as is a tendency for leathery or hard end-feel. Knees hurt with compression and traction. Most other joints show resistance to traction, indicating binding. Client indicates that most joints are stiff, but not painful. Most of the pain is in the knees.
Bones: Increased bony development around area of ankle break. Bump noted in right clavicle (client

had forgotten he had broken it falling out of a tree when he was a child).

Abdominal viscera: Difficult to palpate because of internal abdominal fat distribution

Body rhythms: Strong and fast. Client breathes with his chest but does not necessarily display breathing pattern disorder symptoms other than talking loudly and mild evidence of sympathetic arousal. Pulses are even.

Muscle Testing

Strength: Client pushes hard against resistance and finds it difficult to use 50% effort. No areas of weakness are noted. The client was unable to isolate a muscle pattern and continually recruited and contracted muscles in areas other than the test area during assessment.

Neurologic balance: Antagonist balance at knees is lost. All muscles around joint display a tendency for isometric co-contraction with uneven pull on the knee joint. Synergistic dominance is noted with knee firing patterns.

Gait: Leg muscles do not inhibit as they should against arm activation. Eye reflex patterns do not inhibit movement (phasic) muscles when appropriate. Hip extension and abduction firing patterns are activating together instead of in normal sequence.

Interpretation and Treatment Plan Development

Clinical Reasoning. Osteoarthritis is common and has multiple causal factors. A genetic tendency toward the development of this condition exists. The most common cause is wear and tear on the joint structure, in addition to past trauma and increased weight. The pain is caused by irritation of the synovial membrane and joint capsule and by muscle spasm attempts to guard the area. There is no cure, but management to increase the quality of life is possible. Joint replacement surgery is a last option, and advances in technology have improved outcomes greatly. Muscle spasm usually occurs in all the muscles that cross the joint. Because flexors, adductors, and internal rotators have more mass, when tone increases, the pull is greater from these muscles than from the extensors, abductors, and external rotators. The bone fit at the joint can be pulled out of alignment, creating further irritation in the joint capsule. Also, muscles that cross the joint pull the joint space together. This, coupled with weight bearing at the hips, knees, and ankles, reduces the joint space and increases the

potential for rubbing of the bony structures, increasing the inflammation, swelling, and pain. Arthritic joints are often unstable and have a lax ligament structure. Because the client's knees are affected (closed kinetic chain-hip/knee/ankle), disruption of the knees affects the hips and ankles.

Management includes easing mechanical strain on the knee joint by normalizing the muscle tone without decreasing stability and resourceful muscle guarding. Corresponding muscle shortening and weakening in the hips and ankles need to be addressed. Lymphatic drainage–type methods work well if the fluid is outside the capsule. Edema can increase stiffness and reduce range of motion. Sometimes needle aspiration is necessary if excess fluid builds up inside the capsule. Some increase in synovial fluid in the capsule can be beneficial because an increase in hydrostatic pressure can separate the bone surfaces, easing the rubbing. Correcting posture deviation that contributes to the joint irritation may be possible in younger clients, but in older clients, especially after 75 years of age, this becomes more difficult. Pain management is supported with counterirritation and hyperstimulation analgesia applications, a reduction in sympathetic arousal, and an increase in the pain-modulating chemicals in the system, such as endorphins and enkephalins. The joints must be kept moving, or the condition will worsen. Massage that incorporates passive and active joint movement is supportive for pain management, allowing the client to move with less pain. Joint tractioning can offer temporary relief. Application of hot and cold hydrotherapy to manage pain and encourage circulation is appropriate. Cold is the most effective and can be applied after activity, and heat can be used to warm up before activity or as a counterirritation at night to promote sleep if necessary. Counterirritant ointments would provide symptom management.

This client has a history and posture that give strong indications of the development of osteoarthritis. His body type of long legs with upper body mass strains the knees in general. In addition, he has used his body hard for a long time.

The client is still relatively young and in good health. He is motivated to change, as indicated by his previous diet and exercise alterations. The knee joints and left ankle are likely damaged beyond regeneration.

The following are options for this client:

1. Massage can be beneficial for management of pain, stiffness, and muscle spasm. Also, deterioration may be slowed, prolonging the time before replacement surgery is required. Generally, increasing tissue pliability and circulation, combined with management of sympathetic arousal, could help this client. Short-term symptomatic pain relief or pain reduction is a reasonable expectation, but the massage effects will wear off, and an ongoing appointment schedule is needed.
2. Racquetball may not be the best activity, because the constant running in different directions in short bursts, and the starting and stopping, are hard on the knees. Swimming could be an option.
3. Gradual introduction of a conservative flexibility program would be helpful.

The recreational center where the client plays racquetball has a swimming pool; therefore access is convenient. Swimming does not meet the client's desire for competition. He may try anyway but will not commit. A senior yoga class is available at the recreation center as well. Yoga does not thrill the client, but he is willing to try as long as the class is not full of "old fogies." Massage is available at the same recreation center for convenience. Cost and scheduling are not primary concerns.

Massage has a good likelihood of successful management of his condition as long as the client has regular appointments and realizes that this is a long-term care program. Cardiac medication may alter the amount of pressure tolerated by the client. Regular reports should be sent to his doctor.

He is willing to play less racquetball and more golf, but says golf does not make him sweat like racquetball, and he needs something to make him sweat.

Patience is necessary for everyone: the progress from the massage most likely will be slow, and the effectiveness wears off. The massage therapist needs to realize that under the gruffness is likely an individual who is vulnerable. Awareness and respect of boundary issues are necessary to keep the client empowered.

Decision Making and Treatment Plan Development
Quantitative Goal
1. Reduce sensation of stiffness and pain by 50% as long as regular appointments are scheduled.

Qualitative Goals. The client will be able to participate in moderate low-impact sports exercise activities without being hindered by arthritic pain and joint stiffness.

Treatment Regimen
A long-term massage program is required with an initial schedule of twice a week right after racquetball. This will help reduce some of the strain on the client's knees from racquetball. Because of the client's size and the complex application of massage, 1½-hour sessions are needed. The cost is $70 per session. The appointment schedule will be reduced to weekly as soon as improvement is noted and the client's condition stabilizes.

Full-body massage with multiple goals is needed. The fibrotic and binding connective tissue structure noticed bodywide will need to be addressed systematically but slowly. The focus is to increase the pliability of the ground substance to reduce muscle density and fascial shortening and maintain more flexibility of the body. Effective methods could be myofascial release plus broad-based application of compression with the forearm, and possibly the knee and foot, against the tissue to compress the soft tissue and carry it away from the bone, with the client actively moving the adjacent joint. Side-lying positioning for the legs and working on a floor mat would facilitate this type of application.

The client will likely require varying degrees of pressure and depth of application. The sensation should be on the edge of "good hurt," sufficient to trigger endorphin and serotonin release but not enough to elicit guarding or bracing. Caution for bruising is indicated because of the aspirin. Gliding with drag can stretch the soft tissue. Until the client's muscle tone normalizes, use of active resistance for muscle energy methods may be counterproductive. Direct manipulation of the spindle cell and tendon responses, or having the client make circles with his eyes and head to initiate muscle facilitation and inhibition in the limbs, is likely to be more effective. Kneading can introduce shear, bending, and torsion forces to increase ground substance viscosity, especially around all the scars. The client must drink water so that the connective tissue rehydrates.

The knees can be a primary focus after muscle tone normalizes a bit. The trigger point activity can be addressed, specifically the ones in the quadriceps and gastrocnemius that refer pain into the knees. Traction of the knees can separate joint surfaces temporarily. Surface edema can be moved with lymphatic drainage.

Application of ice between massage sessions will be encouraged.

Questions that need to be answered are the following:

1. What is the process of knee joint replacement?
2. What are the performance demands for golf and racquetball?
3. What is the procedure for using artificial joint lubrication?
4. What are the current treatments for osteoarthritis?

Sessions One to Ten

Massage basically followed the general protocol in this textbook with additional focus on strategies for pain management, managing arthritis, and strategies specific for knees. The sessions changed little from week to week, and his condition really did not improve but did seem to deteriorate more slowly. He was more comfortable if he received massage twice a week. On the rare occasions he missed a session, he could really notice a difference in his stiffness, aching, and mood.

The Rest of the Story

The condition stabilized eventually, except for continued deterioration of the knees. Massage provided enough short-term relief that the client thus far avoided knee replacement but has had the injections of the artificial synovial fluid with moderately successful results. His general stiffness and aching improved moderately. This client became a massage devotee. Luckily finances were not an issue, and he continues with two sessions a week because he was not able to reduce sessions to once a week and remain comfortable. As of this writing, this client is doing well. He has retired but not slowed down much and is still a crusty old Marine with a great big heart. He has been an active supporter of massage for Special Olympics. He also has supported massage at the local Veterans Administration hospital.

CASE TWELVE

JULIA—MARATHON RUNNER

The client is a 22-year-old woman who is a competitive marathon runner. She is currently training for a marathon. She is determined to commit herself to the best performance possible. As an amateur athlete, she coordinates her own training program. She works with a running coach. She had a first-degree ankle sprain 2 years ago, experiences

generalized cramping if she overtrains, and had one experience of shin splints. These symptoms improve if she drinks enough water or sports drinks and stretches. She occasionally gets side stitches. She is a student of the sport and is constantly studying the effects of diet and training protocols to enhance her performance. She is interested in incorporating massage into her program to support recovery and flexibility and to reduce the potential for injury.

Four years ago she lost her left leg below the knee in an automobile accident. She has rehabilitated successfully and has been fitted with a running prosthesis, as well as a prosthesis for general use. She is on a mission to prove to herself and others that she can accomplish this task.

She is a college student, studying exercise science and athletic training. Finances are secure as a result of an insurance settlement from the accident. She has determined that she can afford $150 per month to pay for massage and wants the maximum benefit from the investment.

Assessment

Observation. The client is a slim, muscular, fit woman. Unless she is observed carefully, there is little evidence of the amputation. The client does not attempt to conceal the prosthesis and speaks freely about the accident. She is more concerned about total body performance than the loss of the leg.

Interview and Goals. The client information form indicates minor muscle pain related to training. She experiences mild episodes of phantom pain, usually in response to an increase in training. The pain is managed with rest, massage of the stump, and stretching. Her calf gets tight, she had shin splints in her right leg 8 months ago, and she sprained her right ankle 2 years ago.

She has occasional fatigue and restless sleep if she overtrains or experiences the phantom pain. She has athlete's foot and currently is being treated for that. She takes performance-based supplements that are a well-balanced formula.

The client's goal for massage is support for a training regimen to enhance performance and help prevent injury.

Physical Assessment

Posture: Symmetrical except for highly developed thigh muscles, with increased development on the left and a slightly elevated iliac crest on the left.

Gait: Normal with the prosthesis except for increased arm swing on the right. She indicates that she has experienced extensive rehabilitation to support normal gait after the amputation.

Range of motion: Normal

Palpation

Skin surface: Damp areas are noted at amputation site and on medial calf on the right. There are no areas of inflammation, abrasion, or skin irritation from the prosthesis.

Skin: Smooth and resilient; small area of bind is noted just under right clavicle in the chest.

Skin and superficial connective tissue: Normal

Superficial connective tissue: Small bind and increased tissue density in legs

Vessels and lymph nodes: Normal

Muscles: Normal with hypertrophy in legs. Decreased pliability with slight increase in density and shortening of hamstrings. Tenderness and pain radiate to three areas on stump, two in vastus lateralis, and one in vastus medialis, indicating trigger point activity.

Tendons: Normal except for some shortening in right Achilles tendon

Fascial sheaths: Plantar fascia is slightly short on the right.

Ligaments: Normal

Joints: No evidence of inappropriate end-feel or bind. Slight decrease in dorsiflexion on the right.

Bones: Normal

Abdominal viscera: Normal

Body rhythms: Normal

Muscle Testing

Strength: Normal

Neurologic balance: Normal

Gait: Higher degrees of facilitation between extensors and flexors on right arm and left leg seems appropriate compensation for amputation.

Interpretation and Treatment Plan Development

An understanding of the basic physical concepts involved in exercise and training protocols is important to a massage professional who works with athletes in conditioning, performance enhancement, and injury rehabilitation. To increase a sustainable power output, the athlete must follow a carefully designed training program that will improve the individual's ability to (1) produce metabolic energy by aerobic and anaerobic means; (2) sustain aerobic energy production at high levels before lactic acid accumulates excessively in the blood; (3) recruit more of the efficient slow-twitch muscle fibers in muscle groups used in competition; and (4) become more skillful by recruiting fewer nonessential muscle fibers during competition. Running a marathon requires more than 10,000 repetitions of the running steps and a continuous supply of energy via metabolic mechanisms dependent on the availability of oxygen (aerobic metabolism).

The athlete should get adequate rest—7 to 8 hours of sleep per day. A nap is beneficial.

The athlete should allow 24 hours between exhaustive training sessions to allow for total replenishment of depleted glycogen stores in the muscles before the next training session. Otherwise, the quality of the next training session may be compromised because the athlete's muscles will be depleted easily of one of their main fuels. In addition, training intensity and duration should be reduced gradually during the week before a competitive event so that the athlete's energy reserves are fully loaded before competition.

Shin splints, side stitches, plantar fasciitis, muscle cramps, muscle strains, dehydration, and hyponatremia can quickly make running a painful experience.

Cramping of the abdomen or side is called a side stitch. Several theories attempt to explain what causes this pain: a spasm or cramp in the diaphragm muscle, diminished blood flow as a result of excessive muscle contraction and dehydration, and/or micronutrient imbalances. As with shin splints, the best preventive measures are to stretch and increase flexibility and also to drink plenty of fluids, such as diluted (50% water) sports drinks. One way to ease the pain is to ease the running pace. When the cramping begins, the athlete should slow down and place the arms above the head until the pain subsides.

Recovery is the process the athlete goes through to return to a state of performance readiness. Recovery involves a restoration of nutrient and energy stores, a return to normal physiologic function, a reduction of muscle soreness, and the disappearance of the psychological symptoms associated with extreme fatigue (irritability, disorientation, inability to concentrate). In training, this allows the quality of the workout to be maintained while minimizing the risk of chronic fatigue, illness, and injury. In competition, it means being able to take part in the next round or event and to perform at the same or at a higher level.

The client is in good physical condition, with minor changes that seem appropriate compensation for amputation and use of the prosthesis.

Trigger point activity in the leg with the amputation may be causing the phantom pain. An aggressive training program may be contributing to fatigue and muscle aching.

Massage is indicated for support of sports training programs. Massage can facilitate fluid exchange in the muscles, manage symptoms of delayed-onset muscle soreness, and maintain appropriate pliability in soft tissue structures. Massage can help reduce trigger point activity in the client's left leg, support restful sleep, and encourage well-being.

Quantitative Goals

1. Reduce episodes of phantom pain by 50%.
2. Reduce postexercise aching by 50%.
3. Increase sleep effectiveness to support recovery time.

Qualitative Goals. Client should be able to participate in training program with minimal discomfort.

The massage will be a performance-based, full-body application and will be structured to meet the daily needs of the training regimen. Frequency is once per week with additional sessions if necessary. The massage will support rather than seek to change compensation patterns in gait in response to the amputation because overall posture and performance are good.

Trigger points will be addressed with a variety of methods, and the results will be monitored to see if the phantom pain episodes decrease. The massage will be scheduled in the evening, so the client can go to bed afterward. Sleep will be supported through encouragement of parasympathetic activation.

Appropriate methods that affect the neuromuscular/connective tissue and fluid dynamics of the body will be chosen each session. The client requires various levels of pressure, from very light pressure for lymphatic drainage to deep pressure to address the muscles of stabilization in the layer closest to the bone. The therapist will take care not to increase inflammation in any area. Client will inform the massage therapist what she wants each session. Ongoing extensive assessent is not necessary because the client knows her body and will determine what she needs.

Questions that need to be answered are the following:

1. What are the performance demands of running a marathon?
2. What are the various prostheses for below-the-knee amputation?
3. What are the rehabilitation processes for the amputation?

Session One

S—Client requests general recovery massage—no specific intervention.

O—Full-body massage is given as presented in Unit Two.

A—Client indicates she is fine and will be able to provide more information next session.

P—Session in week two: recovery based

Session Two

S—Client reports that she was satisfied with the results of the massage as provided last week. She would like a bit more attention to her foot; otherwise, repeat the session.

O—Full-body massage is given with increased attention on foot.

A—Client reports she has seen results with the massage.

P—Session in week three: recovery based

Session Three

S—Client reports that she had a difficult night with some phantom pain. Requests that the stump be assessed and treated for trigger point activity or other causal factors.

O—Observation identifies an area on the stump that is warm and a bit discolored like a bruise. Client informs that there seemed to be a fit problem with her prosthesis and she will be getting it checked. Only provide general massage to area because mechanical irritation is likely a causal factor. Used full-body massage: recovery based, with lymphatic drainage on the irritated area of the stump.

A—Client reports that she feels fine.

P—Session next week. Remember to question about the cause of the phantom pain and tissue irritation.

Session Four

S—Client reports that the prosthesis needs some minor fit adjustments. She has had only minor discomfort that is getting better. She requests same massage as previous sessions.

O—Full-body massage: recovery based

A—Client had minor firing pattern issue in shoulders that was corrected easily. Client indicated that she noticed freer shoulder movement.

P—Session next week

Session Five

S—Client requests recovery massage with attention to some aching of her knees and requests additional attention in this area.

O—Vastus lateralis is observably dominant during knee extension. General full-body massage is given with addition of strategies for knees, especially inhibition of vastus lateralis and to encourage appropriate vastus medialis obliquus firing.

A—Firing pattern normalized. Client reports that she is pleased thus far with the massage.

P—Session next week

Session Six

S—Client reports that all is fine. Requests full-body recovery massage.

O—Full-body massage given with focus on recovery.

A—Nothing unusual. Client reports usual results.

P—Session next week

Session Seven

S—Client reports some difficulty with stamina. Requests that her breathing be assessed.

O—Upper chest breathing evident. Shoulder firing is synergistically dominant. General full-body massage with additional strategies for breathing pattern dysfunction. Identified trigger point activity in the serratus anterior. Client could not identify what would have caused the situation.

A—Breathing has improved to normal. Client pleased with results.

P—Reassess breathing. Session next week.

Session Eight

S—Client recalls that she carried some heavy boxes the week before and believes that is what contributed to the breathing problem. She has had no further difficulty. Requests full-body restorative massage.

O—Full-body massage

A—Client falls asleep during massage. She gets up and goes right to bed.

P—Session next week

Session Nine

S—Client reports that she has been overtraining a bit and has reduced training intensity. She requests a general relaxation-based massage.

O—General nonspecific massage

A—Client falls asleep during massage. She gets up and goes to bed.

P—Usual session next week

Session Ten

S—Client has a mild upper respiratory infection. Requests a bit more attention to sinus congestion and relaxation.

O—General massage is given with attention to headache pain. Did specifically address posterior serratus inferior bilaterally because client has been sniffing and coughing.

A—Client is tired and wants to go to bed.

P—Massage next week

The Rest of the Story

This case is typical. The general protocol is used week after week with minor adjustments. The massage benefits are achieved from maintenance and recovery support. This client finished school, continues to run, and receives massage each week. She knows what she wants and expects to get it, regardless of who the massage therapist is.

CAREER OPPORTUNITIES

Now that you have studied all the information in this text and integrated the information into focused massage application presented in the case study examples, what are you going to do with it?

1. Remember there really is not anything special about "sports massage." Therefore these skills, used to help all of your clients, should improve outcomes.

2. Remember that the context of this text is targeted to anyone who is involved in physical activity. Tendonitis in a truck driver, data processor, and professional golfer is still tendonitis.

Career opportunities using this information include physical therapy, orthopedic medicine, occupational rehabilitation, cardiac care, weight management, and sport-specific application.

The general practice massage therapist can incorporate these methods with clients seeking wellness and fitness, which would include exercise. Fitness facilities would be interested in a massage therapist with these skills. High school, collegiate, amateur, and professional athletes also would be interested. Most "athletes" are weekend warriors and recreational participants, not professionals.

The more "elite" the athlete, the more difficult the process for career development. If working with the professional or an Olympic athlete is your goal, then be prepared to have a high level of persistence and commitment. The first question I would ask you is, "Why do you want to do this?" Status is a nonissue because you should not discuss clients and therefore no one would know you work with someone famous.

- It is absolutely unethical to be a superfan or groupie.
- Money: You really do not make enough money to justify the time, flexibility, and often the challenging circumstances.

Let me share why I work with this population:

1. They need help.
2. They are nice people.
3. They challenge my skills and keep me fresh and learning.
4. They keep me young in spirit.
5. They are really good learning subjects for my students.
6. They helped me write this book.
7. They are ambassadors for the acceptance of massage by the general public.
8. I am comfortable with athletes and have enough status of my own and do not have the need to use theirs by association.
9. I enjoy the intensity of the professional relationship.

Once you really understand your motivation, then you can pursue the clients. Most elite athletes find their massage therapist by referral from fellow players, coaches, or trainers. To get on the inside track is not easy. It is hard for me even to tell you how to get there because I did not seek the athletes, they found me. I am very good at therapeutic massage, have a respected reputation, and have worked hard for many years to gain that respect and experience. What are your strengths? What more do you need to learn and practice?

You really have to be good at massage. That is the first step. I suggest you get hands-on experience: at least 3 to 5 years of focused work before even considering working with elite athletes. A chi-

ropractor or sports medicine clinic; high school and collegiate athletes; corporate ball teams; and recreational volleyball, soccer, and bowling leagues are great places for gaining the experience. Working at a gym, golf course, or fitness-focused resort will help you refine your skills. Also target local dance studios, musicians, or other entertainers. Second, it helps to know somebody. Fair or not, it is about who you know. Even if every professional team hired a massage therapist, that would be just a few hundred positions. If you are persistent, become very skilled, and this is truly the path of service for you, then it is likely that you will meet someone who knows someone who will help you make the connection.

The twelve cases in this unit provide models for how to think through each massage session. They also provide a realistic portrayal of what it is like to work with this type of population. The cases describe cardiovascular rehabilitation and maintenance, weight loss, general wear and tear, training support, performance support, recovery, and different ages and genders. It seems possible to write cases like this forever, but other than providing a model for you, they will not address the clients with whom you will work.

The individual cases also present various professional/business practice concepts. The various massage therapists worked in fitness centers, with a team; independently with close communication with the athletic trainer, doctor, or physical therapist; and independently with no support. These massage therapists had individual offices and/or would go to the client's homes for the sessions.

The various schedule modifications are presented, as are situations such as the potential for eating disorders and potential boundary concerns.

None of the cases described typical situations in which third-party insurance payment would be realistic, although in the bursitis case and the presurgical and postsurgical care for the baseball player, it could be possible.

Typically, massage for this population does not qualify for insurance reimbursement; therefore the costs are the responsibility of the client. Currently, sports teams typically do not employ massage therapists, but this may be changing. Teams that do hire massage professionals typically will pay a salary of around $30,000 per year, but this is rare at this time.

Individually, athletes usually seek massage professionals through a word-of-mouth grapevine. Professional athletes can justify the cost of the massage and even may have the finances to support extensive massage care. If you look at the therapeutic change interventions in these various cases, massage was required at least twice a week and often more. The cost burden for this can be extensive. It seems to be the cost of massage at this point that is limiting its use among the general population, including those involved in sports and fitness. These persons appreciate massage and want massage but may not be able to justify the costs.

I personally do not have any quick fixes for this situation but can share that even the most elite and highest paid athletes will notice the cost versus benefit ratio. Most of the elite professional athletes I have worked with (and I have worked with many in various sports) are a bit resistant to using massage extensively if the monthly cost rises above $500 per month, except in special situations where they are injured or getting ready for a competition or the season. Also, most of these athletes play in one location and live off season in another, so the cash flow to the massage therapist is seasonal and erratic.

Again, after working in this area for many years with many athletes, I caution you to be realistic. Do not pay attention to the massage therapists who may work occasionally with one or two professional athletes and indicate that they make $100 or more per hour. This is not really true in the sense of the special accommodations required for elite athletes. They may charge $100 per hour for massage, but it takes a lot of time to work with these athletes and typically the actual amount made per hour is much less. Besides, I only know of a few massage therapists who are truly experienced enough and trained enough to demand that type of reimbursement, and it took them about 20 years to get there.

The clients in the cases in this text were able to pay for the massage because at some level they were financially stable, although some were making major sacrifices to receive massage. Most of your clients may not be able to do this, and this creates various challenges, such as ability to achieve sustained benefits, especially when it is best to receive massage 2 or 3 times per week and the client only can justify paying for a massage every other week. Again, I have no quick fixes or definite answers. You just have to do the best you can, charge reasonable fees, and be really good at what you do.

I also caution you again about the "Status Factor" when working with professional athletes. It is unethical for this to be your motivation or to talk about the clients. Always remember that the elderly lady (Marge), or the old Marine (Sam), or the client struggling with weight maintenance (Laura) is just as important as the professional football, basketball, and golf athletes described.

SUMMARY

Finally, in summarizing these case studies and all the many different pesons I remembered during the writing of each one, I am yet again reminded that the clients also have been my best teachers. Regardless of all the information and strategies in this text, the client is the one who teaches you, if you are willing to learn. May each of you be compassionate and humble enough to learn from them.

In my last few thoughts before ending this text, I want to be your mentor, not teacher.

Massage is an important and valuable career path of service. Most of my clients over the many years I have been a massage therapist have not been famous athletes. Yes, I have worked with hundreds of athletes, understand their world, and appreciate the strain of their lifestyle. The reason these persons are comfortable with me is because to me they are people, just people who benefit from therapeutic massage. I hope the content of this book helps you help people, just people.

The only way I would write this book is because it is about everyday people. All the models used in the illustrations are persons who participate in physical activity, not celebrities. Yes, there is a list of "elite" athletes in the foreword. The list is there for validation. If they support massage, then the everyday people are more apt to be accepting. Their support lends credibility, I hope opening doors that connect massage therapists with all types of sport and fitness situations. I personally have worked extensively with every one of them. They knew I was writing this book and wanted to help because they care about fellow athletes. Just remember, the persons you will touch are just as important.

Please volunteer to support Special Olympics and local fund raising events such as walks and runs for various causes such as cancer research. Pay attention to the senior citizen mall walkers and the kids in Little League. Do not shun the person exercising to manage obesity. They are working just as hard as a football lineman.

Remember those in physical rehabilitation, recovering from accidents, war, and disease. Do not forget the athlete that did not "make it," blew out a knee, or something and really needs massage for the rest of his or her life.

I carry a contentment as I remember all the clients who felt better after the massage. I wish for you the peace of knowing you are of value in a quiet, humble way. Even if no one ever tells you how much you have helped them, you will know because you will have seen clients benefit. They can walk, run, jump, smile or cry, win, lose, try again, and maybe even know when to quit and do something else instead.

Never forget the original "heart tug" that led you to massage in the first place and that it is not about whom you massage, but that you remember to serve each person you touch with expertise and compassion.

Pick five case studies you are especially interested in:

1 For each case study, identify the specific content used to develop and implement the various treatment plans. Include assessment and treatment. List the chapters and page numbers for each.

Example: Case 12

Assessment:

Metabolic energy production:

Running sport movement patterns:

Fitness and sport training recommendations:

Trigger point methods:

Case 1 _____

_____

_____

_____

_____

Case 2 _____

_____

_____

_____

_____

Case 3 _____

_____

_____

_____

_____

Typical sport injury or conditions—ankle sprain shin splints:

_____

_____

_____

_____

_____

_____

_____

_____

Case 4 _____

_____

_____

_____

_____

Case 5 _____

_____

_____

_____

_____

Now choose five different case studies.

2 For each case there are various questions that would need to be answered by research, discussion with the client, or the client's performance or medical support group. For each case, write at least three more questions that you would ask if this were your client.

**Case Study
Questions**

_____

_____

_____

_____

**Case Study
Questions**

_____

_____

_____

_____

**Case Study
Questions**

_____

_____

_____

_____

**Case Study
Questions**

_____

_____

_____

_____

**Case Study
Questions**

_____

_____

_____

_____

**Case Study
Questions**

_____

_____

_____

_____

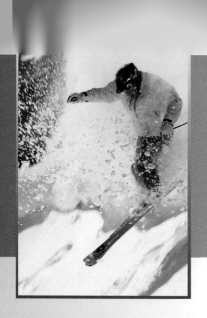

GLOSSARY

abbreviation Shortened forms of words or phrases.

abuse Exploitation, misuse, mistreatment, molestation, neglect.

acquired immunodeficiency syndrome (AIDS) A dysfunction in the body's immune system, which defends the body against disease.

active assisted movement Movement of a joint in which both the client and the therapist produce the motion.

active joint movement Movement of a joint through its range of motion by the client.

active range of motion Movement of a joint by the client without any type of assistance from the massage practitioner.

active resistive movement Movement of a joint by the client against resistance provided by the therapist.

acupressure Methods used to tone or sedate acupuncture points without the use of needles.

acupuncture point Asian term for a specific point that correlates with a neurologic motor point.

acute A term that describes a condition in which the signs and symptoms develop quickly, last a short time, and then disappear.

acute illness A short-term illness that resolves by means of the normal healing process and, if necessary, supportive medical care.

acute pain A symptom of a disease condition or a temporary aspect of medical treatment. Acute pain acts as a warning signal because it can activate the sympathetic nervous system. It usually is temporary, of sudden onset, and easily localized. The client frequently can describe the pain, which often subsides without treatment.

adaptation A response to a sensory stimulation in which nerve signaling is reduced or ceases.

aerobic exercise training An exercise program focused to increase fitness and endurance.

allied health A division of medicine in which the professional receives training in a specific area of medicine to serve as support for the physician.

anatomic barriers Anatomic structures determined by the shape and fit of the bones at the joint.

antagonism Occurs when massage produces the opposite effect, such as with medications.

antagonists The muscles that oppose the movement of the prime movers.

anxiety A feeling of uneasiness, usually connected with an increase in sympathetic arousal responses.

applied kinesiology Methods of evaluation and bodywork that use a specialized type of muscle testing and various forms of massage and bodywork for corrective procedures.

approximation The technique of pushing muscle fibers together in the belly of the muscle.

art Craft, skill, technique, and talent.

arterial circulation Movement of oxygenated blood under pressure from the heart to the body through the arteries.

arthrokinematic movement Accessory movements that occur as a result of inherent laxity or joint play that exists in each joint. The joint play allows the ends of the bones to slide, roll, or spin smoothly on one another. These essential movements occur passively with movement of the joint and are not under voluntary control.

aseptic technique Procedures that kill or disable pathogens on surfaces to prevent transmission.

Asian approaches Methods of bodywork that have developed from ancient Chinese methods.

assessment The collection and interpretation of information provided by the client, the client's family and friends, the massage practitioner, and referring medical professionals.

asymmetric stance The position in which the body weight is shifted from one foot to the other while standing.

athlete A person who participates in sports as an amateur or a professional. Athletes require precise use of their bodies.

autonomic nervous system The body system that regulates involuntary body functions using the sympathetic "fight-flight-fear" response and the restorative parasympathetic "relaxation response." The sympathetic and parasympathetic systems work together to maintain homeostasis through a feedback loop system.

autoregulation Control of homeostasis through alteration of tissue or function.

Ayurveda A system of health and medicine that grew from East Indian roots.

bacteria Primitive cells that have no nuclei. Bacteria cause disease by secreting toxic substances that damage human tissues, by becoming parasites inside human cells, or by forming colonies in the body that disrupt normal function.

balance point The point of contact between the practitioner and client.

beating A form of heavy tapotement involving use of the fist.

benign A term that describes the type of tumor that remains localized within the tissue from which it arose and does not undergo malignant changes. Benign tumors usually grow very slowly.

body mechanics Use of the body in an efficient and biomechanically correct way.

body segment The area of the body between joints that provides movement during walking and balance.

body supports Pillows, folded blankets, foam forms, or commercial products that help contour the flat surface of a massage table or mat.

body/mind The interaction between thought and physiology that is connected to the limbic system, hypothalamic influence on the auto-nomic nervous system, and the endocrine system.

bodywork A term that encompasses all the various forms of massage, movement, and other touch therapies.

boundary Personal space that exists within an arm's length perimeter. Personal emotional space is designated by morals, values, and experience.

burnout A condition that occurs when a person uses up energy faster than it can be restored.

breathing pattern disorders A complex set of behaviors that lead to overbreathing in the absence of a pathologic condition. These disorders are considered a functional syndrome because all the parts are working effectively; therefore, a specific pathologic condition does not exist.

care or treatment plan The plan used to achieve therapeutic goals. It outlines the agreed-upon objectives; the frequency, duration, and number of visits; progress measurements; the date of reassessment; and massage methods to be used.

career A chosen pursuit; a life's work.

centering The ability to focus the mind by screening out sensation.

certification A voluntary credentialing process that usually requires education and testing; tests are administered either privately or by government regulatory bodies.

chakra Energy fields or centers of consciousness within the body.

challenge Living each day knowing that it is filled with things to learn, skills to practice, tasks to accomplish, and obstacles to overcome.

chemical effects The effects of massage produced by the release of chemical substances in the body. These substances may be released locally from the massaged tissue, or they may be hormones released into the general circulation.

chronic A term that describes the type of disease that develops slowly and lasts for a long time, sometimes for life.

chronic illness A disease, injury, or syndrome that shows little change or slow progression.

chronic pain Pain that persists or recurs for indefinite periods, usually for longer than 6 months. It frequently has an insidious onset, and the character and quality of the pain change over time. It frequently involves deep somatic and visceral structures. Chronic pain usually is diffuse and poorly localized.

circulatory Systems that depend on the pumping action of the skeletal muscle (i.e., the arterial, venous, lymphatic, respiratory, and cerebrospinal fluid circulatory systems).

client information form A document used to obtain information from the client about health, preexisting conditions, and expectations for the massage.

client outcome The results desired from the massage and the massage therapist.

client/practitioner agreement and policy statement A detailed written explanation of all rules, expectations, and procedures for the massage.

coalition group formed for a particular purpose.

cognition Conscious awareness and perception, reasoning, judgment, intuition, and memory.

comfort barrier The first point of resistance short of the client's perceiving any discomfort at the physiologic or pathologic barrier.

commitment The ability and willingness to be involved in what is happening around us so as to have a purpose for being.

communicable disease A disease caused by pathogens that is easily spread; a contagious disease.

compensation The process of counterbalancing a defect in body structure or function.

compression Pressure into the body to spread tissue against underlying structures. Also, the exertion of inappropriate pressure on nerves by hard tissue (e.g., bone).

compressive force The amount of pressure exerted against the surface of the body in order to apply pressure to the deeper body structures; pressure directed in a particular direction.

concentric isotonic contraction Application of a counterforce by the massage therapist while allowing the client to move, which brings the proximal and distal attachments of the target muscle together against the pressure.

condition management The use of massage methods to support clients who are unable to undergo a therapeutic change but who wish to function as effectively as possible under a set of circumstances.

confidentiality Respect for the privacy of information.

conflict An expressed struggle between at least two interdependent parties who perceive incompatible goals, scarce resources, and/or interference from the other party in achieving their goals.

connective tissue The most abundant tissue type in the body; it provides support, structure, space, stabilization, and scar formation.

conservation withdrawal A parasympathetic survival pattern that is similar to "playing 'possum" or hibernation.

contamination The process by which an object or area becomes unclean.

contraindication Any condition that renders a particular treatment improper or undesirable.

control The belief that we can influence events by the way we feel, think, and act.

cortisol A stress hormone produced by the adrenal glands that is released during long-term stress. An elevated level indicates increased sympathetic arousal.

counterirritation Superficial stimulation that relieves a deeper sensation by stimulating different sensory signals.

counterpressure Force applied to an area that is designed to match exactly (isometric contraction) or partly (isotonic contraction) the effort or force produced by the muscles of that area.

countertransference The personalization of the professional relationship by the therapist in which the practitioner is unable to separate the therapeutic relationship from personal feelings and expectations for the client.

craniosacral and myofascial approaches Methods of bodywork that work both reflexively and mechanically with the fascial network of the body.

cream A type of lubricant that is in a semisolid or solid state.

credential A designation earned by completing a process that verifies a certain level of expertise in a given skill.

cross-directional stretching Tissue stretching that pulls and twists connective tissue against its fiber direction.

cryotherapy Therapeutic use of ice.

culture The arts, beliefs, customs, institutions, and all other products of human work and thought created by a specific group of people at a particular time.

cupping A type of tapotement that involves the use of a cupped hand; it is often used over the thorax.

cutaneous sensory receptors Sensory nerves in the skin.

database All the information available that contributes to therapeutic interaction.

deep inspiration Movement of air into the body by hard breathing to meet an increased demand for oxygen. Any muscles that can pull the ribs up are called into action.

deep transverse friction A specific rehabilitation technique that creates therapeutic inflammation by creating a specific, controlled reinjury of tissues by applying concentrated therapeutic movement that moves the tissue against its grain over only a very small area.

defensive measures The means by which our bodies defend against stressors (e.g., production of antibodies and white blood cells or through behavioral or emotional means).

denial The ability to retreat and to ignore stressors.

depression A condition characterized by a decrease in vital functional activity and by mood disturbances of exaggerated emptiness, hopelessness, and melancholy or of unbridled high energy with no purpose or outcome.

depth of pressure Compressive stress that can be light, moderate, deep, or varied.

dermatome Cutaneous (skin) distribution of spinal nerve sensation.

direction Flow of massage strokes from the center of the body outward (centrifugal), or from the extremities inward toward the center of the body (centripetal). Direction can be circular motions; it can flow from origin to insertion of the muscle, following the muscle fibers, or can flow transverse to the tissue fibers.

direction of ease The position the body assumes with postural changes and muscle shortening or weakening, depending on how it has balanced against gravity.

disclosure Acknowledging and informing the client of any situation that interferes with or affects the professional relationship.

disinfection The process by which pathogens are destroyed.

dissociation Detachment, discontentedness, separation, isolation.

dopamine A neurochemical that influences motor activity involving movement (especially learned fine movement, such as writing), conscious selective selection (what to pay attention to), mood (in terms of inspiration), possibility, intuition, joy, and enthusiasm. If the dopamine level is low, the opposite effects are seen, such as lack of motor control, clumsiness, inability to decide what to attend to, and boredom.

drag The amount of pull (stretch) on the tissue (tensile stress).

drape Fabric used to cover the client and keep the individual warm while the massage is given.

draping The procedures of covering and uncovering areas of the body and turning the client during the massage.

draping material Coverings that provide the client with privacy and warmth. The most commonly used coverings are standard bed linens because they are large enough to cover the entire body and are easy to use for most draping procedures.

dual role Overlap in the scope of practice, with one professional providing support in more than one area of expertise.

duration The length of time a method lasts or stays in the same location.

dysfunction An in-between state in which one is "not healthy" but also "not sick" (i.e., experiencing disease).

eccentric isotonic contraction Application of a counterforce while the client moves the jointed area, which allows the proximal and distal attachments to separate. The muscle lengthens against the pressure.

effleurage(gliding stroke); Horizontal strokes applied with the fingers, hand, or forearm that usually follow the fiber direction of the underlying muscle, fascial planes, or dermatome pattern.

electrical-chemical functions Physiologic functions of the body that rely on or produce body energy; often called Ch'i, Prana, or meridian energy.

employee A person who works for another for a wage.

end-feel The perception of the joint at the limit of its range of motion. The end-feel is either soft or hard. (See *joint end-feel.*)

endangerment site Any area of the body where nerves and blood vessels surface close to the skin and are not well protected by muscle or connective tissue; therefore deep, sustained pressure into these areas could damage these vessels and nerves. The kidney area is included because the kidneys are loosely suspended in fat and connective tissue, and heavy pounding is contraindicated in that area.

endogenous Made in the body.

endurance A measure of fitness. The ability to work for prolonged periods and the ability to resist fatigue.

energetic approaches Methods of bodywork that work with subtle body responses.

enkephalins and endorphins Neurochemicals that elevate mood, support satiety (reduce hunger and cravings), and modulate pain.

entrainment The coordination of movements or their synchronization to a rhythm.

entrapment Pathologic pressure placed on a nerve or vessel by soft tissue.

environmental contact Contact with pathogens found in the environment in food, water, and soil and on various surfaces.

epinephrine/adrenaline A neurochemical that activates arousal mechanisms in the body; the activation, arousal, alertness, and alarm chemical of the "fight-or-flight" response and all sympathetic arousal functions and behaviors.

essential touch Vital, fundamental, and primary touch that is crucial to well-being.

ethical behavior Right and good conduct that is based on moral and cultural standards as defined by the society in which we live.

ethical decision making The application of ethical principles and professional skills to determine appropriate behavior and resolve ethical dilemmas.

ethics The science or study of morals, values, or principles, including ideals of autonomy, beneficence, and justice; principles of right and good conduct.

exemption A situation in which a professional is not required to comply with an existing law because of educational or professional standing.

experiment A method of testing a hypothesis.

expressive touch Touch applied to support and convey awareness and empathy for the client as a whole.

external sensory information Stimulation from an origin exterior to the surface of the skin that is detected by the body.

facilitation The state of a nerve in which it is stimulated but not to the point of threshold, the point at which it transmits a nerve signal.

fascial sheath A flat sheet of connective tissue used for separation, stability, and muscular attachment points.

feedback A method of autoregulation to maintain internal homeostasis that interlinks body functions; a noninvasive, continual exchange of information between the client and the professional.

fitness A general term used to describe the ability to perform physical work.

forced expiration Movement of air out of the body, produced by activating muscles that can pull down the ribs and muscles that can compress the abdomen, forcing the diaphragm upward.

forced inspiration Movement of air into the body that occurs when an individual is working very hard and needs a great deal of oxygen. This involves not only the muscles of quiet and deep inspiration but also the muscles that stabilize and/or elevate the shoulder girdle in order to directly or indirectly elevate the ribs.

frequency The number of times a method is repeated in a time period.

friction Specific circular or transverse movements that do not glide on the skin and that are focused on the underlying tissue.

fungi A group of simple parasitic organisms that are similar to plants but that have no chlorophyll (green pigment). Most pathogenic fungi live on tissue on or near the skin or mucous membranes.

gait Walking pattern.

gate control theory A hypothetical gating mechanism that functions at the level of the spinal cord; a "gate" through which pain impulses reach the lateral spinothalamic system. Painful impulses are transmitted by large-diameter and small-diameter nerve fibers. Stimulation of large-diameter fibers prevents the small-diameter fibers from transmitting signals. Stimulating (rubbing, massaging) large-diameter fibers helps to suppress the sensation of pain, especially sharp pain.

general adaptation syndrome The process that calls into play the three stages of the body's response to stress (i.e., the alarm reaction, the resistance reaction, and the exhaustion reaction).

general contraindications Factors that require a physician's evaluation to rule out serious underlying conditions before any massage is indicated. If the physician recommends massage, the physician must help develop a comprehensive treatment plan.

gestures The way a client touches the body while explaining a problem. These movements may indicate whether the problem is a muscle problem, a joint problem, or a visceral problem.

goals Desired outcomes.

Golgi tendon receptors Receptors in the tendons that sense tension.

growth hormone A hormone that promotes cell division; in adults it is implicated in the repair and regeneration of tissue.

guarding Contraction of muscles in a splinting action, surrounding an injured area.

hacking A type of tapotement that alternately strikes the surface of the body with quick, snapping movements.

hardening A method of teaching the body to deal more effectively with stress; sometimes called *toughening.*

hardiness The physical and mental ability to withstand external stressors.

healing The restoration of well-being.

health Optimal functioning with freedom from disease or abnormal processes.

heavy pressure Compressive force that extends to the bone under the tissue.

hepatitis A viral inflammatory process and infection of the liver.

histamine A chemical produced by the body that dilates the blood vessels.

history Information from the client about past and present medical conditions and patterns of symptoms.

homeostasis Dynamic equilibrium of the internal environment of the body through processes of feedback and regulation.

hormone A messenger chemical in the bloodstream.

human immunodeficiency virus (HIV) The virus that appears to be responsible for autoimmune deficiency syndrome (AIDS).

hydrotherapy The use of various types of water applications and temperatures for therapy.

hygiene Practices and conditions that promote health and prevent disease.

hyperstimulation analgesia Diminishing the perception of a sensation by stimulating large-diameter nerve fibers. Some methods used are application of ice or heat, counterirritation, acupressure, acupuncture, rocking, music, and repetitive massage strokes.

hyperventilation Deep or rapid breathing in excess of physical demands.

hypothesis The starting point of research; it is based on the statement, "If this happens, then that will happen."

impingement syndromes Conditions that involve pathologic pressure on nerves and vessels; the two types of impingement are compression and entrapment.

indication A therapeutic application that promotes health or assists in a healing process.

inflammatory response A normal mechanism, characterized by pain, heat, redness, and swelling, that usually speeds recovery from an infection or injury.

informed consent Client authorization for any service from a professional based on adequate information provided by the professional. Obtaining informed consent is a consumer protection process that requires that clients have knowledge of what will occur, that their participation is voluntary, and that they are competent to give consent. Informed consent is an educational procedure that allows clients to make knowledgeable decisions about whether they want to receive a massage.

inhibition A decrease in or cessation of a response or function.

initial treatment plan A plan that states therapeutic goals, the duration of the sessions, the number of appointments necessary to meet the agreed goals, costs, the general classification of intervention to be used, and the objective progress measurement to be used to identify attainment of goals.

insertion The muscle attachment point that is closest to the moving joint.

integrated approaches Combined methods of various forms of massage and other bodywork styles.

integration The process of remembering an event while being able to remain in the present moment, with an awareness of the difference between then and now, to bring some sort of resolution to the event.

intercompetition massage Massage provided during an athletic event.

intimacy A tender, familiar, and understanding experience between beings.

intuition Knowing something by using subconscious information.

isometric contraction A contraction in which the effort of the muscle or group of muscles is exactly matched by a counterpressure, so that no movement occurs, only effort.

isotonic contraction A contraction in which the effort of the target muscle or group of muscles is partly matched by counterpressure, allowing a degree of resisted movement.

job A regular activity performed for payment.

joint end-feel The sensation felt when a normal joint is taken to its physiologic limit. (See *end-feel.*)

joint kinesthetic receptors Receptors in the capsules of joints that respond to pressure and to acceleration and deceleration of joint movement. The two main types of joint kinesthetic receptors are type II cutaneous mechanoreceptors and pacinian (lamellated) corpuscles.

joint movement The movement of the joint through its normal range of motion.

joint play The inherent laxity present in a joint.

kinetic chain The process by which each individual joint movement pattern is part of an interconnected aspect of the neurologic coordination pattern of muscle movement.

law A scientific statement that is true uniformly for a whole class of natural occurrences.

lengthening The process in which the muscle assumes a normal resting length by means of the neuromuscular mechanism.

leverage Leaning with the body weight to provide pressure.

license A type of credential required by law; licenses are used to regulate the practice of a profession to protect the public health, safety, and welfare.

longitudinal stretching A stretch applied along the fiber direction of the connective tissues and muscles.

lubricant A substance that reduces friction on the skin during massage movements.

lymph system A specialized component of the circulatory system, responsible for waste disposal and immune response.

lymphatic drainage A specific type of massage that enhances lymphatic flow.

malignant The type of tumor (cancer) that tends to spread to other regions of the body.

manipulation Skillful use of the hands in a therapeutic manner. Massage manipulations focus on the soft tissues of the body and are not to be confused with joint manipulation using a high-velocity thrust.

manual lymph drainage Methods of bodywork that influence lymphatic movement.

marketing The advertising and other promotional activities used to sell a product or service.

massage The scientific art and system of assessment of and manual application of certain techniques to the superficial soft tissue of skin, muscles, tendons, ligaments, and fascia and the structures that lie within the superficial tissue. The hand, foot, knee, arm, elbow, and forearm are used for the systematic external application of touch, stroking (effleurage), friction, vibration, percussion, kneading (pétrissage), stretching, compression, or passive and active joint movements within the normal physiologic range of motion. Massage includes adjunctive external applications of water, heat, and cold for the purposes of establishing and maintaining good physical condition and health by normalizing and improving muscle tone, promoting relaxation, stimulating circulation, and producing therapeutic effects on the respiratory and nervous systems and the subtle interactions among all body systems. These intended effects are accomplished through the physiologic energetic and mind/body connections in a safe, nonsexual environment that respects the client's self-determined outcome for the session.

massage chair A specially designed chair that allows the client to sit comfortably during the massage.

massage environment An area or location where a massage is given.

massage equipment Tables, mats, chairs, and other incidental supplies and implements used during the massage.

massage mat A cushioned surface that is placed on the floor.

massage routine The step-by-step protocol and sequence used to give a massage.

massage table A specially designed table that allows massage to be done with the client lying down.

mechanical methods Techniques that directly affect the soft tissue by normalizing the connective tissue or moving body fluids and intestinal contents.

mechanical response A response that is based on a structural change in the tissue. The tissue change is caused directly by application of the technique.

mechanical touch Touch applied with the intent of achieving a specific anatomic or physiologic outcome.

medications Substances prescribed to stimulate or inhibit a body process or replace a chemical in the body.

mental impairment Any mental or psychologic disorder, such as mental retardation, developmental disabilities, organic brain syndrome, emotional or mental illness, and specific learning disabilities.

mentoring Career support by someone more experienced.

metastasis Migration of cancer cells.

moderate pressure Compressive pressure that extends to the muscle layer but does not press the tissue against the underlying bone.

motivation The internal drive that provides the energy to do what is necessary to accomplish a goal.

motor point The point where a motor nerve enters the muscle it innervates and causes a muscle to twitch if stimulated.

movement cure Term used in the nineteenth and early twentieth centuries for a system of exercise and massage manipulations focused on treating a variety of ailments.

multiple isotonic contractions Movement of the joint and associated muscles by the client through a full range of motion against partial resistance applied by the massage therapist.

muscle energy techniques Neuromuscular facilitation; specific use of active contraction in individual muscles or groups of muscles to initiate a relaxation response; activation of the proprioceptors to facilitate muscle tone, relaxation, and stretching.

muscle spindles Structures located primarily in the belly of the muscle that respond to both sudden and prolonged stretches.

muscle testing procedures An assessment process that uses muscle contraction. *Strength testing* is done to determine whether a muscle responds with sufficient strength to perform the required body functions. *Neurologic muscle testing* is designed to determine whether the neurologic interaction of the muscles is working smoothly. The third type, *applied kinesiology*, uses muscle strength or weakness as an indicator of body function.

musculotendinous junction The point where muscle fibers end and the connective tissue continues to form the tendon; a major site of injury.

myofascial approaches Styles of bodywork that affect the connective tissues; often called deep tissue massage, soft tissue manipulation, or myofascial release.

myofascial release A system of bodywork that affects the connective tissue of the body through various methods that elongate and alter the plastic component and ground matrix of the connective tissue.

needs assessment History taking using a client information form and physical assessment using an assessment form. The information is evaluated to develop a care plan.

nerve impingement Pressure against a nerve by skin, fascia, muscles, ligaments, or joints.

neurologic muscle testing Testing designed to determine whether the neurologic interaction of the muscles is proceeding smoothly.

neuromuscular A term describing the interaction between nervous system control of the muscles and the response of the muscles to the nerve signals.

neuromuscular approaches Methods of bodywork that influence the reflexive responses of the nervous system and its connection to muscular function.

neuromuscular mechanism The interplay and reflex connection between sensory and motor neurons and muscle function.

neurotransmitter A messenger chemical in the synapse of the nerve.

norepinephrine/noradrenaline A neurochemical that functions in a manner similar to epinephrine but that is more concentrated in the brain.

occupation A productive or creative activity that serves as a regular source of livelihood.

oil A type of liquid lubricant.

open-ended question A question that cannot be answered with a simple, one-word response.

opportunistic invasion Infection by potentially pathogenic organisms that are found on the skin and mucous membranes of nearly everyone and that do not cause disease until they have the opportunity, such as in depressed immunity.

origin The attachment point of a muscle at the fixed point during movement.

osteokinematic movements The movements of flexion, extension, abduction, adduction, and rotation; also known as *physiologic movements*.

overload principle A stress on an organism that is greater than the one regularly encountered during everyday life.

oxytocin A hormone that is implicated in pair or couple bonding, parental bonding, feelings of attachment, and care taking, along with its more commonly known functions in pregnancy, delivery, and lactation.

PRICE Acronym for basic first-aid therapy, which stands for *p*rotection, *r*est, *i*ce, *c*ompression, and *e*levation.

pain and fatigue syndromes Multicausal and often chronic nonproductive patterns that interfere with well-being, activities of living, and productivity.

pain-spasm-pain cycle Steady contraction of muscles, which causes ischemia and stimulates pain receptors in muscles. The pain, in turn, initiates more spasms.

palliative care Care intended to relieve or reduce the intensity of uncomfortable symptoms but that cannot effect a cure.

palpation Assessment through touch.

panic An intense, sudden, and overwhelming fear or feeling of anxiety that produces terror and immediate physiologic changes, resulting in immobility or senseless, hysterical behavior.

parasympathetic autonomic nervous system The restorative part of the autonomic nervous system. The parasympathetic response often is called the *relaxation response.*

passive joint movement Movement of a joint by the massage practitioner without the assistance of the client.

passive range of motion Movement of a joint in which the therapist, not the client, effects the motion.

pathogenic animals Large, multicellular organisms called metazoa. Worms that feed off human tissue or cause other disease processes are metazoa.

pathologic barrier An adaptation of the physiologic barrier that allows the protective function to limit rather than support optimal functioning.

pathology The study of disease.

peer support Interaction among those involved in the same pursuit. Regular interaction with other massage practitioners creates an environment in which both technical information and interpersonal dilemmas can be sorted out.

person-to-person contact A method of transmission of pathogens. They can often be carried in the air from one person to another.

pétrissage Kneading; rhythmic rolling, lifting, squeezing, and wringing of soft tissue.

phasic muscles The muscles that move the body.

physical assessment Evaluation of body balance, efficient function, basic symmetry, range of motion, and ability to function.

physical disability Any physiologic disorder, condition (such as cosmetic disfigurement), or anatomic loss that affects one or more of the following body systems: neurologic, musculoskeletal, special sense organ, respiratory (including speech organs), cardiovascular, reproductive, digestive, genitourinary, hemic and lymphatic, skin, and endocrine. Extremes in size and extensive burns also may be considered physical impairments.

physiologic barriers The result of the limits in range of motion imposed by protective nerve and sensory functions to support optimal performance.

piezoelectricity The production of an electrical current by application of pressure to certain crystals such as mica, quartz, Rochelle salt, and connective tissue.

placebo A treatment for an illness that influences the course of the disease even if the treatment is not specifically validated.

polarity A holistic health practice that encompasses some of the theory base of Asian medicine and Ayurveda. Polarity is an eclectic, multifaceted system.

positional release A method of moving the body into the direction of ease (the way the body wants to move out of the position that causes the pain); the proprioception is taken into a state of safety and may stop signaling for protective spasm.

positioning Placing the body in such a way that specific joints of muscles are isolated.

post-event massage Massage provided after an athletic event.

post-isometric relaxation (PIR) The state that occurs after isometric contraction of a muscle; it results from the activity of minute neural reporting stations called the *Golgi tendon bodies.*

post-traumatic stress disorder A disorder characterized by episodes of flashback memory, state-dependent memory, somatization, anxiety, irritability, sleep disturbance, concentration difficulties, times of melancholy or depression, grief, fear, worry, anger, and avoidance behavior.

postural muscles Muscles that support the body against gravity.

powder A type of lubricant that consists of a finely ground substance.

prefix A word element placed at the beginning of a root word to change the meaning of the word.

premassage activities Any activity that is involved in preparation for a massage, including setting up the massage room, obtaining supplies, and determining the temperature of the room.

pressure Compressive force.

prime movers The muscles responsible for movement.

principle A basic truth or rule of conduct.

profession An occupation that requires training and specialized study.

professional A person who practices a profession.

professional touch Skilled touch delivered to achieve a specific outcome; the recipient in some way reimburses the professional for services rendered.

professionalism The adherence to professional status, methods, standards, and character.

prone Lying face down.

proprioceptive neuromuscular facilitation (PNF) Specific application of muscle energy techniques that uses strong contraction combined with stretching and muscular pattern retraining.

proprioceptors Sensory receptors that detect joint and muscle activity.

protozoa One-celled organisms that are larger than bacteria and can infest human fluids and cause disease by parasitizing (living off) or directly destroying cells.

pulsed muscle energy Procedures that involve engaging the barrier and using minute, resisted contractions (usually 20 in 10 seconds), which introduces mechanical pumping as well as post-isometric relaxation and reciprocal inhibition.

qualified Criteria that indicate when the goal is achieved.

quantified Goals measured in terms of objective criteria, such as time, frequency, 1-to-10 scale, measurable increase or decrease in the ability to perform an activity, and measurable increase or decrease in a sensation, such as relaxation or pain.

quiet expiration Movement of air out of the body through passive action. This occurs through relaxation of the external intercostals and the elastic recoil of the thoracic wall and tissue of the lungs and bronchi, with gravity pulling the rib cage down from its elevated position.

quiet inspiration Movement of air into the body while resting or sitting quietly. The diaphragm and external intercostals are the prime movers.

range of motion Movement of joints.

rapport The development of a relationship based on mutual trust and harmony.

reciprocal inhibition (RI) The effect that occurs when a muscle contracts, obliging its antagonist to relax in order to allow normal movement to take place.

reciprocity The exchange of privileges between governing bodies.

recovery massage Massage structured primarily for the uninjured athlete who wants to recover from a strenuous workout or competition.

reenactment Reliving an event as though it were happening at the moment.

referral Sending a client to a health care professional for specific diagnosis and treatment of a disease.

referred pain Pain felt in an area other than the source of the pain.

reflex An involuntary response to a stimulus. Reflexes are specific, predictable, adaptive, and purposeful. Reflexive methods work by stimulating the nervous system (sensory neurons), and tissue changes occur in response to the body's adaptation to the neural stimulation.

reflexive methods Massage techniques that stimulate the nervous system, the endocrine system, and the chemicals of the body.

reflexology A massage system directed primarily toward the feet and hands.

refractory period The period after a muscle contraction during which the muscle is unable to contract again.

regional contraindications Contraindications that relate to a specific area of the body.

rehabilitation massage Massage used for severe injury or as part of intervention after surgery.

remedial massage Massage used for minor to moderate injuries.

resourceful compensation Adjustments made by the body to manage a permanent or chronic dysfunction.

resting position The first stroke of the massage; the simple laying on of hands.

rhythm The regularity of application of a technique. If the method is applied at regular intervals, it is considered even or rhythmic. If it is choppy or irregular, it is considered uneven or not rhythmic.

right of refusal The entitlement of both the client and the professional to stop the session.

rocking Rhythmic movement of the body.

root word The part of a word that provides the fundamental meaning.

safe touch Secure, respectful, considerate, sensitive, responsive, sympathetic, understanding, supportive, and empathetic contact.

sanitation The formulation and application of measures to promote and establish conditions favorable to health, specifically public health.

science The intellectual process of understanding through observation, measurement, accumulation of data, and analysis of findings.

scope of practice The knowledge base and practice parameters of a profession.

self-employment To work for oneself rather than for another.

serotonin The neurochemical that regulates mood in terms of appropriate emotions, attention to thoughts, and calming, quieting, and comforting effects; it also subdues irritability and regulates drive states.

service An action performed for another person that results in a specific outcome.

sexual misconduct Any behavior that is sexually oriented in the professional setting.

shaking A technique in which the body area is grasped and shaken in a quick, loose movement; sometimes classified as rhythmic mobilization.

shiatsu An acupressure and meridian-focused bodywork system from Japan.

side-lying The position in which the client is lying on his or her side.

skin rolling A method that lifts skin.

slapping A form of tapotement that uses a flat hand.

SOAP charting A problem-oriented method of medical record keeping; the acronym SOAP stands for *s*ubjective, *o*bjective, *a*ssessment (analysis), and *p*lan.

soft tissue The skin, fascia, muscles, tendons, joint capsules, and ligaments of the body.

somatic Pertaining to the body.

somatic pain Pain that arises from stimulation of receptors in the skin (superficial somatic pain) or in skeletal muscles, joints, tendons, and fascia (deep somatic pain).

spa treatments Various hydrotherapy methods, application of preparations to the body, and massage applications found in the spa setting.

speed Rate of application (e.g., fast, slow, varied).

spindle cells Sensory receptors in the belly of the muscle that detect stretch.

stabilization Holding the body in a fixed position during joint movement, lengthening, and stretching.

standard precautions Procedures developed by the Centers for Disease Control and Prevention (CDC) to prevent the spread of contagious diseases.

standards of practice The principles that form specific guidelines to direct professional ethical practice and quality care, including a structure for evaluating the quality of care. Standards of practice represent an attempt to define the parameters of quality care.

start-up costs The initial expenses involved in starting a business.

state-dependent memory The encoding and storing of a memory based on the effects of the autonomic nervous system and the resulting chemical levels of the body. The memory is retrievable only during a similar physiologic experience in the body.

sterilization The process by which all microorganisms are destroyed.

stimulation Excitation that activates the sensory nerves.

strain-counterstrain Using tender points to guide the positioning of the body into a space where the muscle tension can release on its own.

strength testing Testing intended to determine whether a muscle is responding with sufficient strength to perform the required body functions. Strength testing determines a muscle's force of contraction.

stress Any substantial change in routine or any activity that forces the body to adapt.

stressors Any internal perceptions or external stimuli that demand a change in the body.

stretching Mechanical tension applied to lengthen the myofascial unit (muscles and fascia); two types are *longitudinal* and *cross-directional stretching*.

stroke A technique of therapeutic massage that is applied with a movement on the surface of the body, whether superficial or deep.

structural and postural integration approaches Methods of bodywork derived from biomechanics, postural alignment, and the importance of the connective tissue structures.

subtle energies Weak electrical fields that surround and run through the body.

suffering An overall impairment of a person's quality of life.

suffix A word element placed at the end of a root word to change the meaning of the word.

superficial fascia The connective tissue layer just under the skin.

superficial pressure Pressure that remains on the skin.

supervision Support from more experienced professionals.

supine The position in which the client is lying face up.

symmetric stance The position in which body weight is distributed equally between the feet.

sympathetic autonomic nervous system The energy-using part of the autonomic nervous system, the division in which the "fight-or-flight" response is activated.

symptoms The subjective abnormalities felt only by the patient.

syndrome A group of different signs and symptoms that usually arise from a common cause.

synergistic The interaction of medication and massage to stimulate the same process or effects.

system A group of interacting elements that function as a complex whole.

systemic massage Massage structured to affect one body system primarily. This approach usually is used for lymphatic and circulation enhancement massage.

tapotement Springy blows to the body at a fast rate to create rhythmic compression of the tissue; also called *percussion*.

tapping A type of tapotement that uses the fingertips.

target muscle The muscle or groups of muscles on which the response of the method is specifically focused.

techniques Methods of therapeutic massage that provide sensory stimulation or mechanical change of the soft tissue of the body.

tendon organs Structures found in the tendon and musculotendinous junction that respond to tension at the tendon. Articular (joint) ligaments contain receptors that are similar to tendon organs and adjust reflex inhibition of the adjacent muscle when excessive strain is placed on the joints.

tensegrity An architectural principle developed in 1948 by R. Buckminster Fuller. The tensegrity principle underlies the design of geodesic domes. An anatomic tensegrity system is characterized by a continuous tensional network (tendons, ligaments, and fascial structures) connected by a discontinuous set of compressive elements, or struts (bones).

therapeutic applications Healing or curative powers.

therapeutic change Beneficial change produced by a bodywork process that results in a modification of physical form or function that can affect a client's physical, mental, and/or spiritual state.

therapeutic relationship The interpersonal structure and professional boundaries between professionals and the clients they serve.

tonic vibration reflex Reflex that tones a muscle with stimulation through vibration methods at the tendon.

touch Contact with no movement.

touch technique The basis of soft tissue forms of bodywork methods.

toughening/hardening The reaction to repeated exposure to stimuli that elicit arousal responses.

traction Gentle pull on the joint capsule to increase the joint space.

training stimulus threshold The stimulus that elicits a training response.

transference Personalization of the professional relationship by the client.

trauma Physical injury caused by violent or disruptive action, toxic substances, or psychic injury resulting from a severe long- or short-term emotional shock.

trigger point An area of local nerve facilitation; pressure on the trigger point results in hypertonicity of a muscle bundle and referred pain patterns.

Tuberculosis (TB) An infection caused by a bacterium that usually affects the lungs but may invade other body systems.

vibration Fine or coarse tremulous movement that creates reflexive responses.

viruses Microorganisms that invade cells and insert their genetic code into the host cell's genetic code. Viruses use the host cell's nutrients and organelles to produce more virus particles.

wellness The efficient balance of body, mind, and spirit, all working in a harmonious way to enhance quality of life.

yang The portion of the whole realm of function of the body, mind, and spirit in Eastern thought that corresponds to sympathetic autonomic nervous system functions.

yin The portion of the whole realm of function of the body, mind, and spirit in Eastern thought that corresponds to parasympathetic autonomic nervous system functions.

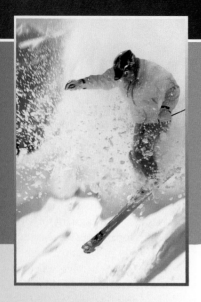

Works Cited

UNIT I

Ahluwalia S: *Distribution of smooth muscle acting-containing cells in the human meniscus.* J Orthopaed Res 19(4):659–664, 2001.

American Psychiatric Association: *Diagnostic and Statistical Manual of Mental Disorders,* ed 4(DSM-IV), Washington, DC, 1994, American Psychiatric Association.

Baechle TR, Roger WE: *Essentials of strength and conditioning,* ed 2, Champaign, IL, 2000, Human Kinetics.

Bandy WD, Irion JM, Briggler M: *The effect of time and frequency of static stretching on flexibility of the hamstring muscles.* Phys Ther 77(10):1090–1096, 1997.

Batson J, Hill M, Satterwhite YE, Watson J: *Strength and Conditioning for Specific Sports.* Sports Science Exchange Roundtable 49, vol 13, no. 3. Barrington, IL, 2002, Gatorade Sports Science Institute.

Berlin JA, Colditz G: *A meta-analysis of physical activity in the prevention of coronary heart disease.* Am J Epidemiol 132:612–628, 1990.

Benardot D, Hartsough C, Engelbert-Fenton K, et al: *Eating disorders in athletes: The dietician's perspective.* Sports Science Exchange Roundtable 18, vol 5, no. 4. Barrington, IL, 1994, Gatorade Sports Science Institute.

Bernasconi P, Kohl J: *Analysis of co-ordination between breathing and exercise rhythms in man.* J Physiol 471:693–706, 1993.

Brownell KD, Rodin J, Wilmore JH: *Eating, body weight and performance in athletes. Disorders of modern society,* Philadelphia, 1992, Lea & Febige.

Bulbena A, Duro JC, Porta M, et al: *Anxiety disorders in the joint hypermobility syndrome*: Psychiatry Res 46:59–68, 1993.

Cafarelli E, Flint F: *The role of massage in preparation for and recovery from exercise.* Sports Medicine 14(1):1–9, 1992.

Clews W: *Making muscles malleable.* Sport Health 14(1):32–33, 1996.

Clews W: *Where does massage draw the line?* Sport Health 11(2):20–21, 1996.

Commerford M, Mottram S: *Movement and stability dysfunction–contemporary developments.* Man Ther 6:15–26, 2001.

Commerford M, Mottram S: *Functional stability retraining. Principles and strategies for managing mechanical dysfunction.* Man Ther 6:3–14, 2001.

Cook G: *Athletic body in balance,* Champaign, IL, 2003, Human Kinetics.

Coombes J, Powers S, Hamilton K, et al: *Exercise intensity and longevity in men. The Harvard Alumni Health Study.* JAMA 273:1179–1184, 1995.

Goats GC: *Massage–the scientific basis of an ancient art: Part 1. The techniques.* Br J Sports Med. 28(3):149–156, 1994.

Gulick DT, Kimura I:. *Delayed onset muscle soreness: What is it and how do we treat it?* J Sport Rehabil 5:234–243, 1996.

Hastreiter D, Ozuna RM, Spector M: *Regional variations in certain cellular characteristics in human lumbar intervertebral discs, including the presence of smooth muscle actin.* J Orthop Res 19(4):597–604, 2001.

Hendrickson T: *Massage for orthopedic conditions.* Philadelphia, 2002, Lippincott Williams & Wilkins.

Hodges P, Heinjnen I, Gandevia S: *Postural activity of the diaphragm is reduced in humans when respiratory demand increases.* J Physiol 537(3):999–1008, 2001.

Knost B, Flor H, Birbaumer N, et al: *Learned maintenance of pain: Muscle tension reduces central nervous system processing of painful stimulation in chronic and subchronic pain patients.* Psychophysiology 36:755–764, 1999.

Kraemer WJ, Adams K, Cafarelli E, et al: *Anerican College of Sports Medicine position stand: Progression models in resistance training for healthy adults.* Med Sci Sports Exerc. 34:364–380, 2002.

Kraemer WJ, Ratamess N, Fry AC, et al: *Influence of resistance training volume and periodization on physiological and performance adaptations in collegiate women tennis players.* Am J Sports Med 28:626–633, 2000.

Marber MS, Mestril R, Chi SH, et al: 1995

Shephard RJ, Balady G: *Exercise as cardiovascular therapy.* Circulation 99(7):963–972, 1999.

The effects of ballistic resistance training. J Strength Cond Res 12:216–221, 1998.

McNair PJ, Stanley SN: *Effect of passive stretching and jogging on the series elastic muscle stiffness and range of motion of the ankle joint.* Br J Sports Med 30(4):313–318, 1996.

Paine T: *The Complete Guide To Sports Massage,* London, 2000, A&C Black, Ltd.

Pope RP, Herbert RD, Kirwan JD, et al: *A randomized trial of preexercise stretching for prevention of lower-limb injury.* Med Sci Sports Exerc 32(2):271–277, 2000.

Sawyer M, Zbieranek CK: *The treatment of soft tissue after spinal injury.* Clin Sports Med 5(2):387–405, 1986.

Shrier I. *Stretching before exercise does not reduce the risk of local muscle injury: A critical review of the clinical and basic science literature.* Clin J Sport Med 9(4):221–227, 1999.

Stark SD. Stretching techniques. In *The Stark Reality of Stretching,* pp 73–80, Richmond, BC, 1997, Stark Reality Publishing, pp 73–80.

Weber MD, Servedio FJ. Woodall WR: *The effects of three modalities on delayed onset muscle soreness.* J Orthop Sports Phys Ther 20(5): 236–242 1994,

Wiktorsson-Möller M, Öberg BA, Ekstrand J, et al: *Effects of warming up, massage, and stretching on range of motion and muscle strength in the lower extremity.* Am J Sports Med 11(4): 249–252, 1983.

Wittink H, Michel T: 2002 *Chronic pain management for physical therapists,* ed 2, Boston, 2002, Butterworth Heinemann.

Yates A: *Compulsive exercise and eating disorders,* New York, 1991, Brunner and Mazel.

Additional Resources

Baechle TR, Roger WE: *Essentials of strength and conditioning,* Champaign, IL, 2000, Human Kinetics.

www.gssiweb.com: The Gatorade Sports Science Institute

National Association of Anorexia Nervosa and Associated Disorders, (Tel: 847-831-3438)

National Anorexic Aid Society, Inc. (Tel: 614-436-1112)

UNIT II

Cantu RI, Grodin AJ: *Myofascial manipulation: Theory and clinical application,* New York, 2001, Aspen Publishers.

Chikly B: *Silent waves: Theory and practice of lymph drainage therapy, with applications,* Scottsdale, AZ, 2001, IHH Publishing.

Chaitow L: *Muscle energy techniques,* ed 2, New York, 2001, Churchill Livingstone.

De Domenico G, Wood EC: *Beard's massage,* ed 4, Philadelphia, 1997, Saunders.

Field T: *Touch therapy,* New York, 2000, Churchill Livingstone.

Freeman LWs: Mosby's *Complementary & alternative medicine: A research-based approach,* ed 2, St. Louis, 2004, Mosby.

Greenman TW, Flynn PE: *Thoracic spine and rib cage: Musculoskeletal evaluation and treatment,* Oxford, 1996, Butterworth-Heinemann.

Kisner C, Colby L: *Therapeutic exercise, foundations and techniques,* ed 3, Philadelphia, 1996, FA Davis.

Kuprian W: *Physical therapy for sports,* ed 2, Philadelphia, 1994, Saunders.

Lederman E: *Fundamentals of manual therapy: Physiology, neurology and psychology,* New York, 1997, Churchill Livingstone.

Rich GJ: *Massage therapy—The Evidence for Practice,* St. Louis, 2002, Mosby.

Miles R, Traub RD, Wong RKS: *Spread of synchronous firing in longitudinal slices from the CA3 region of the hippocampus.* J Neurophysiol 60:1481–1496, 1995.

Additional Resource

Universal College of Reflexology: http://www.universalreflex.com

UNIT III

Arnheim DD, Prentice WE: *Principles of athletic training*, ed 11, New York, 2003, McGraw-Hill.

Bruunsgaard H, Hartkopp A, Mohr T, et al: *In vivo cell-mediated immunity and vaccination response following prolonged, intense exercise.* Med Sci Sports Exerc 29:1176–1181, 1997.

Nieman DC: *Influence of carbohydrate on the immune response to intensive, prolonged exercise.* Exerc Immunol Rev 4:64–76, 1998.

Clements, J.M.; Casa DJ, Knight JC, et al: *Ice-water and cold-water immersion provide similar cooling rates in runners with exercise-induced hyperthermia.* J Athl Train 37:146–150, 2002.

Gonzalez-Alonzo J, Teller C, AndersenSL, et al: *Influence of body temperature on the development of fatigue during prolonged exercise in the heat.* J Appl Physiol 86:1032–1039, 1999.

Latzka WA, Montain SJ: *Water and electrolyte requirements for exercise.* Clin Sports Med 18:513–524, 1999.

Phinney LT, Gardner JW, Kark JA, Wenger CB: *Long-term follow-up after exertional heat illness during recruit training.* Med Sci Sports Exer. 33:1443–1448, 2001.

Roberts WO: *Tub cooling for exertional heatstroke. Phys Sportsmed* 26(5):111–112, 1998.

Shephard RJ, Shek PN: *Heavy exercise, nutrition and immune function: Is there a connection?* Int J. Sports Med 16:491–497, 1995.

Andrews RA, Harrelson, GL: *Physical Rehabilitation of the Injured Athlete,* ed 3, Philadelphia, 2004, Saunders.

Basmajian JV: *Manipulation, traction, and massage,* ed 3. Baltimore, 1985, Williams & Wilkins, pp 135–144.

Cailliet R: *Soft tissue pain and disability,* ed 3, Philadelphia, 1996, FA Davis.

Maitland GD: *Peripheral manipulation,* ed 3, Boston, 1991, Butterworths, pp 25–51, 59–91.

Mennell JMcM: *Joint pain,* Boston, 1964, Little, Brown, pp 32–87.

Additional Resources

Gatorade Sports Science Institute
617 West Main Street
Barrington, IL 60010
U.S.A.International Online:
http://www.gssiweb.com/

The American Academy of Physical Medicine and Rehabilitation*
One IBM Plaza, Suite 2500
Chicago, IL 60611-3604
Tel: 312-464-9700; Fax: 312-464-0227
Online: www.aapmr.org; E-Mail:
info@aapmr.org
American Academy of Orthopedic Surgeons
6300 North River Road
Rosemont, IL 60018-4262
Tel: 847-823-7186, 800-346-2267; Fax: 847/823-8026
Online: http://www.aaos.org; E-mail:
julitz@mac.aaos.org
American Physical Therapy Association
1111 North Fairfax Street
Alexandria, VA 22314-1488
Tel: 703-684-2782, 800-999-2782 ext 3395
Online: http://www.apta.org

Arthritis Foundation
PO Box 7669
Atlanta, GA 30357-0669,
Tel: 404-872-7100 (or call your local chapter)
Online: http://www.arthritis.org

---

*A valuable source of information pertaining to physicians, specific rehabilitation programs, and exercise programs.

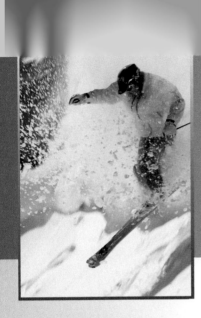

INDEX

Page numbers followed by b indicate boxes; f, figures; t, tables.